SECOND EDITION

INSIDE ULTRASOUND
VENOUS VASCULAR reference guide

Gail P. Size
BS, RPhS, RVS, RVT, FSVU, LAVLS

Laurie Lozanski
BS, RVS, RVT, FSVU

Donna Kelly
RPhS, RVT, RDMS

Linda Antonucci
RPhS, RVT, RDCS

EDITED BY

Nicos Labropoulos, PhD, DIC, RVT
Christopher L. Skelly, MD FACS, RPVI

The complete guide to venous disease, non-invasive testing and interpretation

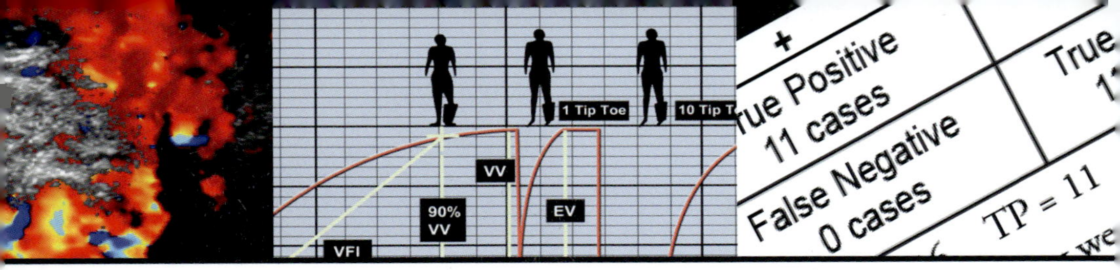

Gail P. Size, BS, RPhS, RVS, RVT, FSVU

Inside Ultrasound Venous Reference Guide

Second Edition 12-06-22

Inside Ultrasound, Inc, 13976 E. Via Cerro Del Molino, Vail, AZ, 85641
Phone 520-838-0011 • www.insideultrasound.com
ISBN: 978-0-974-7694-55

Printed in the United States of America

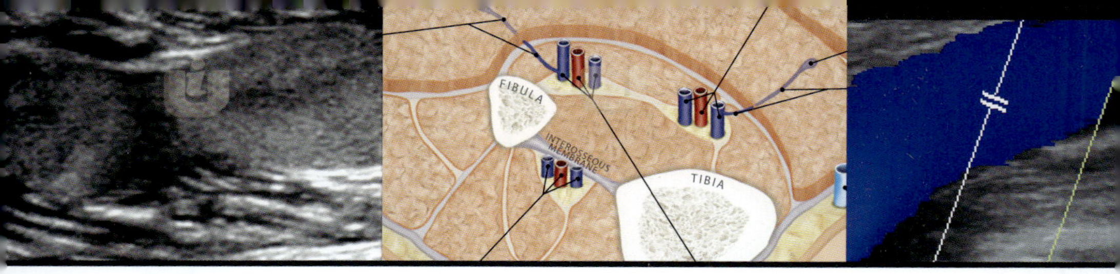

This book is dedicated
to the memory of
Dolores A. Size

To my mother, Dolores A. Size, who keeps looking over me and continues to believe in me and push me forward.

Gail

QR codes can be found throughout this book, which will allow you to view video clips of various pathology or duplex findings using your smartphone or tablet. To access these files, use the camera on your device and a QR code reader. Your device must have internet to use this feature.

There are many free QR code readers available for download, please check your app store for more information.

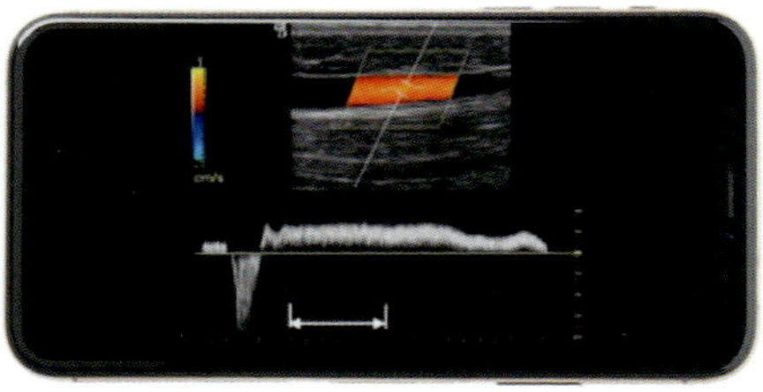

Table of Contents

Table of Contents

List of Tables

List of Tables

Acknowledgements

I am grateful to all my colleagues through the years, especially the wonderful medical and technical staff members at the University of Chicago Vascular Laboratory. Without their help and guidance, this project could not have become a reality. Thank you, to my co-authors Laurie Lozanski, Donna Kelly and Linda Antonucci; editors Nicos Labropoulos and Christopher Skelly; Chellie Buzzeo our graphic designer whose endless dedication and energy made this project happen; and Denise Eggman, our medical illustrator who created the beautiful medical anatomy and graphic drawings.

– Gail

Gail P. Size, BS, RPhS, RVS, RVT, FSVU, LAVLS

President, Inside Ultrasound, Inc.
Vail, AZ

Gail Size has over 40 years of technical and managerial experience in both clinical and private vascular laboratories. She is the founder and president of Inside Ultrasound, Inc. a provider of Basic Training in Non-invasive Vascular Testing and Vascular Interpretation for Physicians and vascular accreditation. Gail is the author of the *Inside Ultrasound's Vascular Reference Guide, Companion Workbook* and the *Venous Reference Guide.*

Laurie Lozanski, BS, RVS, RVT, FSVU

Technical Director, Non-Invasive Vascular Laboratory, University of Chicago Medicine
Faculty, Bachelor of Science Program in Vascular Ultrasound,
Rush University College of Health Sciences
Chicago, IL

Laurie Lozanski has over 33 years of technical and managerial experience in a dedicated vascular laboratory. Currently, Laurie is the Technical Director of the Non-Invasive Vascular Laboratories at the University of Chicago Medicine. Laurie has also been a faculty member of the Bachelor of Science Program in Vascular Ultrasound for over 20 years at Rush University in Chicago, IL. Laurie is serving as the Chair for the Society of Vascular Ultrasound's eLearning Committee

Donna Kelly, RPhS, RVT, RDMS

Technical Director, Non-Invasive Vascular Laboratory,
Middlesex Surgical Associates
Winchester, MA

Donna Kelly is a vascular sonographer with over 28 years of experience. She is currently the technical director of the Middlesex Surgical Associates vascular laboratory as well as a per diem technologist at Massachusetts General Hospital. The majority of her career has been focused on venous disease while working in a dedicated venous vascular lab for Massachusetts General Hospital for 15 years. She is currently on the ultrasound committee for the American Vein and Lymphatic Society (AVLS). Donna is a subject matter expert and Item writer for the Registered Phlebology Sonographer (RPhS) credentialing exam and had previously acted as a site visitor for the IAC vein center division.

Linda Antonucci, RPhS, RVT, RDCS

President, Linda Antonucci Veins, LLC
Technical Director, Non-Invasive Vascular Laboratories,
New York Comprehensive Cardiology and Vein Center, Body Contour and Veins
West Milford, NJ

Linda Antonucci has over 34 years of experience in phlebology ultrasound serving as the technical director for New Jersey and New York Vein Centers since 1988. She is an Internationally recognized educator and speaker and respected phlebology consultant specializing in advanced venous diagnostics. She is currently serving on the Board of Directors for the American Vein and Lymphatic Society and is a subject matter expert (SME) on the Registered Phlebology Sonographer (RPhS) exam committee for Cardiovascular Credentialing International.

Contributors

Matthew Allen MHA, RVS, RVT
Program Director Cardiovascular Sonography
Invasive Cardiovascular Technology
Santa Fe College
Gainesville, FL

Joseph A. Caprini MD, MS, FACS, RVT
Senior Clinician Educator,
Pritzker School of Medicine at the
University of Chicago
Emeritus physician at North Shore University
HealthSystem
Evanston, IL

Mariah Elliot MBA, BS, RVT, RPhS
Vascular Sonographer
University of Washington Medical Centerr
Seattle, WA

Jessy Farris MHS, RVT, RPhS
Coach, Learning and Development Specialist,
and Accreditation Expert
Wilson Farris Consulting
Fort Worth, Texas

Marybeth Georges BS, RVT
Vascular Technologist,
University of Chicago Medicine
Chicago, IL

Paula Heggerick RVT, RDMS, RPhS, FSVU
Vascular Consultant,
Sarasota, FL

Laura Humphries, BS, RVT, RPhS
Director of Accreditation – Vein Center
Intersocietal Accreditation Commission (IAC)
Ellicott City, MD

Janice Hickey Scharf BSc, RDMS, CRGS, FSC
Clinical Applications Specialist, Ultrasound
Philips Healthcare, Canada
Picton, Ontario

Marge Hutchisson LPN, RVT, RDCS
Director of Accreditation – IAC Vascular Testing
Ellicott City, MD

Besnike Kashtanjeva BS, RVT
Vascular Technologist,
University of Chicago Medicine
Chicago, IL

Diana L. Neuhardt RVT, RPhS, LAVLS
Director
Comprehensive Interventional Care Centers
Phoenix, AZ

Richard Palma BS, ACS, RCCS, RCS, RDCS, FACVP, FSDMS, FASE
Program Director and Clinical Coordinator,
Duke School of Medicine Cardiac Sonography
Durham, NC

Jennifer Palombizio, MS
Manager, Environmental, Health and Safety
University of Chicago Medicine
Chicago, IL

Laura J. Phillips BS, RDCS, RVT
Program Director, School of Vascular Sonography
Hoffman Heart and Vascular Institute School of
Cardiovascular Technology Saint Francis Hospital
and Medical Center
Hartford, CT

Sara Skjonsberg BS, RPhS, RVT
Clinical Specialist
EnVVeno Medical
Bend, OR

Allen Tabor RVT
Product Applications Specialist
Philips Healthcare
Seattle, WA

Patrick Washko BSRT, RDMS, RVT, FSVU
Technical Director
Rex Hospital (UNC Healthcare)
Vascular Diagnostic Center
Raleigh, NC

Jeannie White-Melendez
RPhS, RVT, FSVU
President
Quality Medical Imaging, Inc.
ESP Ultrasound
Venice, Florida

Nicos Labropoulos, PhD, DIC, RVT

Professor of Surgery and Radiology
Director, Vascular Laboratory
Department of Surgery
Stony Brook University Medical Center
Stony Brook, NY

Christopher L. Skelly, MD FACS, RPVI

Professor of Surgery
Medical Director, Non-Invasive Vascular Lab
University of Chicago Medicine
Chicago, IL

Illustration and Design

Denise Eggman

Medical Illustrator • Pearce, AZ

Chellie Buzzeo

Graphic Designer • Scottsdale, AZ

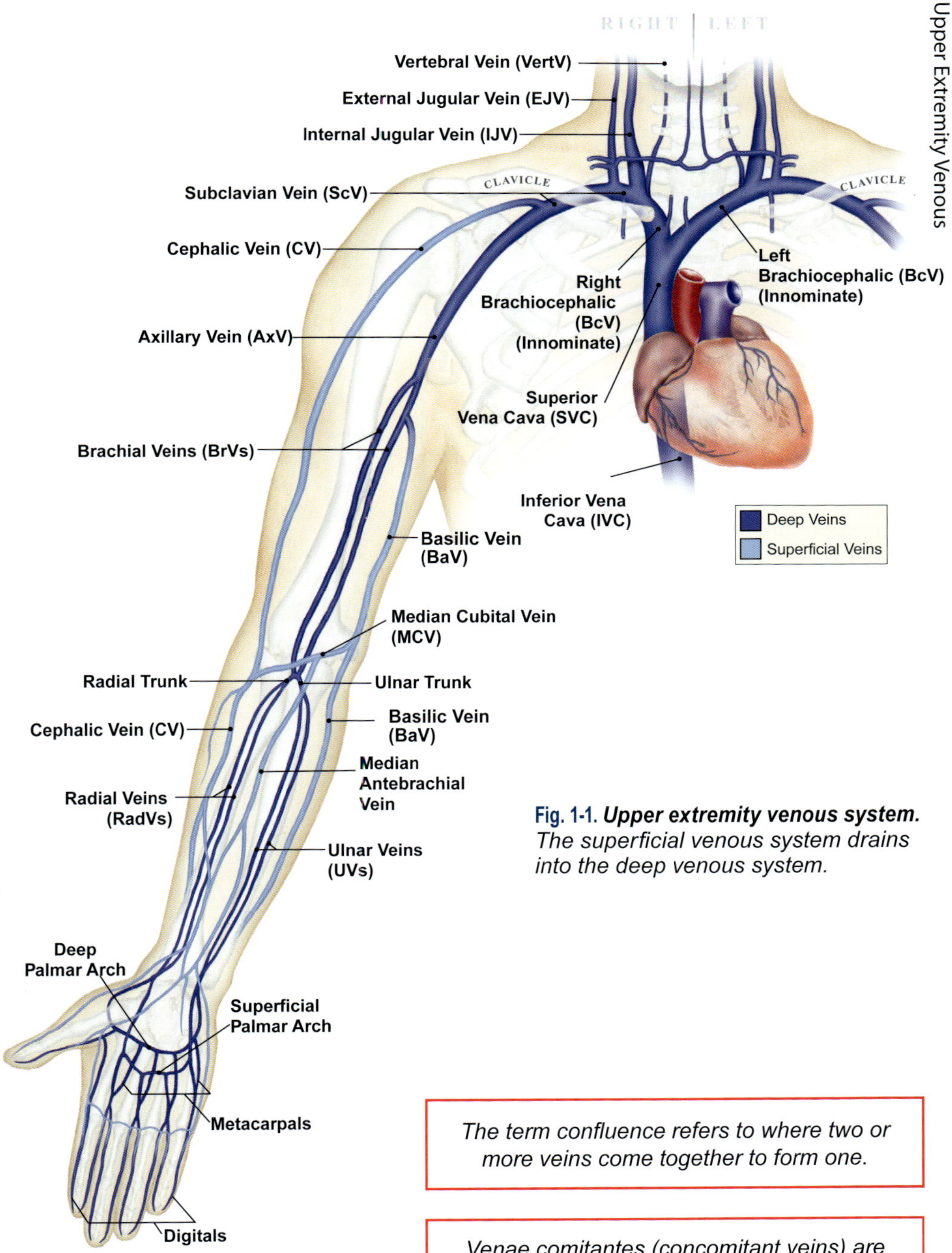

Fig. 1-1. *Upper extremity venous system.* *The superficial venous system drains into the deep venous system.*

The term confluence refers to where two or more veins come together to form one.

Venae comitantes (concomitant veins) are duplicate veins that travel with an artery. Vena comitans is the singular form.

- Deep veins have an accompanying artery.
- The ulnar, radial, anterior, and posterior interosseous and brachial veins are duplicated. The Axillary Veins (AxVs) can also be duplicated.
- Concomitant veins traveling with the same artery communicate with each other via short vessels that transversely cross the accompanying artery.
- Tributaries usually correspond to the AxV: thoracoacromial, lateral thoracic, scapular, anterior circumflex, humeral, and posterior circumflex humeral veins.

Deep Veins of the Upper Extremity *(wrist to chest)*

- The two Ulnar Veins (UVs) arise in the hand from the superficial palmar venous arch, formed by palmar digital veins. They travel along the medial aspect of the forearm (the same side as the fifth digit), joining together to form the ulnar trunk.
- The two Radial Veins (RVs) arise from the deep palmar venous arch, formed by the palmar metacarpal veins. The RVs travel up the lateral aspect of the forearm (the same side as the thumb), joining near the elbow to form the radial trunk.
- The radial and ulnar trunks can continue into the upper arm as the two Brachial Veins (BrVs), or the trunks can join to form one vessel, which splits into the paired brachial veins.
- The anterior and posterior interosseous veins are formed by the carpal venous plexus. In the forearm near the elbow, the posterior interosseous veins drain into the anterior interosseous veins which, drain into the ulnar veins.

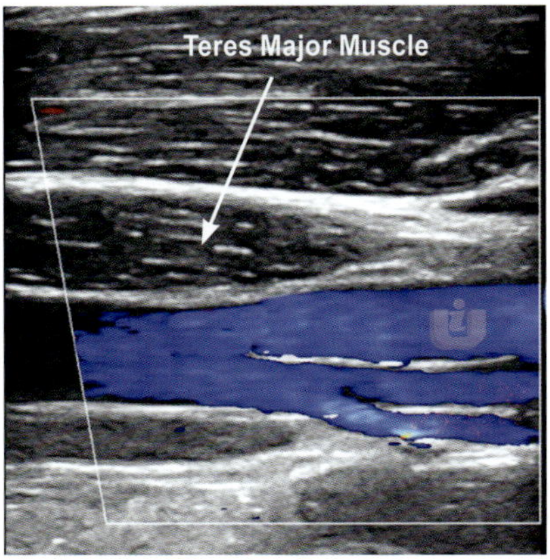

Fig. 1-2. *Confluence of the brachial veins and the AxV*

- The anterior and posterior interosseous veins are rarely examined by ultrasound.
- Landmarks help define the AxV. It begins at the inferior border of the Teres Major muscle. It travels along the shoulder to the lateral border of the first rib, where the cephalic vein terminates and becomes the Subclavian Vein (ScV).
- The formation of the AxV has been described in two ways, and either is acceptable.
  - The AxV is a continuation of the BrVs after they join together near the axilla at the lower margin of the subscapularis muscle. The basilic vein drains into the BrVs at the mid-arm or more proximal.
- Tributaries usually correspond to the AxV: thoracoacromial, lateral thoracic, scapular, anterior circumflex, humeral, and posterior circumflex humeral veins.

Superficial Veins of the Upper Extremity *(wrist to chest)*

Superficial veins run within the superficial compartment above the deep fascia.

- The Cephalic Vein (CV):
  - Is the longest vein in the upper limb.
  - Is formed on the radial (lateral) side of the hand by the radial component of the dorsal venous arch, dorsal veins of the thumb, and the dorsal vein of the radial aspect of the index finger. The dorsal venous arch drains the dorsal metacarpal veins, which drain the dorsal digital veins.
  - Travels around the lateral side of the forearm, ascending first in the groove between the brachioradialis and the biceps brachii in front of the elbow and then in the lateral groove of the biceps brachii. At the shoulder, the CV runs in the deltopectoral groove, between the deltoid and pectoralis major.
  - Dives at the clavicular end of the pectoralis major piercing the fascia and terminates in the AxV of the deep venous system at the junction of the AxV and ScV. *(Fig. 1-1)*
- The Basilic Vein (BsV):
  - Originates in the hand from the ulnar component of the dorsal venous arch and the dorsal vein from the ulnar aspect of the fifth finger.
  - Travels along the posterior side of the arm before wrapping around the medial aspect of the arm to the anterior side below the elbow. In the upper arm, the vein travels medial to the biceps brachii and perforates the deep fascia in the middle of the upper arm.
- Medial Vein (MV) of the forearm:
  - Also known as the Median Antebrachial Vein(MAV), arises from a palmar venous plexus.
  - Travels along the ulnar side of the forearm, starting at the base of the dorsum of the thumb to terminate in the median cubital vein, or the BSV. It can also bifurcate into the median basilic and median cephalic veins, which terminate in the BSV and CV.
- The Median Cubital Vein (MCV):
  - Runs from the CV to the BSV obliquely, crossing the antecubital fossa.

Typical Anatomic Variations of the Veins at the Antecubital Fossa

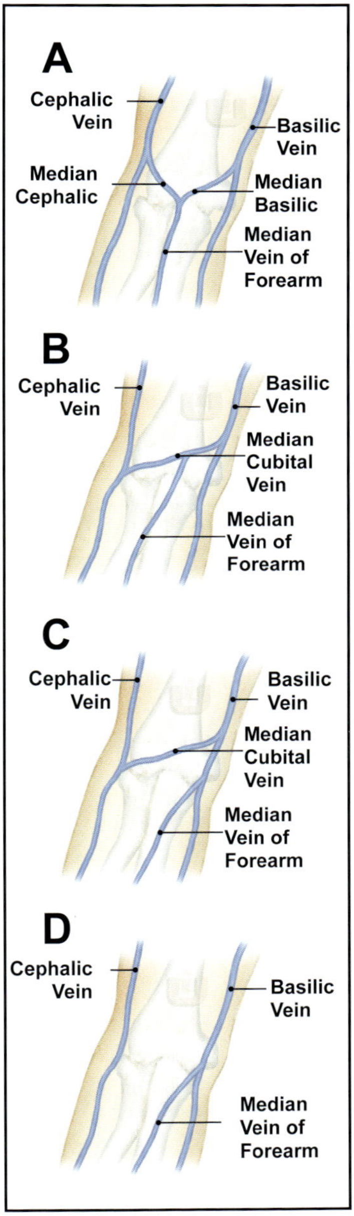

Fig. 1-3. *(A) M-shaped configuration, (B and C) N-shaped configurations with the MCV terminating in CV and BSV, respectively, (D) no communication between the CV and BSV.*

- In the antecubital fossa, there are several anatomical variations of the superficial veins *(Fig. 1-3)* including:
  - M-shaped configuration where the MV branches into the median cephalic and median basilic veins, which terminate in the cephalic and basilic veins, respectively, with no MCV present *(Fig. 1-3A)*.
  - H and N-shaped configurations where the sides of the letters (H and N) are formed by the CV and BSV. The letter N is created when the MCV connects to the cephalic and basilic veins at oblique angles. The letter H is formed when the connections are at right angles. In both cases, the MV can terminate in either the MCV *(Fig. 1-3 B)* or the BSV *(Fig. 1-3 C)*
  - There can be no communication between the BSV and CV *(Fig. 1-3 D)*. In this case, there is no MCV, and the MV will terminate in the BSV.
  - CV is hypoplastic, especially after the MCV tributary.
  - Most common are the M-, H-, and N-shaped configurations.

Neck Veins

- The External Jugular Vein (EJV) receives blood from the cranium, face, and neck via the following veins:
  - Anterior jugular vein
  - Posterior jugular vein
  - Suprascapular vein
  - Transverse cervical vein
- The EJV terminates in the ScV.
- The Anterior Jugular Vein (AJV) is highly variable in size and course. The AJV cross-sectional area varies in size inversely with that of the EJV; if the AJV cross-sectional area is large, the EJV cross-sectional area will be small and vice versa. Typically, right and left AJVs connect via the jugular arch, a transverse trunk that runs just superior to the sternum. There can be just one AJV. In this case, the AJV will usually travel along the midline of the neck.
- The anterior jugular venous system is part of a collateral venous network that sustains venous return when the ScV or brachiocephalic veins thrombose or occlude. [14]
- The AJV terminates in either the EJV (46%) or the ScV (54%).[12, 13]
- The Internal Jugular Vein (IJV) runs adjacent to the common carotid artery and drains the face and neck.
- The IJV can communicate with the AJV via a large branch from the IJV

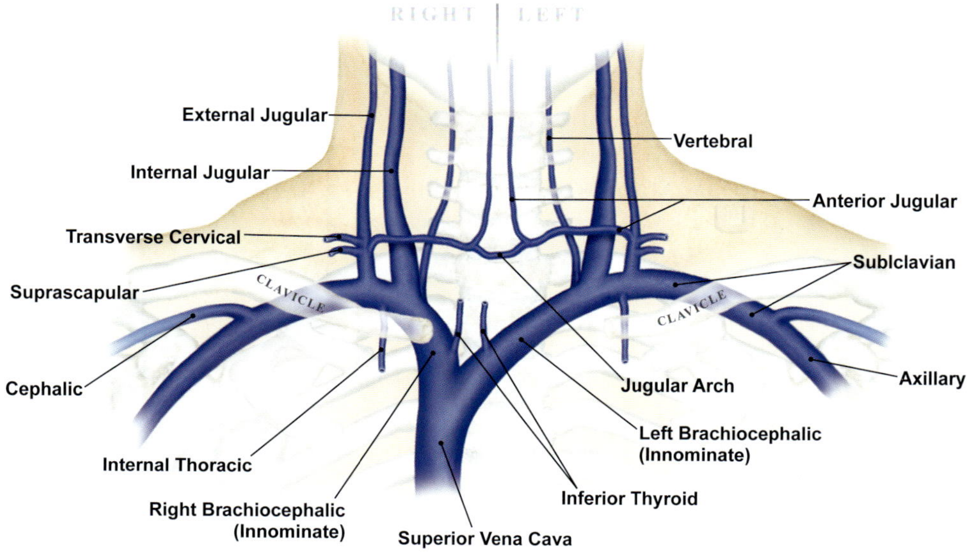

Fig. 1-4. *Neck veins. Venous flow to the heart.*

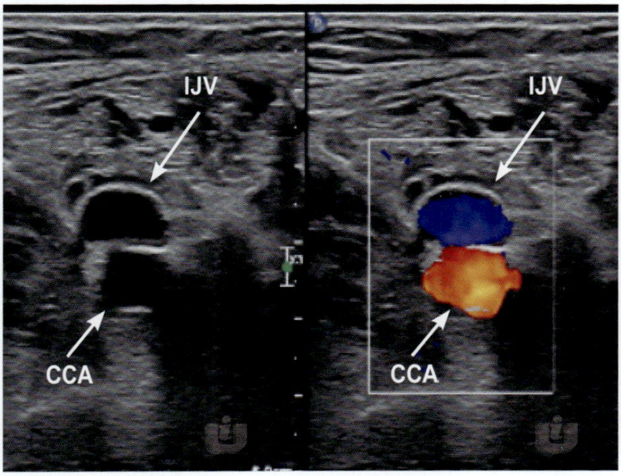

Fig. 1-5. ***Internal jugular vein in transverse.*** *B-mode images of a typical normal IJV.*

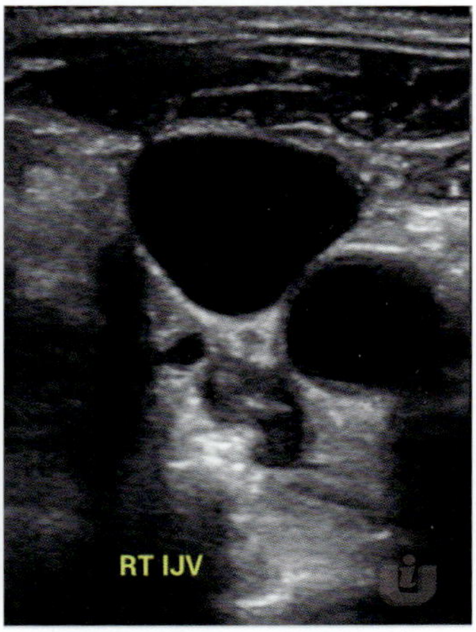

Fig. 1-6. *Transverse image of an enlarged IJV in a patient with congestive heart failure.*

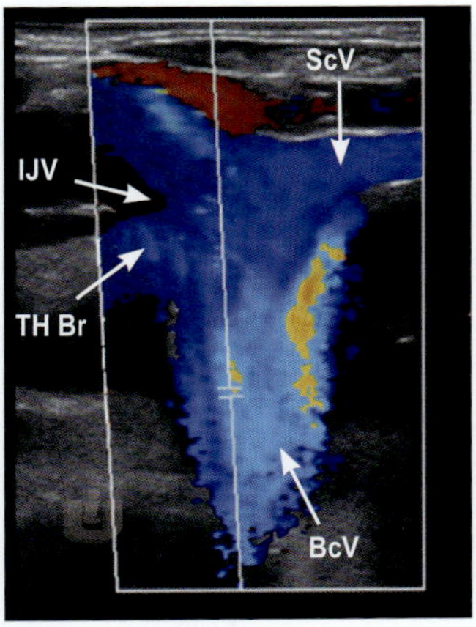

Fig. 1-7. *Confluence of the distal innominate, internal jugular, subclavian and internal thoracic branch.*

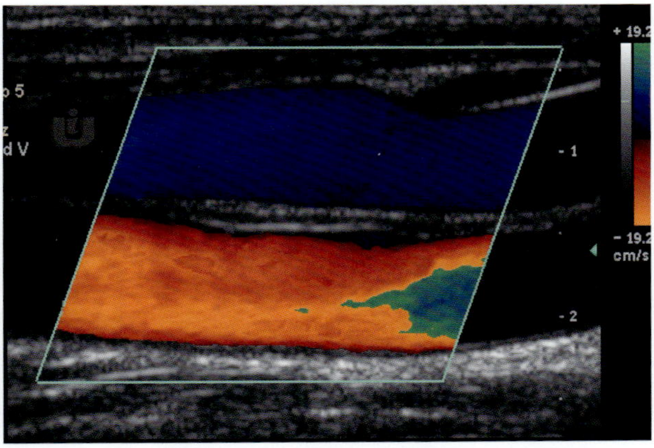

Fig. 1-8. ***Longitudinal image of the internal jugular vein.*** *Color Doppler ultrasound image of the jugular vein (top vessel) and the carotid artery (lower vessel).*

Image courtesy of Philips Healthcare

When imaging the IJV of patients with congestive heart failure, try raising their head with a pillow. This will decrease the pressure in the IJV and subsequently its diameter.

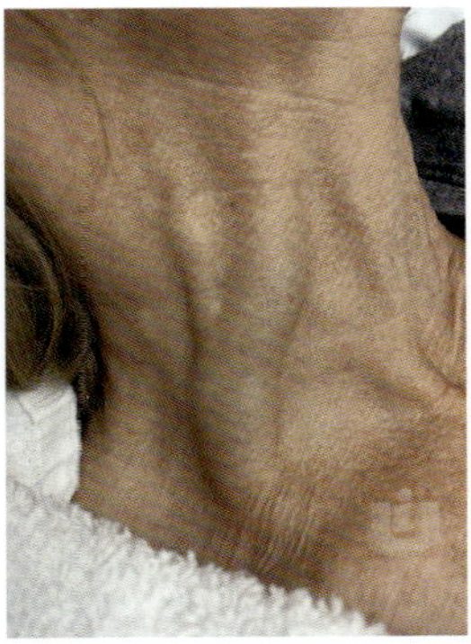

Fig. 1-9. *Patient with distention of the jugular vein.*

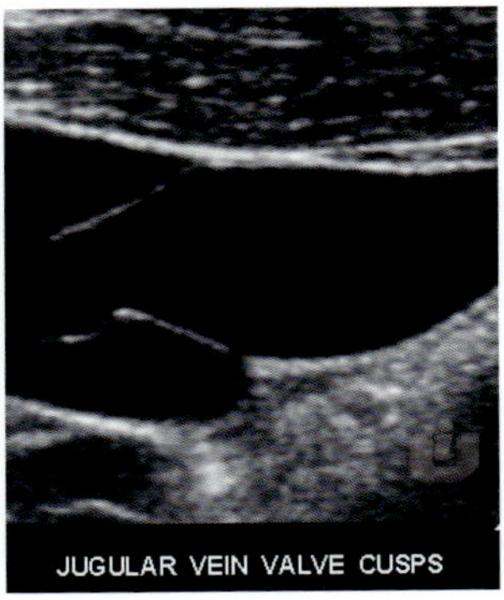

Fig. 1-10. *Jugular vein with valve leaflets extending into the lumen.*

- The ScV is the continuation of the AxV after the lateral border of the first rib joins the IJV at the clavicular level to form the Brachiocephalic/Innominate (BcV/InV).

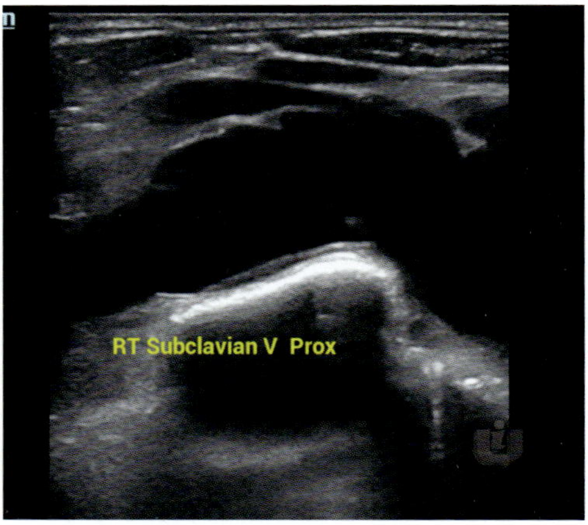

Fig. 1-11. *Longitudinal grayscale image of the subclavian vein at the confluence of the brachiocephalic vein.*

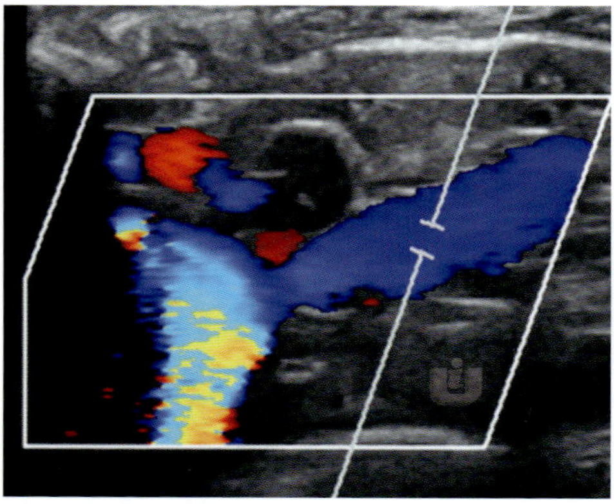

Fig. 1-12. *Color Doppler of the confluence of the subclavian, brachiocephalic vein.*

- The Superior Vena Cava (SVC) terminates at the right atrium of the heart, draining the head, neck, and upper extremities.
- The right and left BcVs join to form the SVC.
- The vertebral vein drains the head and terminates in the posterior aspect of the BcV.
- Veins that drain into the BcVs include:
  - Internal thoracic vein (mammary vein)
  - Inferior thyroid vein
  - Vertebral veins

Venous Valves

- Venous valves are comprised of two leaflets, or cusps (bicuspid valves) formed from the tunica intima. There are bulges at valve sites due to the valve cusps. *(Fig. 1-13)*
- When antegrade flow ceases, you may see a quick period of retrograde flow. However, in competent veins, this retrograde flow quickly ceases as it closes the valve by pushing the valve leaflets together. This flow reversal should not be reported as pathological venous reflux (venous insufficiency).
- Valves can withstand retrograde flow. pressures >200mmHg.
- Upper extremity veins have fewer valves than lower extremity veins.

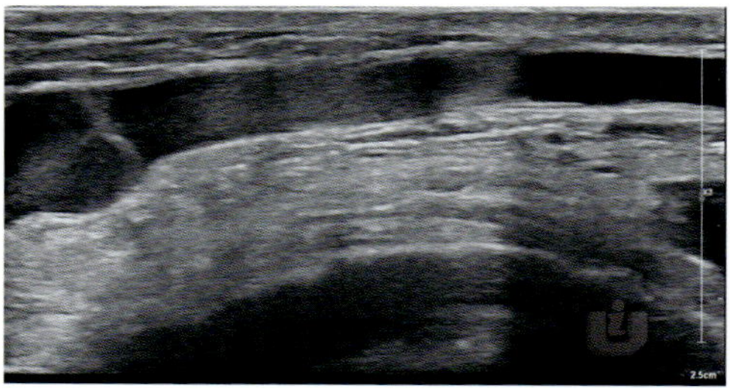

Fig. 1-13. ***Valve leaflets in the cephalic vein.*** *A grayscale image of a CV in which valve leaflets are observed in the lumen. Notice the vein bulge at the cusp site and the rouleaux flow.*

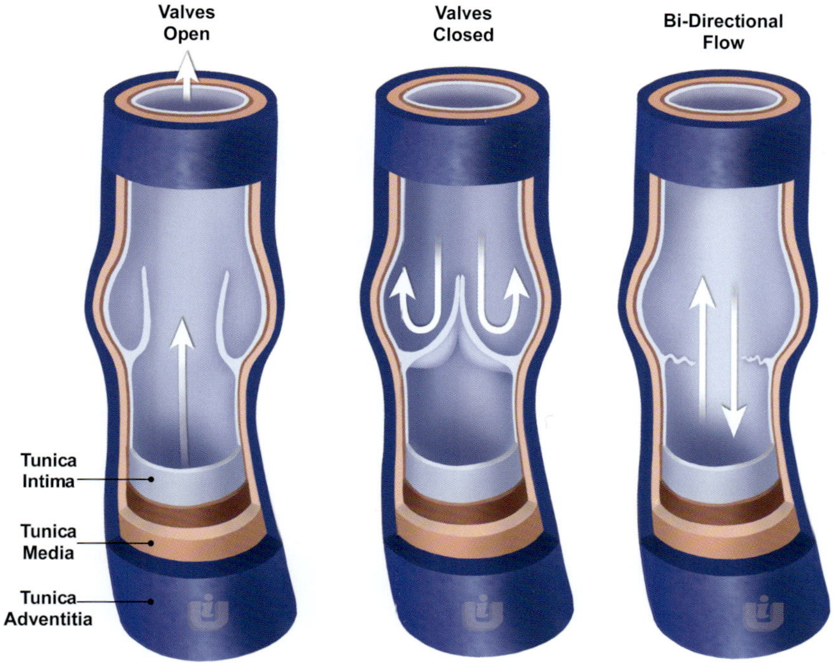

Fig. 1-14. ***Venous valve anatomy.*** *Under normal physiological conditions antegrade flow opens the valves. The valves close to prevent retrograde flow.*

References

1. Gray, H. (1977). The blood-vascular system. In Pick TP & Howden R. (Eds.), *Gray's Anatomy* (551-592). New York: Bounty Books.
2. Gray, H. (1977). The veins. In Pick TP & Howden R. (Eds.), *Gray's Anatomy* (593-614). New York: Bounty Books.
3. Netter FH. (2003). Head and neck. In Atlas of Human Anatomy 3rd ed. (1-144). Terterboro. Icon Learning Systems.
4. Netter FH. (2003). Thorax. In Atlas of Human Anatomy 3rd ed. (174-238). Terterboro. Icon Learning Systems.
5. Netter FH. (2003). Upper limb. In Atlas of Human Anatomy 3rd ed. (401-466). Terterboro. Icon Learning Systems.
6. Tortora, G. J., & Anagnostakos, NP. (Eds.). (1990). The cardiovascular system: vessels and routes. In *Principles of Anatomy and Physiology, 6th ed.* (605-650) New York, NY: Harper & Row Publishers.
7. Uflacker R. (1997). Veins of the head and neck. In Atlas of Vascular Anatomy: An Angiographic Approach. (81-112). Baltimore: Wolters Kluwer Lippincott Williams & Wilkins.
8. Uflacker R. (1997). Veins of the thorax. In Atlas of Vascular Anatomy: An Angiographic Approach. (189-212). Baltimore: Wolters Kluwer Lippincott Williams & Wilkins.
9. Uflacker R. (1997). Veins of the upper extremity. In Atlas of Vascular Anatomy: An Angiographic Approach. (389-399). Baltimore: Wolters Kluwer Lippincott Williams & Wilkins.
10. Zwiebel, WJ (2005). Extremity venous anatomy, terminology, and ultrasound features of normal veins. In Zwiebel WJ, Pellerito JS. (Eds). *Introduction to Vascular Ultrasonography 5th ed. (*415-429). Philadelphia: Elsevier Saunders.
11. Mikuni, Y., et al. (2013). "Topographical anatomy of superficial veins, cutaneous nerves, and arteries at venipuncture sites in the cubital fossa." Anat Sci Int 88(1): 46-57.
12. Deslaugiers B, Vaysse P, Combes JM, et al. Contribution to the study of the tributaries and the termination of the external jugular vein. Surg Radiol Anat 1994;16:173–7.
13. Von Lanz T, Wachsmuth W. Praktische Anatomie. Berlin, Heidelberg, New York: Springer, 1955
14. Schummer, W., et al. (2004). "The anterior jugular venous system: variability and clinical impact." Anesth Analg 99(6): 1625-1629,
15. Gurarie, M .("The Anatomy of the Axillary Vein. Very Well Health (2021) 1-6.

Veins Associated with Pelvic Vein Disorders

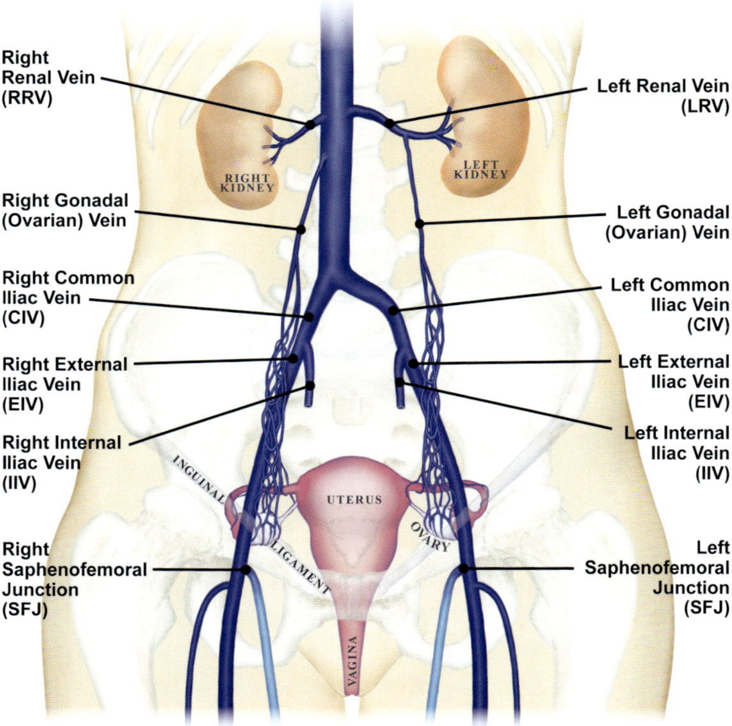

Fig. 2-1. *Primary venous anatomy of the pelvis. Note: Gonadal is a general term for the ovarian or testicular vein.*

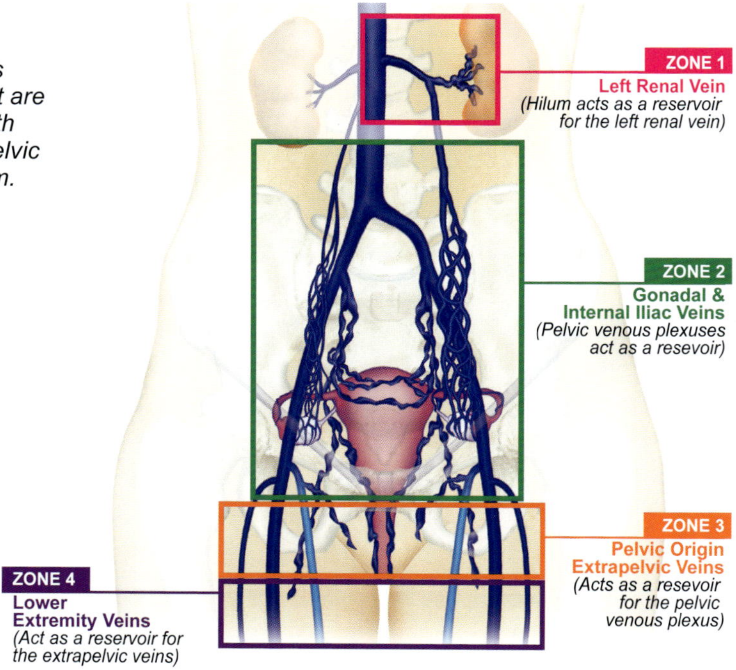

Fig. 2-2. *Venous reservoirs that are associated with the primary pelvic venous system.*

Pelvic venous disorders are a collection of venous pathologies including obstruction and/or reflux within the venous system of the pelvis.

It is essential to have a detailed knowledge of pelvic venous anatomy and physiology to have a complete understanding of pelvic venous disorders.

The venous system of the pelvis can be considered to consist of a group of primary veins (iliacs, gonadals, left renal and inferior vena cava) as well as 4 venous reservoirs where varices may develop;[1] which are described throughout this chapter.

- **Renal hilum** may act as a venous reservoir which is associated with the left renal vein.
- **Venous plexuses of the pelvis** may act as a venous reservoir which is associated with the gonadal and internal iliac veins.
- **Pelvic origin extrapelvic veins** (tributaries of the IIVs that arise outside of the pelvis to drain extrapelvic structures such as the vulva, testicles, buttocks) may act as a venous reservoir for the internal iliac veins.
- **Lower extremity veins** may act as a reservoir for the pelvic origin extrapelvic tributaries.

> *Venous reservoirs are high capacitance venous beds.*

The veins included in the ultrasound assessment for pelvic venous disorders are: [2]

- Inferior Vena Cava (IVC)
- Bilateral Common Iliac Veins (CIV)
- Bilateral External Iliac Veins (EIV)
- Bilateral Internal Iliac Veins (IIV) and their tributaries
- Left Renal Vein (LRV)
- Bilateral gonadal (ovarian or testicular) veins

The significant surrounding anatomy

Possible points of extrinsic venous compression include: [3]

- Bilateral Common Iliac Arteries (CIA)
- Bilateral External Iliac Arteries (EIA)
- Bilateral Internal Iliac Arteries (IIA)
- Superior Mesenteric Artery (SMA)
- Aorta
- Spine

Landmarks used to identify veins relevant to pelvic venous disorders:[2]

- Psoas muscle (gonadal veins)
- Iliac vessels (peripheral gonadal veins)
- Umbilicus (common iliac veins)
- SMA (left renal vein)
- Ovary (IIV using endovaginal approach)

Inferior Vena Cava [4]

- The Inferior Vena Cava (IVC) is the largest vein in the human body.
- The IVC is formed by the confluence of the right and left CIVs.
- The IVC is located at the posterior abdominal wall to the right side of the aorta.
- The IVC carries blood from the lower extremities and the abdominopelvic region to the heart.
- The IVC has multiple tributaries; the most relevant to pelvic venous disorders are:
  - The right gonadal vein
  - The left renal vein

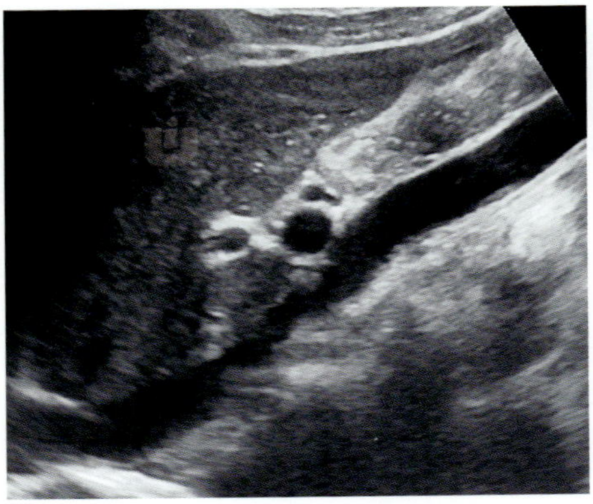

Fig. 2-3. *Longitudinal view of the IVC.*

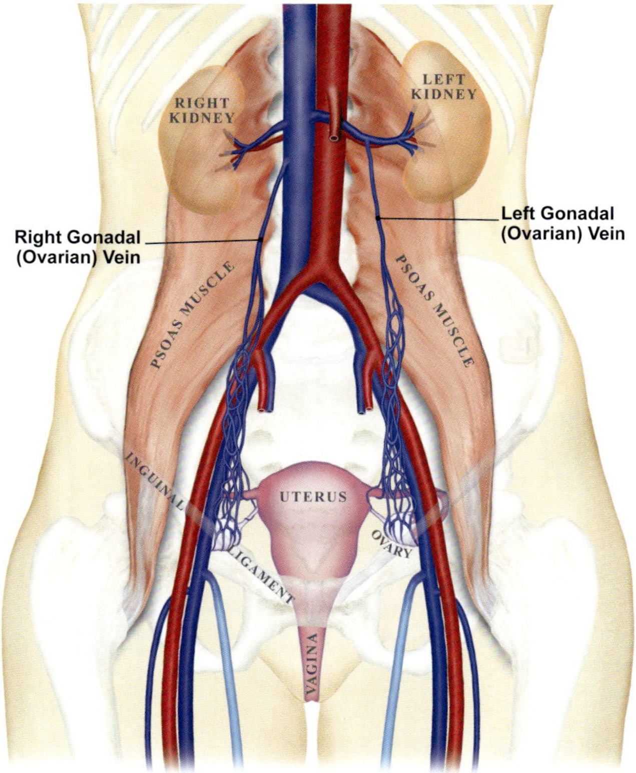

Fig. 2-4. *The anatomical structures surrounding the veins of the abdomen and pelvis can be used as helpful landmarks to identify the veins, but can also affect normal venous function.*

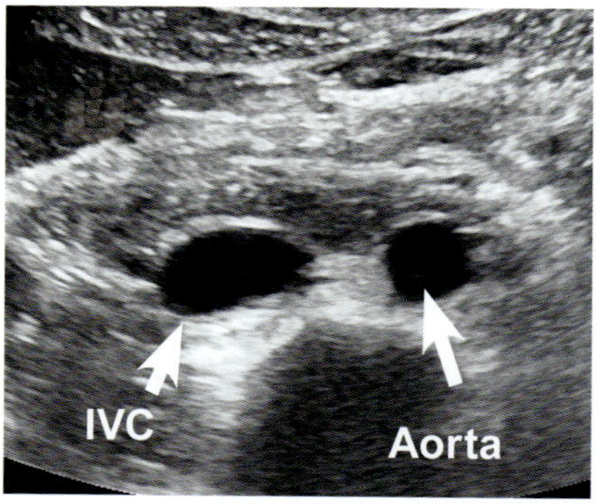

Fig. 2-5. *Transverse view of the IVC and the aorta.*

Iliac Veins

- The CIV is formed at the level of the sacroiliac joint where the IIV confluences with the EIV.
- The CIVs pass upward to the fifth lumbar vertebra to come together to form the IVC [5]
- Tributaries of the CIVs are: [6]
  - Iliolumbar veins
  - Lateral sacral (sometimes)

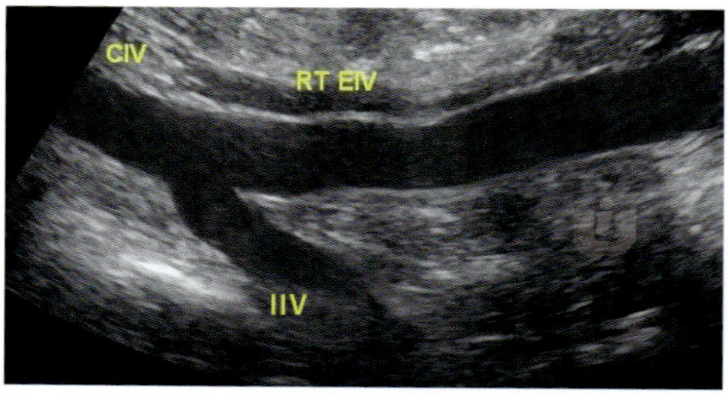

Fig. 2-6. *The confluence of the IIV and EIV to form the CIV.*

External Iliac Veins

- The External Iliac Veins (EIV): [7]
  - Begin above the level of the inferior margin of the inguinal ligament.
  - Enter the pelvis via the vascular lacuna and then ascend medially along the medial side of the psoas major
  - Carry blood away from the lower extremities and the inferior section of the abdominal wall

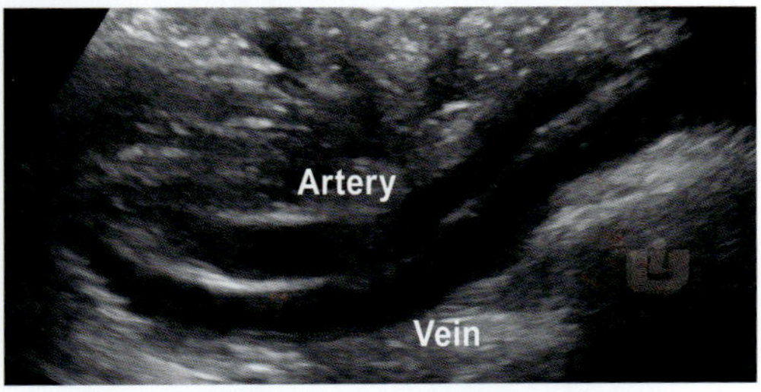

Fig. 2-7. *EIV image demonstrating its "scoop" appearance as it courses toward the EIV-IIV confluence. Note the EIA lying anterior to the EIV. This could be a source of compression.*

- The tributaries of the EIV are:
  - Inferior epigastric
  - Deep iliac circumflex

Iliac vein anatomical landmarks and points of possible extrinsic compression

- Umbilicus
  - The right CIV can be identified by placing the ultrasound transducer just to the right of the umbilicus.
  - The left CIV can be identified by placing the transducer at an oblique angle just below the umbilicus. [9]
- Iliac arteries
  - The common and external iliac arteries can be a source of extrinsic compression on the underlying iliac veins. These forms of extrinsic compression are referred to as Nonthrombotic Iliac Vein Lesions (NIVLs).
- Spine/aorta
  - The left CIV courses just anterior to the spine at the level of the aortic bifurcation.
    - » The left CIV is most likely to have obstructive pathology, however, compression of the right CIV and bilateral EIVs have been documented. *(Table 2-1)*

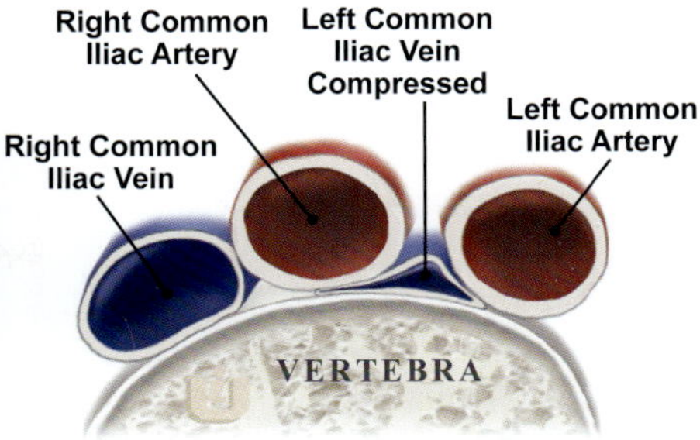

Fig. 2-8. *Cross-section view of the left CIV being compressed by the right and left CIAs.* *Adapted from www.scgvs.com*

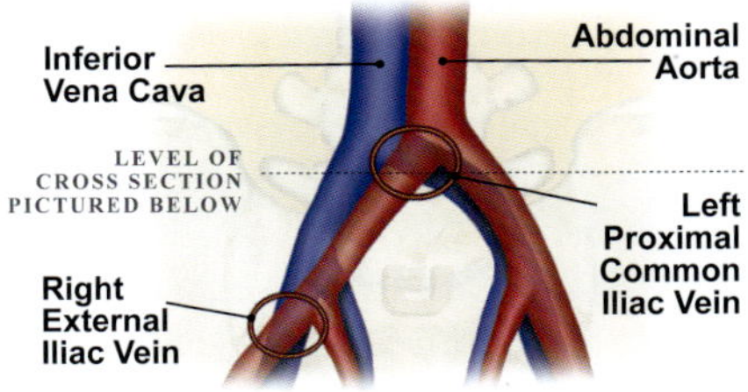

Fig. 2-9. *Most Frequently Occurring NIVLs.*

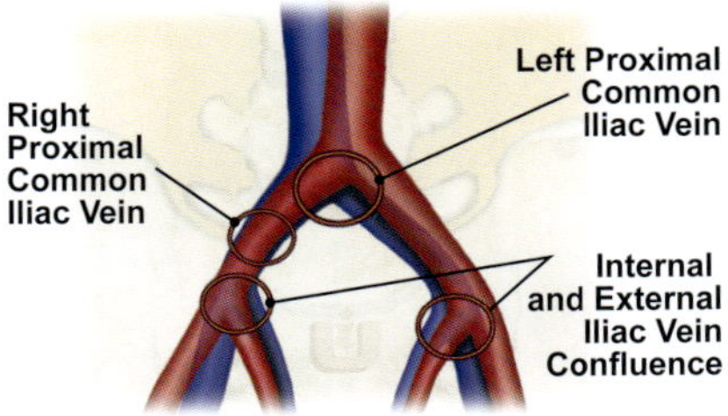

Fig. 2-10. *Less Frequently Occurring NIVLs.*

Note the slight shift in the position (when compared to Fig. 2-9) of the aorta and the IVC creating additional sites of potential obstruction.

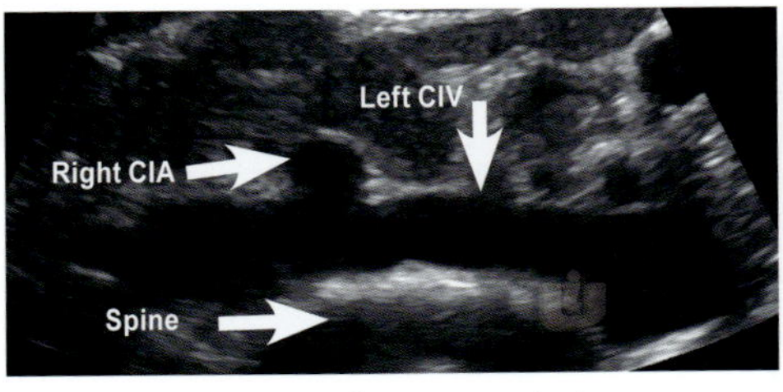

Fig. 2-11. *Left CIV as it courses between the right CIA and spine.*

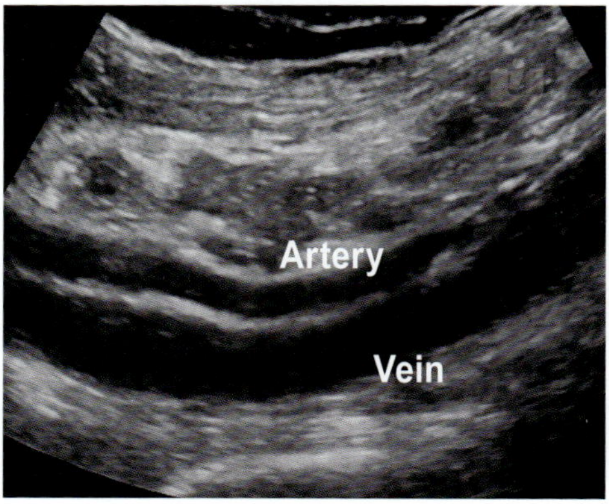

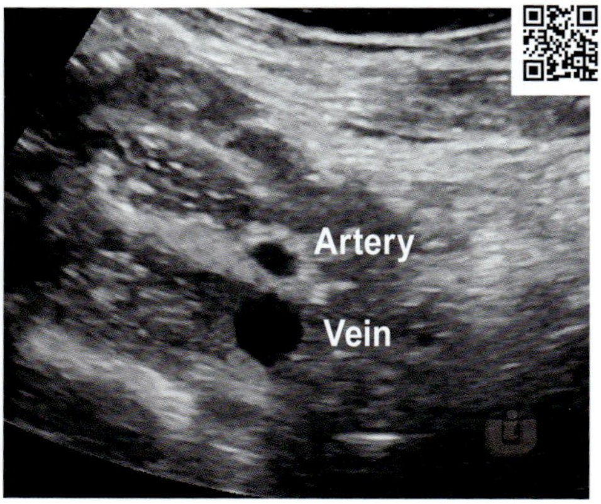

Fig. 2-12. *EIV in longitudinal and transverse views demonstrating pulsatile, repetitive compression of the EIV by the overlying external iliac artery. This repetitive compression can cause damage to the walls of the vein, disrupting flow.*

Table 2-1. **Areas of Iliac Vein Compression***

Common Iliac Veins	External Iliac Veins
• Right common iliac artery on left common iliac vein	• Right external iliac artery on right external iliac vein
• Right common iliac artery on right common iliac vein	• Right internal iliac artery on right external iliac vein
• Left common iliac artery on left common iliac vein	• Left external iliac artery on left external iliac vein
	• Left internal iliac artery on left external iliac vein
	• Inguinal ligament on right external iliac vein
	• Inguinal ligament on left external iliac vein

*More than one type of compression may exist.

Labropoulos Nicos, Diagnosis of Iliac Vein Obstruction with Duplex Ultrasound Criteria used during duplex ultrasound examination to identify iliac vein obstruction. Endovascular Today, July 2018, Vol. 17, No. 7 page 3

Inferior vena cava and iliac vein anatomical variants [3, 10]

- Fourteen anatomical variants have been identified *(See Fig. 2-13 for some examples)*
- Anomalies include:
  - IVC duplication (most common)
  - Left IVC
  - Hypoplasia
  - Aplasia
  - Webs
  - Megacava (diameter of >28-30mm)
- Anomalies like aplasia and hypoplasia are more common in patients with a history of DVT.
- Anomalies related to the iliac veins include:
  - Extra iliac vein(s)
  - Variations in the confluence with the IVC
  - Shortened or absent CIV

When performing an ultrasound for pelvic venous insufficiency, it is important to recognize a double IVC or left IVC, as there have been cases where a left IVC was mistakenly identified as a dilated left gonadal vein.

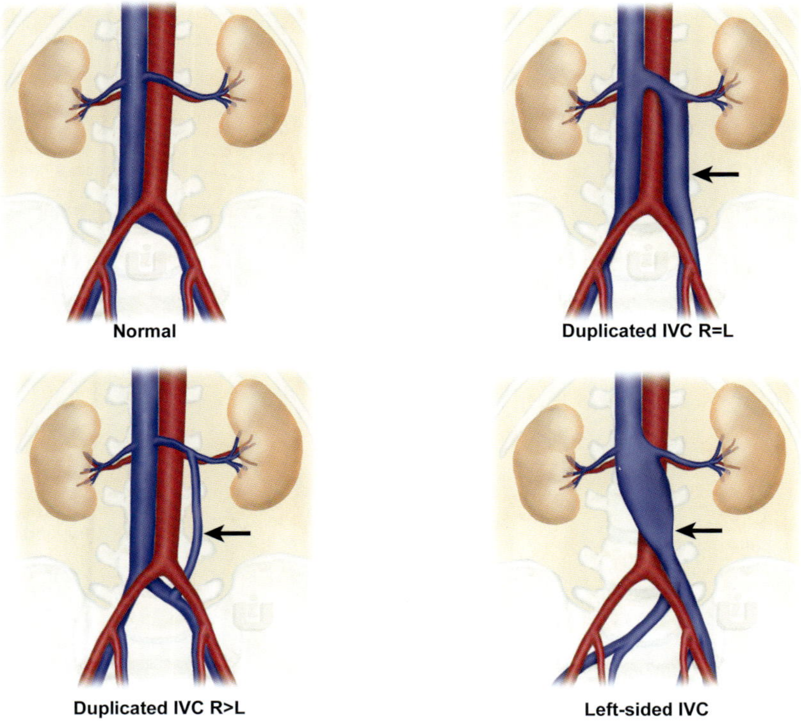

Fig. 2-13. *Most common IVC anatomical variants.* [22]

Internal Iliac Veins

- The IIVs:
  - Also known as the hypogastric veins: [8]
  - Arise at the level of the greater sciatic foramen and run posterior to the internal iliac artery
  - Ascend along the lateral wall of the pelvis
  - The role of the IIVs and their tributaries is to drain the organs within the pelvic cavity as well as the genitalia (vulva and scrotum), buttocks, low back, and hips.
  - Have multiple tributaries, some of which originate within the pelvis and others that originate outside of the pelvis. These tributaries are referred to as extrapelvic tributaries.
- Pelvic tributaries of the IIVs and the areas they drain:
  - Middle rectal veins drain the rectum
  - Vesicle veins drain the bladder
  - Uterine veins drain the uterus
  - Vaginal veins drain the vagina

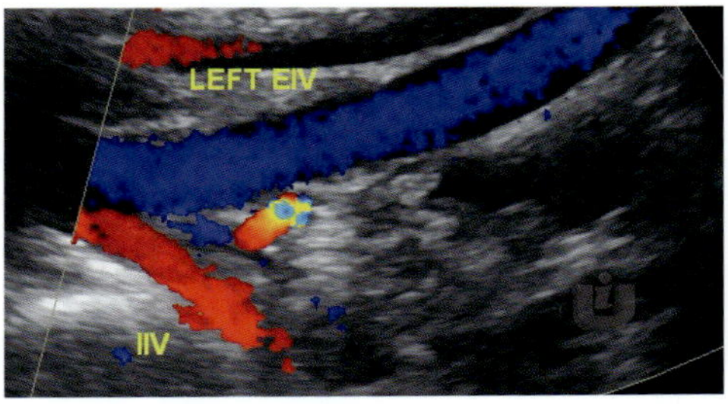

Fig. 2-14. *Internal iliac vein*

- The extrapelvic tributaries are the tributaries of the IIV that originate outside of the pelvis but join the IIVs within the pelvis:
  - Superior and inferior gluteal veins drain the buttocks.
  - Obturator veins drain the low back and hips.
  - Internal pudendal veins drain the external genitalia.
- The round ligament veins are also noteworthy. These veins extend within the round ligament on both sides of the uterus and, in the presence of pelvic vein insufficiency, can become varicosed and contribute to genital varices.

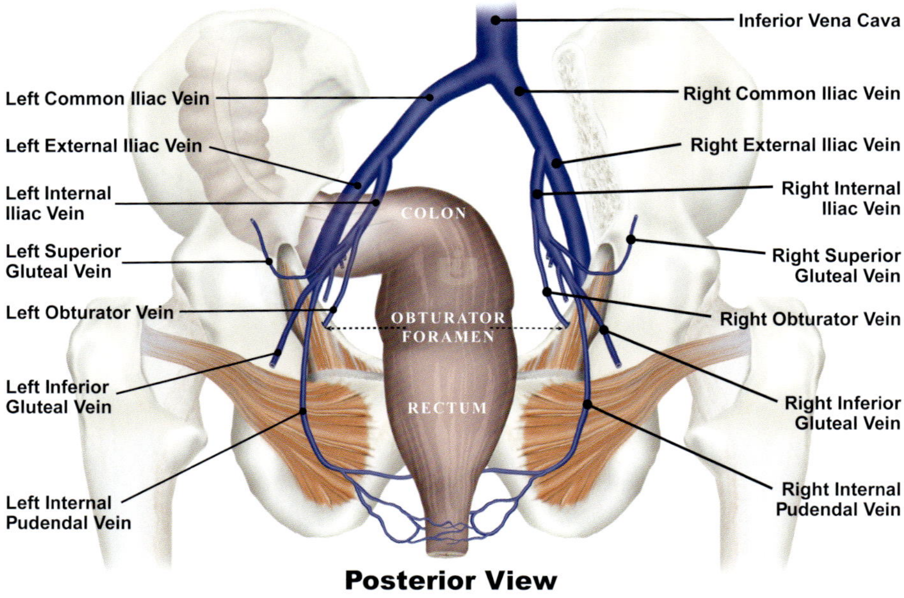

Fig. 2-15. *Extrapelvic tributaries of the IIV connect the pelvis and the lower extremities when reflux is present within the internal iliac and/or gonadal veins.*

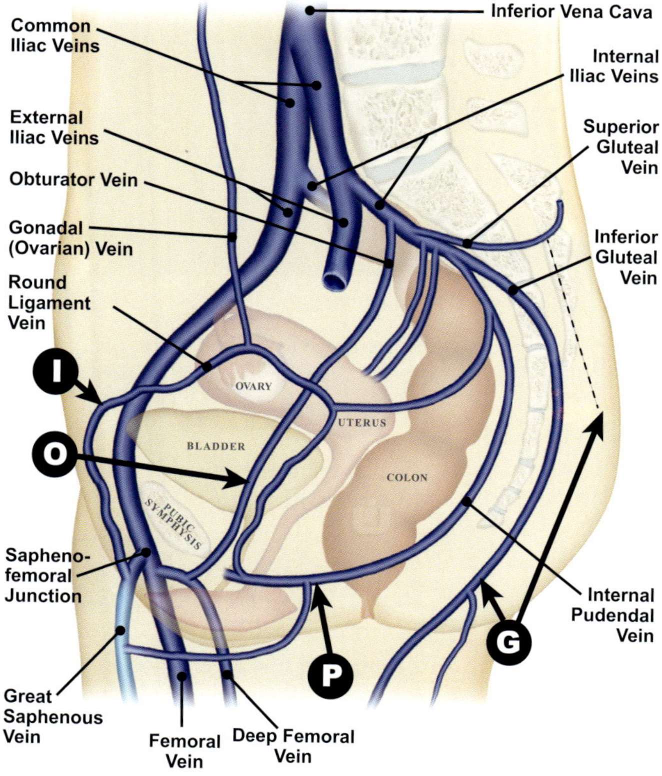

Fig. 2-16. *Four pelvic escape points have been described as connections between the internal iliac tributaries and the lower extremity veins: the inguinal (I) point which is associated with the round ligament veins, the perineal (P) point, which is associated with the pudendal veins, the obturator (O) point which is associated with the obturator veins, and the gluteal (G) points which are associated with the superior and inferior gluteal veins.* [2]

Left Renal Vein

- The Left Renal Vein (LRV) drains the kidney
- Tributaries of the LRV are:
  - Left gonadal vein
  - Left adrenal vein
  - Left inferior phrenic vein
- In the majority of the population, the LRV drains into the IVC by coursing between the SMA and the aorta.

Left renal vein anatomical landmarks and possible points of extrinsic compression:

- SMA/aorta
  - Most left renal veins course between the SMA and the aorta, which could create compression of the LRV between the SMA and the aorta.
- Aorta/spine
  - In a smaller population, the LRV courses posterior to the aorta and anterior to the spine. This could create compression of the LRV between the aorta and spine.
- Left kidney/spine
  - Stretching of the LRV over the aorta can occur due to the left kidney position. This could create a narrowing of the LRV and cause stenosis. *(See chapter 9, pg 148 for diagnostic criteria for the left renal vein)*

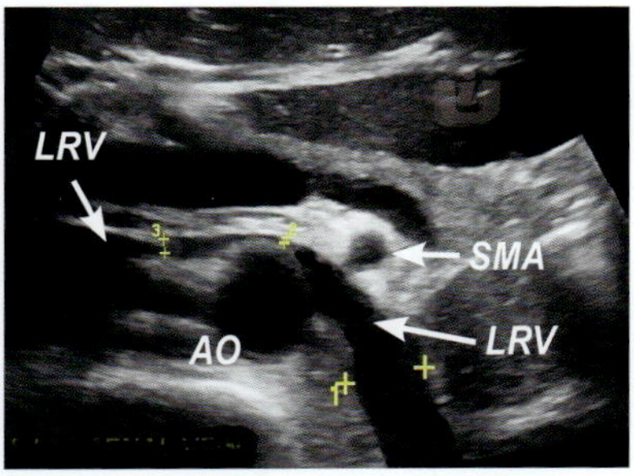

Fig. 2-17. *LRV coursing between the aorta and SMA to its confluence with the IVC*

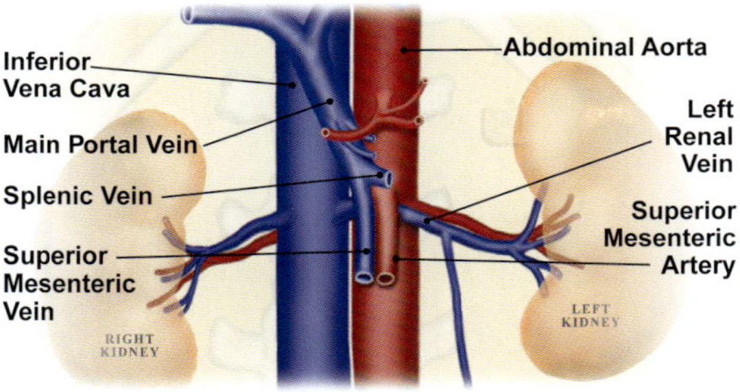

Fig. 2-18. *Mid visceral anatomy. Note how the LRV courses between the aorta and SMA.*

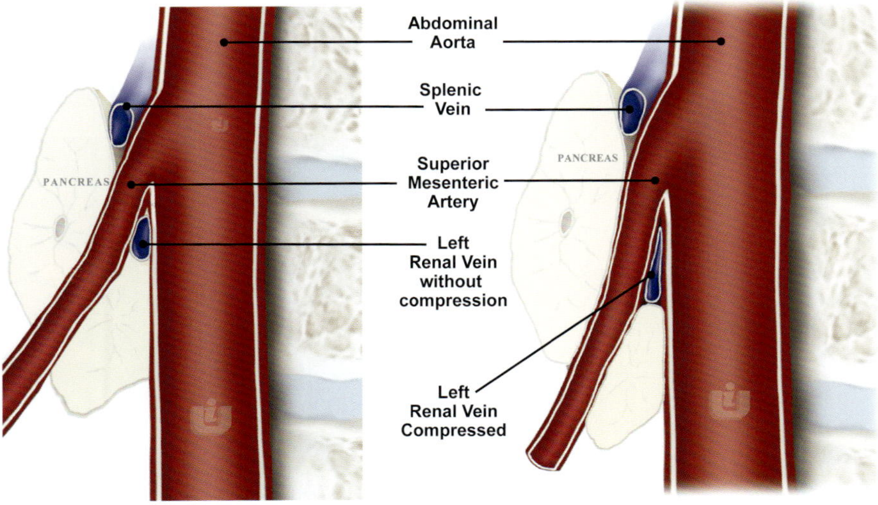

Fig. 2-19. *Longitudinal view demonstrating the LRV coursing between the SMA and aorta without (left) and with (right) compression.*

- The renal hilum may act as a venous reservoir for the left renal vein.
- Left renal vein anatomical variants [11]
  - 3.5% prevalence: Circumaortic LRV where two or more renal veins form a ring around the aorta before entering the IVC.
  - 3% prevalence: Retroaortic LRV, where the LRV courses between the aorta and vertebra before entering the IVC. This variant is the easiest to appreciate with ultrasound.
  - 2.1% prevalence: Multiple left renal veins entering the IVC

Left Renal Vein Anatomy Variants

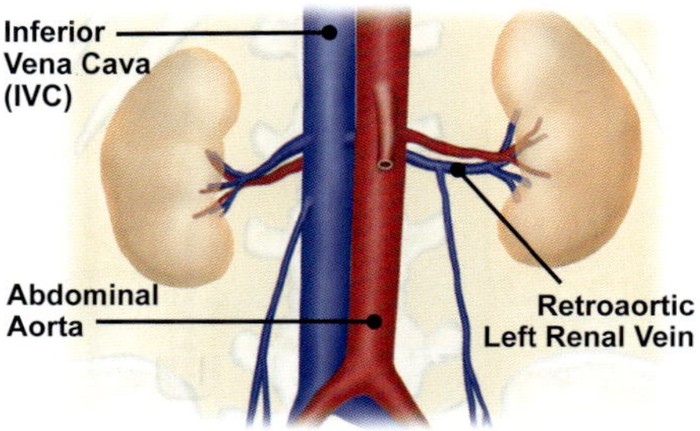

Fig. 2-20. *LRV coursing posterior to the aorta*

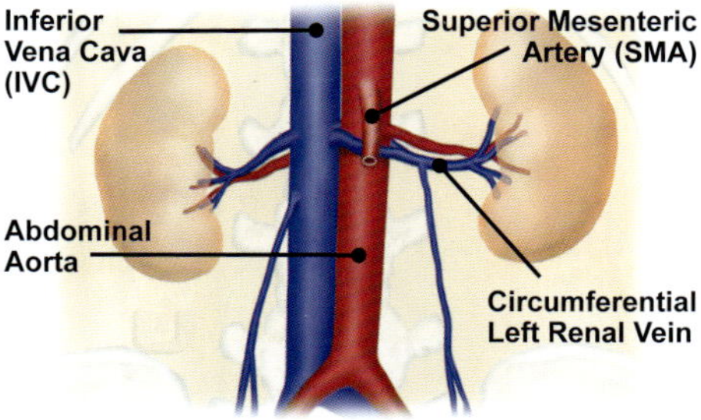

Fig. 2-21. *Two renal vein branches: 1) coursing posterior to the aorta, 2) anterior between the aorta and the SMA*

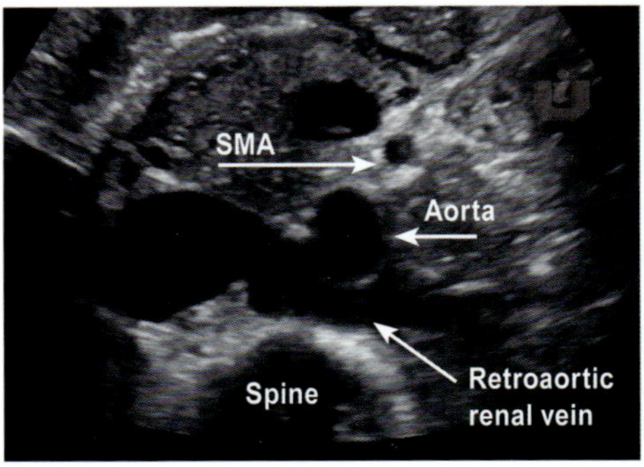

Fig. 2-22. *Retroaortic LRV*

Gonadal Veins

- The right gonadal vein typically drains directly into the IVC.
- The left gonadal vein typically drains into the LRV.
- The normal gonadal vein has a mean diameter of approximately 3mm and usually has two to three valves (which are incompetent in about 50% of women). [13]

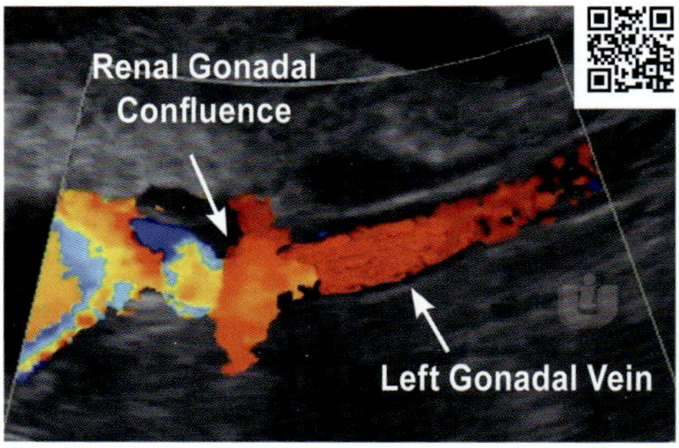

Fig. 2-23. *Color Doppler demonstrating the confluence of the left gonadal vein with the LRV with spontaneous retrograde flow.*

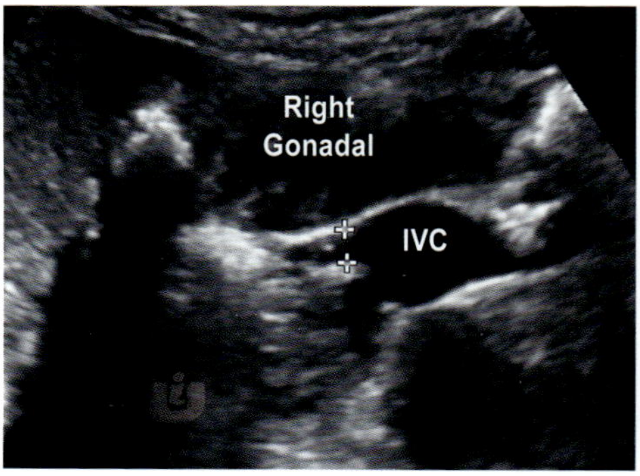

Fig. 2-24. *Transverse view of the confluence of the right gonadal vein with the IVC.*

Female Gonadal Veins

- Also known as ovarian veins
- Are formed by the confluence of multiple pelvic venous plexuses, including the pampiniform plexus.
  - These plexuses form the gonadal vein, which may have two to three trunks before becoming a single trunk at the level of L4.
- Can increase in diameter with pregnancy for the significant increased intravascular volume.

Male Gonadal Veins

- Also known as the testicular veins.
- Are formed by the pampiniform plexus.
- Do not primarily drain the pelvis but pass through the inguinal canal as the testicular vein.

A venous plexus is a complex set of interconnected blood vessels.[16] *The pelvic venous plexuses are described in detail on page 18.*

Gonadal Vein Anatomical Landmarks

- Psoas muscle
  - The gonadal veins course along the anterior wall of the psoas muscle.
- External iliac vein
  - The peripheral (lower abdominal segment) of the gonadal vein crosses over the proximal external iliac vein.

Gonadal Vein Anatomical Variants[12,14,15]

There have been reports of the following variants, although the incidence of occurrence is unclear.

- Right gonadal vein draining to the right renal vein.
- Bilateral duplicated gonadal veins, left > right.

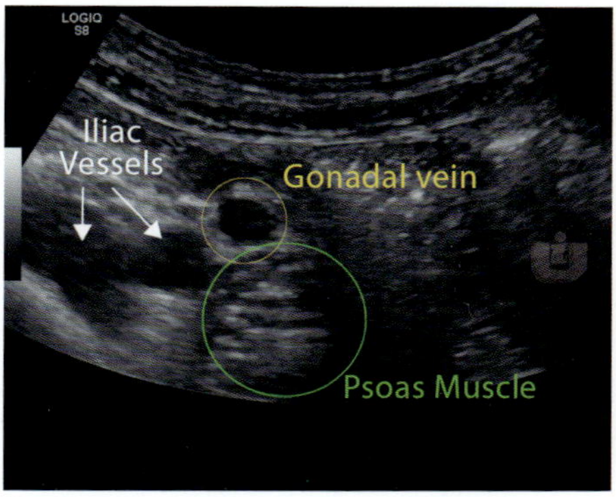

Fig. 2-25. *In transverse view the psoas muscle and iliac vessels can be used as landmarks to help identify the gonadal veins in the distal abdomen.*

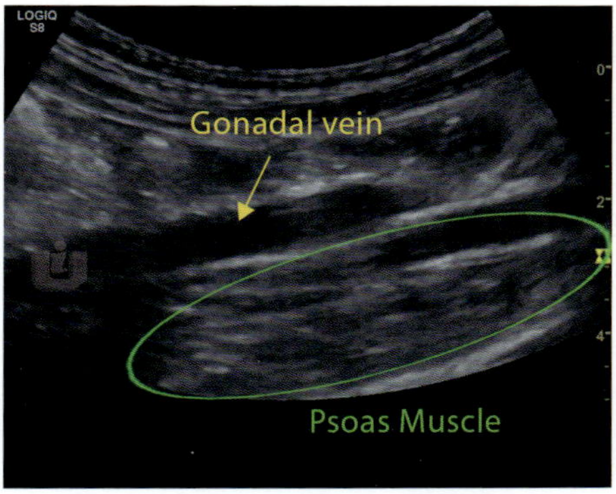

Fig. 2-26. *Longitudinal view of the gonadal vein as it courses over the anterior wall of the psoas muscle.*

Abdominal and Pelvic Veins

Venous Plexuses

A venous plexus is a complex set of interconnected blood vessels.[16]

Female Pelvis

- Uterine venous plexus includes two uterine veins that arise from the sides of the uterus.[16]
- Vaginal venous plexus is comprised of small veins on the sides of the vagina, located near the uterine veins.[16]
- Gonadal venous plexus (pampiniform venous plexus) is located at the top of the ovary and is the origin of the gonadal veins.[17]
- The uterine veins drain into the anterior division of the IIV, draining into the CIV and then into the IVC.[18]
- The uterine veins, vaginal veins, tubal veins, and gonadal tributaries are intimately integrated and interconnected.[19]
- Normal diameter peri- and trans-uterine veins are not always visualized using a transabdominal ultrasound approach.
- Using an endovaginal ultrasound approach, both normal and dilated peri- and trans-uterine veins will be visualized.
- The pelvic venous plexuses act as a venous reservoir for refluxing IIVs or gonadal veins.

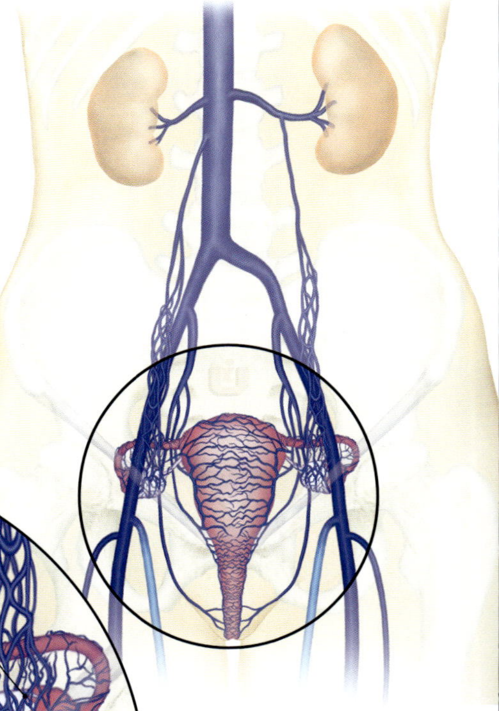

Fig. 2-27. *Pelvic venous plexuses are referred to as peri- and trans-uterine veins.*

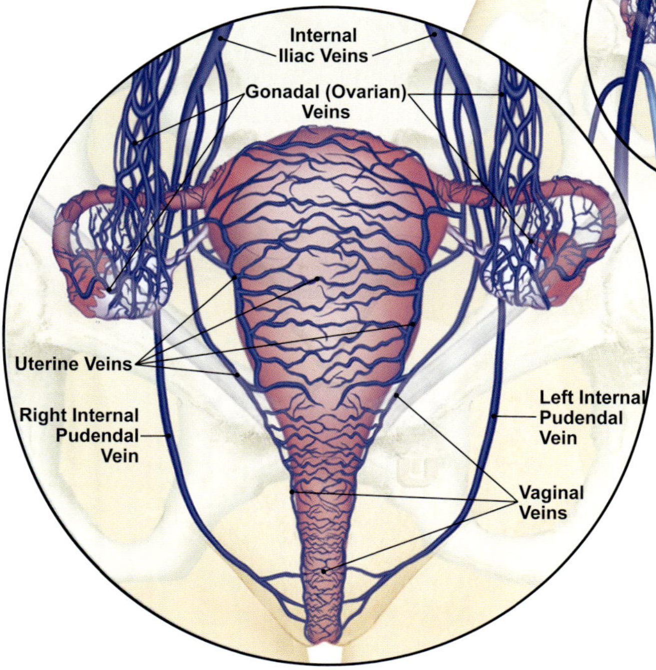

Male Genitalia

- The pampiniform venous plexus is located within the spermatic cord and arise from the mediastinum of the testis. [20]
- The venous vesicle plexus arises. at the neck of the bladder and the base of the prostate gland. [21]

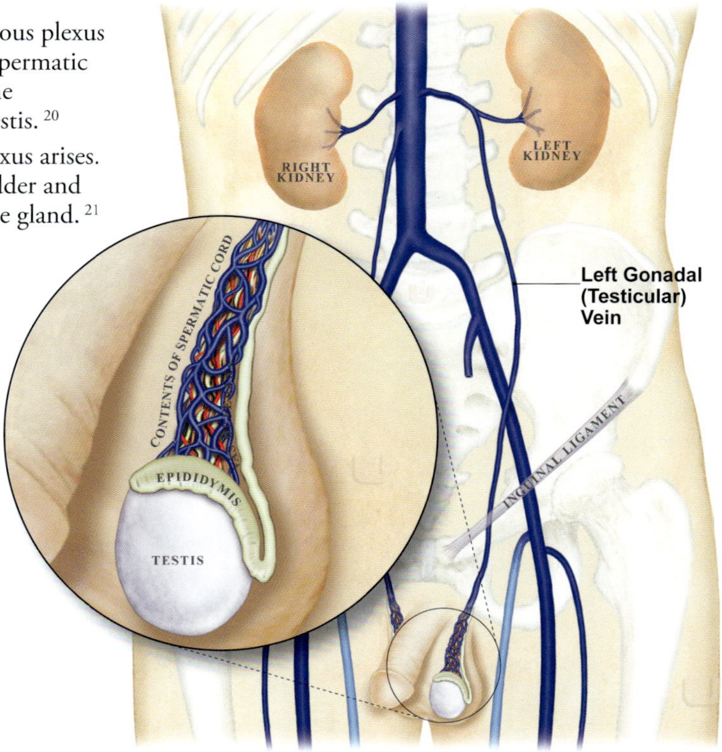

Fig. 2-28. *Male pelvic venous anatomy*

References

1. Meissner, M. H., Khilnani, N. M., Labropoulos, N., et al (2021). The Symptoms-Varices-Pathophysiology classification of pelvic venous disorders: A report of the American Vein & Lymphatic Society International Working Group on Pelvic Venous Disorders. *Journal of Vascular Surgery. Venous and Lymphatic Disorders*, *9*(3), 568–584. https://doi.org/10.1016/j.jvsv.2020.12.084
2. Labropoulos N. (2017). A standardized ultrasound approach to pelvic congestion syndrome. *Phlebology. Oct;32*(9):608-619. doi: 10.1177/0268355516677135. Epub 2016 Oct 31. PMID: 27799418
3. Labropoulos N. (2018). Diagnosis of Iliac Vein Obstruction with Duplex Ultrasound Criteria Used During Duplex Ultrasound Examination to Identify Iliac Vein Obstruction. *Endovascular Today*, *17*(7), 50-52. https://assets.bmctoday.net/evtoday/pdfs/et0718_F2e_Labropoulos.pdf
4. Vaskovic J. (2022, July 6). *Inferior vena cava: Anatomy and Function.* Kenhub. www.kenhub. com/en/library/anatomy/inferior-vena-cava
5. Healthline Medical Network. (2018, Dec. 6). *Common Iliac Vein.* Healthline. www.healthline.com/human-body-maps/common-iliac-vein#1
6. Shahid S. (2022, Feb 14). *Common iliac vein.* Kenhub. www.kenhub.com/en/library/anatomy/iliac-vein
7. External Iliac Vein. (n.d.). *Anatomy App.* Retrieved October 16, 2022, from https://anatomy.app/encyclopedia/external-iliac-vein
8. Vaskovic J. (2022, July 6). *Internal iliac vein.* Kenhub. www.kenhub.com/en/library/anatomy/internal-iliac-vein
9. Brinegar KN, Sheth RA, Khademhosseini A, Bautista J, Oklu R. (2015). Iliac vein compression syndrome: Clinical, imaging and pathologic findings. *World J Radiol*, *7*(11):375-381. doi:10.4329/wjr.v7.i11.375
10. DePietro DM, Carlon T, Trerotola SO, Sudheendra D. (2020). Endovascular Treatment of an Anatomically Complex Iliac Lesion and a Review of Variant Iliac Venous Anatomy, *Journal of Vascular and Interventional Radiology*, *31*(2), 260-264.ISSN 1051-0443, https://doi.org/10.1016/j.jvir.2019.08.032
11. Hostiuc S, Rusu MC, Negoi I, Dorobanțu B, Grigoriu M. (2019). Anatomical variants of renal veins: A meta-analysis of prevalence. *Sci Rep, Jul 25;9*(1):10802. doi: 10.1038/s41598-019-47280-8. PMID: 31346244; PMCID: PMC6658480
12. Maingard, J., Glick, Y. *Gonadal vein.* Reference article, Radiopaedia. org. (accessed on 12 Feb 2022) https://doi.org/10.53347/rID-26030
13. Meissner MH, Gloviczki P. (2019). Pelvic venous disorders. In: J.I. Almeida (Ed.), *Atlas of Endovascular Venous Surgery. 2nd ed.*: (pp. 567-99). Elsevier Philadelphia (PA).
14. Fernandes JR, Strufaldi MB, Machado BDS, Nascimento S, Wafae N, Ruiz CR. (2012). Bilateral duplication of gonadal veins: A case report. *International Journal of Morphology, 30*, 1487-1489.
15. Ghosh A, Chaudhury S. (2019). A cadaveric study of ovarian veins: variations, measurements and clinical significance. *Anat Cell Biol, Dec; 52*(4), 385-389. doi: 10.5115/acb.19.062. Epub 2019 Dec 16. PMID: 31949976; PMCID: PMC6952686
16. Healthline Medical Network. (2018, Jan. 20). *Uterine Venous Plexus.* Healthline. www.healthline.com/human-body-maps/uterine-venous-plexus#1
17. Gibson E, Mahdy H. *Anatomy, Abdomen and Pelvis, Ovary.* [Updated 2021 Jul 26]. In: StatPearls [Internet]. Treasure Island (FL): StatPearls Publishing; 2022 Jan-. Available from: https://www.ncbi.nlm.nih.gov/books/NBK545187
18. Davidoff A. (2010). *Venous Drainage.* The CommonVein.net. https://uterus.thecommonvein.net/the-liver/structure/venous-drainage
19. Davidoff A. (n.d.). *Uterus Part 1.* Applied Anatomy. https://thecommonvein.net/uterus-part-1
20. Healthline Medical Network. (2018, Jan. 23). *Pampiniform Plexus.* Healthline. www.healthline.com/human-body-maps/pampiniform-plexus#1
21. Merriam-Webster, Incorporated. (2022) Vesical. *Merriam Webster.* https://www.merriam-webster.com/medical/vesical
22. Truty, M. J., & Bower, T. C. (2007). Congenital anomalies of the inferior vena cava and left renal vein: implications during open abdominal aortic aneurysm reconstruction. *Annals of Vascular Surgery*, *21*(2), 186–197. https://doi.org/10.1016/j.avsg.2006.10.014

Anatomy of the Veins

A detailed understanding of the lower extremity venous anatomy is the foundation of clinical phlebology, and is essential to the diagnosis and management of venous disorders in the lower extremity. [1, 2, 3, 5, 34, 44]

Similarities between arteries and veins [13, 44, 52]

Veins, like arteries, are composed of 3 layers:

- Tunica Intima or Interna: Innermost layer composed of endothelial cells.
- Tunica Media: Middle layer composed of smooth muscle cells and connective tissue.
- Tunica Adventitia or Externa: Outermost layer composed of collagen fibers, the vasa vasorum and the sympathetic nerve fibers.

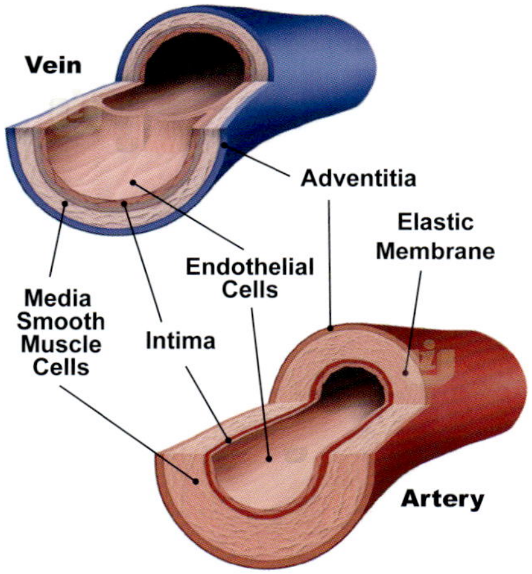

Fig. 3-1. *Wall composition: Vein vs. Artery*

Differences between arteries and veins [13, 44, 52]

Media

- Veins are not as structurally robust as arteries.
- Vein media is ten times thinner than the arterial media.
- Vein media has significantly less elastin than the arterial media.

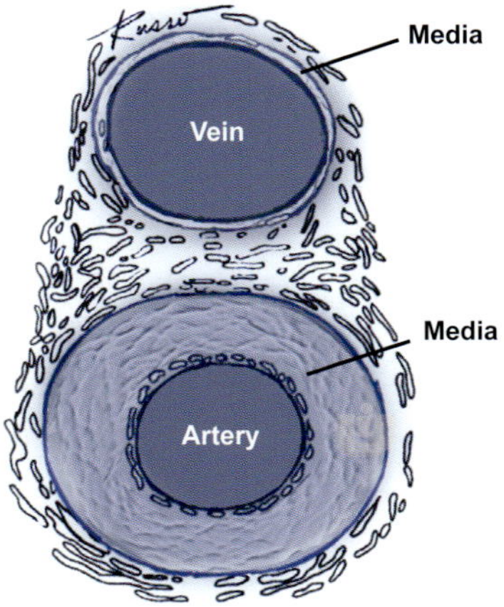

Fig. 3-2. *Vein media is ten times thinner than the arterial media.*

Valves [9, 10, 11, 12, 13, 14, 19, 21, 22, 27, 32, 33, 34, 44, 51, 56]

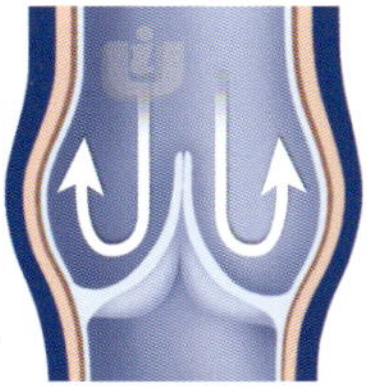

- Venous valves are bicuspid, containing two luminal leaflets.
- Both luminal leaflets or valve cusps are crescent in shape.
- These crescent shaped leaflets are formed by a reduplication of the intima.
- The vein wall is thicker at the base of the valve cusps making it sturdier in this area.
- The lumen is enlarged in the area where the cusps sit, and when closed, creates a pouched appearance. This area is known as a valvular sinus.
- The diameter in the area of the valve sinus is usually two times the diameter of the adjacent segment of vein. The vertical length of the valve sinus is approximately twice its diameter.
- Valves are meant to be unidirectional or one-way and are designed to prevent the backwash of blood.
- Deep, superficial and perforating veins contain valves.
- Perforating veins contain one-way valves that allow blood to flow inward from the superficial veins to the deep veins.

- There are more venous valves in the calf than in the thigh.
- Lower extremity veins have more valves than upper extremity veins. In general, the number of valves is higher in the more peripheral portions of the extremities and decreases centrally.
- Valves can withstand retrograde pressures up to 300mmHg.

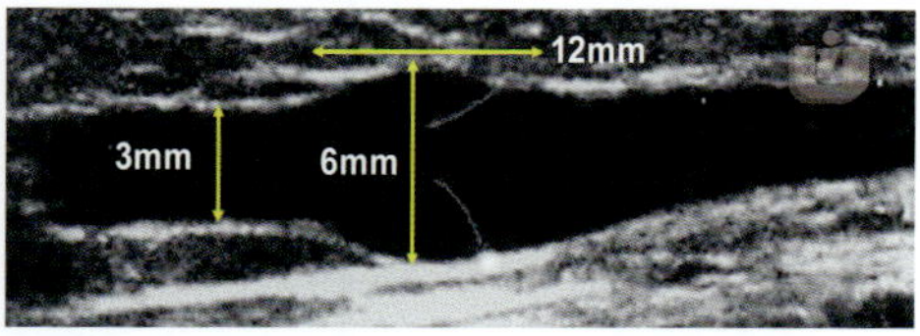

Fig. 3-3. *Valve sinus and adjacent segment of vein: diameter and length relationship.*

> *The diameter in the area of the valve sinus is usually two times the diameter of the adjacent segment of vein. The vertical length of the valve sinus is approximately twice its diameter.*

Competent Valves [9-14, 19, 21, 22, 27, 32, 56, 57]

- In healthy leg veins, these unidirectional valves allow blood to move in one direction: towards the heart. When you walk, your foot, calf and thigh muscles squeeze the veins of your legs, pushing non-oxygenated blood back to the heart. As blood moves toward the heart, it pushes the cusps open. When your leg muscles relax, the valves inside your veins close, preventing the backwash of blood flow down the legs.
- This retrograde flow quickly ceases as it closes the valve by pushing the valve leaflets together. This brief flow reversal is known as the valve closure time (VCT) and should not be reported as venous reflux or venous insufficiency.
- Valve closure time in the femoropopliteal veins is <1sec or <1000ms, and <0.5sec or <500ms in the superficial, perforating and deep calf veins. [31]

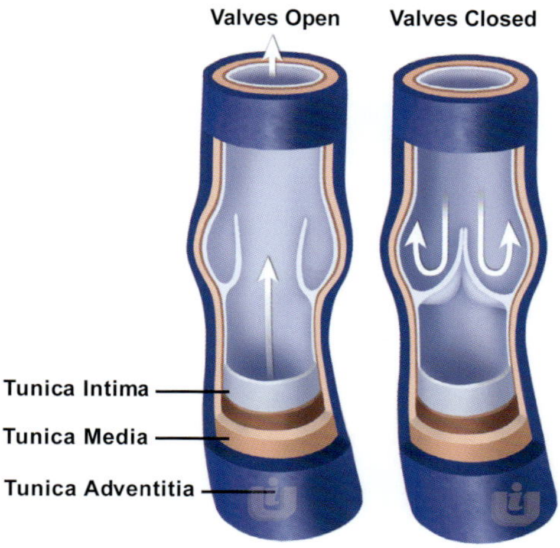

Fig. 3-4. *Under normal physiological conditions antegrade flow opens the valves. The valves close to prevent retrograde flow. This is known as unidirectional flow.*

Incompetent Valves [10-14, 19, 21, 22, 27, 32, 56, 57]

- Weakened, damaged or absent valves allow blood to flow backwards down the lower extremity. This backwash of blood is known as reflux.
- Reflux is defined by retrograde flow >1sec or >1000ms in the femoropopliteal veins and >0.5sec or >500ms in the superficial, perforating and deep calf veins. [31]

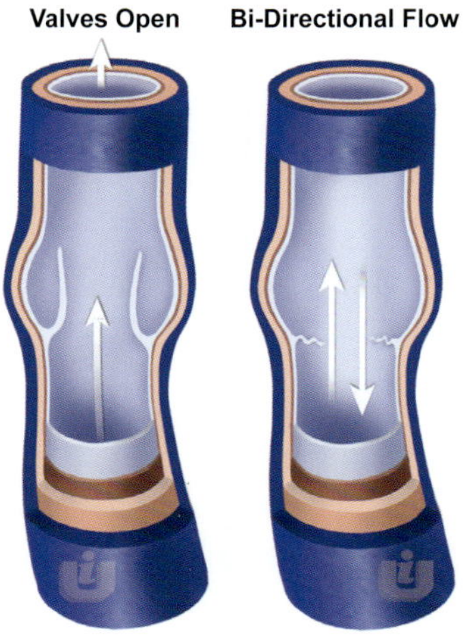

Fig. 3-5. *Under abnormal physiological conditions antegrade flow opens the valves, but the weak, damaged valves allow the blood to flow backwards. This backwash of blood is known as reflux.*

Components of the Lower Extremity Venous System [1, 2, 3, 9, 11, 12, 13, 14, 19]

Three major components of the lower extremity venous system:

- Deep system
- Superficial system
- Communicating system

These systems are located in two main compartments:

- Deep compartment, which is confined by the muscular fascia and contains the deep veins.
- Superficial compartment, which is confined deeply by the muscular fascia and superficially by the dermis.

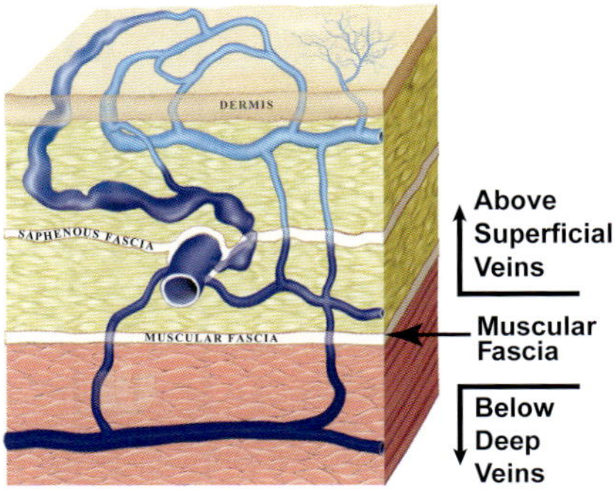

Fig. 3-6. *Deep and Superficial compartments separated by the muscular fascia.*

The superficial compartment is further broken down into two distinct compartments. The interfascial compartment and the epifascial compartment.

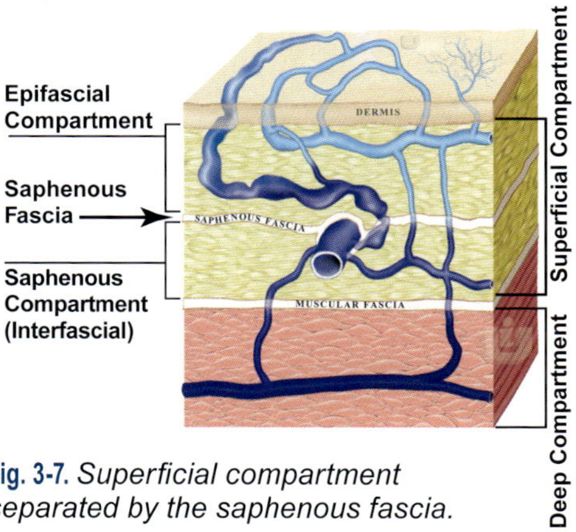

Fig. 3-7. *Superficial compartment separated by the saphenous fascia.*

Interfascial Compartment [1-5, 7, 9, 11-14, 19]

- The interfascial compartment is known as the saphenous compartment.
- The saphenous compartment is bound on the deep side by the muscular fascia and superficially by the saphenous fascia. The two hyperechoic fascial layers come together on the sides to seal the compartment creating what resembles an eye.

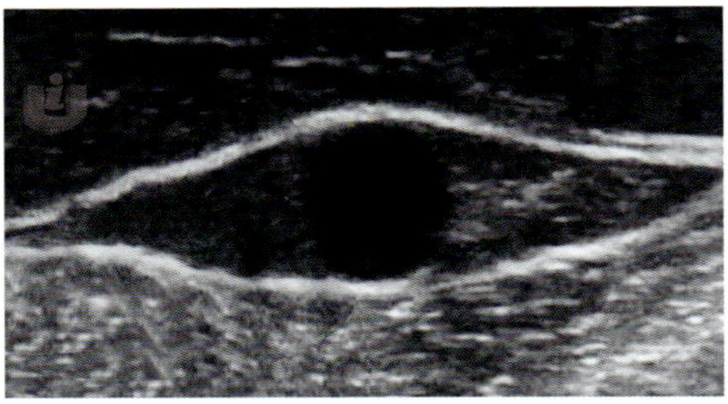

Fig. 3-8. *Fascia is hyperechoic and identifiable on ultrasound: therefore, it is very useful as a landmark.*

- The saphenous fascia is that portion of the membranous layer of the subcutaneous tissue that overlies the saphenous veins.
- The saphenous compartment was first identified by ultrasound. It is an important landmark used to identify the Great Saphenous Vein.
- Interfascial veins lie between the muscular and saphenous fascia within the saphenous compartment.

Epifascial Compartment [1, 2, 9, 11-14, 19]

- The epifascial compartment is bound on the deep side by the saphenous fascia and superficially by the dermis.
- Epifascial veins lie above the saphenous fascia in the superficial subcutaneous compartment.

Saphenous tributaries, and communicating veins, lie external to the saphenous compartment.

The term tributary is used to describe a vein that joins with a superficial axial vein. Axial superficial veins refer to the main trunk of the GSV, AAGSV, and SSV.

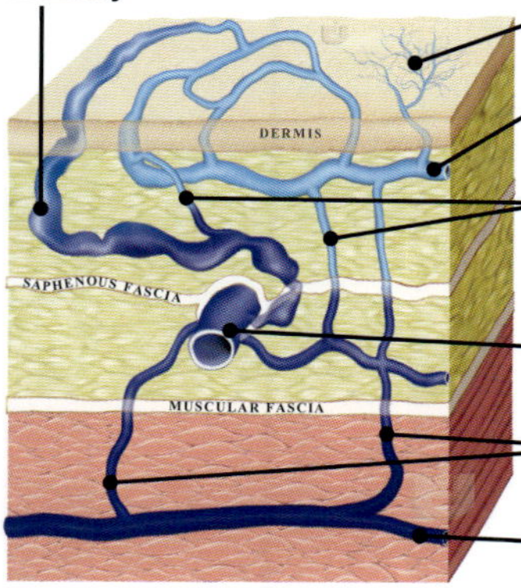

Fig. 3-9. *Named and unnamed veins of the superficial compartments.*

Communicating Veins [1, 2, 3, 13, 33, 34]

- Communicating veins are veins that connect two different points of the venous system. They may communicate the great saphenous vein with the small saphenous vein or the superficial venous system with the deep venous system.
- Perforating veins cross the muscular fascia, connecting the superficial and deep systems.
- Tributaries cross the saphenous fascia, connecting interfascial superficial veins to epifascial superficial veins. The term tributary is used when describing a vein; the term branch is used when describing an artery.
- Unnamed communicating veins connect veins within the same system (i.e., deep to deep, superficial to superficial).

Accessory Veins [1, 2, 3, 5, 8, 9]

- Accessory Great Saphenous Veins are interfascial veins that lie within their own saphenous compartment. They most commonly join with the GSV at or peripheral to the SFJ.

Accessory saphenous veins are venous segments that course in a plane parallel to the saphenous veins. They may be anterior, or posterior to the main trunk.

Table 3-1. **Nomenclature of the Lower Extremity Deep and Superficial Veins** [1-6, 8, 11, 15, 16, 20, 26, 28, 39, 41]

Deep Veins

Thigh

- Common Femoral Vein (CFV)
- Femoral Vein (FV)
- Deep Femoral Vein (DFV)

Knee

- Popliteal Vein (PopV)
- Genicular Venous Plexus (GVP)

Calf

- Anterior Tibial Veins (ATVs)
- Tibial Peroneal Trunk (TPT)
- Posterior Tibial Veins (PTVs)
- Peroneal Veins (PerVs)

Sural Veins

- Soleal veins (SolVs)
- Gastrocnemius veins (GVs)
  - Medial gastrocnemius veins (MGVs)
  - Lateral gastrocnemius veins (LGVs)
- Intergemellar Veins (IntGVs)

Superficial Veins

- Great Saphenous Vein (GSV)
- Anterior Accessory Great Saphenous Vein (AAGSV)
- Posterior Accessory Great Saphenous Vein (PAGSV)
- Anterior Thigh Circumflex Vein (ATCV)
- Posterior Thigh Circumflex Vein (PTCV)
- Small Saphenous Vein (SSV)
- Thigh Extension of the Small Saphenous Vein (TE-SSV)
- Intersaphenous Veins (IntSVs)
- Lateral Venous System (LVS)

In the United States the terms Anterior Accessory Great Saphenous Vein and Posterior Accessory Great Saphenous Vein are used in place of Anterior Accessory Saphenous Vein and Posterior Accessory Saphenous Vein because these terms are recognized by insurance payors.

Comprehensive Venous Anatomy

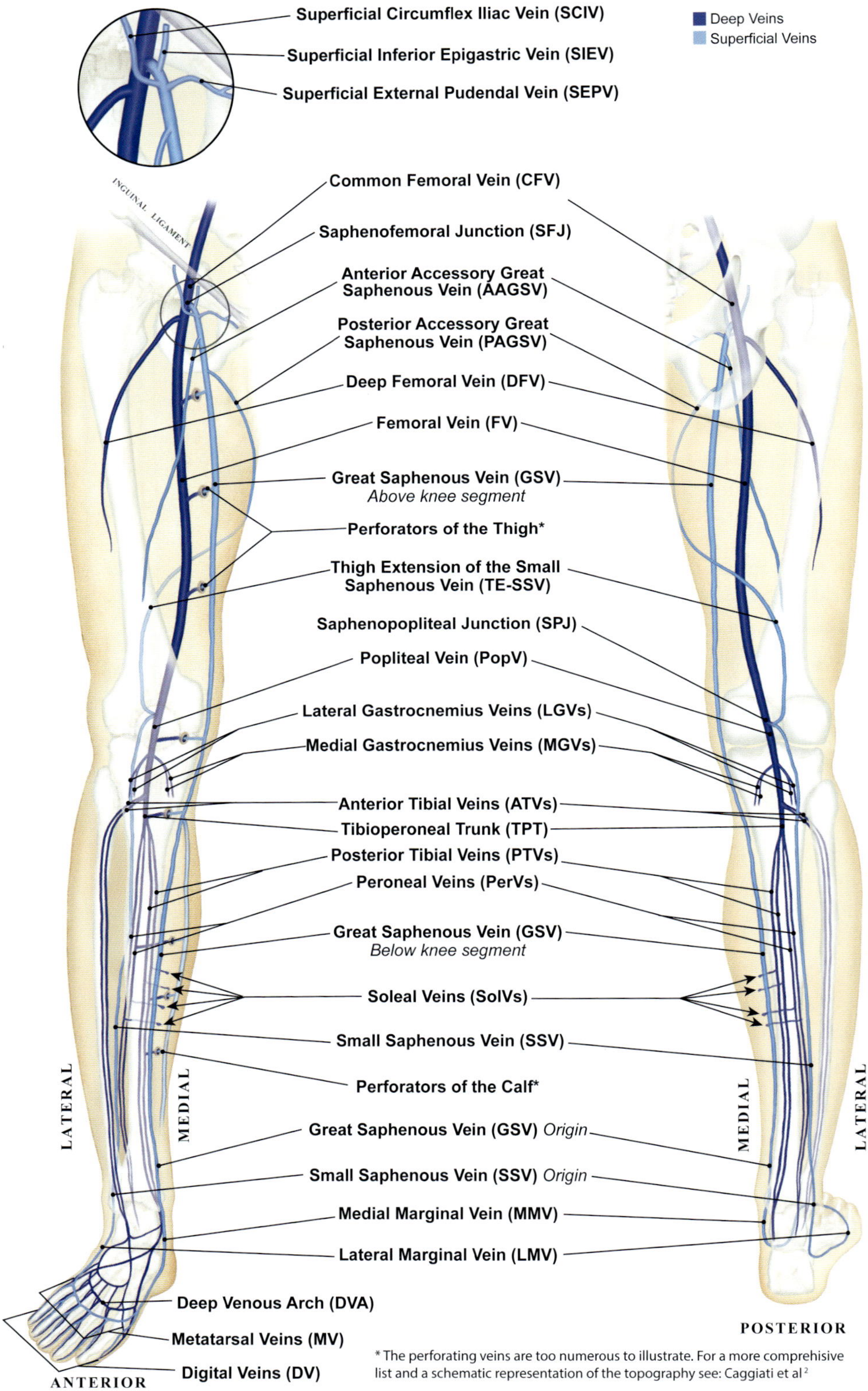

* The perforating veins are too numerous to illustrate. For a more comprehisive list and a schematic representation of the topography see: Caggiati et al[2]

Table 3-2. Nomenclature of the Perforating Veins[1, 2, 3, 6, 11, 12]

Perforators grouped by topography
Thigh Perforators
• Inguinal PV • Medial thigh PV • Anterior thigh PV • Posterior thigh PV • Lateral thigh PV
Knee Perforators
• Popliteal fossa PV • Medial knee PV • Lateral knee PV • Suprapatellar PV • Infrapatellar PV
Medial Calf Perforators
• Medial leg PV • Paratibial PV • Posterior tibial PV
Posterior Calf Perforators
• Medial gastrocnemius PV • Lateral gastrocnemius PV • Intergemellar PV
Ankle Perforators
• Medial ankle PV • Lateral ankle PV

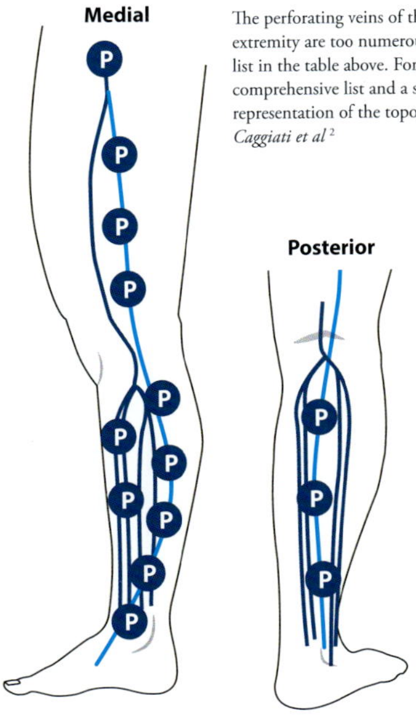

The perforating veins of the lower extremity are too numerous to list in the table above. For a more comprehensive list and a schematic representation of the topography see: *Caggiati et al*[2]

Deep Veins

Venous return or drainage begins at the foot. Therefore, when describing the lower extremity venous anatomy, it will be described from peripheral to central.

- Deep veins have an accompanying artery.
- Deep calf veins are paired.

Deep Veins of the Foot and Calf[9, 15, 16, 17, 35, 51]

- The deep plantar digital veins drain into the deep plantar metatarsal veins. The deep plantar metatarsal veins are drained by the deep plantar venous arch, which runs transversely across the foot from the first interosseous space to the base of the fifth metatarsal bone.
- The medial and lateral plantar veins are a continuance of the medial and lateral ends of the deep plantar arch, respectively. The lateral plantar vein travels across the foot joining with medial plantar veins at the medial malleolus to form the posterior tibial veins (PTVs), which ascend along the medial aspect of the calf.
- The deep dorsal digital veins drain into the deep dorsal metatarsal veins from which the pedal vein originates.
- Anterior tibial veins (ATVs) are a continuance of the pedal vein. They travel superiorly between the tibia and fibula.
- The peroneal veins (PerVs) originate in the foot and ascend behind the fibula along the lateral aspect of the calf.
- The PTVs join to form a common tibial trunk. The PerVs join to form a common peroneal trunk. The common tibial and common peroneal trunks unite to form the origin of the tibioperoneal trunk. The TPT is a short segment of vein in the upper third of the calf.
- The ATVs join to form a common anterior tibial trunk that unites with the tibioperoneal trunk to form the popliteal vein (PopV).

Lower Extremity Venous

The term confluence is used when two or more veins join together to form a single vein.

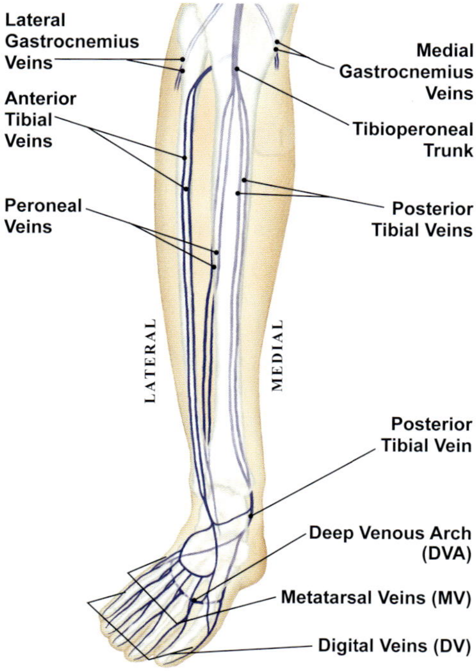

Fig. 3-10. *Deep veins of the foot and calf.*

Intramuscular Veins of the Calf [9, 15, 16, 17]

The gastrocnemius and soleal veins are intramuscular veins of the calf. The gastrocnemius veins are paired with an artery and drain into the popliteal vein. The soleal sinuses are not paired, do not have accompanying arteries and vary in size and extent.

Gastrocnemius Veins (GVs)

- Located within the medial and lateral heads of the gastrocnemius muscle.
- Arise from the venous plexus formed by the venous sinusoids in the gastrocnemius muscle.
- Drain into either the popliteal or posterior tibial veins.
- There are three sets of gastrocnemius veins:
  - Medial gastrocnemius veins: located in the medial head of the gastrocnemius muscle. The medial gastrocnemius veins are typically larger than the lateral gastrocnemius veins.
  - Lateral gastrocnemius veins: located in the lateral head of the gastrocnemius muscle.
  - Intergemellar gastrocnemius vein (IGV): when present, lie between the two heads of the gastrocnemius muscle below the small saphenous vein.

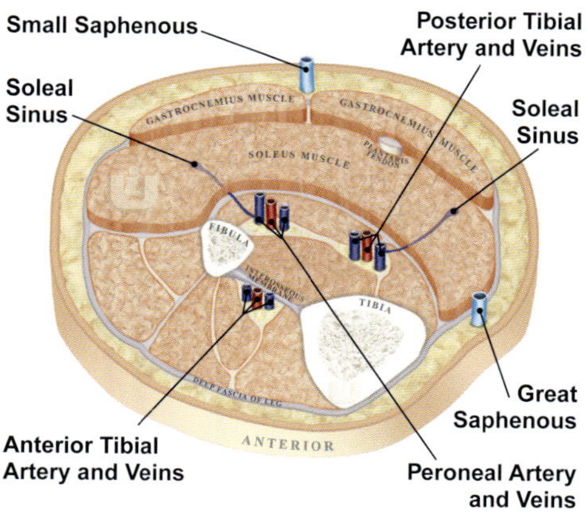

Fig. 3-11. *Deep, superficial, and intramuscular veins of the calf.*

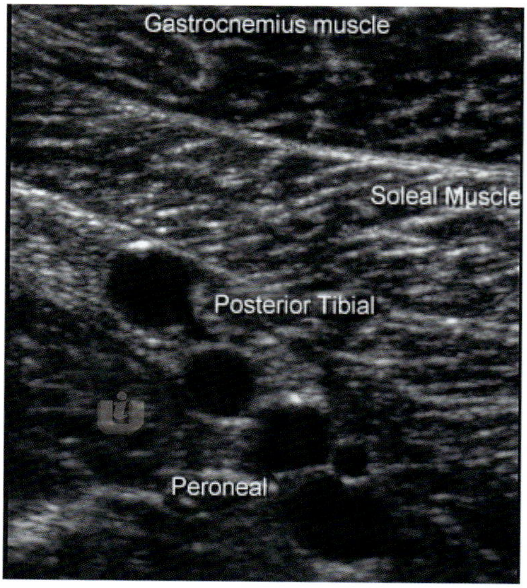

Fig. 3-12. *Gastrocnemius and soleal muscles along with the peroneal and posterior tibial veins*

Soleal Veins (SolVs)

- Located within the soleal muscle.
- Drain into the posterior tibial and peroneal veins.
- Function as reservoirs for blood and thus are sometimes referred to as soleal sinuses.
- Typically, soleal veins only have valves where they connect with other veins. These valves will frequently stop functioning (valvular incompetence) when blood pools in the soleal veins, causing them to dilate. This makes the veins very susceptible to thrombosis.

Genicular Venous Plexus

- A complex venous plexus of interconnecting veins found at the knee region.
- Drain into the popliteal vein.

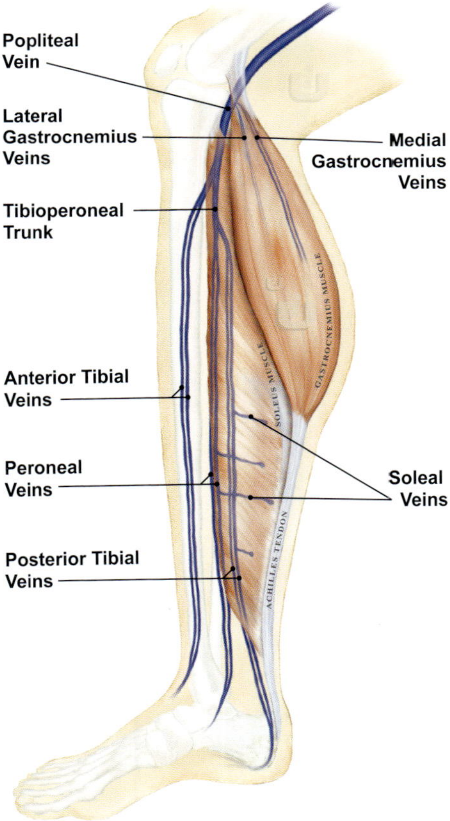

Fig. 3-13. *Deep and intramuscular veins of the calf.*

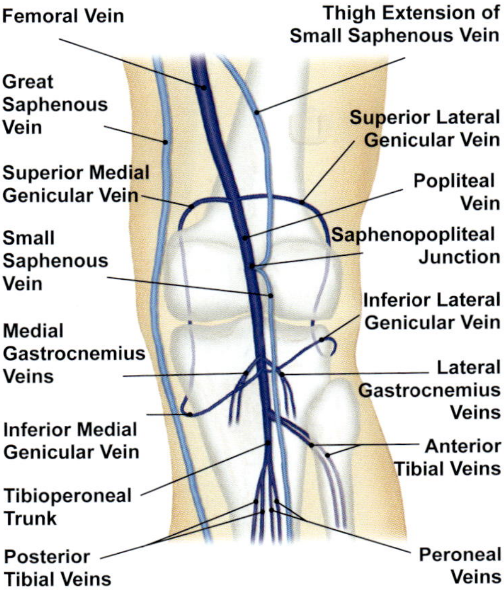

Fig. 3-14. *Veins of the popliteal fossa region.*

Deep Venous System of the Thigh

- At the level where the PopV passes through the adductor hiatus (the opening in the adductor magnus) it becomes the femoral vein (FV).
- The FV travels in the adductor canal to the level of the adductor magnus muscle. It lies medial and slightly deep to the superficial femoral artery.
- The deep femoral vein (DFV) drains the posterior and lateral thigh muscles terminating into the common femoral vein at its confluence with the femoral vein. It lies medial to the deep femoral artery. It is usually only seen at the proximal portion.
- The FV joins the DFV at approximately 9cm below the inguinal ligament to form the common femoral vein (CFV).
- The CFV is approximately 2 to 4cm in length and continues as the external iliac vein (EIV) at the inferior margin of the inguinal ligament. The EIV dives deep at the inguinal ligament and drains the legs and the inferior part of the abdomen.

Femoral Triangle [36, 37, 38]

An anatomical wedge-shaped region located in the upper third of the thigh. It appears as a triangular depression below the inguinal ligament when the limb is flexed, and the hip is externally rotated. It acts as a conduit for structures entering and leaving the anterior thigh.

The femoral triangle consists of three borders, a floor and a roof:

Borders

- Superior – inguinal ligament (a ligament that runs from the anterior superior iliac spine to the pubic tubercle).
- Lateral – medial border of the sartorius muscle.
- Medial – medial border of the adductor longus muscle. The rest of this muscle forms part of the floor of the triangle.

Floor

- Pectineus, iliopsoas, and adductor longus muscles.

Roof

- Fascia lata

The inguinal ligament acts as a flexor retinaculum, supporting the contents of the femoral triangle during flexion at the hip.

Some sources consider the lateral border of the adductor longus to be the medial border of the femoral triangle. However, the majority state that it is the medial border of the adductor longus – and this is the definition used in this book.

Contents

- The femoral triangle contains a number of vital structures. Its contents include (lateral to medial):
  - Femoral nerve
  - Femoral artery
  - Femoral vein
  - Femoral canal
    - » Lymph nodes
    - » Lymph vessels
- The femoral artery, vein and canal are contained within a fascial compartment – known as the femoral sheath.

The great saphenous vein drains into the femoral vein within the triangle.

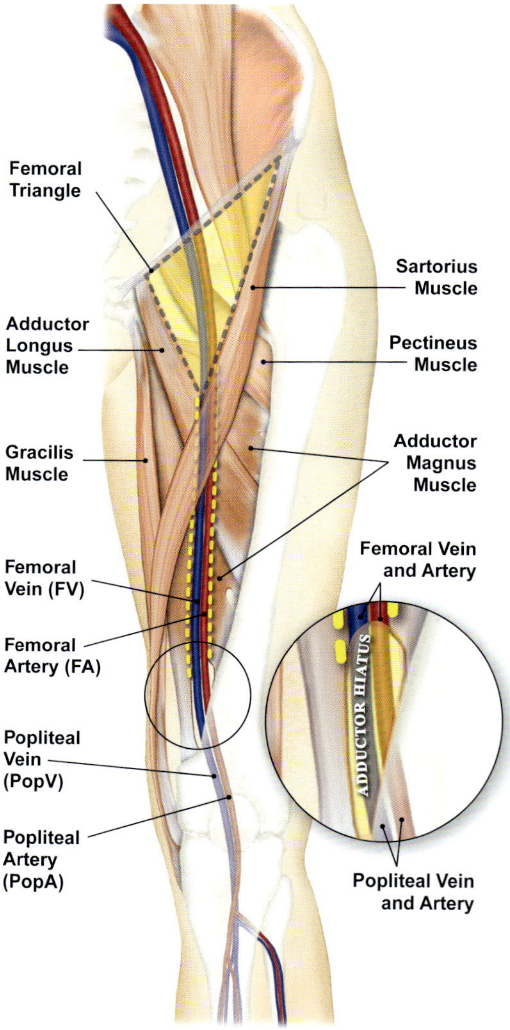

Fig. 3-15. *The adductor canal is a tunnel in the middle of the thigh. It extends from the apex of the femoral triangle to the adductor hiatus.*

Communicating Systems

Perforating Veins[1, 2, 3, 9, 33, 34]

- Perforating veins (PVs) are variable in size, distribution, connection and arrangement.
- Perforating veins are located in the foot, calf and thigh.
- There are approximately 100 - 150 perforators in each leg, most are located below the knee.
- Perforating veins pierce the muscular fascia as they travel from the superficial compartment to the deep compartment.
- Perforating veins connect the superficial and deep venous systems.
- Most perforating veins do not join directly with the saphenous trunks. However, in the thigh and proximal calf region, there are perforating veins which directly connect the great saphenous vein with the deep veins.
- The function of perforating veins is to return venous blood from the superficial venous system to the deep venous system, except in the foot where the blood typically flows from the deep to the superficial venous system.
- In the calf and thigh, the major perforating veins have 1-3 valves to prevent retrograde flow (reflux) from the deep system to the superficial system.

The mid-thigh perforating vein is often times enlarged and may be pathologic; however, most of the important pathological perforating veins in the calf are connected to the posterior arch vein.

There are two types of perforating veins, direct and indirect:

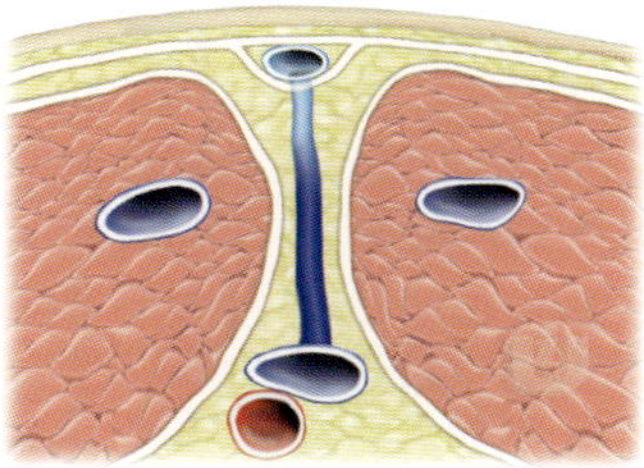

Fig. 3-17. *Direct perforating veins directly connect the deep and superficial systems.*

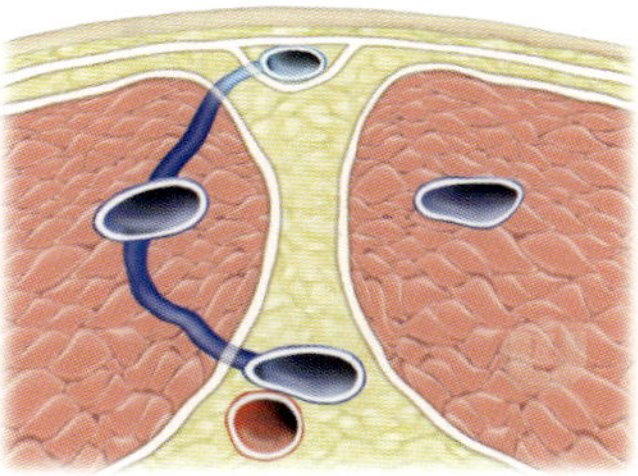

Fig. 3-18. *Indirect perforating veins will connect the deep and superficial systems by way of an intermediary vein (most commonly a gastrocnemius vein).*

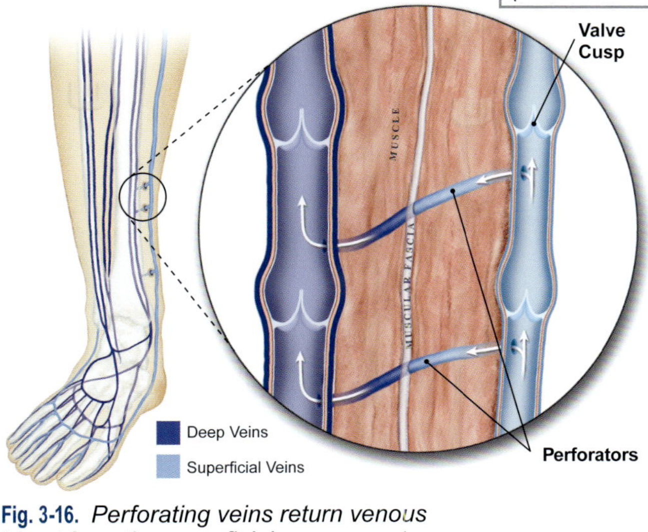

Fig. 3-16. *Perforating veins return venous blood from the superficial venous system to the deep venous system.*

The majority of perforating veins have not been found to be clinically significant.

Superficial Axial Veins [1, 2, 5, 9, 49]

- The superficial system is composed of the great and small saphenous veins, the accessory great saphenous veins and their tributaries.
- Superficial veins do not have a corresponding artery, which allows them to be easily distinguished from deep veins.
- Saphenous veins are located within the saphenous compartment.
- Saphenous tributaries travel in the superficial compartment above the saphenous fascia.
- The dorsal venous arch and the medial and lateral marginal veins are the anatomic origins of the great and the small saphenous veins.
- The medial marginal vein is contiguous with the great saphenous vein, and the lateral marginal vein is contiguous with the small saphenous vein.

Great Saphenous Vein [1, 2, 9, 14]

- The great saphenous vein is an interfascial vein that lies within the saphenous compartment.
- The great saphenous vein is the longest vein in the body.
- The great saphenous vein originates on the medial aspect of the dorsum of the foot where it is a continuum of the medial marginal vein.
- It courses anteriorly over the medial malleolus, ascending along the medial side aspect of the calf and thigh, draining into the common femoral vein, terminating at the inguinal crease just inferior to the inguinal ligament.
- The saphenous hiatus is an opening in the deep fascia. The GSV travels through the hiatus joining the CFV approximately 3-4cm below the inguinal ligament.
- The area where these veins join is known as the saphenofemoral junction (SFJ). The SFJ is located 1 to 4cm lateral to and 0 to 3cm below the pubic tubercle.
- The average diameter of the great saphenous vein is 3 to 5mm at the level of the saphenofemoral junction and 1 to 3mm at the level of the ankle.
- A varying number of veins may join the great saphenous vein to form the confluence of the superficial inguinal veins.

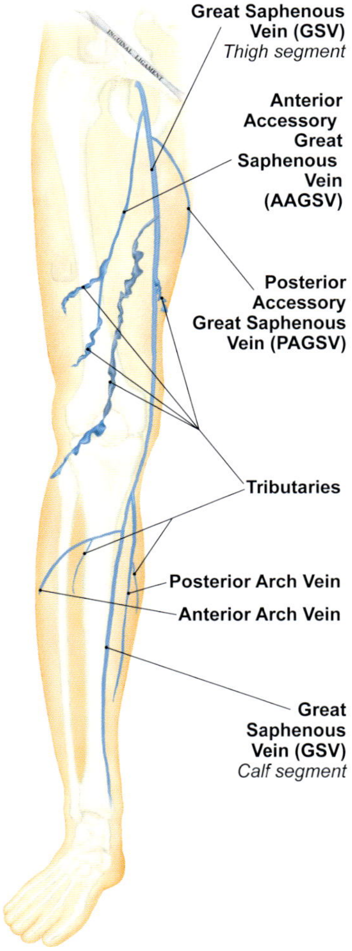

Fig. 3-19. *Superficial veins of the lower extremity anterior view.*

These tributaries may or may not have smaller tributaries or varicosities attached to them.

Familiarizing yourself with the course of great saphenous vein is crucial. Many times patients will have had prior interventions and the great saphenous vein compartment will still require interrogation. If you are not familiar with the trajectory this vein takes you may veer off track.

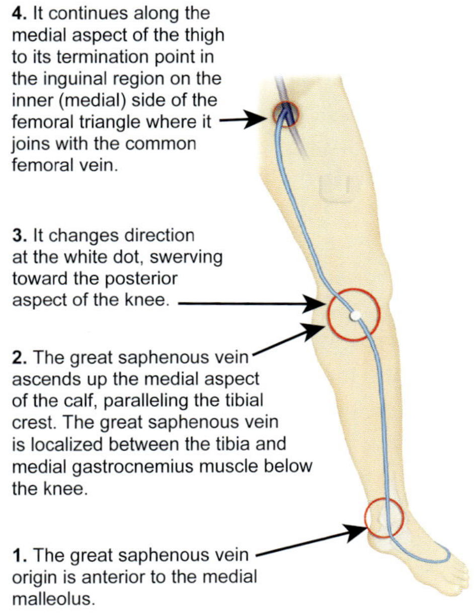

Fig. 3-20. *The great saphenous course from its origin at the medial malleolus (#1) to its termination point at the SFJ (#4).*

Additional Veins that form the confluence of the superficial inguinal veins. [1, 2, 8]

- Superficial Circumflex Iliac Vein
- Superficial Inferior Epigastric Vein
- Superficial External Pudendal Vein
- Anterior Accessory Great Saphenous Vein
- Posterior Accessory Great Saphenous Vein

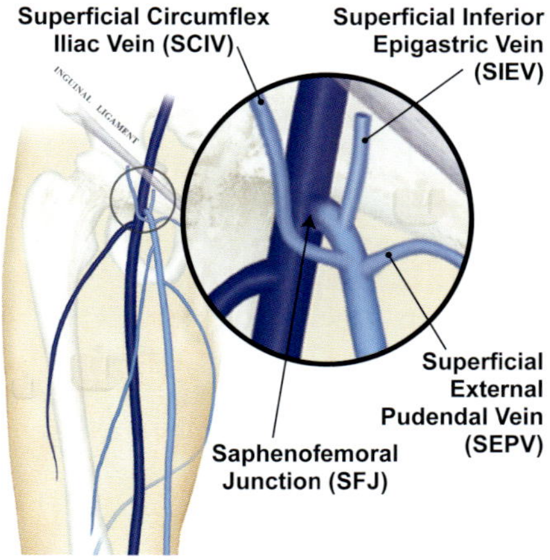

Fig. 3-21. *The superficial circumflex iliac veins, superficial inferior epigastric vein, and superficial external pudendal drain into the GSV at the junction.*

Some of these veins, or all of these veins, may or may not be present.

Tributaries of the Great Saphenous Vein [1, 2, 5, 9, 25]

- The term tributary refers a vein that joins with a superficial axial vein.
- Multiple tributaries join the great saphenous vein in the proximal to mid-thigh region in variable locations.
- In the proximal calf region there are two main tributaries that join the great saphenous vein. They are known as the anterior and posterior arch veins.

Tributaries become easily recognizable when they are diseased.

The term confluence of superficial inguinal veins corresponds to the veins of the saphenofemoral junction (SFJ).

Small Saphenous Vein [1, 2, 9, 53]

- The small saphenous vein is an interfascial vein that lies within the saphenous compartment.

- The small saphenous vein is the primary superficial vein of the posterior aspect of the lower limb.
- The small saphenous vein originates on the lateral aspect of the dorsum of the foot where it is a continuum of the lateral marginal vein.
- It originates posterior to the lateral malleolus, ascending along the posterolateral aspect of the calf between the two heads of the gastrocnemius muscle, terminating at the popliteal crease where it drains into the popliteal vein.
- The small saphenous vein extends into the subcutaneous tissues from the level of the ankle to the posterior aspect of the popliteal vein.
- The average diameter of the small saphenous vein is 2 to 4mm at the level of the saphenopopliteal junction and 1 to 2mm at the level of the ankle.

The termination point of the small saphenous vein is highly variable.

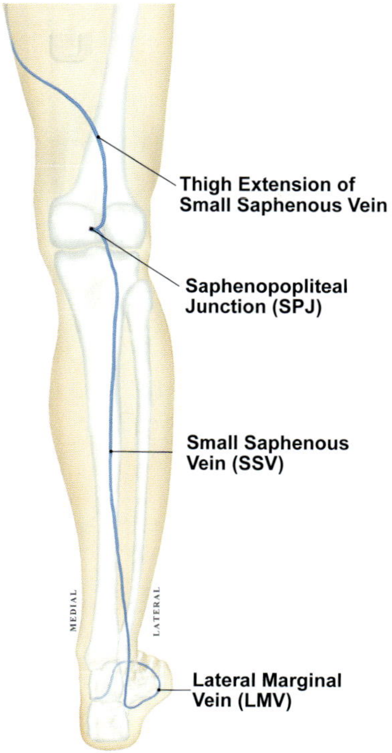

Fig. 3-22. *Superficial veins of the lower extremity posterior view.*

Accessory Veins

Anterior Accessory Great Saphenous Vein [1, 2, 5, 7, 8, 9, 26, 39, 41]

- The AAGSV is an interfascial superficial axial vein.
- The termination point is variable, but it usually joins the GSV between 0.5cm and 2cm peripheral to the SFJ.
- It lies lateral to the great saphenous vein as it ascends the thigh.
- It aligns itself over the deep system and is distinguished from the GSV by this 'alignment' sign.
- It is present in approximately 50% of patients.
- It has a relatively short course (5 to 20cm from the SFJ) and it never reaches below the knee.

Posterior Accessory Great Saphenous Vein [1, 2, 5, 9, 20]

- The PAGSV is an interfascial superficial axial vein.
- The origin is variable, most commonly arising from the thigh extension of the small saphenous vein.
- It joins the great saphenous vein about 5–10cm peripheral to the saphenofemoral junction.

The PAGSV is not present as often as the AAGSV.

Circumflex Veins [1, 2, 5, 20, 41]

Circumflex veins are tributaries of the accessory great saphenous veins.

- The anterior thigh circumflex vein is a tributary of the AAGSV that ascends obliquely in the anterior thigh. It may originate from the lateral venous system.
- The posterior thigh circumflex vein is a tributary of the PAGSV that ascends obliquely in the posterior thigh. It may originate in the SSV, its thigh extension, or the lateral venous system.

At times the posterior thigh circumflex vein forms a connection between the great saphenous vein and the small saphenous. This intersaphenous connection is often referred to as Giacomini's anastomosis.

Intersaphenous Veins [1, 2, 3, 5, 20, 48]

- Intersaphenous anastomoses (confluences) can connect the great and small saphenous veins in the thigh or the leg.
- The thigh extension of the small saphenous vein has multiple connections in the thigh or in the pelvis but the most common is near the saphenofemoral junction.
- The great and small saphenous networks are very close at the knee and may communicate through an intersaphenous vein at this level. The small saphenous trunk can become secondarily incompetent as a result of this overload. Inversely, reflux of the small saphenous vein can induce overload of the great saphenous vein below the knee.

Anatomic Variants [18]

There are many variations of the lower extremity venous anatomy. For practical purposes only the more common variations will be mentioned.

Deep Vein Variants [14]

- Duplication [54, 55]
  - FV (25%)
  - PopV (25%)

Superficial Vein Variants

- Duplication [9,13, 25, 40]
  - Great Saphenous Vein
    - True duplication of the GSV is extremely rare (<2%).
    - It usually only affects a segment of vein.
    - The length of the duplication may vary greatly.
  - Small Saphenous Vein
    - True duplication of the SSV is rare (<2%)
    - Only occurs when both veins are connected for the entire length of the duplication.
    - Occurs predominately in the middle third of the calf.

Hypoplasia and Aplasia [9, 29]

- Great saphenous vein hypoplasia is defined by Caggiati as any segment less than 3mm in luminal diameter.
- Small saphenous vein hypoplasia can also occur in limbs.
- The great saphenous vein is aplastic or absent between the mid thigh and knee in 15% of limbs.
- Aplasia has not been described in the small saphenous vein.

> *Superficial venous anatomy is highly variable.*

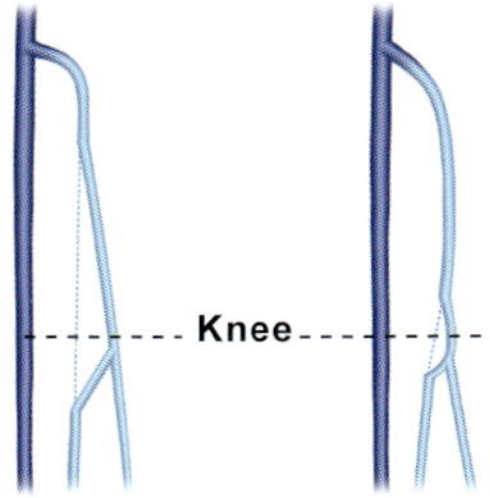

Fig. 3-23. *Aplastic great saphenous vein between the mid thigh and knee (Left). Aplastic great saphenous vein at the knee (Right).*

Nerves [9, 30, 31, 34, 43, 53]

Saphenous Nerve

- The saphenous nerve and the great saphenous vein merge approximately 8-10cm below the knee crease.
- The saphenous nerve is responsible for the sensitivity of the distal inner calf and the inside of the foot.

Sural Nerve

- The medial sural cutaneous nerve is a branch of the tibial nerve that adheres to the small saphenous vein in the lower third of the calf at the descent of the tail end of the gastrocnemius muscle.
- This nerve is responsible for the sensitivity of the back of the distal calf and the outer side of the foot.

Nerves of the Lower Extremity

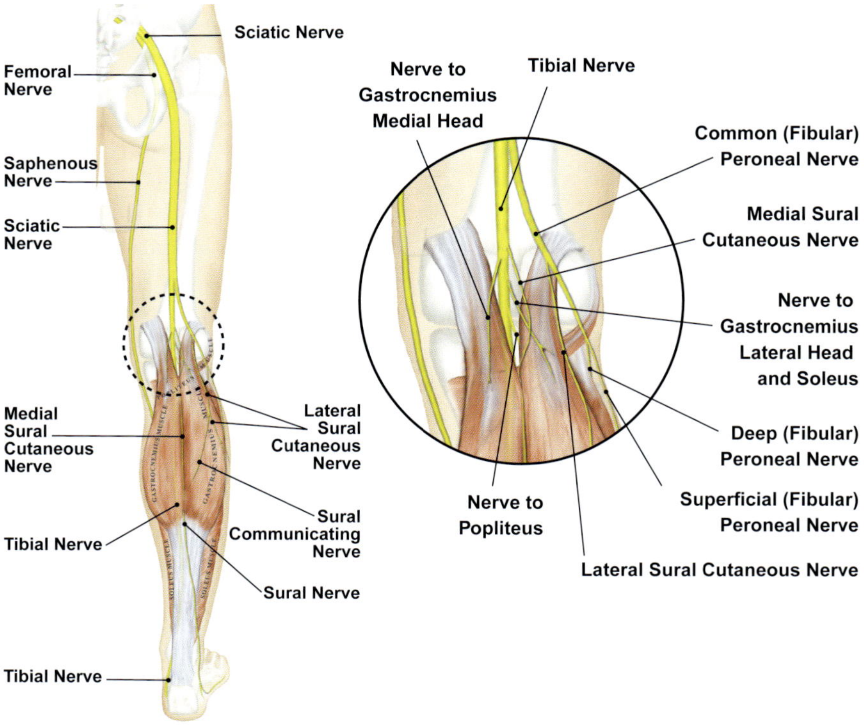

Point of Contact Between Nerves and Saphenous Veins

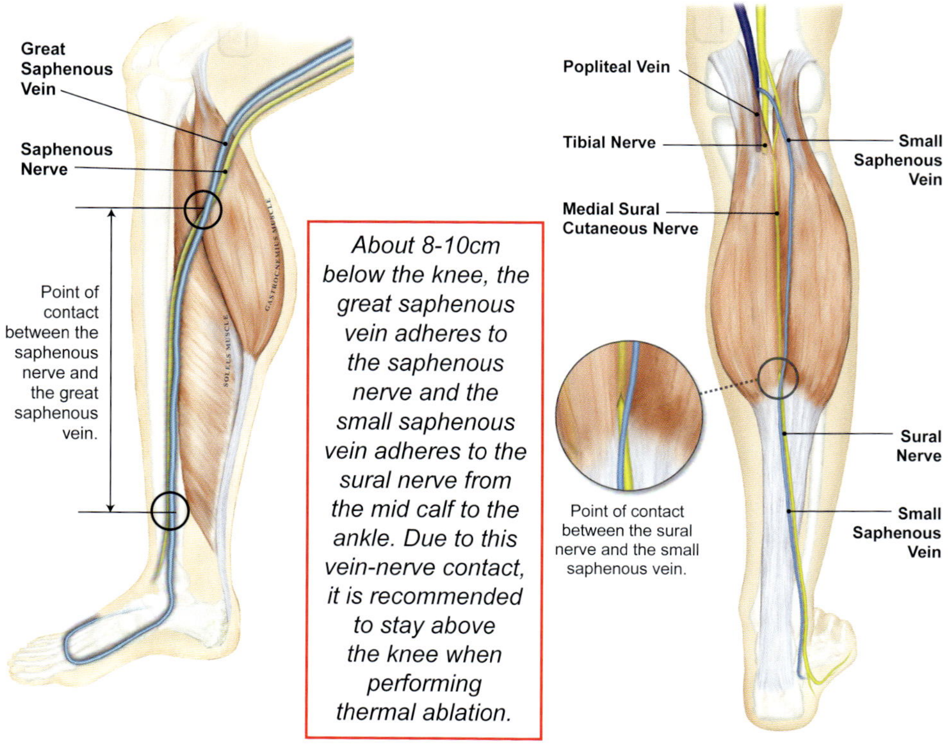

About 8-10cm below the knee, the great saphenous vein adheres to the saphenous nerve and the small saphenous vein adheres to the sural nerve from the mid calf to the ankle. Due to this vein-nerve contact, it is recommended to stay above the knee when performing thermal ablation.

Other Important Nerves

The sciatic nerve bifurcates into the tibial and common peroneal (fibular) nerves. The sciatic nerve is a mixed nerve, containing both motor and sensory fibers. The common peroneal nerve is a branch of the sciatic nerve. It supplies movement and sensation to the lower leg, foot and toes. The tibial nerve, a mixed motor and sensory nerve, supplies motor function to the intrinsic foot muscles, as well as sensation of the medial heel and plantar foot.

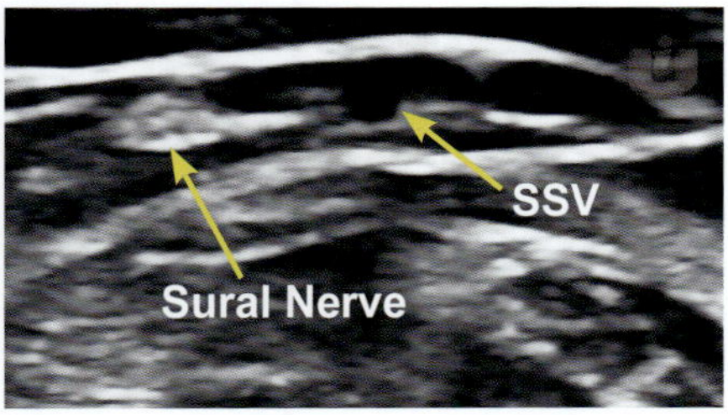

Fig. 3-24. *SSV and sural nerve displayed using B-mode.*

Saphenous Eye [1, 2, 4, 5, 7, 9, 18, 49]

- The compartment, where saphenous trunks course, resembles an eye when scanning in the transverse view. The saphenous lumen is the iris, the superficial fascia the upper eyelid, and the deep fascia the lower eyelid.
- Bailly was the first to describe the "eye sign" to identify the GSV in the thigh by ultrasound.
- The GSV is bound within this compartment which resembles an eye. The "eye sign" allows the saphenous vein to be clearly identified and distinguished from parallel subcutaneous tributaries.
- The saphenous compartment is larger and better defined in the thigh than below the knee.
- The saphenous compartment will vary in size depending on the BMI of the patient.

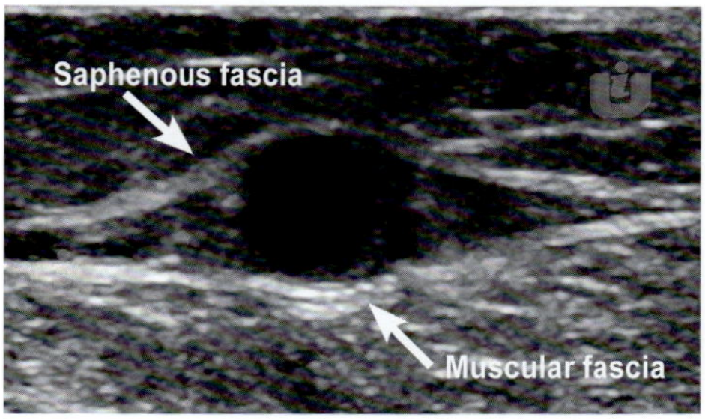

Fig. 3-25. *B-Mode image of the saphenous compartment. The compartment is bound superiorly by the saphenous fascia and inferiorly by the muscular fascia. The GSV is bound within this compartment which resembles an eye.*

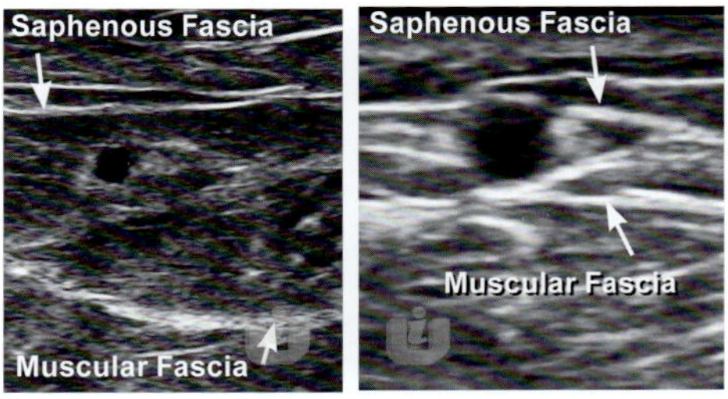

Fig. 3-26. *Saphenous compartment with a high BMI (left) and low BMI (right).*

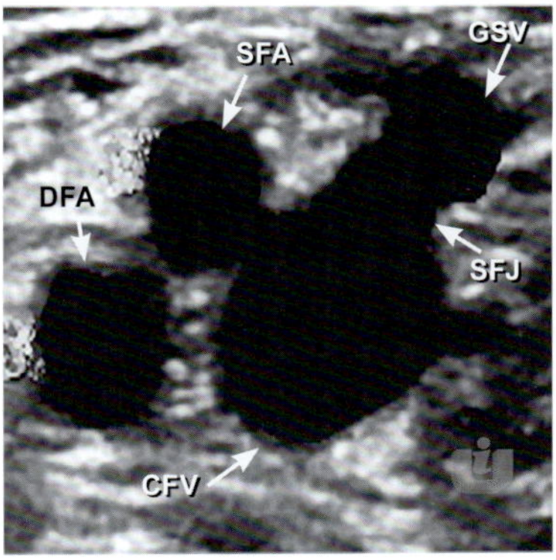

Fig. 3-27. *Cross-sectional view of the saphenofemoral junction (SFJ).*

The anatomy at the Saphenofemoral junction in the transverse view is often referred to as the "Mickey Mouse sign". and consists of the GSV, SFA and the CFV.

Saphenofemoral Junction [9, 10, 32]

The anatomic clinical concept of the saphenofemoral junction includes the valves of the deep vein central and peripheral to the ostium and the terminal segment of the great saphenous vein from the preterminal valve to the ostium.

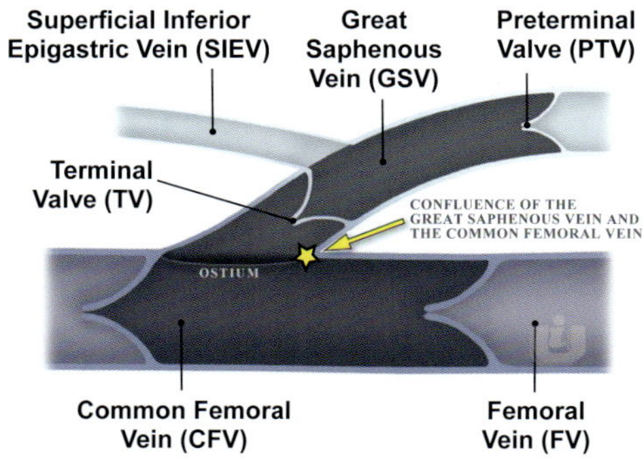

Fig. 3-28. *Anatomy of the SFJ.*

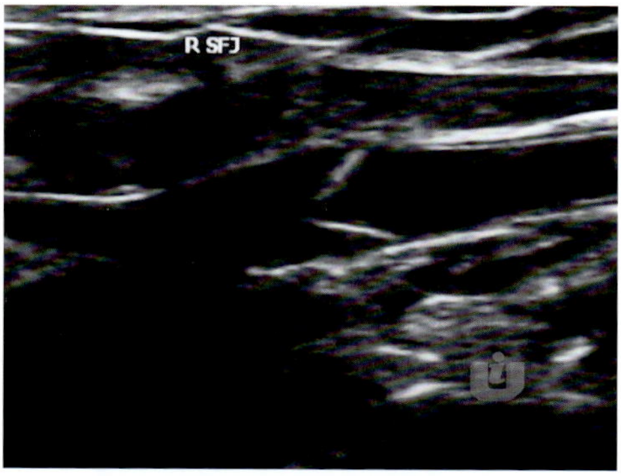

Fig. 3-29. *Grayscale image of the SFJ displaying a patent junction.*

Valves of the Saphenofemoral Junction [10, 22, 23, 27, 32, 45]

Venous valves have been classified into parietal and ostial valves. Parietal valves are located within the lumen of veins; ostial valves are located directly at the confluence of two veins.

> *The GSV terminal and pre-terminal valves are not always present at the SFJ. This may result in reflux from the deep system (CFV) to the superficial system (GSV and its tributaries in the SFJ).*

Ostial Valve

The ostial valve of the saphenofemoral junction is located directly at the confluence of the common femoral and great saphenous veins and usually consists of only a single leaflet.

Parietal Valves

- Terminal valve is situated between 1–2mm peripheral to the ostium.
- Pre-terminal valve is located between 3–5cm peripheral to the ostium.
- The mean distance between terminal and preterminal valves is approximately 2.5cm. Between these valves, major superficial tributaries join the GSV.
- Terminal and preterminal valves are present in approximately 90% of limbs.
- The terminal valve is situated at the termination of the GSV to prevent reflux from the femoral vein.
- The pre-terminal valve prevents venous reflux from the tributaries of SFJ into the GSV trunk while the terminal valve is closed.
- The terminal valve and the preterminal valve are the most important parietal valves in the GSV.

Saphenopopliteal Junction

Valves of the SPJ. [23, 46]

- Venous valves are not as easily identified in the small saphenous vein.
- The terminal valve is found in about 95% of limbs, while the preterminal valve is found in only 64%.

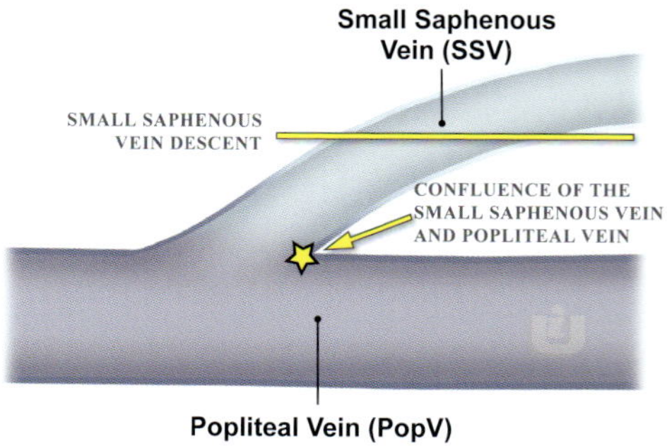

Fig. 3-30. *Anatomy of the Saphenopopliteal Junction.*

Junctional Variants [25, 50, 58]

Saphenofemoral Junction

- Ectasia: The saphenofemoral junction may be dilated near its confluence with the common femoral vein. It may remain dilated for a centimeter or two then it usually tapers off.
- Independent junction of the great saphenous vein and an accompanying accessory vein. Both veins will independently drain into the common femoral vein.
- Occasionally the great saphenous veins and an accompanying accessory saphenous vein will share a short common trunk creating one SFJ.

Saphenopopliteal Junction

- Ectasia: The saphenopopliteal junction may be dilated near its confluence with the popliteal vein.
- Termination point: The small saphenous vein terminates directly into the thigh extension, gastrocnemius veins, or popliteal vein.
- Absent saphenopopliteal junction: Sometimes the SSV does not have a direct relationship with the popliteal vein at all.

Anatomy of a Varicose Vein [23, 24]

Venous hypertension in the superficial venous system causes dilated tortuous structures.

- Superficial veins are predisposed to dilatation and damage due to their thin, weak media.
- Dilatation of the venous wall and/or valvular dysfunction.
- When the valvular function of the veins fail, there is increasing pressure in the superficial venous system.
- Increased pressure in the venous system leads to more venous dilatation.
- Valvular incompetence will progress over time, increasing venous pressure and the cycle continues.

In contrast to the deep veins, the superficial veins are prone to dilatation because they have less muscle support than deep veins.

References

1. Caggiati A, Bergan JJ, Gloviczki P, Eklof B, Allegra C, Partsch H; International Interdisciplinary Consensus Committee on Venous Anatomical Terminology. Nomenclature of the veins of the lower limb: extensions, refinements, and clinical application. *J Vasc Surg. 2005 Apr;41*(4):719-24.
2. Caggiati A, Bergan JJ, Gloviczki P, Jantet G, Wendell-Smith CP, Partsch H; International Interdisciplinary Consensus Committee on Venous Anatomical Terminology. Nomenclature of the veins of the lower limbs: an international interdisciplinary consensus statement. *J Vasc Surg. 2002 Aug;36*(2):416-22. doi: 10.1067/mva.2002.125847. PMID: 12170230
3. Caggiati A. The nomenclature of the veins of the lower limbs, based on their planar anatomy and fascial relationships. *Acta Chir Belg. 2004 Jun;104*(3):272-5. doi: 10.1080/00015458.2004.11679553. PMID: 15285536
4. Coleridge-Smith P, N, Partsch H, Myers K, Nicolaides A, Cavezzi A. (2006). Duplex ultrasound investigation of the veins in chronic venous disease of the lower limbs: UIP consensus document. Part I. Basic principles. *Eur J Vasc Endovasc Surg .31*, 83–92.
5. Cavezzi A, Labropoulos N, Partsch H, Ricci S, Caggiati A, Myers K. Nicolaides A. Smith PC. (2006). Duplex ultrasound investigation of the veins in chronic venous disease of the lower limbs: UIP consensus document. Part II. Anatomy. *Eur J Vasc Endovasc Surg 31*, 288–299.
6. Lurie F, Passman M, Meisner M, Dalsing M, Masuda E, Welch H, Bush R, Blebea J, Carpentier P, Maeseneer M, Gasparis A, Labropoulos N, Marston W, Rafetto J, Santiago F, Shortell C, Uhl JF, Urbanek T, van Rij A, Wakefield T. (2020). CEAP classification system and reporting standard, revision 2020. *Journal of Vascular Surgery: Venous and Lymphatic Disorders*. 8. 10.1016/j.jvsv.2019.12.075
7. Ricci S, Moro L, Ferrini A, Rossi Bartoli I, Antonelli Incalzi R. The E point: A New Echographic great saphenous identification sign in specific anatomical variants and applications. *Phlebology. 2017 Mar;32(2)*:120-124. doi: 10.1177/0268355516633381. Epub 2016 Jul 9. PMID: 26908639
8. De Maeseneer M. (2019). What a phlebologist should know about the anterior accessory saphenous vein? *Phlebolymphology. 26*(2):68–72.
9. Caggiati, Alberto & Mendoza, Erika & Murena-Schmidt, Renate & Lattimer, Christopher. (2014). *Anatomy of the Superficial Veins*. 10.1007/978-3-642-40731-4_2.
10. D. Mühlberger, L. Morandini, E. Brenner. (2008). An anatomical study of femoral vein valves near the saphenofemoral junction. *J Vasc Surg, 48,* 994-999.
11. Caggiati A, Mendoza E, Murena-Schmidt R, Lattimer CRMendoza E, Lattimer CR, Morrison N. (2014). Duplex Ultrasound of Superficial Leg Veins. (19–47). USA Salmon Tower Building New York City Springer.
12. Uhl, JF, Gillot C. (2020). *Atlas of venous anatomy.* Anatomieunesco.org. https://anatomieunesco.org/3155/atlas-of-venous-anatomy-by-j-f-uhl/
13. Almeida JI. (2019). Venous Anatomy. In J.I. Almeida (Ed.), *Atlas of Endovascular Venous Surgery* (2nd ed., pp.1-20). Elsevier.,https://doi.org/10.1016/B978-0-323-51139-1.00001-2
14. Lo Vuolo, M.L.(2014). Venous Ultrasound: A Comprehensive Approach; Lower Extremities and Pelvis; Atlas and Texts. 9789873343599 https://books.google.com/books?id=akPksw EACAAJ
15. Akayo R, Kageyama N. (2016). Clinical Significance of the Soleal Vein and Related Drainage Veins, in Calf Vein Thrombosis in Autopsy Cases with Massive Pulmonary Thromboembolism. *Annals of vascular diseases, 9*(1), 15–21. https://doi.org/10.3400/avd.oa.15-00088

16. Aragão JA, Reis FP, Pitta G, Miranda F, Poli de Figueiredo LF. (2006) Anatomical Study of the Gastrocnemius Venous Network and Proposal for a Classification of the Veins, *European Journal of Vascular and Endovascular Surgery, 31*(4), Pages 439-442, ISSN1078-5884, https://doi.org/10.1016/j.ejvs.2005.10.022. (https:// www.sciencedirect.com/science/article/pii/S1078588405006556)

17. Kageyama N., Ro A., Tanifuji T., Fukunaga T. (2008). Significance of the soleal vein and its drainage veins in cases of massive pulmonary thromboembolism. *Annals of vascular diseases, 1*(1), 35–39. https://doi.org/10.3400/avd.AVDoa07004

18. Caggiati A, Bergan, JJ. (2002). "The saphenous vein: derivation of its name and its relevant anatomy". *Journal of Vascular Surgery. 35* (1): 172–5. doi:10.1067/ mva.2002.118826. PMID 172–5. doi:10.1067/ PMID 11802151

19. Parsi, K. (2007). Anatomy for the Phlebologist. Retrieved October 7, 2022, from http://www.conferencematters.co.nz/pdf/ParsiAnatomy%20and%20physiology%202007.pdf

20. Georgiev M, Myers KA, Belcaro G. (2003). The thigh extension of the lesser saphenous vein: From Giacomini's observations to ultrasound scan imaging, *Journal of Vascular Surgery, Volume 37*(3), 558-563. ISSN 0741-5214, https://doi. org/10.1067/mva.2003.77

21. Caggiati A. (2009) International Interdisciplinary Consensus Committee on Venous Anatomical Terminology. Regarding "Venous valves and major superficial tributary veins near the saphenofemoral junction". *J Vasc Surg. Dec; 50*(6):1547; author reply 1547-8. doi: 10.1016/j.jvs.2009.07.125. PMID: 19958997

22. Dickson, R., Hill, G., Thomson, I. A., & van Rij, A. M. (2013). The valves and tributary veins of the saphenofemoral junction: ultrasound findings in normal limbs. *Veins and Lymphatics, 2*(2), e18. https://doi.org/10.4081/vl.2013.e18

23. Jindal R., Wadhawan B., Chaudhary P. Anatomy, Physiology & Classification of Varicose Veins. www.scribd.com/document/413130775/mu-188

24. Goldman MP, Fronek A. (1989). Anatomy and pathophysiology of varicose veins. *J Dermatol Surg Oncol. Feb;15*(2):138-45. doi: 10.1111/j.1524-4725. 1989.tb03020. x. PMID: 2644324

25. Souroullas P, Barnes R, Smith G, Nandhra S, Carradice D, Chetter I. (2017). The classic saphenofemoral junction and its anatomical variations. *Phlebology. Apr;32*(3):172-178. doi: 10.1177/0268355516635960. Epub 16 Jul 9. PMID: 26924361

26. Laredo J, Lee BB, Neville RF. (2010). Endovenous Thermal Ablation of the Anterior Accessory Great Saphenous Vein. *Endovascular Today.* Retrieved October 7, 2022, from https://assets.bmctoday.net/evtoday/pdfs/et0310_SF_laredo.pdf

27. Caggiati A, Rippa Bonati M, Pieri A, Riva A. (2004). 1603-2003 Four centuries of valves. Eur *J Vasc Endovasc Surg. 2004 Oct;28*(4):439-41. doi: 10.1016/j.ejvs.2004.04.004. PMID: 15350570

28. Caggiati, A. (2015). Clinical Anatomy of the Venous System of the Lower Extremity. In Lanzer, P. (Ed.) *PanVascular Medicine.* Springer, Berlin, Heidelberg. https://doi.org/10.1007/978-3-642-37078-6_158

29. Caggiati A, Mendoza E. (2004). Segmental hypoplasia of the great saphenous vein and varicose disease. *Eur J Vasc EndovascSurg. 28* (3):257-61.

30. Labropoulos N, Tassiopoulos AK, Gasparis AP, Phillips B, Pappas PJ. (2009). Veins along the course of the sciatic nerve. *J Vasc Surg. Mar;49*(3):690-6. doi: 10.1016/j.jvs.2008.09.061. Epub 2009 Jan 9. PMID: 19135832

31. Labropoulos N, Tiongson J, Pryor L, Tassiopoulos AK, Kang SS, Mansour MA, Baker WH. (2001). Nonsaphenous superficial vein reflux. *J Vasc Surg. Nov;34*(5):872-7. doi: 10.1067/mva.2001.118813. PMID: 11700489

32. Mühlberger D., Morandini L., Brenner E. (2007). Frequency and exact position of valves in the saphenofemoral junction. *Phlebologie. 36.* 3-7. 10.1055/s-0037-1622161

33. Labropoulos N. (2020). Current Views on the Management of Incompetent Perforator Veins. *Ann Phlebology. 18*:1-3. https://doi.org/10.37923/phle.2020.18.1.1

34. Meissner MH. (2005). Lower extremity venous anatomy. *Semin Intervent Radiol. Sep;22*(3):147-56. doi: 10.1055/s-2005-921948. PMID: 21326687; PMCID: PMC3036282

35. Ricci S., Moro L., Antonelli IR. (2014). The foot venous system: anatomy, physiology and relevance to clinical practice. *Dermatol Surg. Mar;40*(3):225-33. doi: 10.1111/dsu.12381. Epub 2013 Dec 23. PMID: 24372905

36. Pellerito, J., & Polak, JF. (2019). *Introduction to Vascular Ultrasonography* (7th Edition). Elsevier - OHCE. https://bookshelf.health.elsevier.com/books/9780323625258

37. Krishna G. (2010). Front of the thigh. BD Chaurasia's Human Anatomy (Regional and Applied Dissection and Clinical) Volume 2 - Lower limb, abdomen, and pelvis (5th ed., p.56). India: CBS Publishers and Distributors Pvt Ltd. ISBN 978-81-239-1864-8

38. Basinger H., Hogg JP. *Anatomy, Abdomen and Pelvis, Femoral Triangle.* [Updated 2021 Jul 26]. In: StatPearls [Internet]. Treasure Island (FL): StatPearls Publishing; 2022 Jan-. Available from: https://www.ncbi.nlm.nih.gov/books/NBK541140/

39. Schul MW., Vayuvegula S., Keaton TJ. (2020). The clinical relevance of anterior accessory great saphenous vein reflux. *J Vasc Surg Venous Lymphat Disord. Nov;8*(6):1014-1020. doi: 10.1016/j.jvsv.2020.02.010. Epub 2020 Mar 21. PMID: 32205127

40. Ricci S., Caggiati A. (1999). Does a double saphenous vein exist? *Phlebology,* 14:59–64.

41. Welch HJ., (2022). Combined Treatment of the Anterior Accessory Saphenous Vein and the Great Saphenous Vein, *Vascular & Endovascular Review*;5:e01. https://doi.org/10.15420/ver.2021.07

42. Laredo J., Byung BL., Neville RF. (2010). Laredo J., Byung BL., Neville RF. (2010). *Endovenous Thermal Ablation of the Anterior Accessory Great Saphenous Vein: Clinical aspects of ablating the incompetent anterior accessory great saphenous vein.* Endovascular Today. https://evtoday.com/*Endovascular Today.* https://evtoday.com

43. Hyland S., Sinkler MA., Varacallo M. Anatomy, Bony Pelvis and Lower Limb, Popliteal Region. [Updated 2021 Jul 31]. *In: StatPearls [Internet].* Treasure Island (FL): StatPearls Publishing; 2022 Jan. Available from: https://www.ncbi.nlm.nih.gov/books/NBK532891/

44. Moore, KL. (13 February 2013). *Clinically oriented anatomy* (7th ed.). Philadelphia: Wolters Kluwer/Lippincott Williams & Wilkins Health. ISBN 978-1451119459

45. Tasch C., Brenner E. (2012). The ostial valve of the great saphenous vein. *Phlebology.27*, 179-83.

46. Schweighofer G., Mühlberger D., Brenner E. (2010). The anatomy of the small saphenous vein: fascial and neural relations, saphenofemoral junction, and valves. *J Vasc Surg, 51*, 982-9.

47. Pieri A., Vannuzzi A., Duranti A., Michelagnoli S., Marcelli F., Santini M., et al. (1997). Colour-flow duplex investigation in superficial venous insufficiency of the lower limbs. [Article in French]. *Phlébologie,* 50, 343-50

48. *Intersaphenous Communications.* Phlebolgia; Atlas of Anatomy of the Superficial Veins of the Lower Limbs. www.phlebologia.com/long-saphenous-territory/intersaphenous-communications

49. Caggiati A., Ricci S., (1997). The Long Saphenous Vein Compartment. *Phlebology, 12.* 107-111. 10.1177/026835559701200307

50. Kachlík D., Varga I., Baca V., Musil V. (2020). Variant Anatomy and Its Terminology. *Medicina. 56.* 713. 10.3390/medicina56120713

51. Ludbrook, J. (1966). The musculovenous pumps of the human lower limb. *American Heart Journal, 71* (5), 635-641. https://doi.org/10.1016/0002-8703(66)90313-9

52. Tucker WD., Arora Y., Mahajan K. Anatomy, Blood Vessels. [Updated 2021 Aug 11]. In: StatPearls [Internet]. Treasure Island (FL): StatPearls Publishing; 2022 Jan-. Available from: https://www.ncbi.nlm.nih.gov/books/NBK470401/

53. Caggiati A. (2001) Fascial relationships of the short saphenous vein. *J Vasc Surg 34*:241–246.

54. Khan AA., Asari MA., Hassan A, Aiman N. (2013). An interconnected duplicated femoral vein and its clinical significance. *Folia Morphol (Warsz),* Feb;*72*(1), 82-5. doi: 10.5603/fm.2013.0014. PMID: 23749717

55. Sadowska A., Spodnik JH., Wójcik S. (2013). Variations in popliteal fossa venous anatomy: implications for diagnosis of deep-vein thrombosis. *Folia Morphol (Warsz). Feb;72*(1), 51-6. doi: 10.5603/fm.2013.0008. PMID: 23749711

56. Andersson J,. et al. (1996) Valvular function of peripheral veins after hyperemic dilation. *J Vasc Surg. Apr;23*(4), 611-5. doi: 10.1016/s0741-5214(96)80040-1. PMID: 8627896

57. Labropoulos N., Tiongson J., Pryor L., Tassiopoulos AK., Kang SS., Mansour MA., Baker WH. (2003). Definition of venous reflux in lower-extremity veins. *J Vasc Surg. Oct;38*(4), 793-8. doi: 10.1016/s0741-5214(03)00424-5

58. Labropoulos N., Giannoukas AD, Delis K., Kang SS., Mansour MA, Buckman J, Katsamouris A, Nicolaides AN, Littooy FN, Baker WH. (2000). The impact of isolated lesser saphenous vein system incompetence on clinical signs and symptoms of chronic venous disease. *J Vasc Surg. Nov;32*(5):954-60. doi: 10.1067/mva.2000.110349. PMID: 11054227

Cardiovascular Circulation

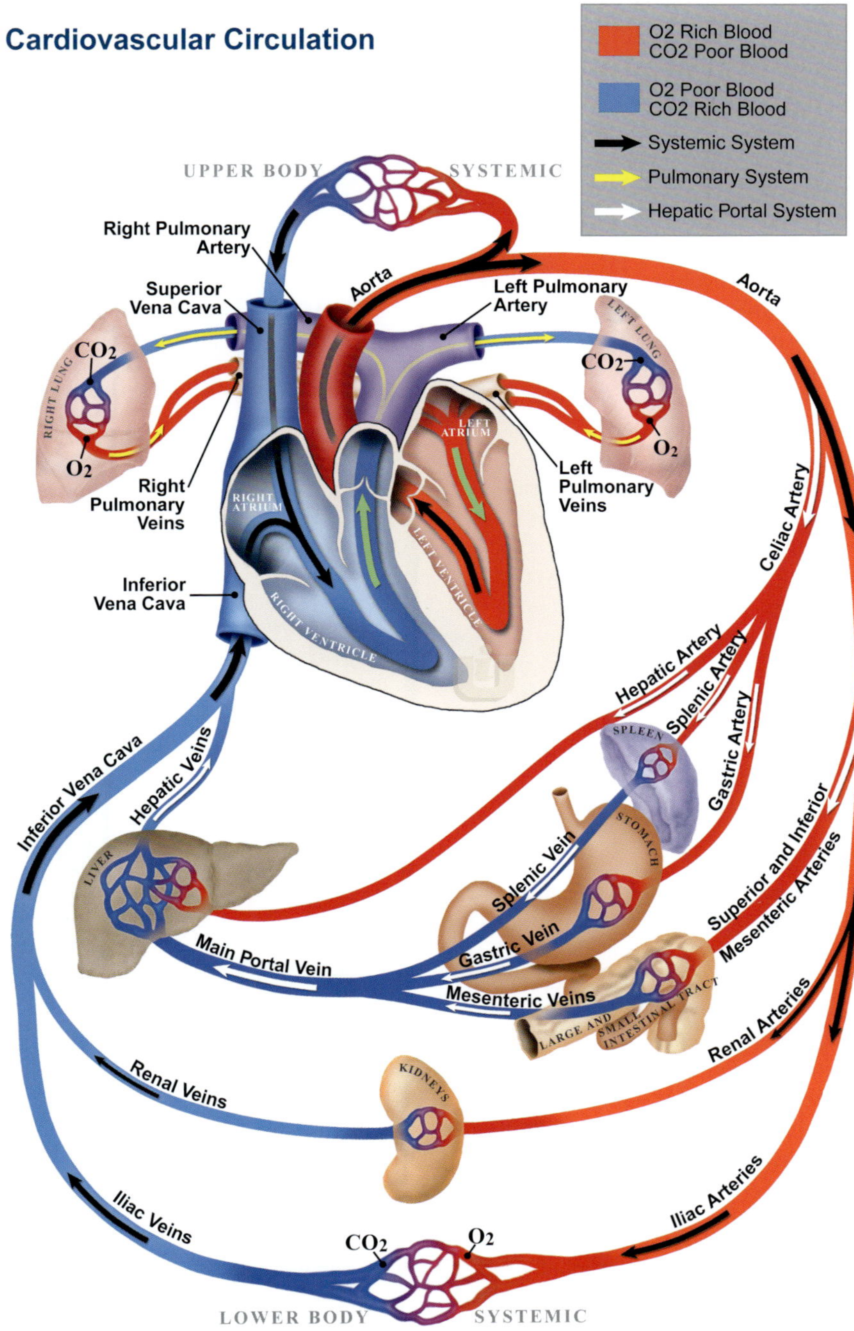

Fig. 4-1. *Cardiovascular Circulation. Blood circulates through the following pathway; from the left ventricle of the heart to the arteries, arterioles, capillaries, venules, veins, to the right atrium, right ventricle, pulmonary artery, lung capillaries, pulmonary vein, back to the left atrium and to the left ventricle.*

Venous Hemodynamics

Two primary functions of the venous system are:

- Transporting blood from the capillaries to the heart
- Being the blood reservoir of the body and maintaining the filling pressure of the right heart by increasing or decreasing the volume of blood circulating through the body. [1-7]

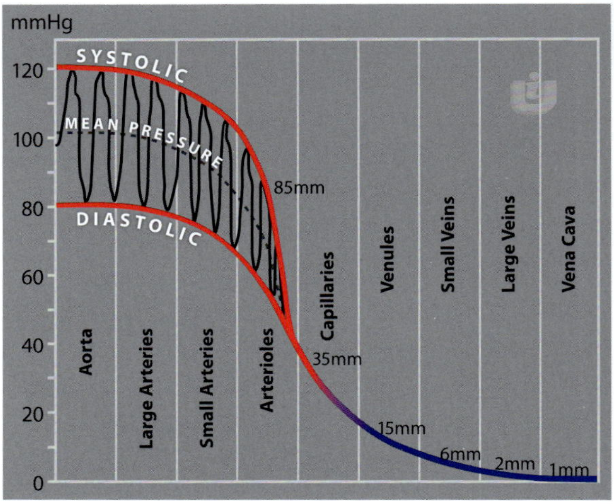

Fig. 4-2. *Pressure drop across different levels of the circulation.*

Blood flow is caused by pressure gradients, with blood flowing from higher pressure regions to lower pressure regions. The contraction of the left ventricle causes blood to flow along the artery in a wave, and it also causes a wave of pressure to travel with it. The contraction increases the pressure within the ventricle, and because the pressure is greater in the ventricle than in the aorta, blood flows from the ventricle into the aorta. This increases the volume of blood in the aorta, causing an increase in the aortic pressure. As the pressure increases, it pushes the blood further along the artery, down the pressure gradient. And as the amount of blood increases in a region of the artery, so does the pressure. Thus, as a wave of blood travels along the artery, so does a pressure wave.

As the ventricle relaxes and fills with blood from the left atrium, blood does not flow from the heart into the aorta. Thus, as the wave of blood flows distally, the amount of blood proximal to the wave decreases. This decrease in blood volume causes the pressure to decrease to a baseline value. Cycling the left ventricle between contraction and relaxation causes pressure waves in the arteries, which propels the blood to travel in a series of waves (pulsatile flow).

As a wave of blood travels through the vessels, it loses energy, thus eventually the ability to increase pressure. Energy is lost due to 1) the resistive frictional force caused by the blood flowing along the vessel's surface that must be overcome. 2) the work required to stretch the vessel wall as the wave passes by temporarily increasing local blood volume. Both of these increase as the blood travels distally. [1] As the wave of blood moves distally through the body, the energy it uses rapidly increases for two primary reasons:

- As the arteries branch, the number of vessels carrying the blood increases, and they become smaller and smaller. This increases vessel surface area per unit volume of blood, increasing the resistant frictional force, which requires more energy to keep the blood moving.
- The vessels' compliance decreases; thus, the amount of energy required by the wave of blood to expand them as they pass through increases.

As a blood wave moves through the vessels, it causes smaller and smaller pressure increases, and the size of the wave decreases. In the arterioles, the wave will cease to exist when it no longer has the energy required to expand the vessel wall. The flow is then no longer pulsatile. The flow pattern in microcirculation is different as blood velocity is significantly reduced. Patients with chronic venous disease may have altered flow patterns in the microcirculation, reflecting, the inflammatory changes in the area. [13,14]

Because the resistance for a unit volume of blood flow in small vessels is greater than in large vessels, the force required to move the same volume of blood through them is greater than the force needed for the aorta and large arteries. Thus, the pressure gradient, the driving force moving the blood, is greater in the arterioles and capillaries than in the aorta and large arteries. The pressure gradient across the arterioles and capillaries is about 15mmHg, while the pressure drops across the aorta and large arteries are approximately 1mmHg.

Hydrostatic Pressure

The hydrostatic pressure caused by gravity upon standing increases venous pressure, which must be overcome for blood to flow back to the heart. Other physiologic forces facilitate venous return to the heart and reduce the high venous pressure at the ankle, including respiratory changes, skeletal muscle contraction, venous valves, temperature control, and motor tone.

- All fluids need a pressure gradient to flow. Since the pressure in the capillaries is about 15mmHg and the central venous pressure in the heart's right atrium is much lower (2 to 6mmHg), a pressure gradient exists.
- When a person stands upright, gravity resists blood flow from the ankle and wrist to the heart. A 6-foot-tall individual who is standing has a venous pressure of approximately 117mmHg.

The vein wall stiffens with standing.

- The additional 102mmHg pressure is called *hydrostatic pressure*, which is caused by the weight of the column of blood from the ankle to the heart, where the hydrostatic pressure is zero.
- The pressure is highest in the lower portion of the body
- The further the distance from the right atrium, the greater the force of gravity.
- In an arm that is lifted, the dependent wrist is closer to the heart than the ankle, making the column shorter and the hydrostatic pressure lower. Capillary pressure increases in the arm, so vessels do not collapse.

Compliance and Capacitance[3,4]

- Approximately 2/3 of systemic blood is located in the veins. The vein walls are very compliant and collapse or expand depending on the internal (intramural) and external pressures (tissue pressure) placed on the vein.
- The shape of the venous wall depends upon the pressure, volume, and flow.
- This ability to collapse and expand is referred to as capacitance and allows the venous system to easily adapt to variations in blood volumes. Extra fluids can be stored or adjusted for blood loss.
- This compliance allows for a large increase in venous flow without a significant increase in venous pressure. A wide range of venous volume changes can occur without changing the central venous pressure.
  - This variable amount of blood capacitance is dependent upon the limb's position, muscle pump activity, integrity of the venous valves, and blood volume.
  - Veins are less elastic than arteries but more compliant.

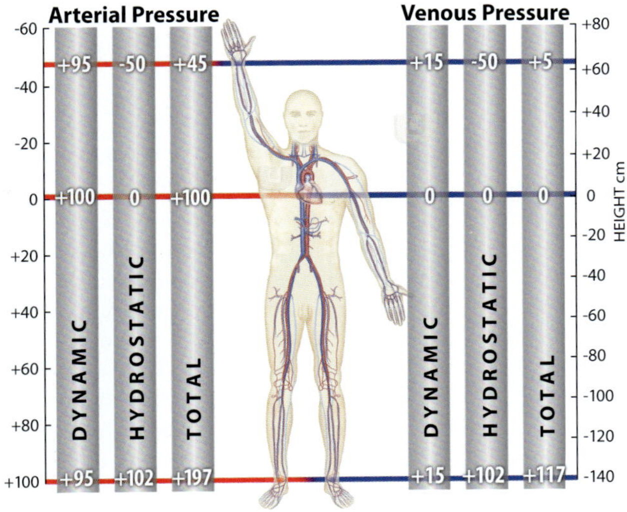

Fig. 4-19. *Systemic and hydrostatic pressure within the vascular system.*

Veins act similarly to rubber bands and can be stretched and collapsed in a wide range of sizes.

- Extremes of fluid overload or severe blood loss will affect the central venous pressure.

Compliance decreases at higher pressures and volumes.

- By changing the cross-sectional area, the vein can change its resistance. Veins can distend 3-4 times that of the corresponding artery [1]
- The greatest resistance occurs when the vein is elliptical. The least resistance exists when the vein is distended.

Flow/Pressure and Volume Relationships

- As venous flow increases, pressure and volume decrease and as venous flow decreases, pressure and volume increase.
- The shape of the vein wall depends upon the pressure, volume, and flow.

Table 4-1. **Flow/Pressure and Volume Relationships**
↑ Blood back to the heart ↓ Venous pressure ↓ Blood volume
↓ Blood back to the heart ↑ Venous pressure ↑ Blood volume

Transmural Pressure

- Different pressure forces surround blood vessels. The force occurring from outside the vein is the tissue pressure. The force occurring within the walls of a vessel is called intraluminal pressure. The pressure difference between the forces pushing on the inside and outside of the vessel wall is called transmural pressure.
  - **Low transmural pressure:** as volume and pressure decrease, the vein wall collapses and becomes elliptical in shape.
  - **High transmural pressure:** as volume and pressure increase, the vein wall becomes circular and may distend at higher venous pressures.

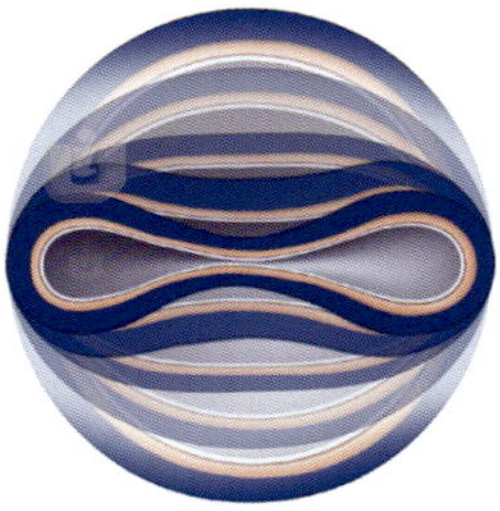

Fig. 4-3. *Transmural pressure. (intraluminal vs. tissue pressure)*

The more blood a vein contains the more pressure within the vein, making the vein more circular in shape.

A high blood volume may be stored in the vein with only a small change in pressure.

$$c = \frac{\Delta V}{\Delta P}$$

c = Vessel compliance
(ΔV) = Change in volume
(ΔP) = Change in pressure

Pressure While Supine [2,3,4,6]

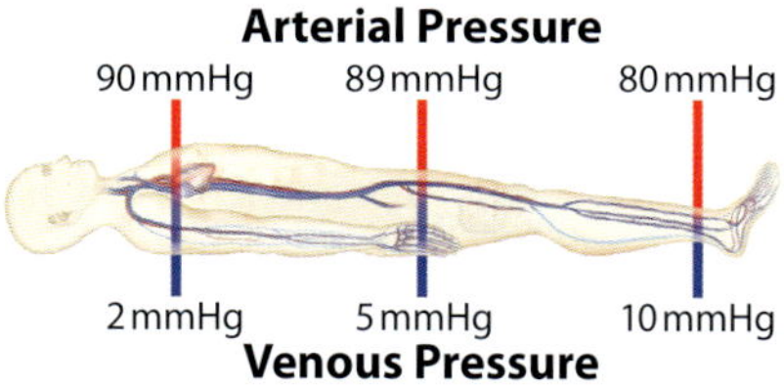

Fig. 4-4. *When supine, the venous pressure is approximately 10-15mmHg*

During inspiration, the intrathoracic cavity pressure is less than the abdominal cavity pressure; this causes a pressure gradient in the inferior vena cava. The intrathoracic pressure decreases, the intra-abdominal pressure increases, and blood moves from the abdomen into the chest, but the outflow from the peripheral veins stops. During inspiration, inflow is allowed from the upper extremities.

Table 4-2. **Pressure and Flow Relationships of Inspiration and Expiration**

Inspiration	Expiration
Intrathoracic pressure decreases ↓	Intrathoracic pressure increases ↑
Diaphragm moves down ↓	Diaphragm moves up ↑
Intra abdominal pressure increases ↑	Intra abdominal pressure decreases ↓
Outflow from peripheral veins decreases ↓	Outflow from peripheral veins increases ↑

Venous Return

Respiratory Function at Rest

- Respiration creates large changes in intrathoracic and intra-abdominal pressures.[2]
- During inspiration, intra-abdominal pressure increases by lowering the diaphragm, which causes the vena cava to collapse and reduces or stops the venous flow from the lower extremities.
- During expiration, intra-abdominal pressure decreases by lifting the diaphragm, the vena cava opens, and flow resumes in a phasic pattern from the lower extremities.
- During expiration, there is a decrease in venous flow into the thorax.
- The presence of respiratory variation is a major indicator of normal venous flow.
- Respiratory function has a lesser effect on the upper extremity veins than on the lower extremities:
  - During inspiration, the intra-thoracic pressure decreases, resulting in increased flow from the upper extremity veins, increasing venous flow. Sometimes we ask the patient to perform a quick sniff, which results in a pressure drop and an increase in venous flow.
  - During expiration, the intra-thoracic pressure increases in the upper extremity veins decreasing venous flow.
  - Augmentation is less and sometimes not seen because of the smaller vein size and lower blood volume.
  - Venous flow in the upper extremities is more pulsatile because of the close proximity to the heart.
  - Respiration has a small effect on venous flow when standing.

Table 4-3.
Inspiration/ Expiration Flow Changes

Upper Extremities	Lower Extremities
↑ Flow increases with inspiration	↓ Flow decreases with inspiration
↓ Flow decreases with expiration	↑ Flow increases with expiration

Skeletal Muscle Contraction[6]

- There are three veno-muscular pumps in the leg; the thigh-pump, the calf muscle pump and foot (plantar) pump. The calf muscle is the main pump.
- During muscle contraction, venous flow in the deep and superficial veins is toward the heart. On relaxation of the muscles, a small amount of flow occurs in the perforators, from the superficial to the deep veins.
- The foot pump (plantar pump) assists with filling the calf with venous flow.
- **Calf muscle pump:** contraction of the gastrocnemius and soleus muscles is the most efficient of the pumps. The calf has a high capacitance and generates great pressure (about 200mmHg during contraction), while 40 - 60% of the venous volume is ejected with a single contraction.
  - The calf muscles act as a venous "heart" when contracted and squeeze the calf veins, propelling the blood in the calf veins toward the heart. The venous valves are very important for the effective work of the calf muscle pump, stopping the blood from flowing toward the foot and directing it to the heart.
  - The calf muscle pump lowers venous pressure, reduces venous volume in the leg, and facilitates venous return to the heart.

- The thigh pump has an ejection fraction of approximately 15%.[5]
- Chronic venous disease occurs from venous hypertension or the failure to reduce venous pressure with exercise.
- There is abnormally high venous pressure on standing with ambulatory venous hypertension. When the calf muscle pumps the blood, it is expelled in any direction due to dysfunction of the valves. Subsequently, venous pressures do not decrease normally.[3] *(See Chronic Venous disorders, page 49)*

Table 4-4. Calf Muscle Pump Dynamics

1. High venous pressure on standing
2. Muscles squeeze veins on walking
3. Blood is expelled toward heart due to valve direction
4. Venous pressure and volume are lowered in the legs

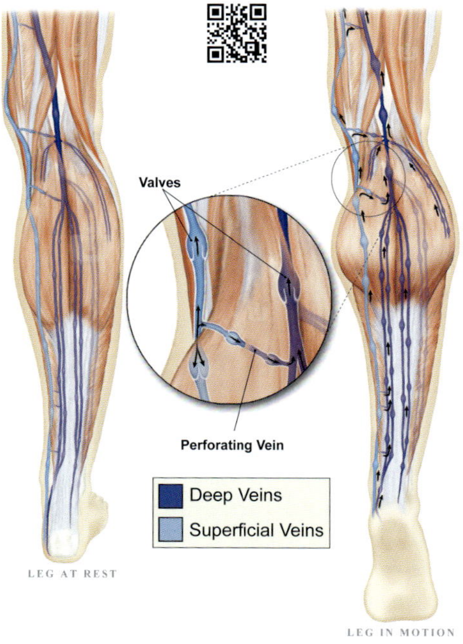

Fig. 4-5. *When the leg is in motion (walking), muscle contractions squeeze the veins, forcing blood past the open valves of the deep, superficial, and perforating veins upward towards the heart. After the muscle relaxes, valves close to prevent backflow (reflux).*

Venous Valves

Venous valves assist blood flow back toward the heart and prevent retrograde flow (*reflux*) back down the venous segment.[3]

- The valves are bicuspid and function to divide the column of blood into segments. This reduces hydrostatic pressure.
- There are more venous valves in the calf veins, possibly due to high hydrostatic pressure in the distal limb. The calf has a valve approximately every 2-5cm.
- Valves in the perforating veins prevent deep to superficial venous flow.
- Valves can withstand retrograde pressures up to 300mmHg.
- UE veins have fewer valves than LE veins. Gravity has a lesser effect in UE flow due to the shorter column of blood and the closer proximity to the heart.
- Valvular damage and dysfunction (valvular incompetence) result in venous reflux and subsequent venous hypertension. Ambulatory Venous Pressure (AVP) is the "gold standard" test for evaluation of the efficiency of the calf muscle pump. It is performed by placing a small needle into one of the foot veins and connecting a needle to a blood pressure unit.
- Air Plethysmography (APG)® has widely replaced the AVP exam by measuring changes of the calf in response to positional changes and exercise, by measuring absolute volume changes. *(See APG chapter, page 222).*

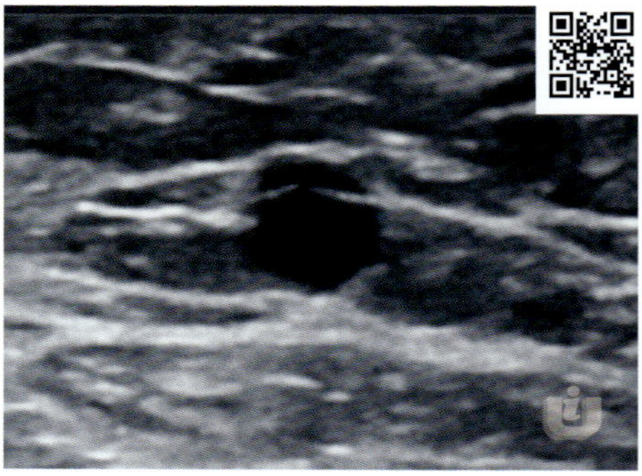

Fig. 4-6. *Normal venous valves with no evidence of thrombus.*

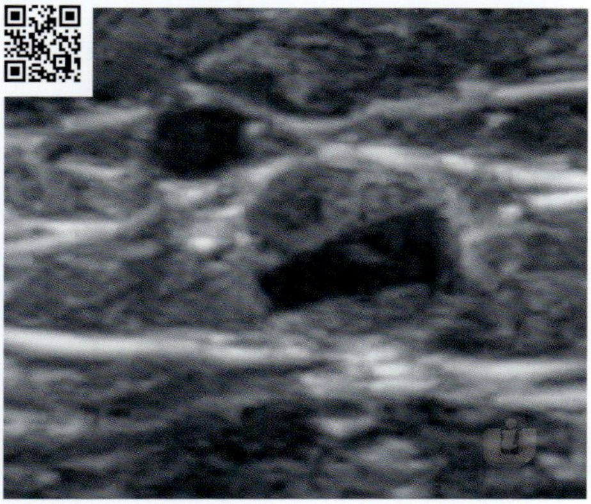

Fig. 4-7. *Abnormal venous valves with thrombus*

Vasomotor Tone

- Veins contain sympathetic-adrenergic constrictor nerves, which control contraction of smooth muscle.[7]
- Vasodilation increases venous blood volume at a lower pressure so that cardiac output can be reduced.[7]
- Veins react to physical and emotional stress, creating vasoconstriction.
- Vasoconstriction increases blood flow to the heart, increasing cardiac output.

Effect of Cardiac Contraction

- With cardiac contraction and relaxation, there is a suction effect on venous blood flow.
- Because of the strong respiratory variation in the legs, cardiac contraction does not affect the blood flow from the lower extremities.
- In the presence of congestive heart failure, central venous pressure increases, creating pulsatile waveforms in the lower extremities.

Thermal Regulation

- Thermal regulation is controlled by the sympathetic nerves.
- Vasoconstriction occurs in response to cold. Vasodilatation occurs in response to heat.
- Superficial veins are sensitive to cold and vasoconstriction.
- Venous blood flow in the superficial veins is slow, allowing heat to be transferred from the body to the skin to increase heat loss.

Normal Flow Characteristics

Phasicity with Respiration: cyclical increase and decrease in the venous PW Doppler waveform is directly associated with respiration and movement of the diaphragm.

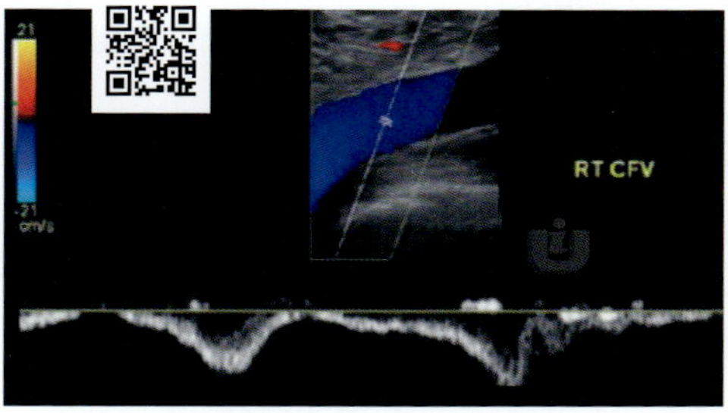

Fig. 4-8. *Normal PW Doppler waveform in a common femoral vein.*

Distal Augmentation: A distinct pattern in the PW Doppler waveform produced by a sudden surge and increased flow through the vein. The augmentation is directly related to the patency of the vein, usually when the limb veins are manually compressed distal to the transducer or upon muscle contraction.

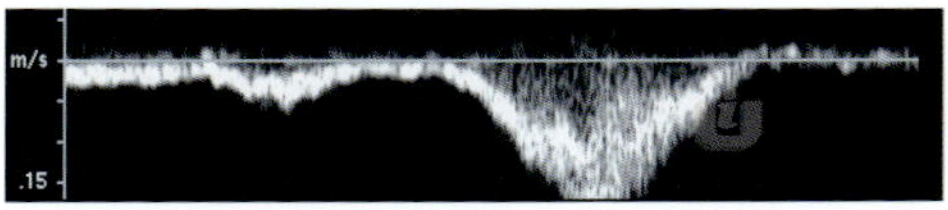

Fig. 4-9. *Distal compression producing augmentation.*

Valsalva Maneuver or Proximal Compression: Demonstrates competency of the venous valves. Normal flow will stop on proximal compression of veins or a Valsalva maneuver, returning on release of the maneuver.

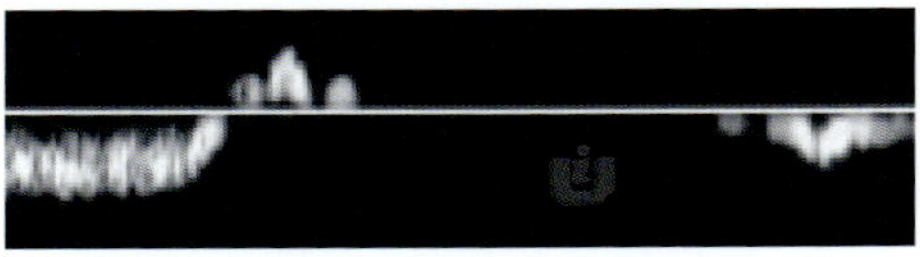

Fig. 4-10. *Normal venous PW Doppler waveform from a Valsalva maneuver which stops flow momentarily.*

Pulsatility: A finding expected in the upper extremity veins due to their proximity to the heart and the upper thigh in patients with congestive heart failure (CHF).

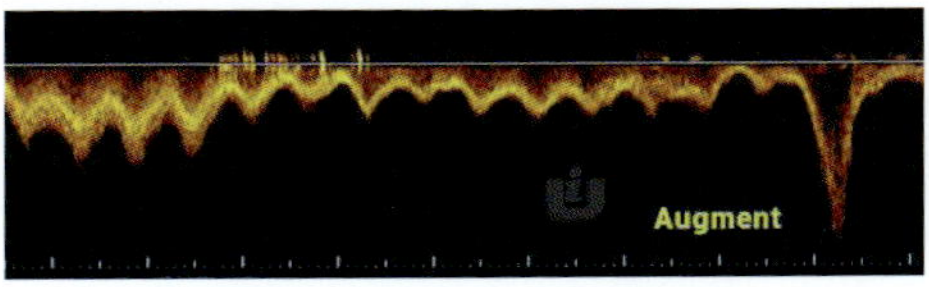

Fig. 4-11. *Pulsatile venous PW Doppler signal.*

Abnormal Flow Characteristics

Venous Incompetence can increase venous pressure due to the lack of unidirectional flow back to the heart. While distal augmentation also helps confirm the patency of the vein of interest, this maneuver can also elicit venous incompetence and demonstrate the inability of the venous valves to function properly.

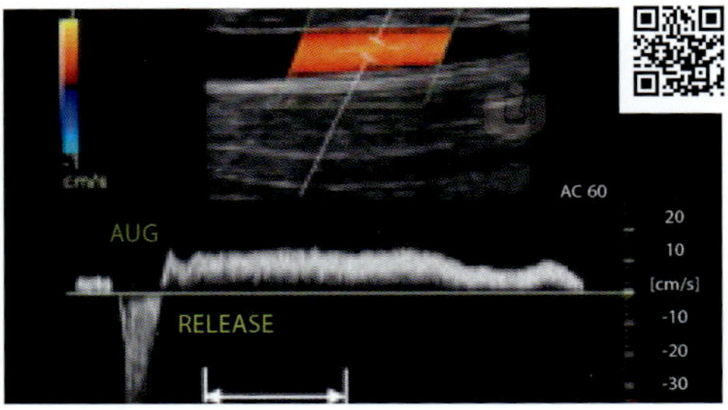

Fig. 4-12. *Venous reflux by PW Doppler upon release of distal compression. Image courtesy of GE Healthcare*

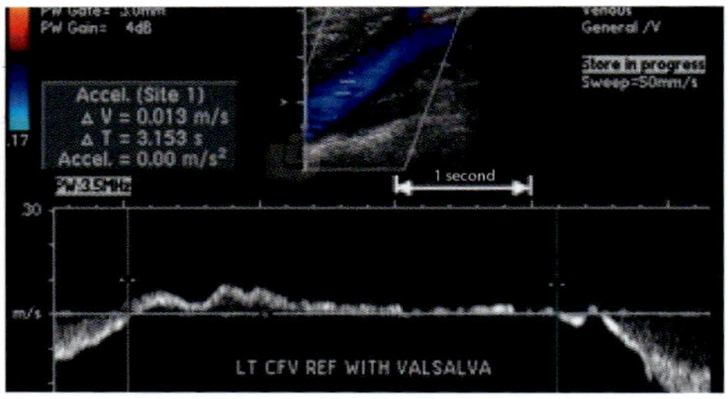

Fig. 4-13. *Venous reflux with a Valsalva maneuver.*

Continuous flow takes on a steady and consistent appearance with little to no variability during normal respiration. It is suggestive of significant proximal obstruction, occlusion, or extrinsic compression, impeding the venous outflow and causing the continuous appearance in the PW Doppler.

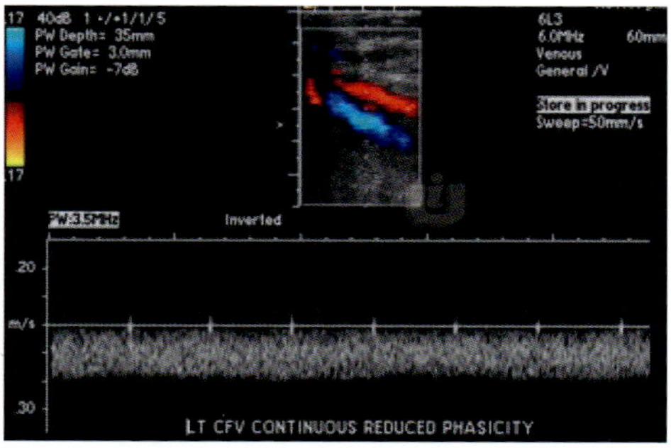

Fig. 4-14. *Continuous venous PW Doppler flow.*

Augmentation: reduced augmentation indicating an obstruction proximal to the transducer.

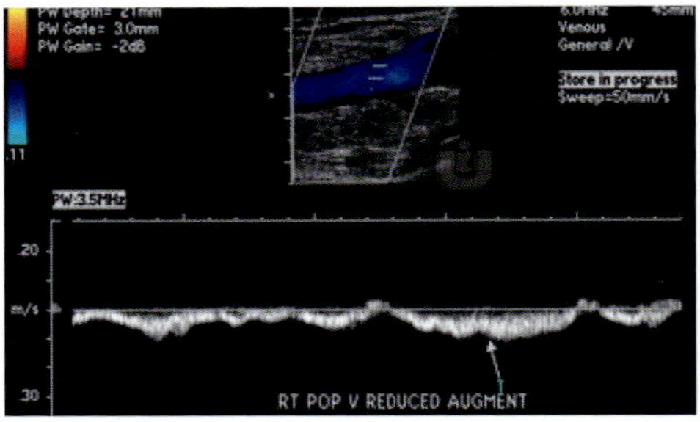

Fig. 4-15. *No increase in augmentation with compression of the distal limb.*

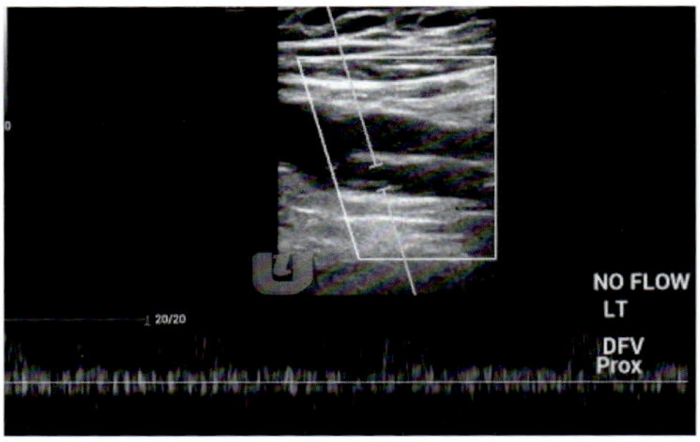

Fig. 4-16. *No flow due to thrombosis.*

Pulsatility: This finding is abnormal in the lower extremity veins and could suggest congestive heart failure.

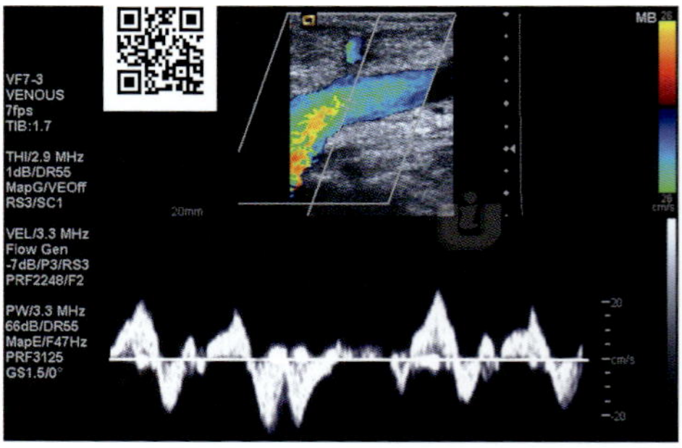

Fig. 4-17. *Pulsatile venous flow demonstrated with PW Doppler.*

Soft Tissue Edema[3,4]

- **Edema** is a common finding in patients with venous disease and is usually associated with elevated venous pressures.[3] Fluid shifts from intravascular compartments (heart and blood vessels) to the extravascular ones (interstitial space, cells, and cerebrospinal fluid) with inadequate absorption from the lymphatic vessels leading to edema.[15,16]
- Causes of edema include venous reflux, obstruction (DVT, chronic post-thrombotic luminal changes, compression), and organ failures. Right heart failure, lymphedema, vascular malformations, and drugs are most common.
- Venous hypertension increases fluid filtration leading to edema. Fibrinogen and red blood cells (RBC) escape into the tissues, thus promoting an inflammatory cascade responsible for skin discoloration and fibrosis. Some patients eventually will develop an ulcer.[3,5,11,12]
- Elevating the legs causes a drop in hydrostatic pressure which will reduce the intracapillary pressure, thus decreasing the swelling.

> *The forces between the pressures are usually balanced with any remaining fluid absorbed by the lymphatics.*

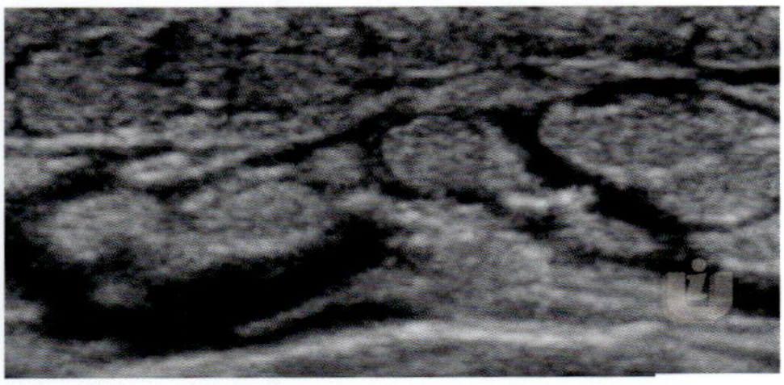

Fig. 4-18. *Soft tissue edema in the lower extremity.*

Ambulatory Venous Pressure (AVP)

Ambulatory venous pressure is the lowest pressure reached during exercise.[7] The AVP functions as a calf muscle pump venous capacitance, amount of reflux, and outflow resistance. The normal AVP equals 30mmHg, and the pressure is greater when venous reflux is present. Pressures of >40mmHg are associated with venous ulceration. (*Fig. 4-20)*

Points to Remember

- Two-thirds of the blood is within the venous system.
- As we age, the arteries become stiffer, increasing systolic pressure.
- Circulation is controlled by the nervous system and the state of the tissue bed.
- The amount of volume moving past a point at a given time (volume per unit of time) is measured in flow units (e.g., L/min, ml/min or cc/hour).
- Blood flow moves from one point to another in response to differences in the energy across the system. Blood will move from an area of high pressure to an area of lower pressure (energy).
- Small changes in the vessel's radius can result in large changes in flow volume.
- During exercise, the flow and pressure gradient increase.
- Flow resistance is higher in smaller vessels.
- A longer vessel has more wall surface for flow to drag on, which can create higher resistance.
- Vein diameter varies with muscle contraction (vasomotor tone).
- The normal venous system is a compliant, low-pressure, non-pulsatile flow system which is responsive to positional changes, cold, respiratory variation, and muscle contraction.

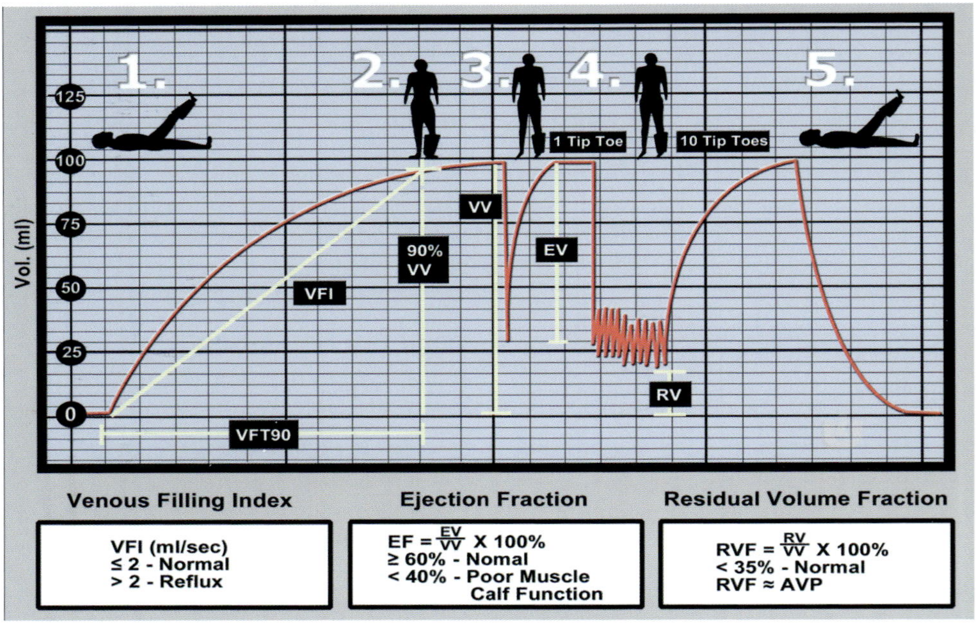

Fig. 4-20. *An example of an APG report which can assess for reflux, calf muscle pump function and venous hypertension.*

References

5. Owen, C, Robers, M. Arterial Vascular Hemodynamics .Journal of Diagnostic Medical Ultrasound 23:129-140, May/June 2007.
6. M Boron,WF and Boulpaep, EL Medical Physiology, A Cellular and Molecular Approach. Elsevier, 2005.
7. Cardiovascular Physiology Concepts, Richard E. Klabunde, Ph.D., Lippincott, Williams and Wilkins 2011 Chapters 5,7,& 8.
8. Needham, T, Needham, A. Characteristics of Pressure and Flow in Arteries and Veins: The Application to Noninvasive Peripheral Vascular Testing. The journal for Vascular Ultrasound 35(4):229-236, 2011.
9. Sumner DS, Zierler RE. (2005). Vascular physiology: essential hemodynamic principles. In Rutherford Vascular Surgery 6th edition. Philadelphia. Elsevier Saunders.
10. Kupinski, Anne Marie (2013) In The Vascular System 1st edition (p 66, 81), Philadelphia. Wolters Kluwer/
11. Miele, FR: Ultrasound Physics and Instrumentation. 4th edition, Forney, TX, Miele enterprises, 2006
12. Meissner MH. (2010). Chronic venous disorders. In Zierler RE (Ed.), Strandess's duplex scanning. disorders in vascular diagnosis 4th ed. (223-229). Philadelphia Wolters Kluwer Lippincott Williams & Wilkins.
13. Size, Gail, Introduction to Venous testing, Inside Ultrasound, Pearce, AZ, Inside Ultrasound 1995.
14. Gianni Belcaro, Andrew N. Nicolaides, M. Veller, A Manual of Diagnosis and Treatment W.B. Saunders, 1995.
15. Sumner DS, Zierler RE. (2005). Vascular physiology: essential hemodynamic principles. In Rutherford *Vascular Surgery 6th edition.* (75 - 123). Philadelphia. Elsevier Saunders.
16. Meissner MH. (2010). Chronic venous disorders. In Zierler RE (Ed.), Strandess's duplex scanning disorders in vascular diagnosis 4th ed. (223 - 229).Philadelphia Wolters Kluwer Lippincott Williams & Wilkins. Oklu et al. (2012). J Vasc Interv Radiol; 23:33-39.
17. Labropoulos N. How Does Chronic Venous Disease Progress from the First Symptoms to the Advanced Stages? A Review. Adv Ther. 2019 Mar;36(Suppl 1):13-19.
18. Labropoulos N, Wierks C, Golts E, Volteas SK, Leon M, Volteas N, et al. Microcirculatory changes parallel the clinical deterioration of chronic venous insufficiency. Phlebology. 2004;19(2):81–86.
19. Levick JR, Michel CC. Microvascular fluid exchange and the revised Starling principle. Cardiovasc Res. 2010;87(2):198–210.
20. Mortimer PS, Rockson SG. New developments in clinical aspects of lymphatic disease. J Clin Invest. 2014 Mar;124(3):915-21.

Chronic Venous Disorders

The term "Chronic Venous Disorder (CVD) includes the full spectrum of morphologic and functional abnormalities of the venous system, from telangiectasias to venous ulcers. [1,2]

Some of these, such as telangiectasias, are highly prevalent in the healthy adult population, and in many cases, the term "disease" is inappropriate. [3]

The term "chronic venous insufficiency" implies a functional abnormality of the venous system and is usually reserved for more advanced disease, including edema (C3), skin changes (C4), or venous ulcers (C5-6). *(See Table 5-1)* [2]

CEAP Classification System [3,4,5]

To distinguish the different manifestations of CVD, the CEAP classification system is used.

In 1994, a comprehensive classification system (CEAP) was developed to allow for uniform diagnosis and comparison of patient populations. The CEAP classification system was updated in 1996, revised in 2004, and most recently updated in 2020.

The fundamentals of the CEAP classification include a description of the following:

- (C) Clinical class based upon objective signs
- (E) Etiology (cause of the condition)
- (A) Anatomical distribution of reflux and obstruction in the superficial, deep, and perforating veins
- (P) Pathophysiology (whether due to reflux or obstruction)

- To further define the clinical class (C), a subscript can be added indicating the presence of symptoms (subscript s) or the absence of symptoms (subscript a). [5]
- Symptoms include aching, pain, tightness, skin irritation, heaviness, muscle cramps, and other complaints attributed to venous dysfunction.
- For example, a patient with:
  - Varicose veins with symptoms would be classified as $C2_s$
  - Telangiectasias without symptoms would be classified as $C1_a$

Table 5-1. CEAP: Summary of Clinical (C) Classifications

C0	No visible or palpable signs of venous disease
C1	Telangiectasias or reticular veins
C2	Varicose veins
$C2_r$	Recurrent varicose veins
C3	Edema
C4	Changes in skin and subcutaneous tissue secondary to CVD
$C4_a$	Pigmentation or eczema
$C4_b$	Lipodermatoscerosis or atrophie blanche
$C4_c$	Corona Phlebictatica
C5	Healed venous ulcer
C6	Active venous ulcer

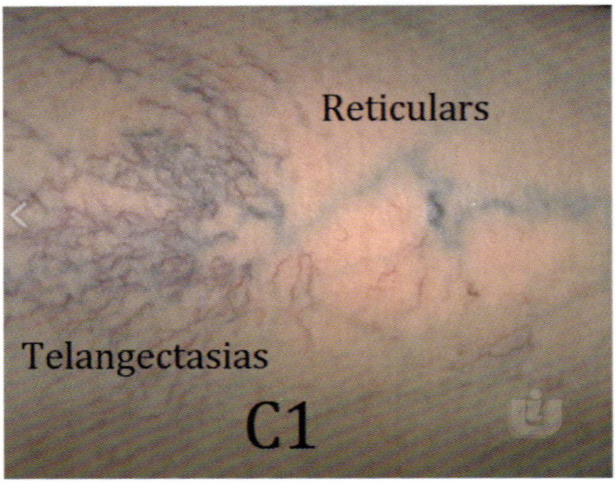

Fig. 5-1. ***C1 Telangiectasias and Reticulars:*** *Telangiectasias are multiple dilated intradermal venules of <1mm in diameter joined together. Reticulars are dilated intradermal veins that are often 1 - 3mm in diameter.*

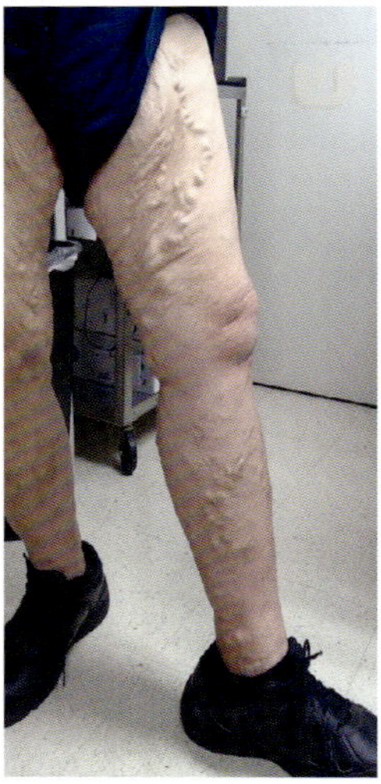

Fig. 5-2. ***C2 and C2r:*** *Subcutaneous dilated veins that are >3mm in diameter. Varicose veins occur because of a degenerative process of the vein wall leading to venous dilation and valvular incompetence.*

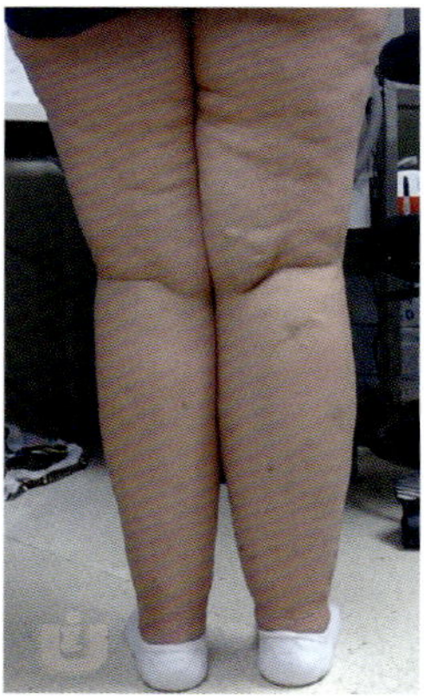

Fig. 5-3. ***C3 Swelling:*** *Edema is caused by increased capillary hydrostatic pressures secondary to venous hypertension leading to extraction of fluid and proteins.*

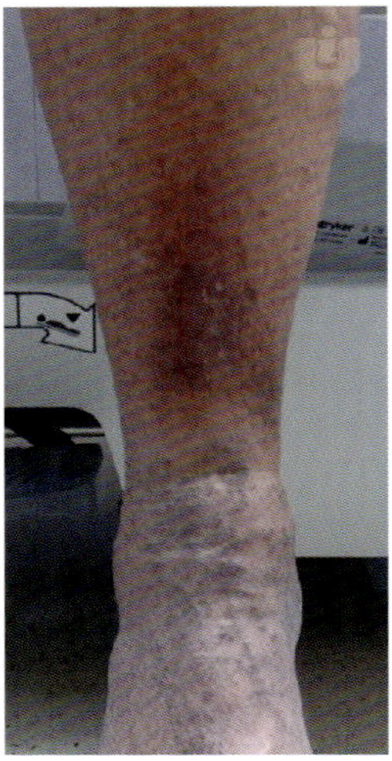

Fig. 5-4. ***C4a Pigmentation:*** *A brownish pigmentation (hemosiderin deposition) that typically occurs in the gaiter area resulting from extravasation and break down of the red blood cells, which have escaped from the capillaries into the surrounding tissue in response to the high venous pressure.*

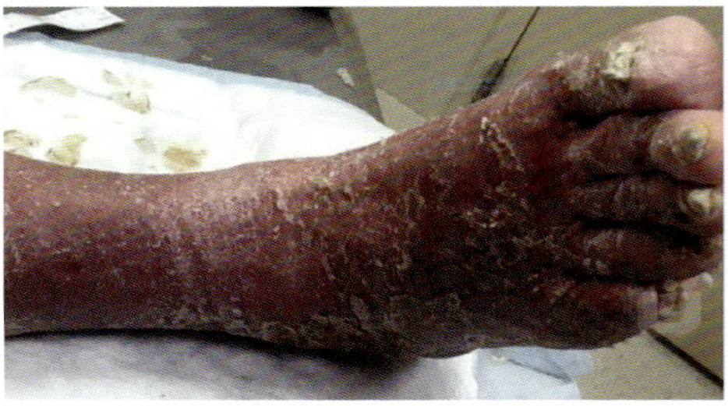

Fig. 5-5. ***C4a Eczema:*** *As capillary fluid leaks into the skin, oxygen is blocked from reaching the skin surface, causing dry, itchy, sensitive skin, which appears as scaly patches.*

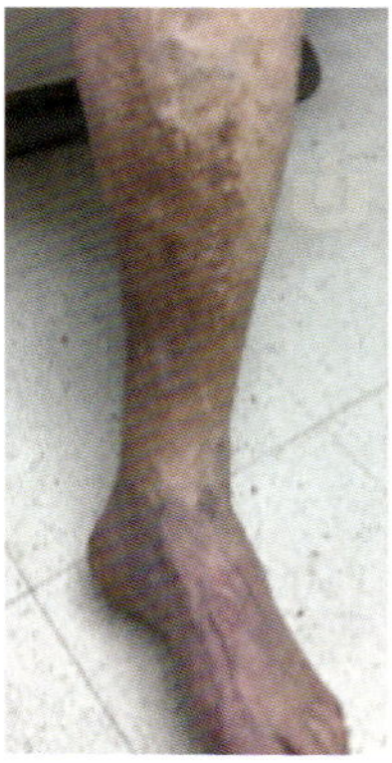

Fig. 5-6. ***C4b Lipodermatosclerosis:*** *Localized chronic inflammation and fibrosis of the skin and subcutaneous tissues as fibrin escapes into the tissue.*

Photo courtesy of Dr. William Breckwoldt

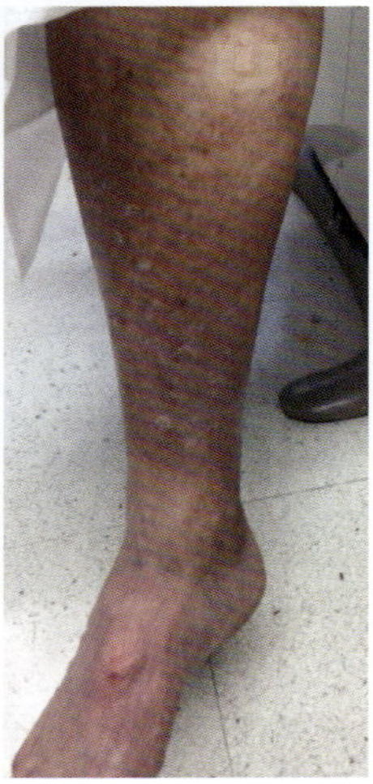

Fig. 5-7. *C4b Atrophie Blanche:* *Localized, often circular whitish, and atrophic skin areas surrounded by dilated capillaries and sometimes hyperpigmentation caused by thrombosis within dermal blood vessels and endothelial proliferation.*

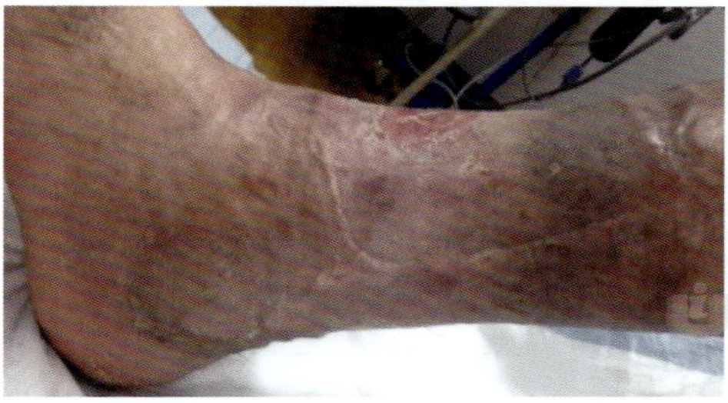

Fig. 5-9. *C5 Healed Ulcer:* *A healed venous leg ulcer usually shows skin damage around the ankle or lower leg typical of CEAP C4 with a patient history of an open ulcer (C6) in the area.*

Photo courtesy of Dr. Joseph Caprini

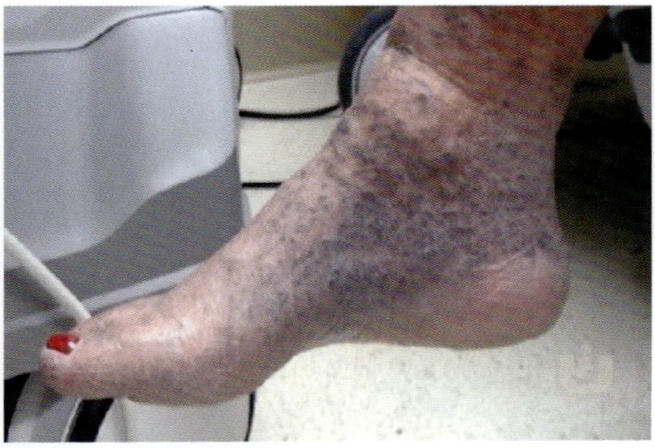

Fig. 5-8. *C4c Corona Phlebectatica* *Abnormally visible fan-shaped pattern of numerous small intra-dermal veins on medial or lateral aspects of the ankle and foot where deoxygenated blood flows upstream toward the heart.*

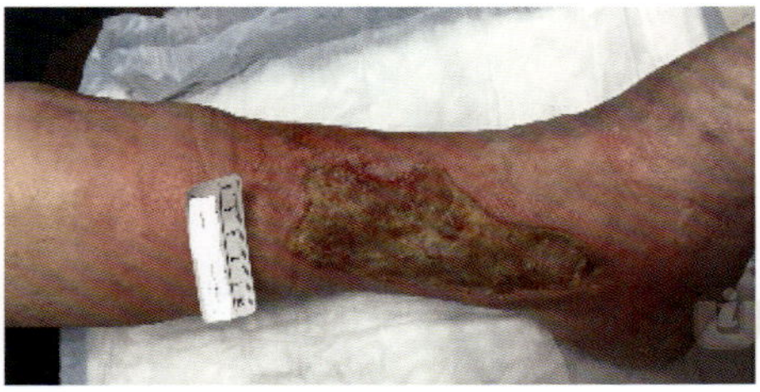

Fig. 5-10. *C6 and C6r Active Ulcer:* *Ulcers appear as open sores with no skin covering the underlying tissue. This is caused by the disruption of the diffusion of oxygen, thereby contributing to local tissue hypoxia. The result is open, draining wounds with overlying slough and surrounding induration. The surrounding skin is usually red as the body uses inflammation to heal the ulceration.* [6]

Table 5-2. Ulcers [6,7,8]

	Venous	Arterial
Cause	Venous hypertension	Arterial obstruction
Location	Between the knee and the ankle. The medial or lateral malleoli are the most common sites, but other sites can be involved.	Prominent bony areas between the toes, tips of the toes, over phalangeal heads, lateral malleolus, and points subjected to repetitive trauma
Ulcer appearance	Variable ulcer bed appearance	Even sharply demarcated and punched-out ulcer margins
Surrounding tissue appearance	Eczematous, presenting with erythema, scaling, weeping, induration, and crusting	Blanched or purpuric skin that is often shiny and tight
Symptoms	Itchy, painful if infected	May be localized to the ulcer or more generalized to the foot

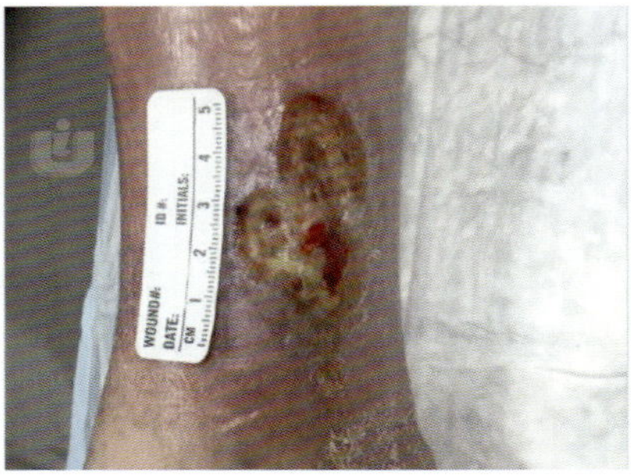

Fig. 5-11. *Venous ulcer lateral malleolus*

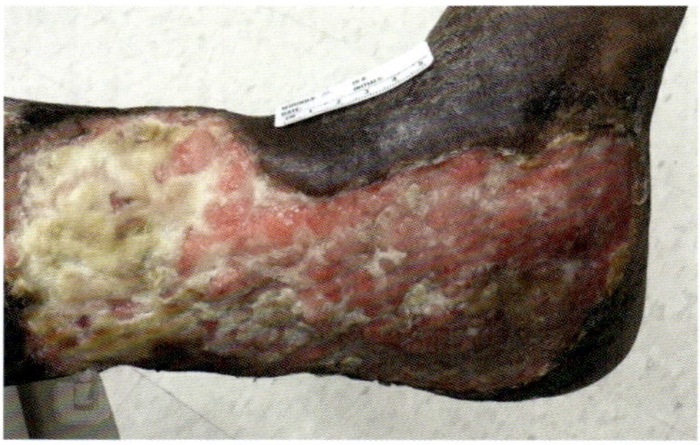

Fig. 5-12. *Venous ulcer on the medial malleolus*

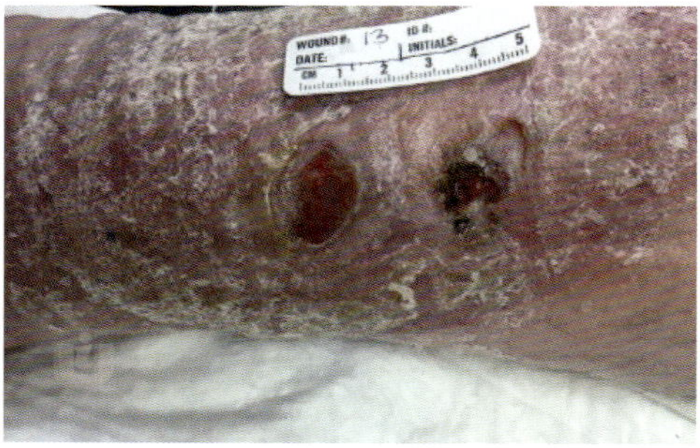

Fig. 5-13. *Venous ulcer lateral malleolus with stasis dermatitis and eczema*

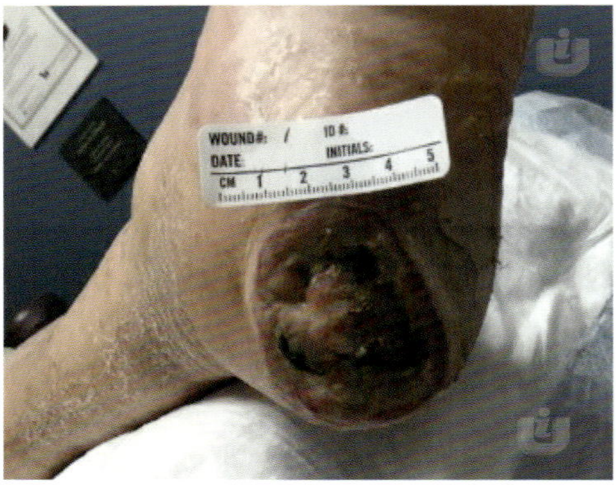

Fig. 5-14. *Arterial ulcer of the heel*

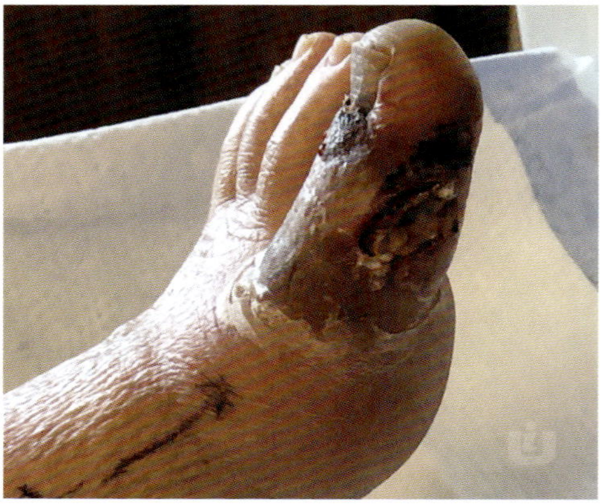

Fig. 5-15. *Arterial ulcer & gangrene of the great toe*

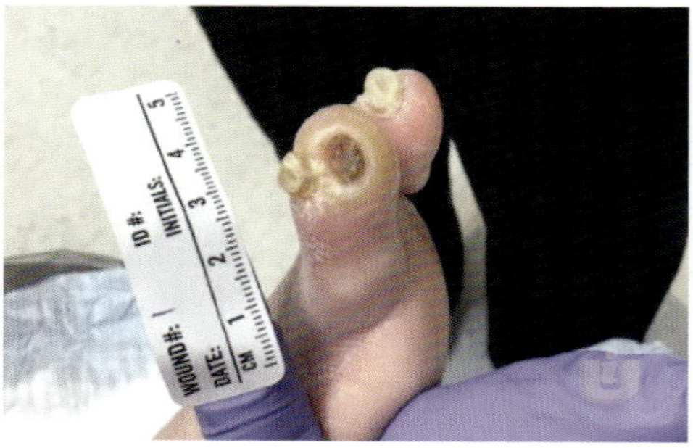

Fig. 5-16. *Arterial ulcer-toe*

Etiology

The etiology or the cause of the disease is divided into three categories:

- Primary
  - The most common causes of venous insufficiency are often under-recognized or poorly defined. [9]
  - The pathogenesis remains unclear. Initially, it was thought that varicose veins were due to valvular incompetence.
  - A current hypothesis states that the structural changes in the vein wall as they become varicosed cause valvular dysfunction. [10]
- Secondary
  - DVT is the most common cause of chronic deep venous obstruction or valvular insufficiency. [9]
  - Post-thrombotic valvular damage may result from initial thrombus adherence to the valve cusp or trauma to the vein wall. [11]
  - Valvular insufficiency may also develop following venous recanalization or pregnancy and progesterone-induced venous wall and valve weakness. [9]
- Congenital
  - Congenital causes include venous malformations.
  - Examples include Klippel-Trenaunay variants and avalvulia (absence of valves). [9]

Risk Factors

- Age (greater with advanced age)
- Previous deep vein thrombosis (DVT)
- Female
- Pregnancy
- Obesity
- Family history
- Occupations requiring extended periods of standing or sitting
- Congenital abnormalities (e.g., Klippel-Trenaunay)

Mechanism of Disease

Normal Venous Valve Function [11-18]

- Venous blood typically flows towards the heart and from the superficial to the deep venous system.
- In the perforating veins, blood flows from the superficial to deep veins.
- When standing still, with the calf muscle relaxed, the veins in the calf fill with blood. Pressure on the valves from retrograde flow forces the valves to close, preventing blood flow toward the feet.
- While walking, muscle contractions squeeze the veins initiating venous blood flow. Venous flow opens the venous valves allowing the blood to flow towards the heart. As the muscle relaxes, the valves close to prevent the backflow of blood (reflux).
- Multiple components facilitate effective venous return from the lower extremities.
  - **Cardiac pump:** During cardiac contraction and relaxation, there is a passive push from the arterial system and a mild suction from the cardiac valves that assist venous blood flow.
  - **Respiratory pump:** During inspiration and expiration pressure changes occur in the thoracic and abdominal cavities. These pressure changes compress the nearby veins and assist blood return to the heart.
  - **Peripheral muscle pumps:**
    - » **Foot:** During flexion, the plantar venous plexus is compressed, and it primes the calf muscle pump.
    - » **Calf:** Gastrocnemius and soleus muscles eject 40-60% of venous volume with a single contraction.
    - » **Thigh:** Although the thigh-level veins are surrounded by muscle, the contribution to venous return is less when compared to the calf.

> *The calf muscle pump is the most important of the three muscle pumps. It is highly efficient, has the most significant capacitance, and generates the highest pressures (mmHg during muscular contraction)* [14,17,19]

- **Pressure gradient and muscle pumps:** the muscle pumps drive blood into the popliteal and femoral veins.
  - » The valves prevent retrograde flow (reflux) during relaxation, generating negative pressure and drawing blood from the superficial to the deep system through perforating veins.
  - » Venous pressure is lowered until arterial inflow equals venous outflow.
  - » When exercise ceases, the veins slowly fill from the capillary bed, causing a slow return to the resting venous pressure.
- **Competent venous valves:**
  - » Are unidirectional
  - » Function to divide the hydrostatic column of blood into segments
  - » Prevent retrograde venous flow

Venous Disease

> *The manifestations of the chronic venous disease result from a complex interaction of anatomy and hemodynamic failure.* [10]

Venous Obstruction [20, 21]

- There are three factors responsible for the formation of venous thrombosis. A combination of any of these events may result in venous thrombosis.
  - » Vein wall injury
  - » Hypercoagulability
  - » Stasis of blood flow
- Obstruction of the iliac veins can directly affect the lower extremities. This should be considered when assessing the lower extremities for venous disease, particularly when the signs and symptoms are out of proportion with the lower extremity ultrasound findings.
- Compression, although most often found in the left common iliac vein, may be observed in the right common iliac and both external iliac veins.
- There can also be a combination of obstruction and reflux.

Venous Reflux

- Reflux is defined as retrograde flow of blood caused by incompetent valves and, in rare cases, absent valves.
- Reflux or pathologic retrograde flow occurs when the valves are absent or rendered incompetent either by degenerative processes (primary venous disease) or an episode of DVT (secondary venous disease). [10]
- Along with reflux, there can also be a component of obstruction.

Dysfunction of the Muscular Pump

- Retrograde flow during calf muscle relaxation prevents the usual reduction in pressure, and rapid venous refilling occurs from the retrograde flow of blood, as well as slow capillary inflow [10]
- Normally, when walking (contracting and relaxing the calf muscles), the calf muscle pump is activated and propels blood upwards toward the heart, reducing blood volume and venous pressure.
  - When venous valves are incompetent, blood flows backward during calf muscle relaxation, which can cause a significant increase in venous pressure.
- Increased venous pressure may also be transmitted from the deep to the superficial veins through incompetent perforators. [10]

Less Common Venous Disorders

- Malformations
- Aneurysms

> *The function of the calf muscle pump may be impaired in patients with chronic venous disease, an observation that is at least partially related to reduced ankle range of motion.* [10]

Location of Disease

Incompetent valves may be located anywhere within the deep, superficial, or perforating venous systems, including:

- Common femoral vein
- Femoral vein

- Popliteal vein
- Saphenofemoral Junction (SJF)
- Saphenopopliteal Junction (SPJ) if present
- Saphenous veins
- Superficial tributaries
- Perforating veins, most commonly those in the gaiter area.

Differential Diagnosis

- Deep venous thrombosis
- Stasis dermatitis
- Contact dermatitis
- Nerve compression
- Arterial disease
- Lymphedema
- Cellulitis
- Skin cancer
- Inguinal hernia

Diagnostic Modalities

- Duplex ultrasonography
- Air plethysmography
- Descending venography
- Intravascular Ultrasound (IVUS)
- MR venogram
- CT venogram

Medical/Conservative Treatment

Elastic compression (graduated compression stockings)

- Elastic compression therapy conforms to leg size changes and thus sustains compression during activity and at rest. The most common type of elastic compression is graduated compression stockings.
- These stockings work by exerting the greatest degree of compression at the ankle, with the level of compression gradually decreasing up the garment.
- The pressure gradient ensures that blood flows upward toward the heart instead of refluxing downward to the foot or laterally into the superficial veins.
- Different degrees of compression are available, and the level of compression is chosen based on the severity of the venous disease.

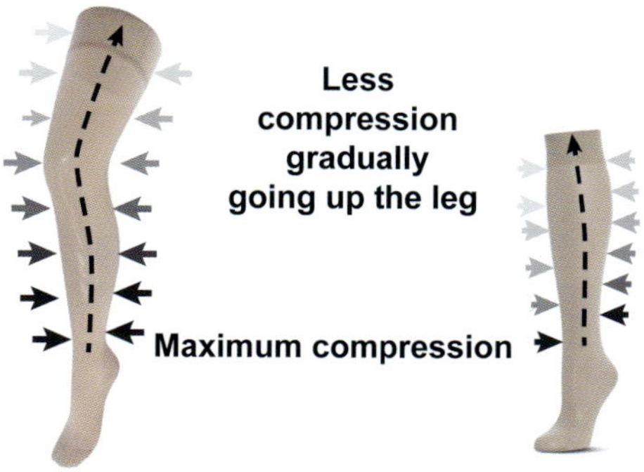

Fig. 5-17. *Compression stockings are used to decrease distal swelling.*

Inelastic compression (bandages, Velcro wraps)

- Inelastic compression therapy does not conform to leg size changes; the degree of compression is not sustained at rest.
- Provides a high working pressure with muscle contraction, and therefore during ambulation, but no resting pressure
- Inelastic bandages do not accommodate changes in leg volume if edema increases during prolonged standing or decreases when the legs are elevated.
- The most common type of inelastic compression, particularly for patients with venous ulcers, is the Unna boot- an inelastic single-component moist bandage that is impregnated with zinc oxide or calamine (with or without glycerin) that hardens after application.
  - A well-trained provider is needed to apply the bandage.
  - The dressing needs to remain dry and be changed 1-3 times per week, depending on the amount of drainage
- A Velcro wrap is another type of inelastic compression
  - A series of overlapping, interlinked straps are fastened using Velcro.
  - Recommended for use with patients who have difficulty donning or doffing (putting on or taking off) a compression sock. (Age, weakness, arthritis, obesity)

Venous Diseases

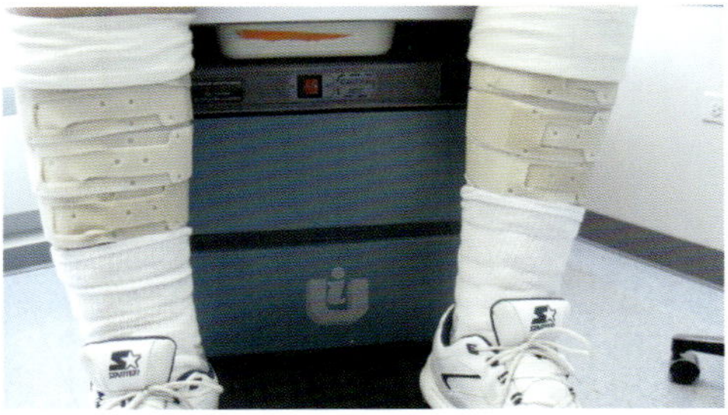

Fig. 5-18. Velcro wrap

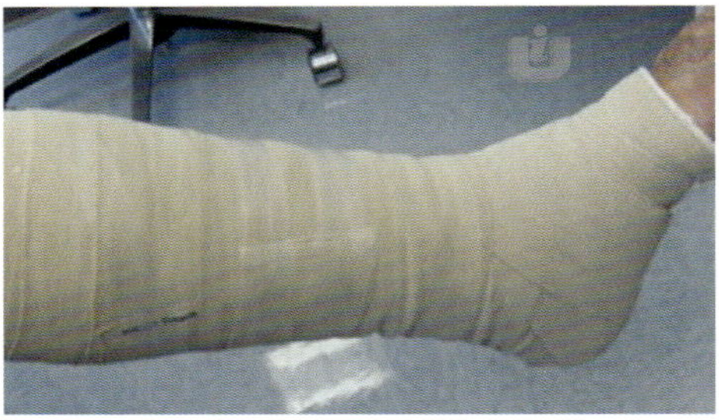

Fig. 5-19. Unna boot *Photos courtesy of Dr. Caprini*

Non-compression conservative treatment options

- Periodic elevation of legs during the day
- Anti-inflammatory medication

Surgical Treatment

- Ligation and Stripping
  - The proximal portion of the vein is ligated
  - Stripping of the vein may be performed concomitantly
- Ambulatory Phlebectomy
  - The removal of large tortuous varicose veins through small incisions in the skin.

Endovascular Treatment

- **Thermal Ablation:** A procedure using heat to remove tissue or destroy its function. Two types of thermal ablation methods are used:
  - Endovenous LASER Ablation
  - Radiofrequency Ablation (RFA)
- **Chemical Ablation:** A procedure using a chemical to remove tissue or destroy its function. Sclerotherapy is the targeted chemical ablation of a varicose vein by intravenous injection of a liquid or foam sclerosant. [22]
- **Adhesive Ablation:** A procedure using cyanoacrylate to close a vein. Cyanoacrylate (Superglue) is a strong, biodegradable tissue adhesive that polymerizes upon contact with tissues. [23]

For more detailed descriptions of treatment for chronic venous disorders refer to *Chapter 11 Venous Ablation*.

Points to Remember

- An estimated 40% of people in the United States have CVD: [24]
  - Occurring more often in women than in men. [24]
  - Occurring more frequently in people over age 50
  - Approximately 50% over the age of 50 have VVs [24]
- If both parents had VVs, their children are estimated to have a 90% chance of developing VVs. If only one parent had VVs, the son has a 25% chance, and the daughter has a 62% chance of developing VVs. If neither parent had VVs, there is still a 20% chance of developing VVs. [25]
- Varicose veins can occur anywhere in the body, though most often occur in the legs.
- There are terms used to describe venous issues that are sometimes misused.
  - **Thrombophlebitis:** An inflammation of a vein associated with a thrombus.
  - **Phlebitis:** Venous inflammation and can occur in the absence of a thrombus.
  - **Superficial venous thrombosis:** Thrombosis within a superficial vein can occur with or without inflammation.

- Studies estimate that 69% of patients with a history of DVT will develop chronic venous insufficiency within one year. [26]
- Dilatation of the lower extremity venous system can be due to venous or portal hypertension.
- Birth control pills can increase the risk of varicose/spider veins. [28]
- There are multiple options available for the treatment of chronic venous disorders.
- A complete understanding of the disease process and the treatment options are needed to make a well-informed decision when choosing a treatment modality.

Iliac Vein Compression
(Previously May-Thurner Syndrome)

- **Iliac vein compression syndrome** is the pathologic compression of an iliac vein by an overlying iliac artery causing lower extremity venous hypertension and/or the development of pelvic varices.
- This syndrome was previously known as May-Thurner syndrome and was specific to the compression of the left common iliac vein by the overlying right common iliac artery.
- The left common iliac vein is the most likely to have obstructive pathology. However, compression of the right common iliac and bilateral external iliac veins has been documented. *(Table 5-3)*
- These iliac vein lesions are referred to as Nonthrombotic Iliac Vein Lesions (NIVLs).
- Obstruction of the iliac veins results in high outflow resistance, venous claudication, and a higher deep vein thrombosis recurrence. It also causes more prevalent and severe post-thrombotic symptoms, impairing the quality of life for patients. [21]
- Symptomatic iliocaval obstruction of NIVL or thrombotic etiology can present with a wide range of clinical features, including all clinical CEAP classes. Specific correction is seldom warranted unless patients present with advanced symptoms (CEAP clinical class 3 or greater) or significant pain. [29]

It is critical that anatomic stenosis alone not be considered a criterion for intervention and that any measurement of stenosis be interpreted in the context of the patient's clinical presentation. [7]

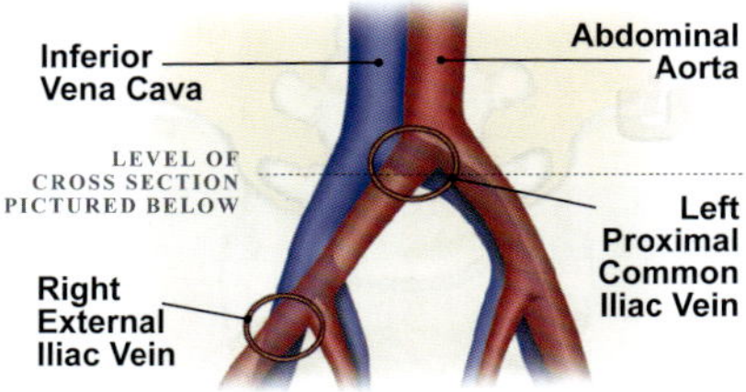

Fig. 5-20. *Most frequently occurring NIVLs typical mid-line anatomy.*

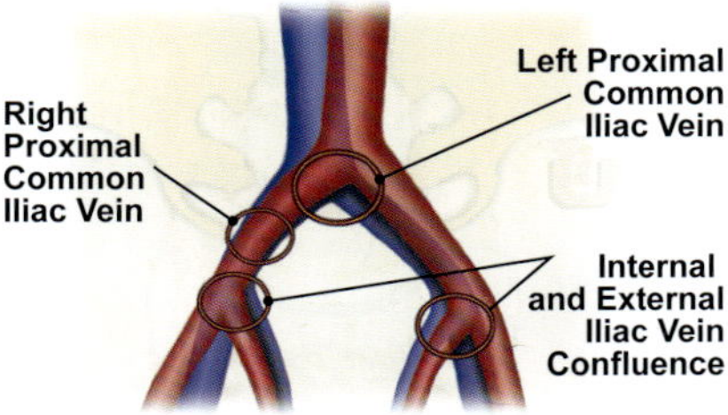

Fig. 5-21. *Less frequently occurring NIVLs. Notice that a slight shift in the mid-line anatomy will create additional areas of potential extrinsic compression.*

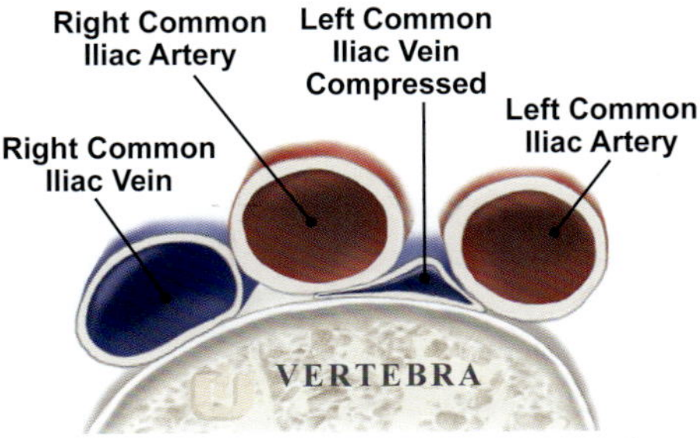

Fig. 5-22. *Cross-sectional view of the left common iliac vein being compressed by the right and left common iliac arteries* *Adapted from www.scgvs.com*

Table 5-3. **Areas of Iliac Vein Compression***
Common Iliac Veins
• Right common iliac artery on left common iliac vein
• Right common iliac artery on right common iliac vein
• Left common iliac artery on left common iliac vein
External Iliac Veins
• Right external iliac artery on right external iliac vein
• Right internal iliac artery on right external iliac vein
• Left external iliac artery on left external iliac vein
• Left internal iliac artery on left external iliac vein
• Inguinal ligament on right external iliac vein
• Inguinal ligament on left external iliac vein
*More than one type of compression may exist.

Labropoulos N. (2018). Diagnosis of iliac vein obstruction with duplex ultrasound criteria used during duplex ultrasound examination to identify iliac vein obstruction. Endovascular Today, 17(7), 3.

Etiology

- Congenital
- A traumatic etiology from pulsations of the adjacent artery [29]

Mechanism of Disease

- **Extrinsic obstruction**
  - Compression of an iliac vein by an overlying artery (NIVL)
  - Could be a partial compression or a complete occlusion of the vein
  - Anatomical structures surrounding the veins, including the inguinal ligament may also cause obstruction of a vein. [21]
- **Intrinsic obstruction**
  - Wall fibrosis and intraluminal changes caused by the pulsations of an overlying artery. (NIVL) [7, 29]

Location of Disease

- Common iliac vein
- External iliac vein

Differential Diagnosis

- Unilateral deep venous thrombosis not caused by iliac compression
- Lymphedema
- Cellulitis
- Hematoma
- Adenopathy
- Vascularized mass

Diagnostic Modalities

- Duplex ultrasonography
- CT venography
- MR venography
- IVUS
- Venography

Medical Treatment

- Anticoagulation
- Thrombolysis

Surgical Treatment

With the improvement of endovascular procedures to treat iliac vein obstruction, these surgical procedures are rarely utilized:

- Iliocaval bypass
- Transposition of the right CIA
- Iliac vein disobleration (opened to remove webs/spurs)

Endovascular Treatment

- Iliac vein angioplasty
- Iliac vein stenting (common and external)
- Vena cava filters (in cases of thrombus and risk of PE)

Points to Remember

- Iliac vein compression is the updated terminology for May-Thurner Syndrome.
- Iliac vein compression can involve the bilateral common and external iliac veins.
- NIVL are defined as venous reflux or obstruction arising from complex lesions involving not only external compression of an iliac vein but also wall fibrosis and intraluminal changes caused by the pulsations of an overlying artery. [7,29]

- Symptomatic iliocaval obstruction of NIVL or PTS etiology can present with a wide range of clinical features, including all clinical CEAP classes [29]
- ≥50% iliac stenosis may be present in 25 – 33% of the general population; it is critical that anatomic stenosis alone not be considered a criterion for intervention and that any measurement of stenosis be interpreted in the context of the patient's clinical presentation. [7]

Lymphedema [30,31,32]

An accumulation of interstitial fluid develops due to obstruction or abnormal lymphatic system development (vessels or lymph nodes). There are two types of lymphedema:

- **Primary lymphedema:** Occurs independently (less common).
- **Secondary lymphedema:** Secondary to a disease or another condition (most common).

Etiology

- Congenital
- Surgery (post-op complication)
- Infection
- Cancer
- Radiation
- Trauma

Risk Factors

- Family history
- Female
- Cancer, with a history of surgery or radiation for the condition (e.g., breast cancer with mastectomy)
- History of lymph node dissection
- Exposure to infectious bacteria, especially in tropical regions
- Trauma

Mechanism of Disease

- Primary lymphedema is an inherited condition that affects the development of the lymph vessels. During the embryonic stage, there is a malformation of lymph nodes or an absence of valves in the lymph vessels. This can occur during infancy (Milroy disease), in childhood or puberty (Meige disease), or later, after the age of 35 (lymphedema tarda).
- Certain conditions or interventions can damage your lymph vessels and cause lymphedema (secondary lymphedema). Lymph nodes are often removed during surgery to biopsy and assess for the spread of cancer. If the remaining lymph nodes/vessels do not compensate for this loss, the limb will swell.
- Scarring and inflammation of the lymph nodes/vessels after radiation treatment can restrict flow in the lymphatic system.
- Cancerous tumors can block lymphatic pathways and prevent flow. Infections and parasites can access the lymphatic system and restrict lymphatic flow.

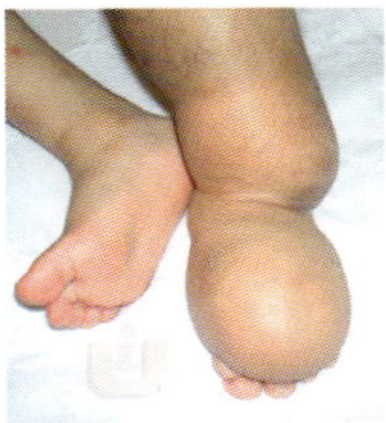

Fig. 5-23. *Physical presentation of primary lymphedema*

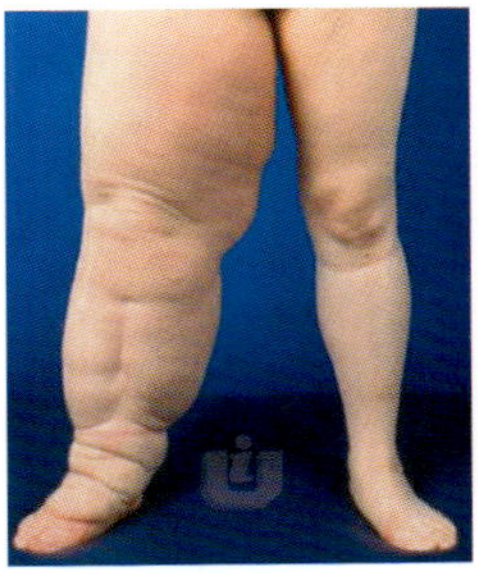

Fig. 5-24. *Physical presentation of secondary lymphedema*

Images courtesy of Byung-Boong Lee MD Ph.D. FACS

Location of Disease

- Lower and upper extremities

Differential Diagnosis

- Vascular conditions such as venous insufficiency, congenital malformation, or arteriovenous fistula
- Infection
- Cardiac failure (edema is usually bilateral)
- Insect bites
- Renal failure
- Liver failure
- Rheumatoid arthritis
- Side effects of certain drugs, hormones

Diagnostic Modalities

- Duplex ultrasonography
- CT angiogram
- MR angiography
- Contrast lymphangiography
- Lymphoscintigraphy

Medical Treatment

- Leg elevation
- Compression stockings
- Manual lymph drainage
- Intermittent pneumatic compression
- Prompt treatment of cellulitis
- Exercise

Surgical Treatment

- Microsurgical lymphatic reconstruction (lymphatic grafting)
- Liposuction (reduce edema)

Points to Remember

The lymphatic system serves to balance intracellular and extracellular environments. Some of the components of this system include lymph nodes, spleen, thymus, nasopharyngeal tonsils, lymphocytes, and macrophages. This unidirectional system transports fluid throughout the tissues and collects bacteria, viruses, and waste products. There are numerous communications between the blood and lymph streams. For example, lymph from the upper extremities enters the bloodstream at the junction of the subclavian and jugular veins.

- **Lymphedema** is a common differential diagnosis for lower extremity edema and is aggravated by repetitive attacks of cellulitis, which scar the existing lymphatic channels.
- **Elephantitis** is a complication of lymphedema where the skin becomes extremely hard and thick. These patients are at risk for chronic ulcers and infection.
- **Lymphangiosarcoma** is a rare soft tissue cancer resulting from severe cases of untreated lymphedema that originate in the lymph nodes and vessels.

Pelvic Venous Disorders *Previously Pelvic Congestion Syndrome*

The term Pelvic Venous Disorders (PeVD) describes a group of related clinical findings with overlapping clinical presentations ultimately leading to venous hypertension (high pressure within a venous system) of the pelvic veins and/or other peripheral venous beds. The signs and symptoms of PeVD may vary depending on the venous bed(s) affected by the underlying venous hypertension. The symptoms may include chronic pelvic pain, pelvic, lower extremity and genital varices, lower extremity pain, swelling, and left flank pain and hematuria. [33]

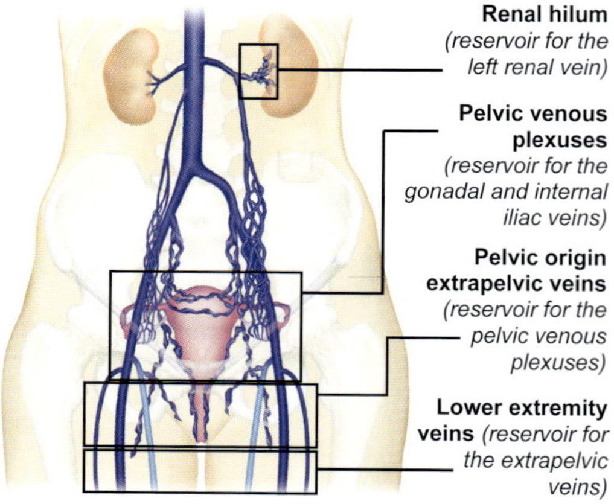

Fig. 5-25. *Diagram depicting the peripheral venous reservoirs affected by venous hypertension of the abdominal and pelvic veins.*

Etiology [7, 33]

- **Thrombotic**
  - Reflux arising from a previous DVT
  - Obstruction arising from a previous DVT
- **Nonthrombotic**
  - Reflux arising from a degenerative process of the vein wall
  - Reflux arising from a proximal obstruction due to an extrinsic compression
- **Congenital**
  - Venous malformation
  - Mixed vascular malformation

Mechanism of Disease

Increased central venous pressure of the pelvic veins leads to the development of peri-uterine and trans-uterine varicosities. [7] This increased pressure occurs due to a more central obstruction and/or reflux. These may occur concurrently or independently.

Obstruction

Obstruction is most likely to occur in the left renal vein and the left common iliac vein.

- **Extrinsic pathology**

  Non thrombotic iliac vein lesions (NIVL)
  - Mechanical compression of a vein due to an overlying artery or other anatomic structure, which results in obstruction.
- **Intrinsic pathology**

  Development of an obstruction within the vein.
  - Chronic pulsatile compression of an iliac vein by an overlying iliac artery stimulates the formation of fibrotic adhesions that can cause partial or complete iliac vein obstruction over time. This finding is associated with NIVLs. [34,35,36]
  - Changes associated with previous DVT

Reflux

Reflux is most likely to occur in the following:

- Gonadal veins
- Internal iliac veins and their tributaries

Based upon anatomic patterns and patients' symptoms, reflux within the pelvic veins has been described as compensated or uncompensated. [37]

- **Uncompensated reflux** [7,33,37]
  - Venous pressure is transmitted directly to the peripheral venous reservoirs (renal hilar, pelvic venous plexus, pelvic origin extrapelvic veins, and the lower extremity)
  - Will result in the development of symptoms at the location of the pathology
- **Compensated reflux** [7,33,37]
  - Venous pressure is decompressed via collaterals into more peripheral venous reservoirs.
  - Will result in the development of symptoms in the peripheral venous reservoir, not at the direct site of the pathology

For a complete list of reflux patterns and associated symptoms, see the pelvic venous duplex chapter.

Location of Disease

- Gonadal vein, left more often than right
- Left renal vein
- Iliocaval
- Pelvic venous plexus (peri-uterine and/or trans-uterine)
- Extrapelvic tributaries of the IIVs. These tributaries originate outside of the pelvis and then join the IIV in the pelvis. Branches of the internal iliac vein include:
  - Round ligament
  - Obturator
  - Perineal
  - Gluteal (superior and inferior)
- Scrotal pampiniform plexus reflux

Differential Diagnosis

- Endometriosis
- Adhesions
- Adenomyosis
- Malignancy
- Uterine prolapse
- Ovarian cysts
- Cystitis
- Irritable bowel

Diagnostic Modalities

- Duplex ultrasonography
- CT venography
- MR venography
- IVUS
- Venography

Medical/Surgical Treatment

Left Renal Vein

- Nephropexy
- External renal vein stenting
- Aortomesenteric transposition
- Renal autotransplantation
- Gonadal vein transposition
- Left renal vein transposition

Ovarian and iliac veins

- Endovascular approaches to primary ovarian and internal iliac venous reflux have largely replaced medical and surgical approaches.

Endovascular Treatment

- Coil embolization of the refluxing trunk (gonadal)
- Combination of coil embolization and sclerotherapy
- Sclerotherapy of the pelvic venous plexus
- Iliac vein angioplasty
- Iliac vein stenting (common and external)
- Left renal vein stenting (not considered the gold standard of treatment, more research is needed)

Points to Remember

- It is useful to consider the venous circulation of the pelvis to consist of multiple interconnected venous systems—the left renal and ovarian veins, the iliac veins (common, external, and internal), and the lower extremity veins.
- Communications between these three systems frequently allow for crossover from one side to the other within the pelvis.
- Nonsaphenous origin lower extremity varicose veins are often caused by pelvic varicose veins via the pelvic escape/pelvic leak points.

Phlegmasia Alba Dolens [38,39]

Decreased venous drainage due to thrombosis of extremity deep veins, without collateral vein involvement.

Etiology

- Hypercoagulable state
- Massive venous thrombosis

Risk Factors

- Female > male
- Middle-aged
- Pregnancy (esp. during the last trimester)

Mechanism of Disease

- Extensive edema (usually due to iliofemoral thrombosis) obscures capillary circulation causing a "white" discoloration of the skin.
- Arterial spasms similar to those in phlegmasia cerulea dolens may also be a contributing factor.

Location of Disease

- Iliofemoral deep veins; iliac, common femoral, deep femoral, and femoral veins
- Upper extremity deep veins (rare)

Differential Diagnosis

- Arterial embolism
- Aortic dissection
- Lymphedema

Diagnostic Modalities

- Duplex ultrasonography
- Arteriography
- Venography

Medical Treatment

- IV heparin and Coumadin
- Graduated compression stockings

Surgical Treatment

- Venous thrombectomy
- Compartment fasciotomy
- Cross pubic vein-vein reconstruction with PTFE

- Creation of an arteriovenous fistula between the femoral artery and great saphenous vein
- Amputation

Endovascular Treatment

- Mechanical thrombectomy
- Thrombolytic therapy

Points to Remember

- Phlegmasia alba dolens can progress to phlegmasia cerulea dolens

Phlegmasia Cerulea Dolens [38,39]

Massive venous occlusion due to multi-segment thrombosis of extremity deep veins; iliofemoral, lower leg veins, and collaterals.

Etiology

- Malignancy
- Hypercoagulable state
- Trauma

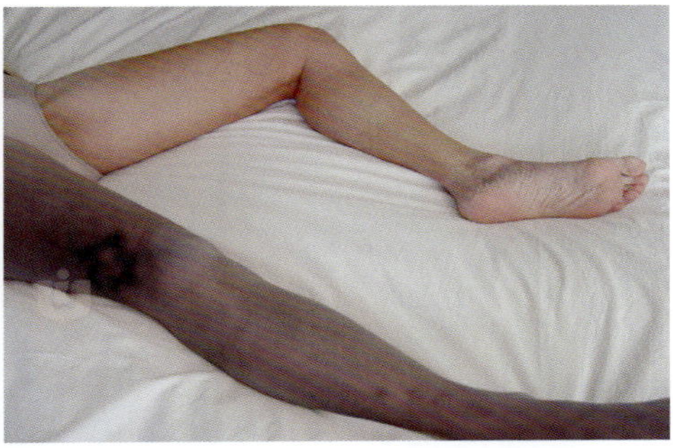

Fig. 5-26. *Phlegmasia cerulea dolens of the right leg.*

Risk Factors

- Female > male
- Middle-aged
- Post-operative
- Vena cava insertion
- Ulcerative colitis
- Gastroenteritis
- Heart failure
- Mitral valve stenosis
- Iliac vein compression syndrome

Mechanism of Disease

- Massive obstruction of venous outflow reduces arterial inflow to the limb and causes arterial vasoconstriction, and may cause arterial thrombosis.
- Venous congestion results from significant iliac vein thrombosis and causes a "blue" discoloration of the skin.

Location of Disease

- Iliofemoral deep veins; iliac, common femoral, deep femoral, and femoral veins (along with their collaterals).
- Upper extremity deep veins (only 2-5% of cases)

Differential Diagnosis

- Arterial ischemia/thrombosis
- Aortic dissection
- Toxic shock syndrome
- Superficial phlebitis of the upper extremity

Diagnostic Modalities

- Duplex ultrasonography
- Arteriography
- Venography

Medical Treatment

- Maximize limb elevation
- Correct any hypovolemia
- Aggressive anticoagulation
- Graduated compression stockings

Surgical Treatment

- Venous thrombectomy
- Compartment fasciotomy
- Cross pubic vein-vein reconstruction with PTFE
- Creation of an arteriovenous fistula between the femoral artery and great saphenous vein
- Amputation

Endovascular Treatment

- Mechanical thrombectomy
- Thrombolytic therapy

Points to Remember

Venous gangrene can occur with phlegmasia cerulea dolens because of substantial venous outflow and arterial inflow obstructions. All toes and part of the foot will be gangrenous, instead of only one or two toes, typically occurring in cases of gangrene caused by arterial disease.

Pulmonary Embolism [40-43]

Definition

The occlusion of a pulmonary artery by a thromboembolism.

Etiology

- Venous sites that may thrombose and be the source of the embolus include:
  - Lower extremity deep veins (90%)
  - Pelvic deep veins
  - Upper extremity deep veins

Risk Factors

- Age (greater with advanced age)
- Immobilization (e.g., long-distance air travel, paraplegia)
- Genetic prothrombotic conditions (clotting disorders, such as Factor V Leiden)
- Post-operative phase (especially after orthopedic surgery)
- Central venous or femoral catheters
- Cancer/malignancy
- Pregnancy
- Medications (e.g., oral contraceptives)
- Estrogen replacement therapy
- Previous DVT
- Heart complications
- Obesity
- Family history
- Smoking
- Chronic Obstructive Pulmonary Disease (COPD)
- Blood type (highest risk with type-A, the lowest risk with type-O)
- Trauma
- Antiphospholipid antibodies (lupus, etc.)
- Varicose veins
- Inflammatory bowel disease

Mechanism of Disease

- Embolization occurs when a piece of a blood clot (embolus) breaks free from a venous thrombus and travels centrally to the pulmonary arterial circulation.
- An embolus can pass through the right side of the heart to the lungs, where it obstructs one of the pulmonary arteries. As a result, lung tissue is deprived of blood, which can be fatal.

Location of Disease

- Pulmonary artery
- Pulmonary artery branches

Differential Diagnosis

- Bronchitis pneumonia
- Pleurisy
- Myocardial ischemia (MI)

Diagnostic Modalities

- CT angiography
- Ventilation-perfusion (VQ) Scan
- Chest x-ray
- Pulmonary angiogram

Medical Treatment

- Heparinization
- Long-term anticoagulation

Surgical Treatment

- Caval filter placement
- Pulmonary embolectomy

Endovascular Treatment

- Thrombolytic therapy
- Pulmonary suction embolectomy

Points to Remember

- Pulmonary embolism (PE) is a complication of venous thrombosis.
- PE is the third most common cause of death in the US, with approximately 630,000 cases/per year. It is one of the top causes of "unexpected death" in any age group.
- Venous duplex exams do not rule out a pulmonary event; they can only suggest a source of emboli for an episode of PE.

- A normal, negative VQ scan excludes PE. False positive VQ results may occur in patients for other reasons, such as lung disease.
- Studies have indicated that approximately one-third of PE cases are asymptomatic.
- The source of emboli is usually iliofemoral thrombus. Calf thrombi rarely result in pulmonary emboli, though they often propagate above the knee, becoming a greater risk for embolus.
- To decrease the risk of a PE, an IVC filter is placed via a catheter (typically using CFV, EIV, or jugular access). This procedure aims to "catch" any thrombi floating in the bloodstream, lowering the risk of PE.

Superior Vena Cava (SVC) Syndrome [44,45]

Obstruction of the superior vena cava due to thrombosis or extrinsic compression.

Etiology

- Central venous interventions (e.g., central catheters, pacemakers)
- Malignancy, with or without lymphadenopathy (esp. of lung and thorax)
- Histoplasmosis (fungal disease)
- Genetic prothrombotic conditions (clotting disorders, such as Factor V Leiden)
- Radiation therapy to the thorax

Risk Factors

- Cancers/lymphoma of the head, neck, and thorax regions
- Central catheterization
- Cardiac pacemaker

Mechanism of Disease

- Decreased venous return from the head, neck, and upper extremities can result in extremity edema, headaches, facial swelling, dilated torso veins, and in extreme cases, respiratory "embarrassment" or difficulty.

Location of Disease

- Superior vena cava

Differential Diagnosis

- Acute respiratory distress
- COPD/emphysema
- Aortic dissection
- Mediastinitis (tissue inflammation in the mid-chest or mediastinum)
- Pericarditis
- Pneumonia
- Syphilis
- Tuberculosis

Diagnostic Modalities

- X-ray
- Duplex ultrasonography
- CT angiography
- MRI
- Venography
- IVUS

Medical Treatment

- Elevation of patient's head during night-time hours
- Limit daily episodes of bending over
- Clothing: wear loose collars
- Diuretics to reduce edema
- Anticoagulation

Surgical Treatment

- SVC reconstruction (using femoral vein, spiral saphenous, PTFE, allograft, or cryopreserved homografts)
- Removal of external compression (e.g., tumor resection)

Endovascular Treatment

- Thrombolysis
- Angioplasty and stenting

Points to Remember

- Malignancies are the chief cause of SVC syndrome.
- The severity of symptoms depends on the degree of collateral circulation.
- Chemotherapy and radiotherapy may relieve symptoms in patients suffering from SVC syndrome caused by malignancies (extrinsic compression).

Venous Malformations [46-49]

Venous Malformations (VM) are developmental anomalies (birth defects) of the venous system. Together with arterial, capillary, and lymphatic malformations, they are a part of a large group of Congenital Vascular Malformations (CVM), which are developmental anomalies of the peripheral vascular system.

Etiology

- Congenital

Mechanism of Disease

Arrested development of the venous system during the various stages of embryogenesis may result in venous malformation.

Extratruncular Lesions

- Developmental arrest occurs before the main vascular trunks are formed.
- May produce symptoms due to compression of the surrounding structures (muscles, nerves).
- May have a significant hemodynamic impact on the involved vascular system.
- There is a high risk of re-occurrence after treatment.

Truncular Lesions

- Defects of fully formed and often named vessels
- Developmental arrest occurs during the "later" stages of vascular trunk formation
- Risk of re-occurrence after treatment is minimal to none.
- Associated with more serious hemodynamic consequences. Incomplete, abnormal development of the main axial veins results in:
  - Aplasia, hypoplasia, or hyperplasia of the vessel (e.g., agenesis/rudimentary femoral vein)
  - Obstruction (e.g., vein web, spur, annulus, or septum)
  - Dilation (e.g., popliteal or iliac vein ectasia or aneurysm)
- These lesions also manifest as persistent embryonic veins (marginal or sciatic) when a fetal (truncal) vessel fails to undergo normal involution
  - A **persistent marginal vein** courses along the lateral aspect of the thigh and calf just under the skin.
    - It is incompetent along its entire length because it lacks valves.
    - Drainage is either into a lateral branch of the deep femoral vein or the internal iliac vein.
    - The vein sometimes crosses anterior in the thigh and joins the femoral vein next to the great saphenous vein
  - A **persistent sciatic vein** may either:
    - Run within the main trunk of the nerve, surrounded by the nerve fibers
    - Or have a spiral course around the main trunk of the nerve, inside the epineurium.

> *Prior to treatment of any superficial veins, it is essential to include a complete duplex ultrasound assessment of the deep venous system to ensure that it is intact. In patients with venous malformations, the superficial system may act as the primary outflow for the lower extremity.*

Differential Diagnosis

- Hemangioma (vascular tumors that have a distinctly different etiology, genetics, presentation, prognosis, and treatment)
- Peripheral nerve sheath tumors
- PTEN hamartoma syndrome
- Fibroadipose vascular anomaly
- Spindle cell hemangioendothelioma
- Congential fibrosarcoma

> *Venous malformations should be differentiated from hemangiomas. Hemangiomas are vascular tumors that present on ultrasound as a soft tissue mass. A venous malformation is a collection of abnormal vessels.*

Location of Disease

- Venous Malformations (VMs) most commonly appear on the skin but can be present in other tissues and organs as well.
- Lateral lower extremity with the appearance of a varicosity (persistent marginal vein)
- Posterior thigh along the sciatic nerve (persistent sciatic vein)

Patient History

- Pain
- Disfiguration
- Functional impairment

Physical Examination

- Lesion(s)
- Presence of dilated vessels/varicosities
- Lymphatic system
- Edema
- Skin changes
- Limb size and symmetry
- Soft tissue or bony hypertrophy or atrophy

Diagnostic Modalities

- Duplex ultrasound
- CT
- MRI
- Angiogram/Venogram

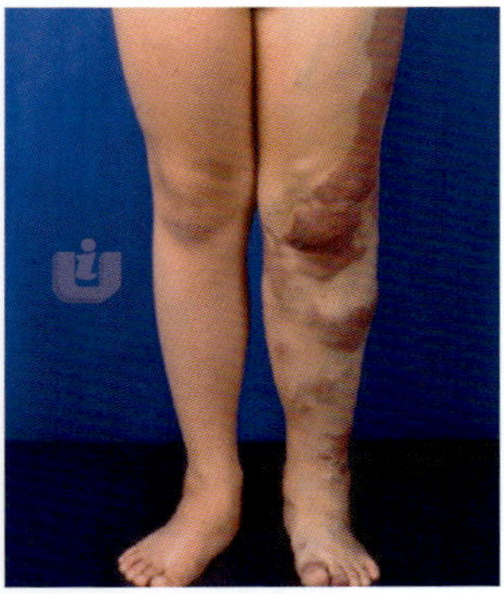

Fig. 5-27. *Klippel-Trenaunay Syndrome (KTS) is a syndrome that affects the development of blood vessels, soft tissues, and bones. This syndrome has three characteristic features: a red birthmark called a port-wine stain, overgrowth of soft tissues and bones, and vein malformations such as varicose veins or malformations of deep veins in the limbs.* [46] *Image courtesy of Byung-Boong Lee MD Ph.D. FACS*

Venous Thrombosis

The obstruction of venous outflow within a deep or superficial vein by thrombus.

Etiology

The theory of Virchow's Triad states that venous thrombosis is caused by: venous stasis, vein wall injury, or a hypercoagulable state. Varicose veins and extrinsic compression can lead to one or more of these.

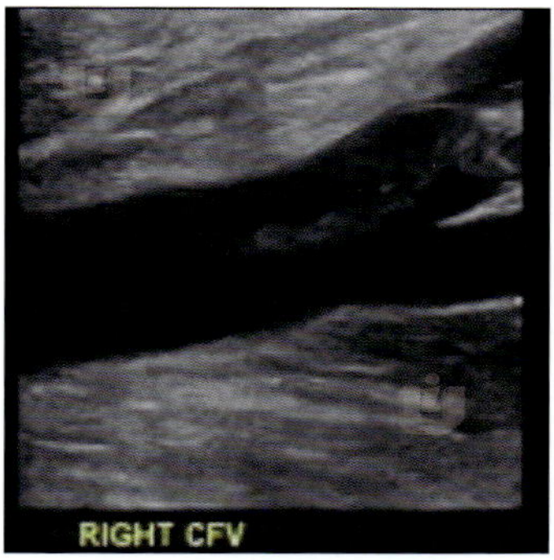

Fig. 5-28. *Free-floating thrombus: free-floating tail located in the common femoral vein.*

Risk Factors

- Age (greater with advanced age)
- Immobilization
- Prothrombotic gene mutations (clotting disorders such as Factor V Leiden)
- Post-operative phase (especially after orthopedic surgery)
- Central venous or femoral catheters
- Female
- Pregnancy
- Oral contraceptives
- Estrogen replacement
- Cancer/malignancy
- Previous DVT
- Heart complications (myocardial infarction, congestive heart failure, etc.)
- Obesity
- Family history
- Smoking
- COPD
- Blood type (highest risk with type-A lowest risk with type-O)
- Trauma

- Antiphospholipid antibodies (e.g., lupus, etc.)
- Occupations requiring extended periods of standing or sitting
- Varicose veins
- Congenital abnormalities (e.g., Klippel-Trenaunay)
- Inflammatory bowel disease
- Drug abuse
- Cerebrovascular events (stroke, TIA)
- Iliac vein compression syndrome

Mechanism of Disease

- There are three factors responsible for the formation of venous thrombosis, as outlined in Virchow's Triad: vein wall injury, hypercoagulability, and stasis of blood flow. A combination of any of these events may result in venous thrombosis.
- In blood, coagulation factors are balanced by anticoagulation factors. This allows blood coagulation to occur where and when vessels are severed to stop bleeding and prevent exsanguination (bleeding to death) and blood coagulation in the lumens of blood vessels that leads to blood flow obstruction.
- Endothelial cells that line the lumen of blood vessels provide an antithrombotic surface inhibiting blood coagulation and thrombus formation. The endothelial cells also prevent the adhesion of platelets to the vessel's wall.
- The body is designed so that when a blood vessel is severed or cut, a fibrin clot will form to plug the hole. In a severed vessel, endothelial cells are injured, exposing the thrombotic surface below them. Platelets can now attach to the vessel wall where they will aggregate, forming a platelet plug that stops the bleeding. Blood coagulation pathways are also instantly activated by the injury, leading to fibrin formation. The fibrin will be incorporated into the platelet plug, forming a fibrin clot.
- The coagulation pathways are a series of reactions requiring the sequential activation of numerous enzymes. Anticoagulation factors work by inhibiting these reactions and thus blocking the pathway. At the end of the coagulation pathway, the plasma protein prothrombin is converted to thrombin by the enzyme "prothrombin activator." The enzyme thrombin then converts fibrinogen to fibrin. Once bleeding has ceased, and the fibrin clot has formed, the coagulation pathway is blocked by anticoagulation factors. If the pathways are not blocked, the clot will continue to obstruct blood flow.
- Hypercoagulable states result from genetic mutations or acquired deficiencies in anticoagulation factors that accompany certain diseases (e.g., liver disease). In such cases, naturally occurring anticoagulants (antithrombin, protein C, protein S, etc.) are deficient or unable to function. For example, a genetic mutation in the gene encoding coagulation factor V results in the synthesis of factor V Leiden instead of factor V. Factor V Leiden functions like factor V in the coagulation pathway. However, protein C, the anticoagulation factor that inhibits factor V, cannot inhibit factor V Leiden. Therefore, once factor V Leiden is activated, it functions when it should not, producing a hypercoagulable state. Individuals with this mutation are at increased risk for venous thromboembolism (VTE).
- There are several mechanisms through which blood stasis can increase one's risk of thrombosis. Stasis never actually occurs in blood vessels. Although, the velocity can become extremely low and the flow very sluggish.
- Under very low blood flow conditions, the tendency for platelets to become trapped behind valve cusps is believed to increase. Behind the valve cusps are a small region in which blood flow is turbulent. As this is where venous thrombi form in the valve, it is thought that the turbulent flow injures the local endothelial cell layer activating the coagulation pathway and leading to venous thrombosis. These two factors, (an increased number of platelets and injured endothelial cells due to turbulent flow) combine to increase the risk of pathological thrombosis in these regions.

- Cancer is thought to increase the formation of venous thrombi by activating coagulation factors and decreasing the levels of coagulation inhibitors (e.g., proteins C and S) in the blood.
- Thrombosis in pregnancy is attributed to a prothrombotic state [50], along with decreased venous outflow due to the weight of the fetus. [51]
- The use of estrogen (in replacement therapy or contraceptives) alters coagulation and may predispose an individual to thrombosis. [51]
- Once a thrombus is formed, it can remain stable, propagate, or shed/embolize:
  - **Stabilize:** Stabilized thrombi firmly adhere to the vessel wall and do not move, change location or propagate. If a thrombus has formed, the most favorable occurrence would be stabilization. This reduces the risk of embolization for the individual.
  - **Propagate:** Propagation includes "growth of thrombus" in size or location. Likely examples of propagated thrombi are:
    - Thrombus can start in the superficial system and "grow" into the deep venous system.
    - A thrombus that extends from a calf vein into the popliteal vein. It probably first formed in the calf vein and grew into the popliteal vein.
  - **Embolize:** A portion of a thrombus breaks free and is carried by the flowing blood through the vessel until it becomes lodged in a smaller vessel, obstructing it. Because emboli can and do become wedged in pulmonary vessels, a thrombus releasing emboli is an extremely high-risk factor for pulmonary embolism.

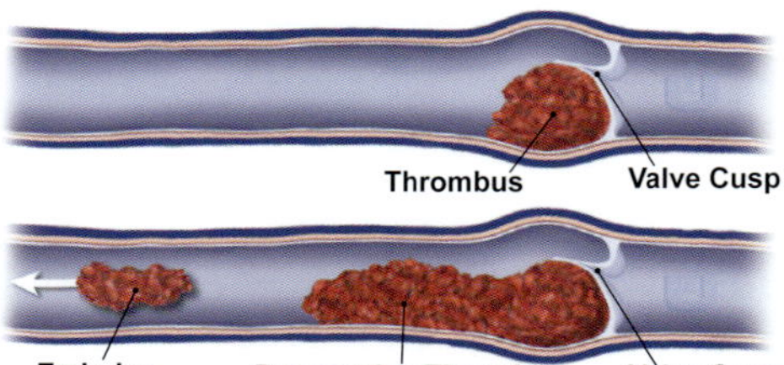

Fig. 5-29. *Venous thrombosis and propagation. In the top vessel, a thrombus has formed behind the valve cusp. This thrombus can stabilize, or as depicted in the bottom vessel, it can propagate. A piece of the thrombus can break off and cause a pulmonary embolism.*

Location of Disease

Although a thrombus can develop at any venous site, the more common sites are the:

- Muscular veins (gastrocnemius and soleal sinus)
- Behind venous valves
- Venous confluences
- Deep venous system (common femoral, deep femoral, femoral, popliteal, peroneal, posterior tibial, anterior tibial, jugular, innominate, subclavian, axillary, brachial, radial, ulnar, inferior vena cava and iliac veins)
- Superficial venous system (great saphenous, small saphenous, basilic, cephalic, median cubital veins)

Differential Diagnosis

- Arterial disease
- Lymphedema
- Cellulitis
- Cysts (popliteal, Baker's, etc.)
- Extrinsic compression
- Hematoma
- Muscle tear
- Joint effusion
- Adenopathy
- Arteriovenous fistula
- Heart failure (edema)
- Direct injury to an extremity
- Vascularized mass
- Collagen vasculitis
- Abscess

Diagnostic Modalities

- Duplex ultrasonography
- Venogram
- MRI
- CT angiography
- IVUS

Medical Treatment

- Serial venous duplex exams to monitor for change
- Anticoagulation therapy (e.g., heparin, low-molecular-weight heparin, or warfarin)
- DVT prophylaxis (e.g., intermittent pneumatic cuff compression)
- Limit long periods of inactivity
- Promote venous drainage (e.g., elevate legs, wear elastic stocking/support hose)

Surgical Treatment

- IVC filter
- Iliofemoral venous thrombectomy
- Bypass grafting (caval occlusion)
- SVC reconstruction (using femoral vein, spiral saphenous, PTFE, or cryopreserved grafts)

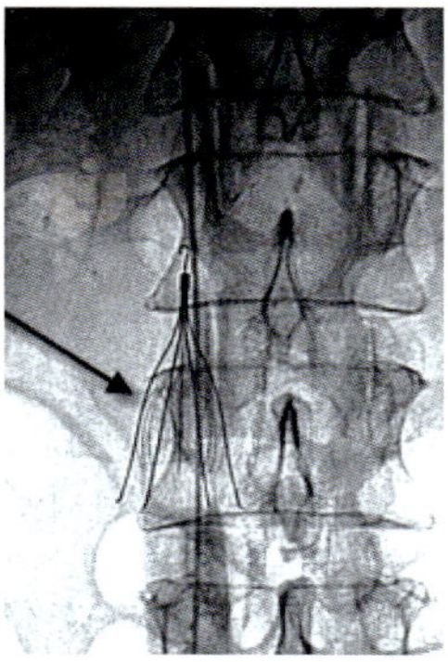

Fig. 5-30. *Inferior vena cavagram showing an IVC filter*

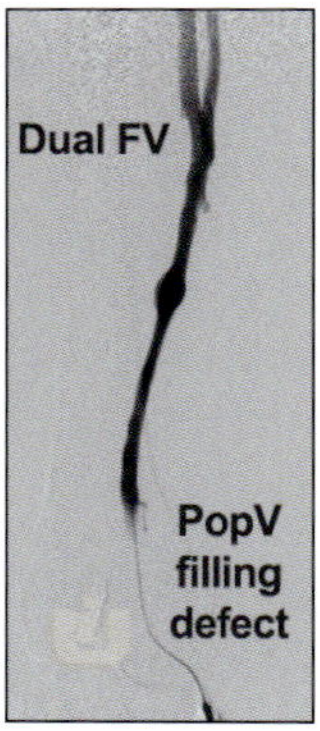

Fig. 5-31. *Venogram of partial popliteal vein thrombosis*

Endovascular Treatment

- Catheter-directed thrombolysis with Urokinase, etc. (acute DVT)
- Balloon venoplasty and stenting (chronic iliofemoral DVT)
- Mechanical catheter-directed thrombectomy (acute DVT)
- Percutaneous transluminal angioplasty and stenting (SVC syndrome)

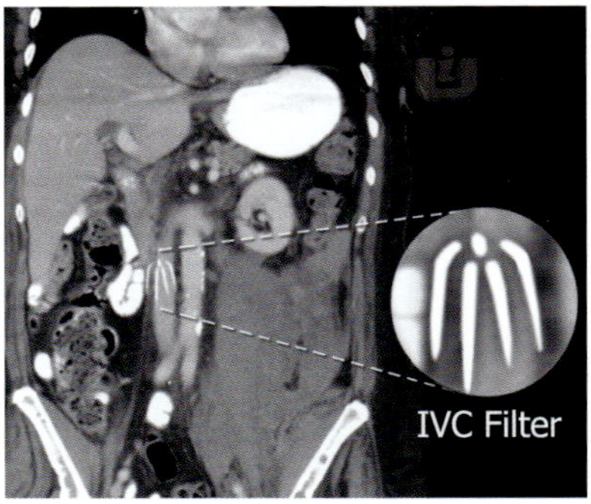

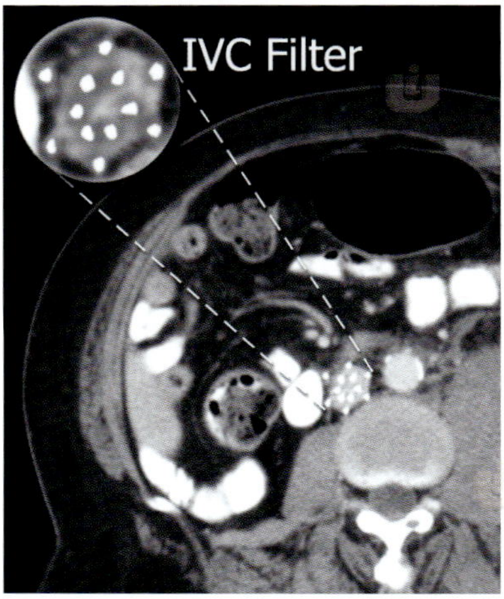

Fig. 5-32. *IVC filter on CT angiogram*

Points to Remember

- Clinical diagnosis of DVT based on patient's symptoms and history is not very reliable (<50%).[52]
- A thrombus frequently originates at a valve cusp site or in the soleal veins.[51]
- The length of the thrombosed segment, the number of veins involved, and the degree of collateralization all affect the presentation of venous symptoms.[52]
- "Economy class syndrome," where travel passengers have been exposed to cramped positions for extended periods, can result in venous thrombosis. Venous stasis during travel may increase the incidents of clot formation for those already at risk for venous thrombosis due to other risk factors.[51]

- Von Willebrand Factor (vWF) is a blood protein activated by thrombin early in the coagulation process to help promote clotting by binding with platelets. [50,53] Patients with vWF deficiency or dysfunction (Von Willebrand Disease) have bleeding complications (GI bleeds, nosebleeds, etc.). This disease can be inherited or acquired and occurs in approximately 1 - 2% of the population. [53]
- A pulmonary embolism can occur when a portion or an entire thrombus breaks loose and travels to the lungs.
- Differentiation of chronic DVT versus acute DVT may be difficult.

References

1. Partsch, H. Varicose veins and chronic venous insufficiency. (2009). *Vasa. 38.* (4), 293-301. doi: 10.1024/0301-1526.38.4.293. PMID: 19998250
2. Eklof, B., Perrin, M., Delis, K. T., Rutherford, R. B., Gloviczki, P., American Venous Forum, European Venous Forum, International Union of Phlebology, American College of Phlebology, & International Union of Angiology (2009). Updated terminology of chronic venous disorders: the VEIN-TERM transatlantic interdisciplinary consensus document. *Journal of Vascular Surgery, 49*(2), 498–501. https://doi.org/10.1016/j.jvs.2008.09.014
3. Eklof et al., (2004). Revision of the CEAP classification for chronic venous disorders: Consensus statement. *J Vasc Sur. 40*, 1248-1252.
4. Porter, J.M., Moneta, G.L. (1995). Reporting standards in venous disease: an update. International Consensus Committee on Chronic Venous Disease. *J Vasc Surg. 21*, 635-645.
5. Fedor Lurie, M., De Maeseneer, G.R., (2020). The 2020 Update of the CEAP Classification: What is New? *European Journal of Vascular and Endovascular Surgery, 59*(6), 859-860.
6. Singer, A. J., Tassiopoulos, A., & Kirsner, R. S. (2017). Evaluation and Management of Lower-Extremity Ulcers. *The New England Journal of Medicine, 377*(16), 1559–1567. https://doi.org/10.1056/NEJMra1615243
7. Meissner, M.H., et al. (2021). The Symptoms-Varices-Pathophysiology Classification of Pelvic Venous Disorders: A Report of the American Vein & Lymphatic Society International Working Group on Pelvic Venous Disorders. *Journal of Vascular Surgery: Venous and Lymphatic Disorders, 9*(3), 568-584.
8. Moneta, G. (2021). *Classification of Lower Extremity Chronic Venous Disorders.* UpToDate. https://www.uptodate.com/contents/classification-of-lower-extremity-chronicvenous-disorders#
9. Lew, W.K., (2021, August 19). Varicose Vein Surgery. eMedicine. https://emedicine. medscape.com/article/462579-overview
10. Meissner, M.H. (2005). Lower extremity venous anatomy. *Semin Intervent Radiol. 22*(3), 147-156. https://doi:10.1055/s-2005-921948
11. Labropoulos, N., et al. (2009). Secondary chronic venous disease progresses faster than primary. *Journal of Vascular Surgery, 49*(3), 704–710. https://doi.org/10.1016/j.jvs.2008.10.014
12. Sumner, D.S., Zierler, R.E. (2005). Vascular physiology: essential hemodynamic principles. In *Rutherford Vascular Surgery* (6th ed., pp.75-123). Philadelphia. Elsevier Saunders.
13. Venous return. (n.d.). howMed. Retrieved April 1, 2022 from http://howmed.net/physiology/venous-return/#.YdcaV7YJqns
14. Ludbrook, J. (1996) The Musculovenous Pumps of The Human Lower Limb. *Am Heart J. 71*(5), 635-641.
15. Lejars, F., (1890). Les veines de la plante du pied. *Archives de Physiologie.* 5° série.
16. Uhl, J.F., Gillot, C. (2010). *The plantar venous pump: Anatomy and physiological hypotheses.* Phlebolymphology.org. https://www.phlebolymphology.org/the-plantar-venous-pump-anatomy-and-physiological-hypotheses
17. Meissner, M. H., et al. (2007). The hemodynamics and diagnosis of venous disease. *Journal of Vascular Surgery, 46* Suppl S, 4S–24S. https://doi.org/10.1016/j.jvs.2007.09.043
18. Goldman, M.P., Fronek, A. (1989). Anatomy and pathophysiology of varicose veins. *J Dermatol Surg Oncol, 15,* 138-145.
19. Burnand K.G. (2001). The physiology and hemodynamics of chronic venous insufficiency of the lower limb. In: P. Gloviczki, P & Yao. J.S.T. (Eds.), *Handbook of Venous Disorders Guidelines of the American Venous Forum.* (2nd ed., pp. 49-57). London Arnold.
20. Kushner, A., West, W.P., Pillarisetty, L.S. (Updated 2021 Sep 14). *Virchow Triad.* StatPearls Publishing, Treasure Island FL. https://www.ncbi.nlm.nih.gov/books/NBK539697/
21. Labropoulos N. (2018). Diagnosis of iliac vein obstruction with duplex ultrasound: Criteria used during duplex ultrasound examination to identify iliac vein obstruction. *Endovasc Today, 17*(7), 50–52.
22. E Rabe et al. (2014). European guidelines for sclerotherapy in chronic venous disorders. *Phlebology, 29*(6), 338–354
23. Calık, E.S. et al. (2019). Ablation therapy with cyanoacrylate glue and laser for refluxing great saphenous veins – a prospective randomized study. Vasa, *48*, 405–412.
24. Joseph, D. (2019, May 14). *Chronic Venous Insufficiency (CVI).* Cleveland Clinic. https://my.clevelandclinic.org/health/diseases/16872-chronic-venous-insufficiency-cvi
25. Cornu-Thenard, A., et al. (1994). Importance of the familiar factor in varicose disease. Clinical study of 134 families. *J Dermatol Surg, 20*(5), 318-326.
26. Labropoulos, N., Leon, L.R. (2005) Evaluation of chronic venous disease. In Mansour MA & Labropolos N. (Eds.), *Vascular Diagnosis,* (pp. 447-461). Philadelphia: Elsevier Saunders.
27. Size, G.P., et al. (2013). Cardiac Effects on Spectral Doppler. In C. L. Skelly & E.F. Sherry (Eds.), *Inside Ultrasound Vascular Reference Guide* (pp. 336-344). Inside Ultrasound Inc.
28. Min, R.J., Rosenblatt, M. (2010). *Varicose Veins and Spider Veins.* US Department of Health and Human Services, Office on Women's Health. Retrieved April 23, 2022 from http://www.womenshealth.gov/faq/varicose spider veins.cfm
29. Raju, S. (2013). Best management options for chronic iliac vein stenosis and occlusion. *J Vasc Surg, 57*, 1163-1169.
30. Gloviczki, P., Wahner, H.W. (2005). Clinical diagnosis and evaluation of lymphedema. In *Rutherford Vascular Surgery* (6th ed., pp. 2396-2415). Philadelphia. Elsevier Saunders.
31. Jobst Publication. (2002). Lymphedema; its cause and how to manage it. Charlotte. BSN-Jobst, Inc. Retrieved May 2022
32. Witte, C.L., Witte, M.H. Lymph circulatory dynamics, lymphangiogenesis and pathophysiology of the lymphovascular system. In *Rutherford Vascular Surgery* (6th ed., pp. 2379-2396). Philadelphia. Elsevier Saunders.
33. Khilnani, N.M., et al. (2021). Clinical Presentation and Evaluation of Pelvic Venous Disorders in Women. *Tech Vasc Interventional Rad, 24*(1), 100730. https://doi.org/10.1016/j.tvir.2021.100730
34. Brinegar, K.N., et al. (2015). Iliac vein compression syndrome: Clinical, imaging and pathologic findings *World J Radiol , 7*(11), 375-381.
35. McDermott, S., et al. (2013). May-Thurner Syndrome: Can It Be Diagnosed by a Single MR Venography Study? *Diagn Interv Radiol, 19,* 44-48. 22801870 https://doi.org/10.4261/1305-3825.DIR.5939-12.1
36. Heijmen, R.H., Bollen, T.L., Duyndam, D.A., Overtoom, T.T., Van Den Berg, J.C., Moll, F.L. (2001). Endovascular venous stenting in May-Thurner Syndrome. *The Journal of Cardiovascular Surgery, 42*(1), 83–87.
37. Meissner, M.H., Gloviczki, P. (2019). Pelvic venous disorders. In J.L. Almeida (Ed.), *Atlas of Endovascular Venous Surgery.* (2nd ed., pp.567-599). Philadelphia (PA), Elsevier.
38. Dardik, A., Rahhal, D. (2009-9-10). *Phlegmasia alba and cerulea dolens.* eMedicine. Retrieved December 10, 2021, from http://emedicine.medscape.com/article/461809-overview.
39. Browse, N.L., Burnand, K.G., Thomas, M.L. (1988). Disease of the Veins; Pathology, Diagnosis and Treatment, (pp. 674). London. Edward Arnold, a division of Hodder & Stoughton.

40. Tortora, G.J., Anagnostakos, N.P. (1990). The respiratory system. In *Principles of Anatomy and Physiology* (6th ed., pp. 689 - 730). New York. Harper Row Publishers.
41. Feied, C.F., Handler, J.A. (2004-12-23). *Pulmonary Embolism.* eMedicine. Retrieved (4-22-2022) from http://www.blueguitar.org/new/misc/pe_copd.pdf.
42. Stein, P.D., Matta, F., Musani, M.H., Diaczok, B. (2010). Silent pulmonary embolism in patients with deep venous thrombosis: A systematic review. *Am J Med. 123*(5), 426-431.
43. Torbicki, A., et al. (2000). Guidelines on diagnosis and management of acute pulmonary embolism. *European Heart Journal. 21*, 1301-1336.
44. Gloviczki, P., et al. (2005). Surgical treatment of superior vena cava syndrome. In *Rutherford Vascular Surgery* (6th ed., pp. 2357- 2371). Philadelphia. Elsevier Saunders.
45. Dake, M.D. (2005). Endovascular treatment of vena caval occlusions. In *Rutherford Vascular Surgery* (6th ed., pp. 2352 - 2344). Philadelphia. Elsevier Saunders.
46. Lee, B. B., et al. (2015). Diagnosis and Treatment of Venous Malformations. Consensus Document of the International Union of Phlebology (IUP): International angiology: *A Journal of the International Union of Angiology, 34*(2), 97–149.
47. Huegel, U., & Baumgartner, I. (2019). Implementation of new endovenous treatments in therapy for lateral embryonic veins. *Journal of vascular surgery cases and innovative techniques, 5*(3), 243–247. https://doi.org/10.1016/j.jvscit.2018.12.016
48. Olivieri, B., White, C. L., Restrepo, R., McKeon, B., Karakas, S. P., & Lee, E. Y. (2016). Low-Flow Vascular Malformation Pitfalls: From Clinical Examination to Practical Imaging Evaluation--Part 2, Venous Malformation Mimickers. *AJR. American journal of roentgenology, 206*(5), 952–962. https://doi.org/10.2214/AJR.15.15794
49. *Klippel-Trenaunay Syndrome.* (2021, February 1). National Center for Advancing Translational Services. Retrieved April 22, 2022, from https://rarediseases.info.nih.gov/diseases/3122/klippel-trenaunay-syndrome
50. Fareed J., et al. (2005). Normal and abnormal coagulation. In *Rutherford Vascular Surgery* (6th ed., pp. 493 - 511). Philadelphia. Elsevier Saunders.
51. Meissner, M.H., Strandess, D.E. (2005). Pathophysiology and natural history of acute deep venous thrombosis. In *Rutherford Vascular Surgery* (6th ed., pp. 2124 - 2142). Philadelphia. Elsevier Saunders.
52. Cook J., Meissner, M.H. (2005). Clinical and diagnostic evaluation of the patient with deep venous thrombosis. In *Rutherford Vascular Surgery* (6th ed., pp. 2143 - 2156). Philadelphia. Elsevier Saunders.
53. Eagleton, M., Ouriel, K. (2005). Perioperative considerations: coagulation and hemorrhage. In *Rutherford Vascular Surgery* (6th ed., pp. 545 - 567). Philadelphia. Elsevier Saunders.

6. ABI and Pedal Artery Waveforms

Definition

A non-invasive physiological test compares the systolic pressure at the ankle level to the systolic pressure at the brachial artery level. Continuous-wave (CW) Doppler waveforms are recorded to support the pressure information.

This exam should be completed to ensure there is no concomitant PAD when testing venous systems.

Indications for Exam

- Claudication (exercise-related limb pain)
- An abnormal ABI
- Limb pain at rest
- Absent peripheral pulses
- Extremity ulcer
- Gangrene
- Pre-operative assessment of healing potential
- Digital cyanosis
- Cold sensitivity
- Arterial aneurysm
- Trauma to an artery
- A revascularization procedure (follow-up)

Contraindications/Limitations

- Calcified vessels will falsely elevate pressure measurements (typically encountered in patients with diabetes or end-stage renal disease).
- Significant lesions with excellent collateral circulation may result in normal distal pressures and waveforms at rest.
- Acute venous thrombosis in the lower extremities as pressure cuffs should not be inflated over thrombi.
- Extensive bandages or casts that are not removable.
- A pressure cuff should not compress trauma, surgery, ulceration, or graft placement.
- An ipsilateral mastectomy or dialysis graft/fistula. Pressure measurements are typically prohibited in these cases.

Mechanism of disease

The supply of arterial blood to the lower extremity is frequently compromised by atherosclerotic plaques and emboli. Of these, atherosclerotic plaques are the most common. The following are pathologies that can cause a reduction in lower extremity blood flow:

- **Atherosclerosis:** The most common arterial disease. Atherosclerotic plaque forms in the artery and either partially blocks blood flow by narrowing the lumen (arterial stenosis) or totally blocks flow by occluding the artery (arterial occlusion). The term "hemodynamically significant obstruction" refers to an obstruction that significantly decreases blood flow. A significant decrease in blood flow is typically defined as a decrease corresponding to diameter reduction of at least 50%. An arterial occlusion is defined as an obstruction that completely inhibits blood flow. These typically occur in the ostia (origin) of branches.
- **Embolization:** A piece of plaque or thrombus (the embolus) breaks off, flows through the vessels, and becomes lodged in a smaller vessel.[2] The culprit plaques and thrombi are commonly located in the heart or at a proximal aneurysm.
- **Extrinsic compression:** Tumors, hematomas, etc., can result in stenosis or occlusion if the pressure they apply squeezes the vessel and compromises blood flow.[1]
- **Vasospasm:** A temporary constriction of arteries (typically digital arteries). This may cause the patient significant discomfort (uncommon).[3]

- **Aneurysmal disease:** a weakening of the medial layer of the arterial wall due to changes in structural proteins (elastin and collagen) and smooth muscle cells, resulting in pathological stretching of the arterial wall. Aneurysmal disease typically does not obstruct flow, but the resulting aneurysm may be the source of an embolus.[4]

Patient History

- Claudication (exercise related)
- Rest pain
- Paralysis (weakness)
- Paresthesia ("pins and needles")
- Poikilothermia (ice-cold limbs)
- Previous ulceration/gangrene in the feet or toes
- Previous therapeutic vascular procedures (e.g., bypass, stenting)

Physical Examination

- Pulselessness
- Pallor
- Cyanosis
- Dependent rubor
- Bruit (abnormal sound heard through auscultation and caused by tissue vibration due to turbulent flow)
- Marked temperature difference between extremities
- Gangrene/necrosis (tissue death)
- Palpable thrill (turbulent blood flow-induced vibration that can be detected by palpation)

Location of Disease

- Arterial disease can be focal or diffuse and can affect any or all levels of the arterial system.
- The most common locations of obstructions in the lower extremities are arterial bifurcations and the superficial femoral artery at the adductor canal.

Ankle-Brachial Indices Protocol

Pressure measurements should be taken with the patient in the supine position with the extremity at heart level. If the patient sits, the pressures recorded will be falsely elevated due to the effects of hydrostatic pressure.

- This protocol can be used with an automatic blood pressure cuff or a standard manometer.
- Rest the patient for 5-10 minutes before beginning the exam. This allows their blood pressure to stabilize and recover from walking into the exam room. You may use this time to obtain the patient's history, including their symptoms and risk factors. Cuffs may also be placed at this time.
- Appropriately wrap blood pressure cuffs around the limbs. The cuffs should be placed "straight" rather than angled. The fit should be snug, so applied pressure increases as the bladder inflates. If it is not snug, the expanding bladder will fill the gap between the bladder and the limb before it applies pressure to the limb. This produces falsely elevated readings.
  - Place blood pressure cuffs with a 10-12cm (width) bladder bilaterally at the ankle, 2-3cm above the medial malleolus to obtain pedal pressures.
  - Place blood pressure cuffs with a 10-12cm (width) bladder bilaterally on the upper arms to obtain brachial pressures.
- Locate the Posterior Tibial Artery (PTA), which lies posterior to the medial malleolus using a high frequency (8MHz) CW Doppler transducer. Use a lower frequency transducer (e.g., 4MHz) when the vessels are deep.

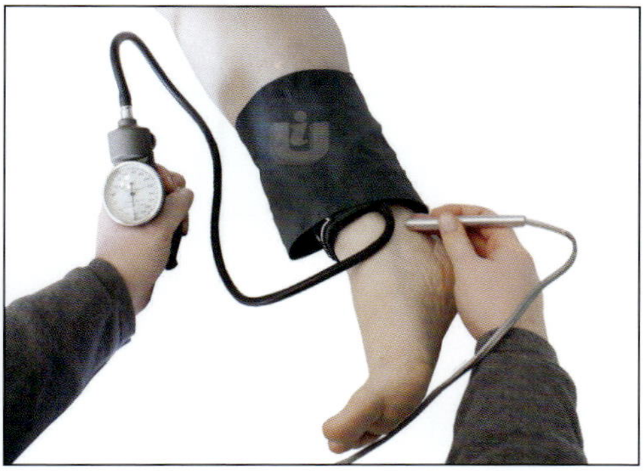

Fig. 6-2. *Pressure measurement at the PTA.*

- Position the CW Doppler transducer to point toward the heart. The insonation angle is between 45-60°. Apply pressure on the transducer to keep it in place, but avoid compressing the artery.

- Manipulate the transducer until the strongest arterial signal is obtained. Gently rest on the patient's foot so your hand will be stable during cuff inflation.
- Record several representative PTA waveforms. If no arterial signal is detected at the ankle, you should move the transducer proximally along the medial calf for a short distance and determine if arterial blood flow is detectable in this region of the PTA. You may also have to reposition the pressure cuff higher on the leg. In such cases, document what level the pressure was taken.
- Inflate the blood pressure cuff 20-30mmHg above the pressure that coincides with the PTA's last audible arterial Doppler signal.
- Deflate the cuff slowly, 2-4mmHg per second. Upon hearing the first audible arterial Doppler signal, record the coinciding cuff pressure (mmHg) as the systolic pressure. Continue to monitor the Doppler pulse. It must be present. This ensures that you have detected the patient's pulse, not motion artifact.

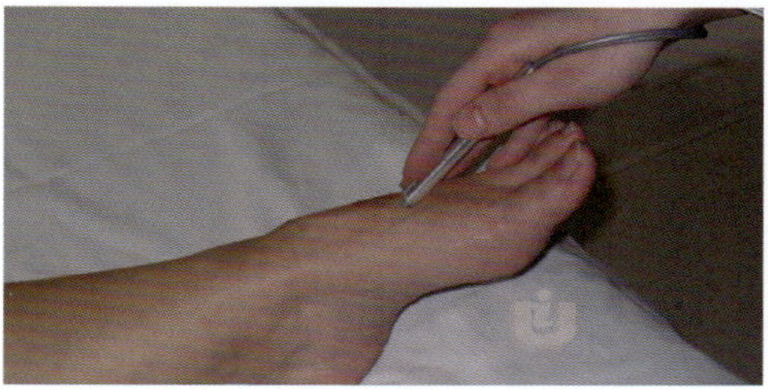

Fig. 6-3. *Placement of CW Doppler at the DPA.*

For patients with irregular heartbeats decrease deflation speeds.

- Locate the Dorsalis Pedis Artery (DPA) on the dorsum of the foot (halfway between the toes and ankle) using the CW Doppler. Examine the DPA using the same procedure used for the PTA.
  - Avoid sampling too close to the toes, or you could error and record the waveforms and pressures of the plantar arch or digital vessels. Be aware that blood flow can be detected in these vessels when there is none in the DPA because they receive blood from the PTA instead.
  - If the signal is damped, retrograde, or absent, move to the anterior aspect of the ankle and determine if blood flow in the ATA is detectable by CW Doppler.
  - If blood flow in the ATA is undetectable, move to the Peroneal Artery (PerA), located slightly anterior to the lateral malleolus, and determine if blood flow in the PerA is detectable by CW Doppler.
- Obtain Bilateral Brachial Artery (BrA) pressures.

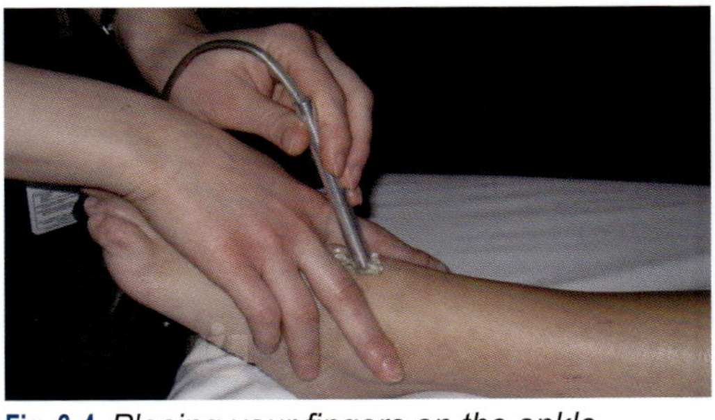

Fig. 6-4. *Placing your fingers on the ankle bones will help you locate the DPA.*

If brachial pressures differ by >20mmHg or if the brachial waveforms are different, the vertebral arteries should be examined for flow direction. Retrograde flow in the vertebral artery ipsilateral to the arm with the lower brachial pressure indicates subclavian steal syndrome.

- Calculate the ABI on each side by dividing the highest pedal pressure by the highest of the two brachial pressures:

$$ABI = \frac{\text{highest pedal pressure}}{\text{highest brachial pressure}}$$

Table 6-1. ABI Protocol Summary

- Wrap pressure cuffs around arm and leg-ankle level
- Using CW/PW Doppler, record representative waveforms
  - DPA
  - PTA
  - BrA
- Inflate cuff 20-30mmHg beyond the last audible arterial signal using a Doppler transducer on the appropriate artery distal to the cuff.
- Deflation of the cuff should be at a rate of 2-4mmHg per second. The pressure is recorded as soon as the first audible arterial Doppler signal returns.
- Calculate the ABI:

$$\frac{\text{highest pedal pressure}}{\text{highest brachial pressure}} = ABI$$

- Determine classification of disease according to laboratory diagnostic criteria.

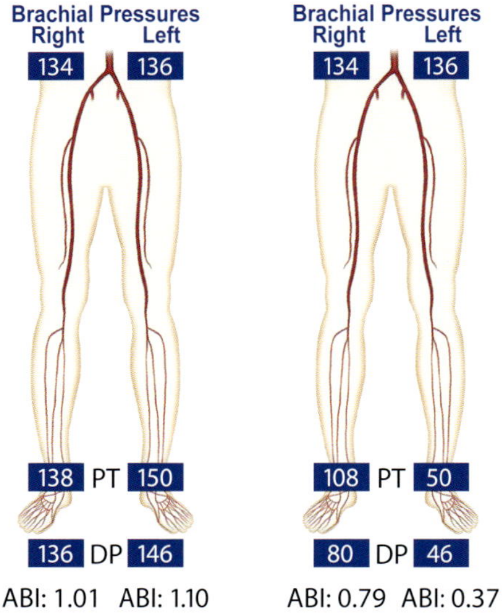

Fig. 6-5. Ankle-Brachial pressures. *The pressures on the left indicate that the patient has normal ABIs. The pressures on the right indicate that the patient has abnormal ABIs.*

The diagnostic criteria used to determine the severity of abnormal ankle-brachial indices varies across laboratories.

Principles of Interpretation

Pressures

Leg pressures are normally higher than the highest brachial pressure. The difference between the pressures at the arm and at the ankle is normally between 12 (±8) and 24 (±9)mmHg. [5]

Waveforms

There is controversy among vascular professionals regarding the terminology used to describe CW Doppler analog waveforms.

- Essentially, all vascular professionals agree that a waveform that consists sequentially of a sharp, quick upstroke with forward flow, a reverse flow phase, and a forward third phase, is termed "triphasic". This is considered a normal finding in the peripheral arteries.

- A waveform with a reversed flow second phase that is missing the forward flow third phase may be referred to as either "triphasic" or "biphasic". However, nearly all will interpret this as normal. Recently, some laboratories have adopted terminology that recognizes that the reverse flow phase is sufficient for the waveform to be considered normal. They use the term "Normal Reversed" (NR). This avoids the use of the misused terms "triphasic" and "biphasic".
- Some laboratories reserve the term biphasic only for waveforms that have a reverse flow component but no third phase. It is likely that these biphasic waveforms would be considered normal due to the presence of the reversed component.
- Monophasic arterial Doppler waveforms are characterized by a slow upstroke that slopes to the right, a low amplitude, and a broad peak with no evidence of a reverse flow component in late systole. Continuous forward flow is typical in diastole, but diastolic flow may be absent if there is distal resistance from a high-grade distal obstruction. Some laboratories will refer to any waveform without a reverse flow component as monophasic. Monophasic waveforms are typically present proximal to occlusions and very high-grade stenoses.

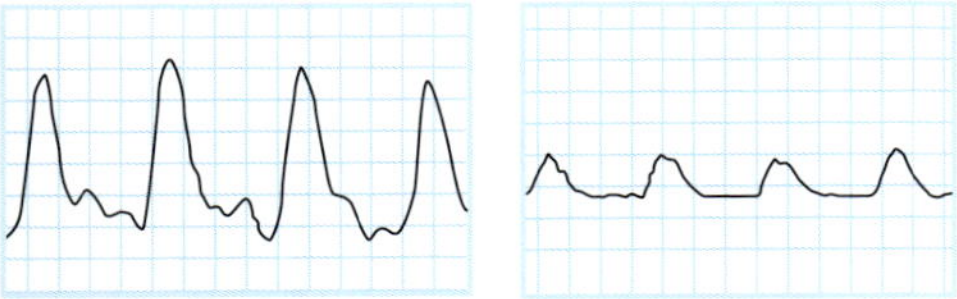

Moderately abnormal waveforms *Severely abnormal waveforms*

Fig. 6-6. *Abnormal CW Doppler arterial waveforms. Triphasic, biphasic, and monophasic waveforms have multiple definitions throughout the vascular ultrasound community. Although these two waveforms may be labeled differently in different laboratories, most would identify the left waveform as moderately abnormal, and the right as severely abnormal.*

Interpretation-Diagnostic Criteria

Normal

Pressures

- If the ABI is ≥1.0, the presence of an occlusion or hemodynamically significant stenosis between the heart and ankle cuffs is unlikely. The upper and lower limits for normal ABIs vary in literature and are thought to depend on whether the patient is hypertensive or hypotensive.[6]
- An ABI >0.97 is often considered normal.[7]
- In a non-stenotic limb, the ABI is typically no less than 0.92.[5]

CW or PW Doppler

A normal triphasic signal consists of three phases: a strong forward flow in late systole (sharp upstroke; first phase), flow reversal in early diastole (below the baseline; second phase) and forward flow in late diastole (above the baseline; third phase).[7] Many laboratories will accept a waveform with a reversed flow component as normal even if the third phase is missing.

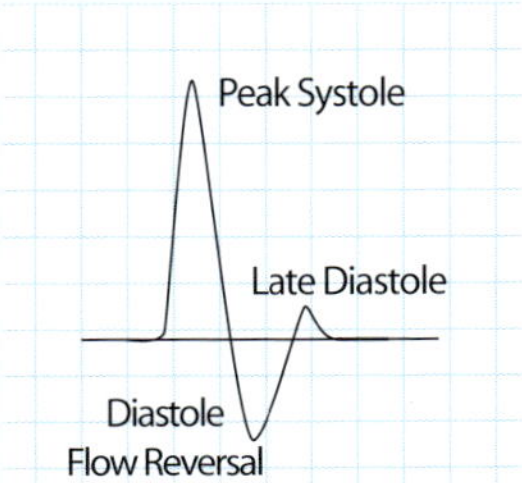

Fig. 6-7. *Normal, triphasic Doppler waveform.*

Abnormal

Pressures

- An ABI of <1.0 suggests that a hemodynamically significant obstruction may exist somewhere between the heart and the ankle cuff. [5]
- When the pedal pressure is 90% of the arm pressure (0.90), it is likely that a hemodynamically significant obstruction has developed in the lower extremity above the level of the ankle. [8]

- The difference in the DPA and PTA pressures at the level of the ankle, in the same limb should be <10 mmHg.[5] An ABI difference >15mmHg suggests a proximal obstruction. [5,7,9]
- A change in the ABI of ≥0.15 from one study to the next is considered significant. [5,7,8]
- An ABI of >1.3 suggests calcific disease and is considered non-diagnostic. In these cases, an alternative is to use the toe/brachial index to estimate disease severity. [5,7] It is acceptable to base a diagnosis of disease severity (normal, mild, moderate, severe, critical) on waveform analysis alone when calcific disease is present. [7]

CW or PW Doppler

- Biphasic waveforms have a reverse flow component, but no third phase. As outlined in the "Principles of Interpretation" section in this chapter, please note the controversies regarding biphasic waveforms in particular and discuss what your lab considers to be "biphasic."
- Monophasic arterial Doppler waveforms are characterized by a slow upstroke that slopes to the right, a low amplitude, and a broad peak with no evidence of a reverse flow component in late systole. Continuous forward flow is typical in diastole, but diastolic flow may be absent if there is distal resistance from a high-grade distal obstruction.
- Monophasic waveforms are typically present proximal to occlusions and very high-grade stenoses.
- An absent or non-pulsatile Doppler signal suggests arterial occlusive disease at the site of interrogation. [5] Absent Doppler signals in all the pedal arteries of a limb suggest there is a critical decrease in the perfusion of the lower extremity, particularly if the Volume Pulse Recording (VPR) or Photoplethysmography (PPG) waveforms at the toe are flat. Be aware that extensive calcification will obscure the Doppler signal and decrease the amplitude, but the VPR and PPG waveforms are typically not affected.

In 2022 a Consensus Statement from the Society for Vascular Medicine and Society for Vascular Ultrasound was published. The consensus statement proposes a standardized nomenclature for arterial and venous Doppler waveforms. [14]

The writing committee recommends that:

Arterial Doppler waveforms should be reported using major key descriptors: direction of flow, phasicity, and resistance.

- Direction of flow can be described using the terms:
  - **Antegrade** blood flows in the normal direction for the artery being evaluated.
  - **Retrograde** blood flows opposite the normal direction for the artery being evaluated.
  - **Bidirectional** blood flows in a combination of the normal and abnormal direction for the artery being evaluated.
- Phasicity be described using the terms:
  - **Multiphasic** waveforms cross the zero-flow baseline and contain both forward and reverse velocity components.
  - **Monophasic** waveforms do not cross the zero-flow baseline and reflect blood that flows in a single direction for the duration of the cardiac cycle.
- Doppler waveforms demonstrate high, intermediate, or low resistance.
  - **High-resistive** waveforms have a sharp upstroke and brisk downstroke and may be either multiphasic or monophasic.
  - **Intermediate-resistive** waveforms reflect a sharp upstroke, brisk downstroke, continuous forward flow through diastole above the zero-baseline with a visible notch in end diastole.
  - **Low-resistive** waveforms contain a prolonged downstroke in late systole with continuous forward flow throughout diastole without an end systolic notch. Low-resistive waveforms are monophasic.

Table 6-2. **Diagnostic Criteria for ABI**

ABI	Comment
≥1.0	Normal
0.90 - <1.0	Mild disease
0.50 - 0.90	Claudication
0.30 - 0.50	Severe occlusive disease
<0.30	Ischemia

Source: AbuRahma AF. (2000). Segmental Doppler pressures and Doppler waveform analysis in peripheral vascular disease of the lower extremities. In AbuRahma AF, Bergan JJ (Eds). *Non-invasive Vascular Diagnosis.* (213-229). London: Springer.

Table 6-3. **University of Chicago Diagnostic ABI Criteria**

ABI	Severity
≥0.95	Normal
0.80 - 0.94	Mild disease
0.50 - 0.79	Moderate disease
0.30 - 0.49	Severe disease
<0.29	Critical disease

Source: Internally validated at the University of Chicago Medical Center Vascular Laboratory.

Table 6-4. **ABI Symptoms**

ABI	Symptom
≥1.0	Normal
<0.80	Claudication
<0.40	Rest pain
<0.20	Impending gangrene

Source: Modified from Yao JST. (1970). Hemodynamic studies in peripheral arterial disease. Br J Surg. 57:761.

Differential Diagnosis

- Spinal stenosis
- Venous thrombosis
- Restless leg syndrome
- Compartment syndrome
- Nocturnal leg cramps
- Neuropathy
- Muscle/tendon strains
- Arthritis
- Abnormalities of the adrenergic receptor/ sympathetic nervous system
- Connective tissue disease (scleroderma)

Correlation

- Duplex ultrasound
- Computed Tomography (CT) scan
- MRA
- Arteriography

Medical Treatment

- Modify risk factors (e.g., reduce cholesterol, manage HTN and DM, smoking cessation)
- Exercise regimen
- Antiplatelet medication (e.g., aspirin)
- Anticoagulation (warfarin)
- Thrombolysis (acute blockage)

Surgical Treatment

- Bypass grafting
- Atherectomy
- Endarterectomy
- Direct focal repair
- Resection (aneurysmal disease)
- Sympathectomy
- Amputation
- Angioplasty
- Stent
- Intra-arterial directed thrombolysis (acute blockage)

Points to Remember

- The ABI only evaluates the presence and severity of disease. The ABI should be combined with segmental pressures, volume pulse recording, Doppler waveforms, or duplex imaging to determine location of disease.

- Pressure measurements:
  - Should be recorded in the supine position with the extremity at the same level as the heart.
  - Recorded while the patient is sitting will be falsely elevated due to the effects of hydrostatic pressure.
  - For every 10 inches that the heart is elevated above the ankle level, pressure increases 18.67mmHg. Since the heart is 34 inches from the ankle on an average person while sitting, the blood pressure at the ankle will be increased by about 63mmHg (3.4 x 18.67mmHg).
  - If pressures can only be obtained in the seated position, use the same method for follow-up exams for accurate comparisons.
- When the extremity is elevated above the heart level, misleadingly low pressure readings will result.
- The systolic pressure is recorded at the return of the first audible arterial Doppler signal. There should be a period of silence after inflation and prior to hearing the first pulse to be sure the cuff was inflated above the local arterial pressure. Continue to monitor the pulse after hearing the first pulse signal to ensure that the transducer is detecting the pulse and not motion.
- If a pressure measurement needs to be repeated, the cuff should be fully deflated for approximately one minute before the next measurement.
- A diabetic patient's foot ulcer is unlikely to heal if the ankle pressure is <80mmHg. [13]
- The ABI examination may be combined with exercise stress testing to detect obstructions that are insignificant at rest and become significant with exercise.
- A patient with claudication is likely to have an ABI <0.80. [12]
- An ABI <0.50 suggests multiple levels of disease. [5,7,8]
- A patient with rest pain is likely to have an ABI <0.40. [7]
- Do not take blood pressure over a bypass graft, dialysis access conduit or fistula without first consulting your medical director. Do not take blood pressure on the arm of a patient with a history of mastectomy.
- Moderate to severely abnormal waveforms typically have a somewhat wider peak and a slightly slower upstroke than normal waveforms
- There are waveforms with a down-stroke that stays above the baseline (no flow reversal) but flow is "multiphasic" in that there is a "notch" or two in the slope of the down-stroke. This is the most difficult waveform to describe due to its very qualitative nature, but it is helpful to distinguish the moderately abnormal Doppler waveform from a severely abnormal one, especially at the common femoral and pedal levels.
- PW Doppler on a duplex scanner can also be used to obtain arterial waveforms when necessary. Be sure to keep the sample volume wide and the image in real-time while measuring pressures to ensure sample volume location during and after cuff inflation.

References

1. Sumner DS, Zierler RE. (2005). Vascular physiology: essential hemodynamic principles. In *Rutherford Vascular Surgery 6th edition.* (75-123). Philadelphia. Elsevier Saunders.
2. Fecteau SR, Darling III RC, Roddy SP. (2005). Arterial thromboembolism. In *Rutherford Vascular Surgery 6th edition.* (971-986). Philadelphia. Elsevier Saunders.
3. Shepard RFJ. (2005). Raynaud's syndrome: vasospastic and occlusive arterial disease involving the distal upper extremity. In *Rutherford Vascular Surgery 6th edition.* (1319-1346). Philadelphia: Elsevier Saunders.
4. Dawson DL, Lee ES, Lindholm K. (2010). Aortic and peripheral aneurysms. In Zierler RE (Ed.), *Strandess's duplex scanning disorders in vascular diagnosis 4th ed.* (157-168). Philadelphia: Wolters Kluwer Lippincott Williams & Wilkins.
5. Zierler RE, Sumner DS. (2005). Physiologic assessment of peripheral arterial occlusive disease. In *Rutherford Vascular Surgery 6th edition.* (197-222). Philadelphia. Elsevier Saunders.
6. Nicolaides AN. (2003). Basic and practical aspects of peripheral arterial testing. In Bernstein EF (Ed.), *Vascular Diagnosis* (481-485). St. Louis: Mosby.
7. Carter SA. (2003). Role of pressure measurements. In Bernstein EF (Ed.), *Vascular Diagnosis* (486-512). St. Louis: Mosby.
8. Zierler, RE, (2005). Nonimaging Physiologic Tests for Assessment of Lower Extremity Arterial Occlusive Disease. In Zwiebel WJ, Pellerito JS (Eds.), *Introduction to Vascular Ultrasonography.* (275-295). Philadelphia: Elsevier Saunders.
9. Nordness PJ, Money SR. (2005). In Mansour MA, Labropoulos N. (Eds.), *Vascular Diagnosis,* (207-214). Philadelphia: Elsevier Saunders.
10. Needham T. (2005). In Mansour MA, Labropoulos N. (Eds.), *Vascular Diagnosis,* (215-222). Philadelphia: Elsevier Saunders.
11. AbuRahma AF. (2000). Segmental Doppler pressures and Doppler waveform analysis in peripheral vascular disease of the lower extremities. In AbuRahma AF, Bergan JJ (Eds). *Non-invasive Vascular Diagnosis.* (213-229). London: Springer.
12. Yao JST. (1970). Hemodynamic studies in peripheral arterial disease. Br J Surg. 57:761.
13. Raines JK, Darling RC, Both K et al. (1976). Vascular laboratory criteria for the management of peripheral vascular disease of the lower extremities. Surgery 79:21-29.
14. Kim ESH, et al.(2020) Interpretation of Peripheral Arterial and Venous Doppler Waveforms: A Consensus Statement From the Society for Vascular Medicine and Society for Vascular Ultrasound. Journal for Vascular Ultrasound. 44(3):118-143. *doi:10.1177/1544316720943099*

Definition

The combination of real time B-mode ultrasonography with PW Doppler and color flow to evaluate the lower extremity veins for evidence of a venous thrombus or aneurysm. Typically, venous compression studies are a component of these exams. Venous aneurysms are very rare.

Indications for Exam

- Edema/swelling (especially when unilateral)
- Limb pain/tenderness
- Symptoms of a pulmonary embolism (PE; shortness of breath, chest pain, hemoptysis)
- Ulceration (especially in gaiter area)
- Discoloration in the gaiter area
- Varicose veins
- Hypercoaguable state
- Pallor (phlegmasia alba dolens)
- Cyanosis (phlegmasia cerulea dolens)
- Positive D-dimer test result

Contraindications/Limitations

- Obesity or severe edema that increases vessel depth to the extent that it prevents vessel visualization by ultrasound.
- Open wounds prohibiting ultrasound transducer placement along the length of the vessels.
- Non-removable casts or tractions that interfere with the placement of the ultrasound transducer.
- Patients who cannot be adequately positioned.

Mechanism of Disease [1,2]

Three factors vein wall injury, hypercoagulability and the stasis of blood flow are responsible for venous thrombosis according to Virchow's Triad theory. The presence of one or more of these three factors increases the risk for venous thrombosis.

In blood, coagulation factors are balanced by anticoagulation factors. This allows blood coagulation to occur where and when vessels are severed, stopping bleeding and preventing exsanguination (bleeding to death), while at the same time preventing blood coagulation in the lumens of blood vessels that leads to blood flow obstruction.

Endothelial cells that line the lumen of blood vessels provide an antithrombotic surface inhibiting blood coagulation and thrombus formation. The endothelial cells also prevent the adhesion of platelets to the vessel's wall.

The body is designed so that when a blood vessel is severed or cut, a fibrin clot will form to plug the hole. In a severed vessel, endothelial cells are injured, exposing the thrombotic surface that lies below them. Platelets can now attach to the vessel wall where they will aggregate, forming a platelet plug that stops the bleeding. Blood coagulation pathways are also instantly activated by the injury, leading to the formation of fibrin. The fibrin will be incorporated into the platelet plug, forming a fibrin clot.

The coagulation pathways are a series of reactions requiring the sequential activation of numerous enzymes. Anticoagulation factors work by inhibiting these reactions and thus blocking the pathway. At the end of the coagulation pathway the plasma protein, prothrombin is converted to thrombin by the enzyme "prothrombin activator". The enzyme thrombin then converts fibrinogen to fibrin. Once bleeding has ceased and the fibrin clot has formed, the coagulation pathway is blocked by anticoagulation factors. If the pathways are not blocked, then the clot will continue to grow obstructing blood flow.

When a vessel wall is injured, the endothelial cells are often damaged exposing the thrombotic surface below them. This activates the coagulation process as if the wall was punctured and the vessel is bleeding. In this case, instead of stopping the vessel from bleeding, an intravenous thrombus will form. If this thrombus continues to grow, the outcome may be detrimental to the patient's health. However, in healthy individuals, under normal circumstances anticoagulation factors are quickly activated, inhibiting thrombogenesis. The thrombus will usually resolve by thrombolysis without symptoms but, there is always the risk that it will go on to be pathological.

Hypercoaguable states are the result of genetic mutations or acquired deficiencies in anticoagulation factors that accompany certain diseases (e.g., liver disease). In such cases, naturally occurring anticoagulants (antithrombin, protein C, protein S, etc.) are deficient or unable to function. For example, a genetic mutation in the gene encoding coagulation factor V results in the synthesis of factor V Leiden instead of factor V. Factor V Leiden functions just like factor V in the coagulation pathway. However, protein C, the anticoagulation factor that inhibits factor V, cannot inhibit factor V Leiden. Therefore, once factor V Leiden is activated, it continues to function when it should not, producing a hypecoaguable state. Individuals with this mutation are at increased risk for Venous Thromboembolism (VTE).

Cancer is thought to increase the formation of venous thrombi by activating coagulation factors and decreasing the levels of coagulation inhibitors (e.g., proteins C and S) in the blood.

There are several mechanisms through which blood stasis can increase one's risk of thrombosis. Stasis never actually occurs in blood vessels. Although, the velocity can become extremely low and the flow very sluggish.

Under very low blood flow conditions, the tendency for platelets to become trapped behind valve cusps is believed to increase. Behind the valve cusps, there is a small region in which blood flow is turbulent. As this is the location where venous thrombi form in the valve, it is thought that the turbulent flow injures the local endothelial cell layer activating the coagulation pathway leading to venous thrombosis. These two factors, (an increased number of platelets and injured endothelial cells due to turbulent flow) combine to increase the risk of pathological thrombosis in these regions.

Thrombosis in pregnancy is attributed to a prothrombotic state along with decreased venous outflow because of the weight of the fetus on the pelvic veins.

The use of estrogen (in replacement therapy or contraceptives) alters coagulation and may predispose an individual to thrombosis.

Aneurysms are rare in veins, but can occur at sites of chronic inflammation. As an aneurysm grows, the vessel's wall becomes thinner. There is significant degradation of the structural fibers elastin and collagen, and there is a decrease in the number of smooth muscle cells, which contribute to the maintenance of the wall's integrity. The degradation of the fibers, especially collagen decreases the wall's tensile strength. As the walls get weaker, the vein expands due to the pressure of the blood. The outward expansion is first minimized by elastin. The load shifts to the stronger collagen fibers as the elastin breaks down. Eventually a breaking point is reached, the collagen fibers are too weak to resist the pressure and the vessel bursts.

Once a thrombus of sufficient size has formed, it can *(Fig. 7-1)*:

- **Stabilize:** Stabilized thrombi firmly adhere to the vessel wall and do not move (change location) or propagate. If a thrombus forms, the most favorable occurrence would be stabilization. This minimizes the risk of embolization and a PE.
- **Propagate:** Propagation occurs when the thrombus continues to enlarge. Likely examples of propagated thrombi are:
  - A thrombus that extends from the superficial venous system into the deep venous system. Probably formed in the superficial system and it grew into the deep venous system.
  - A thrombus that extends from a calf vein into the popliteal vein. Probably first formed in the calf vein and it grew into the popliteal vein.

- **Embolize:** A portion of a thrombus breaks free and is carried by the flowing blood through the vessels until it becomes lodged in a smaller vessel, obstructing it. Because emboli can and do become wedged in pulmonary vessels, a thrombus releasing emboli is an extremely high risk factor for PE.

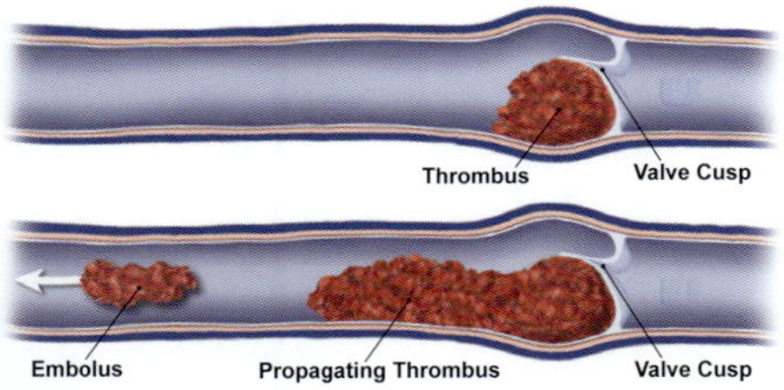

Fig. 7-1. *Venous thrombosis and propagation. In the top vessel, a thrombus has formed behind the valve cusp. This thrombus can stabilize or as depicted in the bottom vessel, or it can propagate. A portion of the thrombus can break off and cause a pulmonary embolism.*

Patient History

- Acute onset of leg pain
- Acute onset of swelling
- Persistent leg/calf swelling (usually unilateral, but can be bilateral)
- Symptoms of PE (e.g., shortness of breath, chest pain, hemoptysis)
- Previous DVT
- Clotting issues (e.g., problems with anticoagulation therapy, malignant cancer)
- Recent periods of immobilization (e.g., bed rest, long plane or car ride)
- Post-operative (e.g., orthopedic or neurosurgery; can occur anytime during surgery or the 6 months thereafter)
- Family history
- Smoking
- COPD
- Blood type, (highest risk with type-A lowest risk with type-O)
- Trauma
- Antiphospholipid antibodies (e.g., lupus)
- Occupations requiring long periods of standing or sitting
- Varicose veins
- Congenital abnormalities (e.g., Klippel-Trenaunay)
- Inflammatory bowel disease
- Drug abuse
- Cerebrovascular events (stroke, transient ischemic attack (TIA))
- Iliac compression syndrome
- Elevated D-dimer levels (D-dimer is a degradation product of fibrin polymers, biomarker for ongoing thrombus formation and fibrinolysis

Physical Examination

- Edema or swelling
- Tenderness
- Limb redness or warmth (superficial thrombophlebitis)
- Varicose veins
- Hyperpigmentation, hardened tissue around the ankles
- Ulceration (especially in the gaiter area)
- Pallor (phlegmasia alba dolens)
- Cyanosis (phlegmasia cerulea dolens)

Location of Disease

A thrombus within the deep veins is referred to as a Deep Venous Thrombosis (DVT). A thrombus within the superficial veins is referred to as a superficial venous thrombosis.

Venous Thromboembolism (VTE) refers to either a deep venous thrombosis or a pulmonary embolism.

Although a thrombus can develop at any venous site, the more common sites are the:

- Valves (behind the cusps)
- Venous confluences
- Inferior vena cava
- Iliac veins
- Deep venous system of the lower extremity (common femoral, deep femoral, femoral, popliteal, peroneal, posterior tibial, gastrocnemius and soleal veins)

- Superficial venous system of the lower extremity (great and small saphenous veins)
- Perforators (lower extremity)

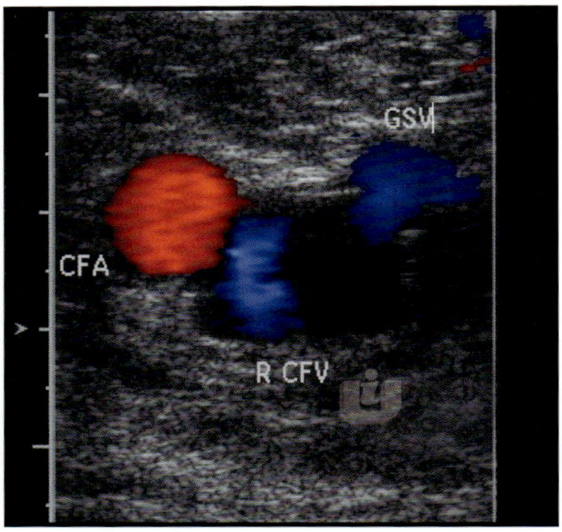

Fig. 7-2. *A thrombus in the common femoral vein at the saphenofemoral junction that partially blocks blood flow.*

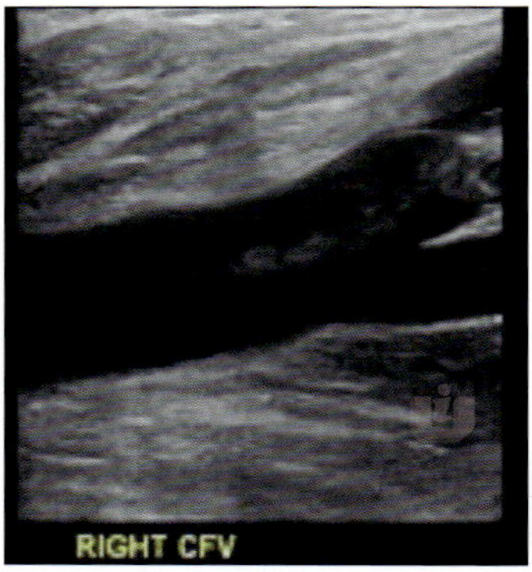

Fig. 7-3. *Free-floating venous thrombus: free-floating tail located in the common femoral vein.*

Lower Extremity Venous Duplex Protocol

- Obtain a patient history that includes symptoms and risk factors for venous thrombosis.
- Assist the patient as they get into a supine position with their head elevated. Placing the bed in a reverse Trendelenburg position may optimize the exam when visualization is difficult, as it increases the size of the calf veins.
- For some patients it may be necessary to use a range of transducers. Typically, two high-frequency (5 - 7MHz) (8 - 15MHz) transducers and one low frequency (1 - 4MHz) transducer is needed.
- It is possible for only one vein of a pair to be thrombosed. For this reason, it is important to make sure all veins are studied carefully *(Fig. 7-4 and 7-5)*.

The best grayscale images are obtained when the transducer is kept at a 90° angle to the skin.

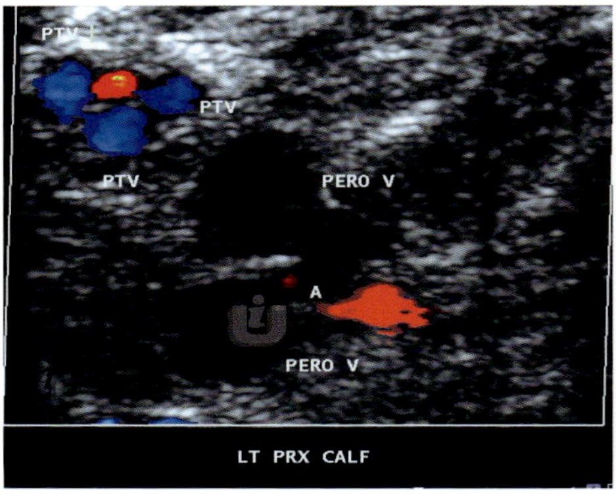

Fig. 7-4. *Color flow is present indicating venous blood flow in the posterior tibial veins. No color is present in the peroneal veins indicating venous occlusion.*

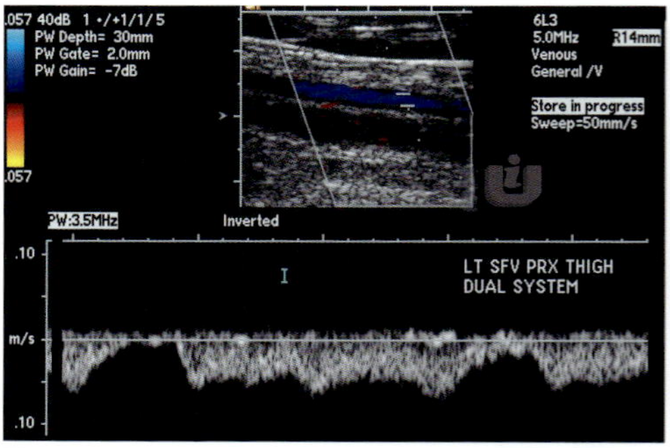

Fig. 7-5. *PW Doppler spectral waveform for a dual venous system. The PW Doppler spectral waveform for the superior vein is typical for venous blood flow. No color flow is present in the inferior vein indicating venous occlusion.*

Transverse Scan and Images

- Locate the common femoral vein and artery at the groin above the saphenofemoral junction in the transverse (short axis) plane. A normal vein will collapse with light to moderate transducer pressure, while the artery remains open. Observe for the vein to completely collapse upon compression *(Fig. 7-6 and 7-7)*.

> *Vein compression at the distal thigh is sometimes difficult. Try placing one hand under the thigh while compressing the vein with the transducer or push your hand up against the transducer to compress the vein*

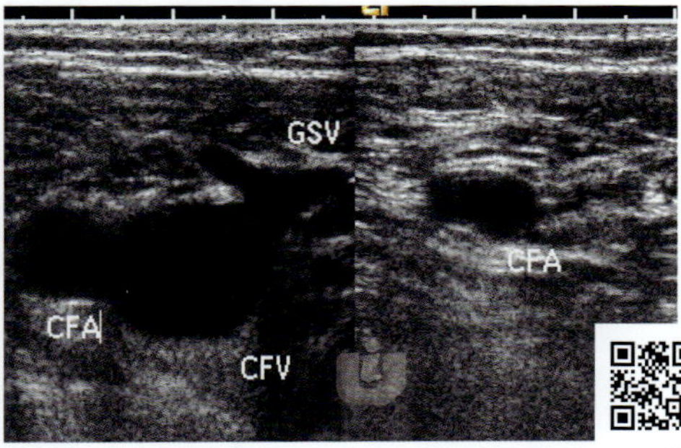

Fig. 7-6. *Compression of the saphenofemoral junction. On the left of the dual screen image is the uncompressed saphenofemoral junction and on the right is the compressed.*

- Veins can usually be imaged from a medial view or "window". Move the transducer distally performing venous compression every 2 - 4cm while watching for the vein to fully collapse.
- Transverse images are to be captured using "dual-screen" on the duplex scanner to allow for comparisons between the compressed and uncompressed vein *(Fig. 7-6 and 7-7)*. Obtain and freeze an image without vein compression on the left side of the screen. Capture an image with vein compression on the right side of the screen. Capture transverse images with and without compressions as described above for the following veins:
  - Common Femoral Vein (CFV): above the saphenofemoral junction
  - Saphenofemoral junction (SFJ): image includes the common femoral vein and proximal end of the great saphenous vein *(Fig. 7-6)*
  - Proximal Deep Femoral Vein (DFV) *(Fig. 7-10)*
  - Proximal Femoral Vein (FV)
  - Mid femoral vein
  - Distal femoral vein: try a medial to posterior window if visualization is difficult with the medial window or change to a lower frequency transducer.
  - Popliteal Vein(PopV): for best visualization move the transducer behind the knee using a posterior approach. To scan the entire popliteal vein, it is often best to start in the middle at the crease of the knee and move proximally to the femoral vein and then distally to the tibial-peroneal confluence *(Fig. 7-11)*.
  - Posterior Tibial Veins (PTV): place the transducer posterior to the medial malleolus and use color flow as a guide to locate these veins alongside their artery *(Fig. 7-12 and 7-13)*.
  - Peroneal Veins (PerV): the peroneal veins can be seen using a medial window superficial to the fibula and deep to the posterior tibial veins. They can also be visualized using a posterolateral approach alongside the fibula.
- Images need to be captured for each of the vein segments listed regardless of whether or not it collapses when compressed.
- Documentation of venous compression can also be obtained for the common and external iliac, great and small saphenous, gastrocnemius, soleal or anterior tibial veins when appropriate.

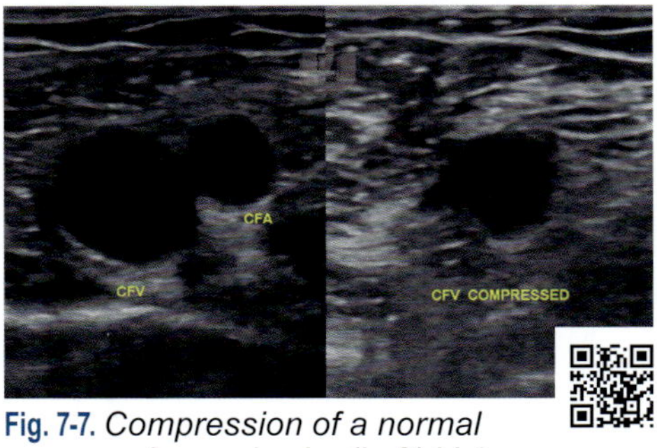

Fig. 7-7. *Compression of a normal common femoral vein. (Left) Vein prior to compression. (Right) The compressed vein has collapsed.*

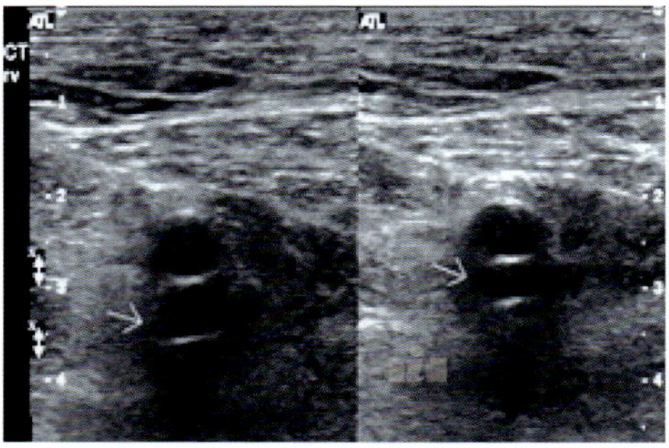

Fig. 7-8. *Compression of a thrombosed femoral vein. The femoral vein is partially incompressible on the right.*

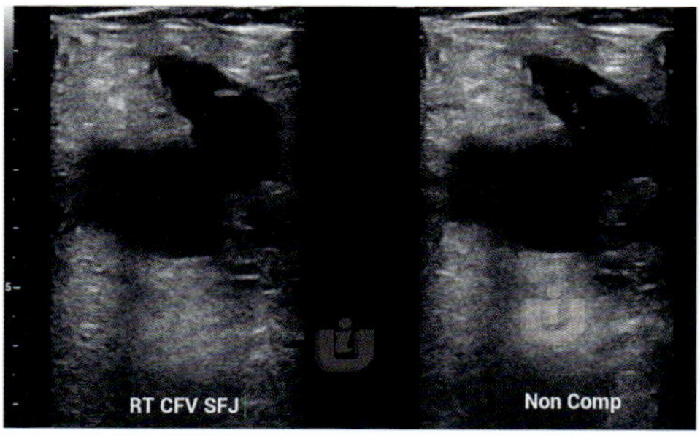

Fig. 7-9. *Compression of the SFJ. (Left) The uncompressed SFJ. (right) The SFJ is non-compressible.*

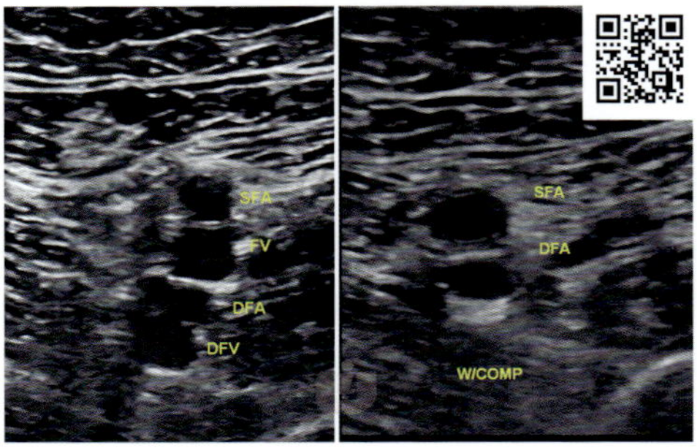

Fig. 7-10. *Compression at the junction of the femoral vein and deep femoral vein. On the left of the dual-screen image is the femoral junction prior to compression. On the right, the femoral junction is compressed.*

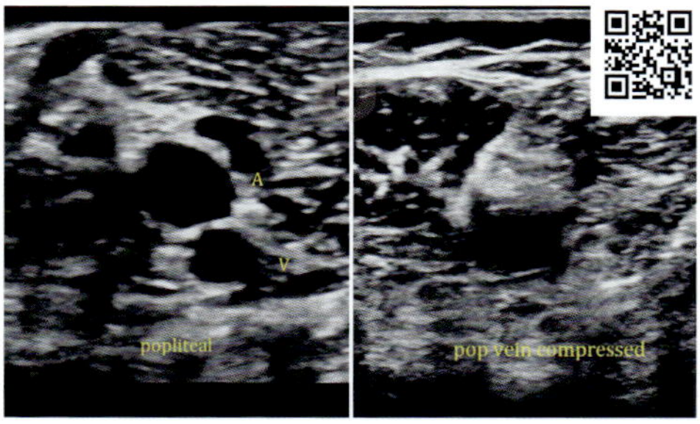

Fig. 7-11. *Compression of the popliteal vein. On the left of the dual screen image is the popliteal vein prior to compression. On the right, the popliteal vein is compressed.*

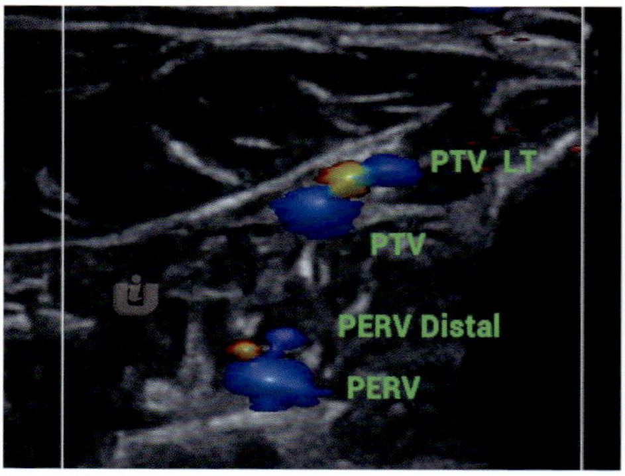

Fig. 7-12. *Color Doppler image of patent tibial veins and arteries.*

Use venous presets on the duplex scanner. Low color and Doppler scales will be needed to detect flow.

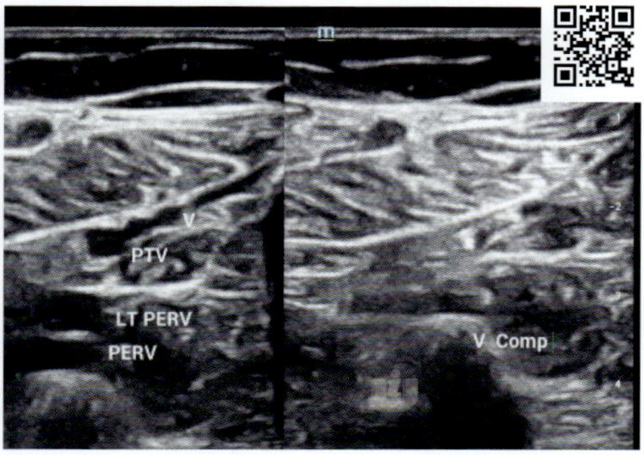

Fig. 7-13. *Compression of the tibial veins. On the left of the dual screen image are the tibial veins prior to compression. On the right, the tibial veins are compressed.*

Some labs record venous PW Doppler waveforms without setting an angle since actual velocities are usually not important in a venous exam. If your lab chooses to set an angle, use a Doppler angle ≤60° with the cursor placed parallel to the vessel walls in the center of the flow stream.

Longitudinal Scan and Images

- On one image, record both color images of the veins in longitudinal and the PW Doppler spectral waveform.
- The Doppler sample gate should be set in the center of the flow stream with the gate set approximately 2 - 4mm wide. Spectral documentation should illustrate spontaneity (hear Doppler signal automatically), respiratory variation and phasicity (flow increases and decreases with respiration).
- The spectral trace needs to show both non-augmented and augmented flow.
- Document venous flow in the following segments:
  - **Common femoral vein:** either above or at the saphenofemoral junction. Augment the signal using a distal compression of the thigh. *(Fig.7-14)*
  - **SFJ:** Augment the signal using a distal compression of the thigh.
  - **Deep femoral vein:** using a medial approach (patient's leg is turned outward), begin at the distal CFV and move the transducer distally to observe the DFV which lies deep to the femoral vein. Augment the signal using a compression of the thigh (not the calf).
  - **Proximal femoral vein:** using a medial approach and color Doppler, capture an image of the femoral vein alone in the proximal thigh or at the junction of the femoral vein and the DFV. Record a FV Doppler waveform, while augmenting the signal using a compression of the calf.
  - **Mid and distal femoral vein:** using a medial approach and color Doppler, capture an image of the femoral vein in the mid and distal thigh. Record a FV Doppler waveforms while augmenting the signal using a compression of the calf.
  - **Mid popliteal vein:** use a posterior approach with the transducer behind the knee. Record a mid PopV Doppler waveform while augmenting the signal using a compression of the calf.
- When necessary, you can document patency of the inferior vena cava, the common and external iliac veins, and the great saphenous, small saphenous and tibial veins.
- If veins are duplicated, PW Doppler waveforms may need to be recorded for each vein individually.
- To confirm absence of flow use PW Doppler. This needs to be done for each vein segment suspected of being thrombosed. Lack of PW Doppler flow, will compliment compression, color flow and B-mode images that indicate the vein is occluded. Arteries that accompany veins can be helpful in locating concomitant veins that have occluded.
- Repeat for the contralateral extremity if a bilateral exam was ordered.

- If a unilateral exam was requested, B-mode and color flow images of the contralateral CFV with and without compression, as well as PW Doppler waveforms, must be recorded for comparison purposes.

Table 7-1. **Lower Extremity Venous Protocol Summary**

Scan transverse (short axis) with and without compression in grayscale and color flow	**Scan longitudinal** (sagittal axis) with PW Doppler and B-mode
• CFV	• CFV
• Saphenofemoral junction	• DFV
• Proximal DFV	• FV
• Proximal FV	• PopV
• Mid FV	
• Distal FV	
• PopV	
• PTV	
• PerV	

- Additional documentation of compression and PW Doppler waveforms may be recorded in additional venous segments.
- If venous compressions are contraindicated due to anatomy or patient discomfort, document patency with color

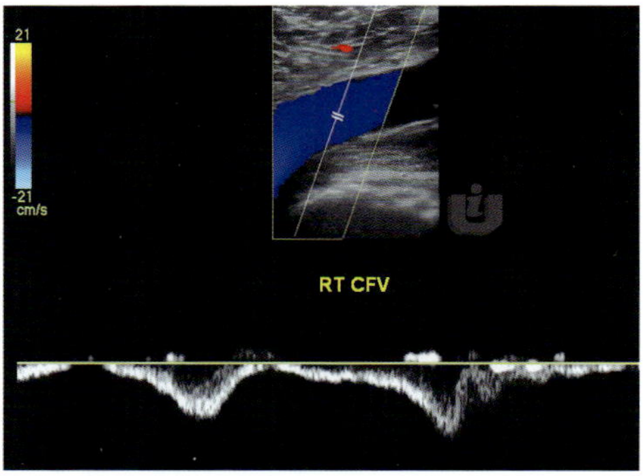

Fig. 7-14. *PW Doppler trace of blood flow in a normal common femoral vein.*

Principles of Interpretation

B-mode Imaging

Use B-mode imaging to determine if a thrombus is present.

- The vein collapses completely with light transducer pressure.
- Echogenic material is present within the lumen of the vein.
- It is possible for only one vein of a pair to be thrombosed. For this reason it is important to make sure all veins are studied carefully. It is possible for only one vein of a pair to be thrombosed.
- Collapse of the artery with transducer pressure can be a confirmation of an incompressible venous segment.

Color Doppler

Use color Doppler to determine if color flow is present wall to wall or if a filling defect is present.

PW Doppler

Use PW Doppler to determine if venous flow is:

- **Spontaneous** (automatically hear a Doppler signal due to blood flow, no compression required)
- **Phasic** (flow increases and decreases with respiration)
- **Augmentable** (flow increases with distal compression)
- **Pulsatile** should be absent normally in lower extremity veins

Interpretation-Diagnostic Criteria

Normal

B-mode Imaging

The vein is free of echogenic material and compresses completely when it is technically possible to compress the vein.

Color Doppler

Wall to wall color flow will fill the vein spontaneously and upon distal compression.

PW Doppler

- **Spontaneity:** The vein demonstrates spontaneous flow, especially in the large veins above the knee. In the calf veins, the absence of spontaneous flow can be a normal finding.
- **Phasicity:** Venous flow is phasic and varies with the respiratory and cardiac cycles. Due to intrathoracic pressure changes during respiration, venous flow decreases during deep inhalation and increases during exhalation. In the calf veins, the absence of phasic flow is a normal finding.
- **Augmentation:** Compression of the limb distal to the transducer augments (increases) venous flow at the transducer.
- **Pulsatility:** Absent in the lower extremity veins.

Abnormal

B-mode Imaging

- Intralumenal echoes are visualized within the vein and the vein is not completely compressible *(Fig. 7-15)*
- The vein is partially compressible when the lumen is partially obstructed and incompressible when the lumen is completely obstructed. *(Fig. 7-25)*

Thrombus

If a thrombus is present, determine

- location (by B-mode)
- whether the thrombus is partially or completely occlusive
- extent (by B-mode and color flow)
- characteristics of the thrombus (echogenicity; acute, chronic, re-canalization; by B-mode)

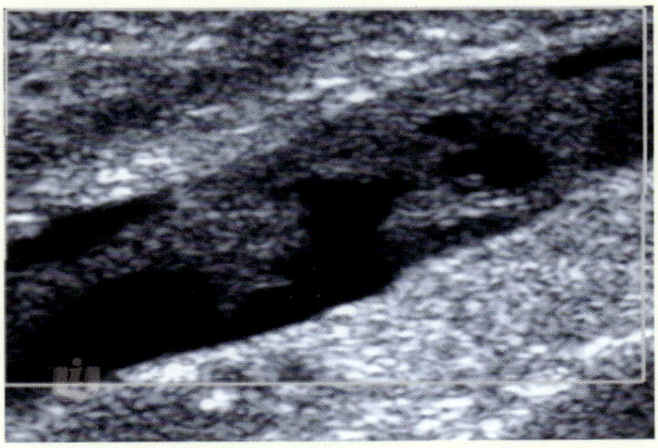

Fig. 7-15. *B-mode image of a venous thrombus which is partially obstructing the vein.*

Age of Thrombus

- Acute thrombus: Typical characteristics include medium to lightly echogenic or anechoic, spongy texture observable, and poor attachment to the vein wall or thrombus is noted to be "free floating" within the lumen *(Fig. 7-3)*. A moving tail may be seen at the end of the thrombus. When a vein is fully thrombosed, the cross sectional area has usually increased, (in an acute event) making it larger than that of the adjacent artery [1,3,7] *(Fig. 7-24 and 7-25)*.

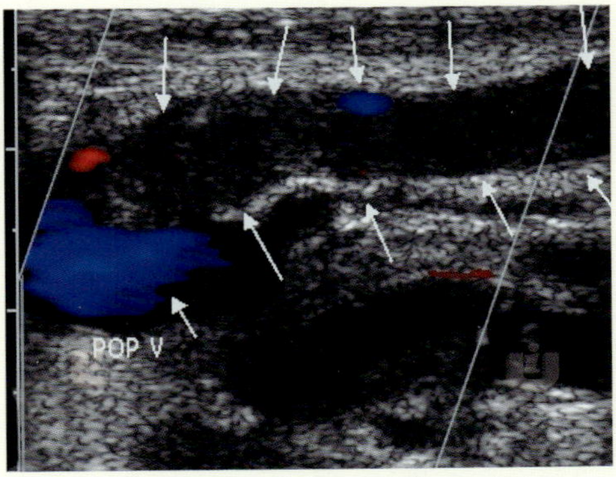

Fig. 7-16. *An acute gastrocnemius vein thrombus extending into the popliteal vein.*

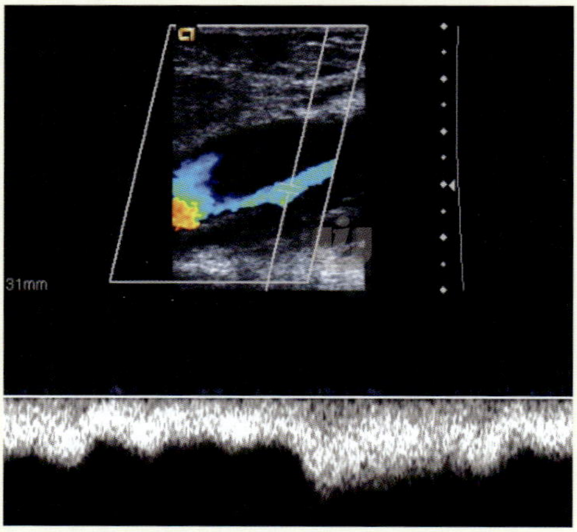

Fig. 7-17. *A longitudinal view of an acute DVT that is partially obstructing blood flow can still produce spontaneous, phasic signal with augmentation.*

- **Chronic thrombus:** Typical characteristics include brightly echogenic or heterogeneous echoes, irregular surface texture and the thrombus is attached to the venous wall with no signs of floating flaps *(Fig. 7-18)*. The vein can stay the same size as the artery, but often contracts in diameter over time. Collateral veins may be observed adjacent to the affected vein(s) and small irregular flow channels within the thrombus can sometimes be seen with color.

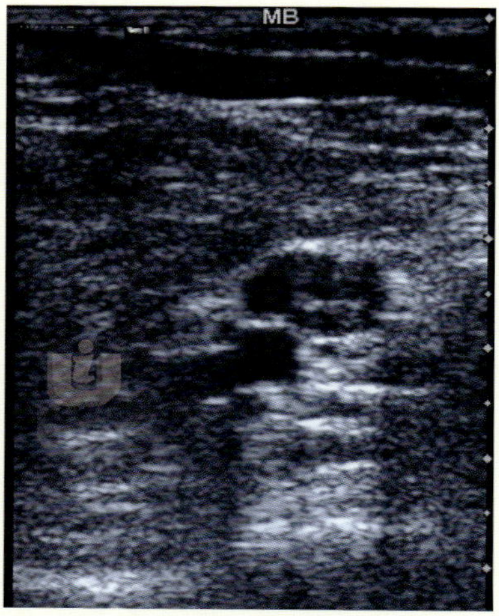

Fig. 7-18. *A transverse view of a partially occlusive chronic DVT in the popliteal vein.*

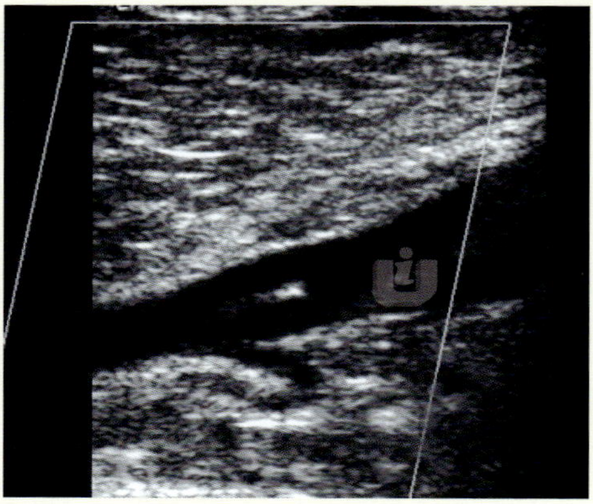

Fig. 7-19. *A longitudinal view of a chronic DVT in the popliteal that is partially obstructing blood flow.*

- **Indeterminate age:** Characteristics of both acute and chronic stages may be present, making age difficult to determine *(Fig. 7-20)*. It is best not to guess.

Table 7-2. **Thrombosis Descriptions and Characteristics**

Acute	Chronic
• Light to medium echogenic/anechoic	• Bright/heterogeneous echoes
• Spongy texture on compression (Homogeneous)	• Irregular texture (Heterogeneous)
• Poorly attached or free floating	• Attached
• Dilated vein (if totally occluded)	• Same or smaller diameter than that of the artery
	• Collateral veins may be observed
• Veins can be partially or totally incompressible in both acute and chronic stages. • Combination of events can occur (e.g., acute thrombus on top of a chronic thrombus). • Chronic thrombus with partial recanalization is seen as a thrombus with small color flow channels. • Age of thrombus is sometimes indeterminate.	

Color Doppler

- If a thrombus does not completely inhibit blood flow, color flow will be seen flowing around echogenic material in the vein spontaneously or with distal compression.
- If a totally obstructive thrombus is present, color flow will not be observed even with distal limb compression using the appropriate low-flow machine settings

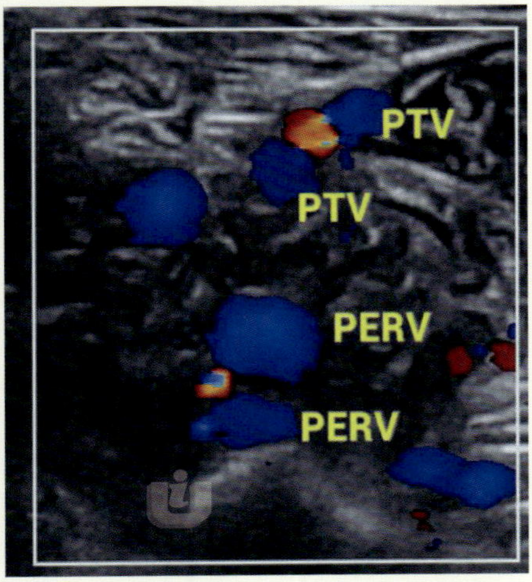

Fig. 7-20. *Transverse view of normal tibial veins with color flow.*

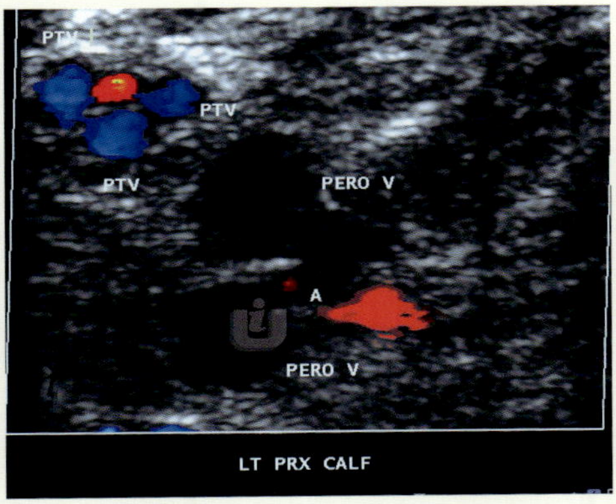

Fig. 7-21. *Transverse view of occluded peroneal veins. The absence of color flow within the vein indicates that the vein has occluded.*

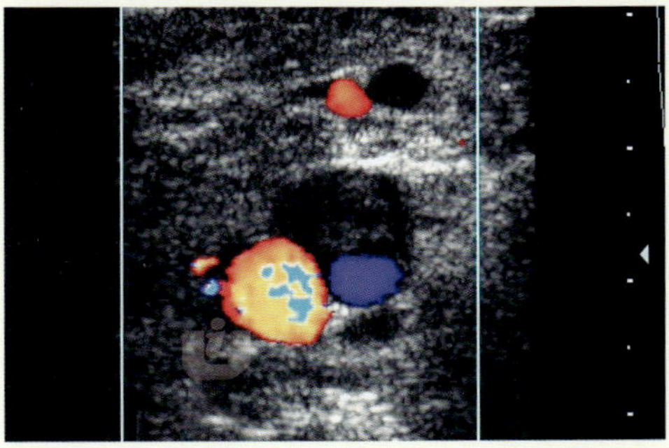

Fig. 7-22. *Color Doppler image of a thrombus in the popliteal vein. Color flows around the thrombus indicating that the thrombus is partially obstructing blood flow.*

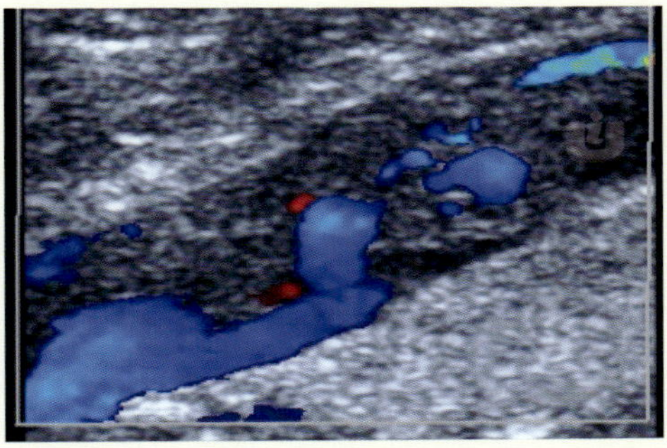

Fig. 7-23. *Color Doppler image of an irregular thrombus in the CFV. Note echogenic material in the CFV by B-mode with color flowing around the thrombus indicating a partial obstruction.*

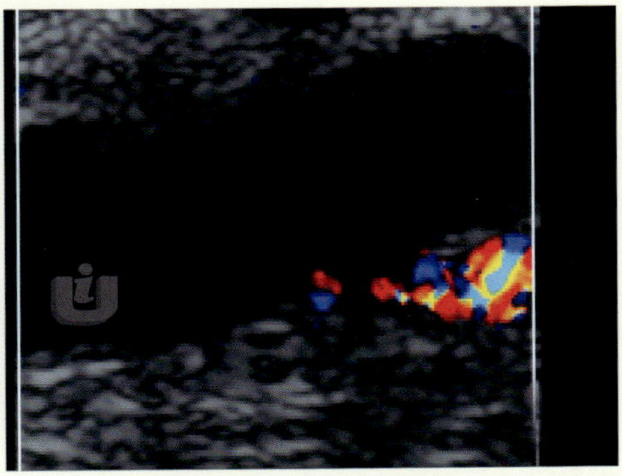

Fig. 7-24. *Color Doppler image of an occluded vein. No color flow indicates that the thrombus has occluded the vein.*

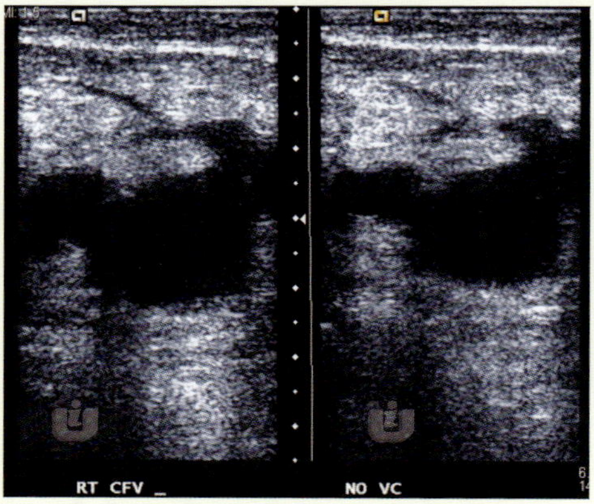

Fig. 7-25. *B-mode image of an incompressible common femoral vein. On the left of the dual screen image is the common femoral vein prior to compression. On the right, common femoral vein compression does not cause the walls to collapse indicating the presence of an obstruction within the lumen.*

PW Doppler

- **Spontaneity:** Absence of flow indicates venous obstruction. Use color flow in the adjacent artery as a guide to identify an occluded vein. But always confirm the absence of flow by placing sample volume in the vessel while using Doppler.
- **Phasicity:** Continuous venous flow (does not vary with respiratory and cardiac cycles) suggests either obstruction from DVT in a proximal venous segment or extrinsic compression of a proximal vein. Partially occlusive thrombus can still produce spontaneous, phasic signal with augmentation.

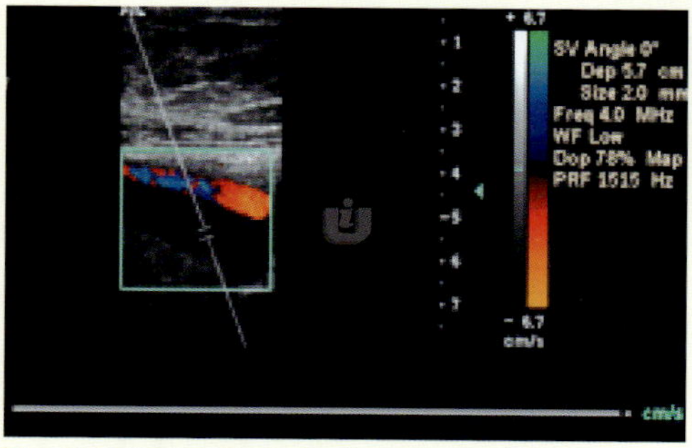

Fig. 7-26. *Color Doppler image and PW spectral waveform of an occluded vein. The absence of color flow and no spectral waveform (no flow) indicates that the thrombus has totally occluded the vein.*

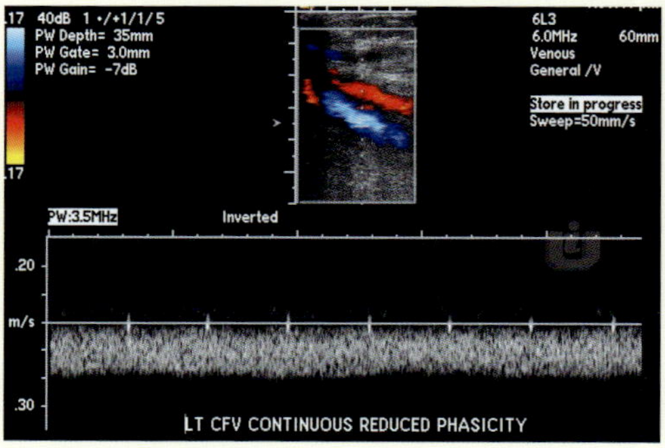

Fig. 7-27. *PW Doppler image of the CFV. Continuous venous flow (reduced phasicity) in the CFV indicating obstruction or extrinsic compression*

- **Augmentation:** If distal compression does not produce augmentation of the venous signal, a total obstruction distal to the transducer is suspected. *(Fig. 7-26)*. A weak or dampened augmentation suggests there is a venous obstruction distal to the transducer, but it does not occlude the vessel. If the augmentation is weak or undetectable, changing the patient's position and/or compressing a more muscular area of the leg may increase the augmentation. Allow time for venous refill before compressing a second time. A normal Doppler signal can be produced proximal to a dual venous system when only one vein is thrombosed, or if large collateral veins are present.

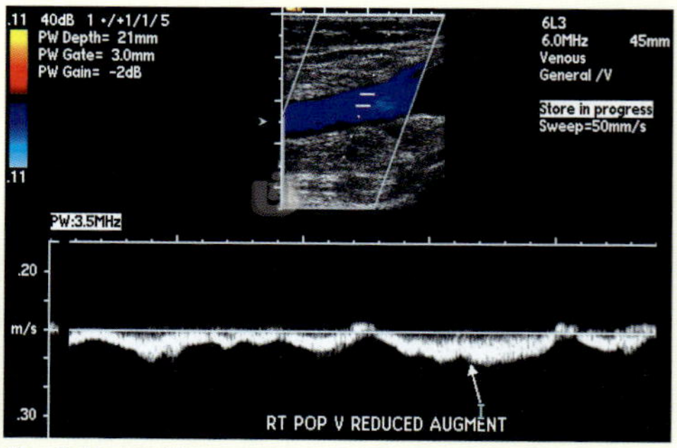

Fig. 7-28. *PW Doppler of the popliteal vein. The flow is not augmented by distal compression indicating venous obstruction distal to the transducer.*

- **Pulsatility:** Pulsatile venous flow is present in the legs when right sided heart disease, a distal fistula and/or a hypervolemic state is present *(Fig. 7-29)*.

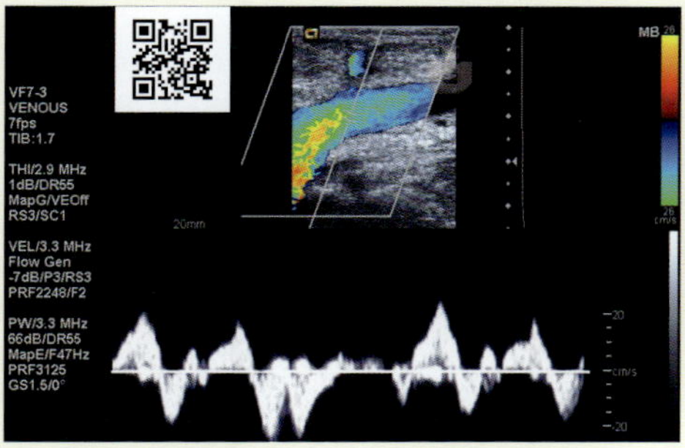

Fig. 7-29. *PW Doppler of the CFV with pulsatile venous flow indicating right sided heart disease, a distal fistula and/or a hypervolemic state is present.*

Table 7-3. **Diagnostic Criteria for Venous Duplex**	
Normal	**Abnormal**
Complete collapse of vein walls with light transducer pressure	Lack of complete vein compression
Absent intralumenal thrombus	Intralumenal echoes present (acute thrombus can be echolucent)
Color flow fills the lumen completely	Decrease or absence of color flow
Normal venous Doppler spontaneity, phasicity and augmentation	Abnormal venous Doppler spontaneity, phasicity or augmentation
No venous dilatation	Dilated or contracted veins noted

Other Pathology

Extrinsic compression

Extrinsic compression by a cell mass or a tumor can cause a venous stenosis. When continuous flow and high venous velocities are present (compared to a proximal segment), a venous stenosis secondary to compression is suspected.

Venous Aneurysms

Venous aneurysm: a region in the vein where the lumen has become significantly larger than that of the proximal segment [3] *(Fig. 7-30).*

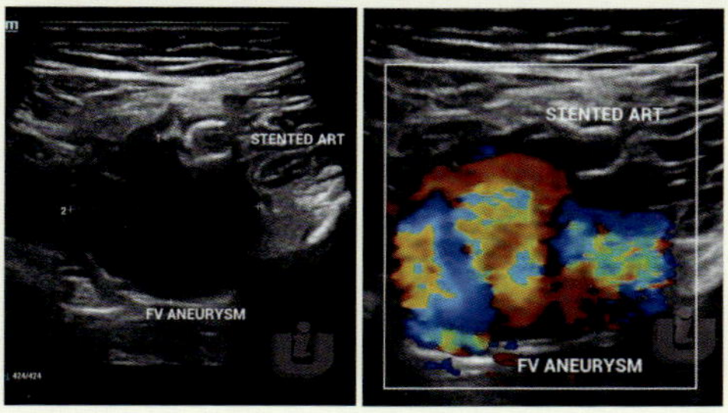

Fig. 7-30. *Venous aneurysm*

Differential Diagnosis

- Arterial disease
- Lymphedema
- Cellulitis
- Cysts (e.g., popliteal, Baker's)
- Extrinsic compression
- Hematoma
- Muscle tear
- Joint effusion
- Adenopathy
- Arteriovenous fistula
- Heart failure (edema)
- Direct injury to extremity
- Vascularized mass
- Collagen vasculitis
- Abscess

Correlation

- Venogram
- MRI
- Computed Tomography (CT) scan

Medical Treatment and Prevention

- Anticoagulation therapy (e.g., heparin, warfarin)
- DVT prophylaxis (e.g., intermittent pneumatic cuff compression)
- Limit long periods of inactivity
- Promote venous return (e.g., elevate legs, wear elastic stockings/ support hose)
- Compression bandaging (for ulceration)

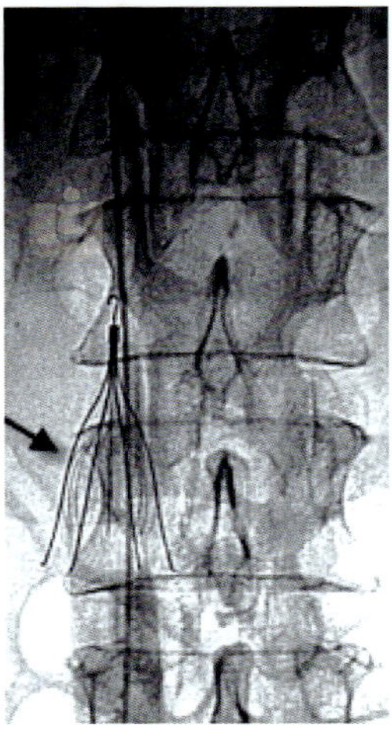

Fig. 7-31. *Inferior vena cavagram showing an IVC filter*

Surgical Treatment

- Iliofemoral venous thrombectomy
- Bypass grafting (caval occlusion)
- Surgical ligation/excision/bypass (aneurysms)

Endovascular Treatment

- IVC filter (acute DVT)
- Catheter-directed thrombolysis with Urokinase, etc. (acute DVT)
- Balloon venoplasty and stenting (chronic iliofemoral DVT)
- Mechanical thrombectomy (e.g., Angiojet; acute DVT)

Points to Remember

- Venous duplex ultrasound can identify the presence, exact location and extent of venous thrombosis. The course of the veins, collaterals and thrombi can be visualized using B-mode and color Doppler, whereas PW Doppler traces can estimate the severity of obstructions.
- The left leg has a higher incidence of DVT than the right leg. The major reason is that the left common iliac vein crosses under the right common iliac artery, which can compress the vein and cause thrombosis. This is known as iliac compression syndrome (formerly May-Thurner). [11]
- Femoral and popliteal veins are commonly duplicated.
- Compressions should always be performed when imaging in the transverse plane to ensure full compression and to avoid missing duplicated veins.
- Dilatation of the lower extremity venous system can be due to portal hypertension.
- When scanning the popliteal vein, the patient may be placed in the prone position.
- Vessel size can be affected by the incline of the bed and room temperature.
- Putting a patient in the reverse Trendelenburg position can improve visibility of small veins (e.g., calf veins).
- Venous aneurysms are less common in the lower extremity than they are in the upper extremity. [9]
- It is helpful to include incidental findings, such as superficial tissue edema or enlarged lymph nodes, in reports to clinicians as these findings may be contributing to the patients' symptoms (e.g., swelling and edema) *(Fig. 7-32 and 7-33).*

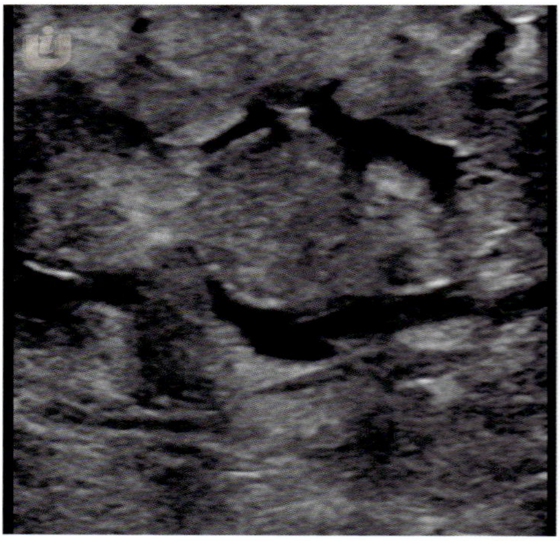

Fig. 7-32. *B-mode image of lower extremity superficial tissue edema.*

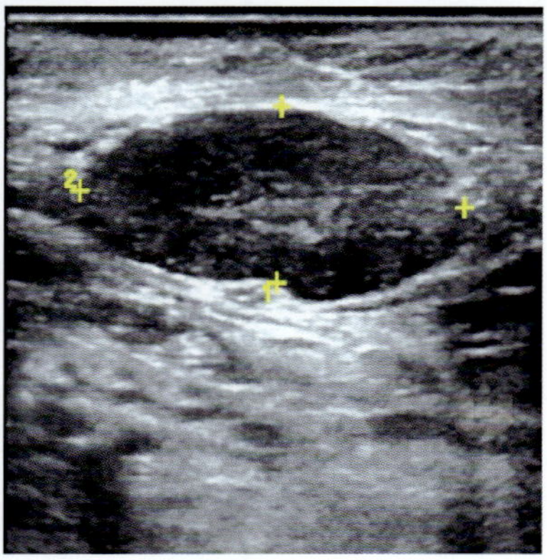

Fig. 7-33. *B-mode image of an enlarged lymph node.*

References

1. Wakefield TW. (2005). Bleeding and clotting: fundamental considerations. In Rutherford Vascular Surgery 6th edition. (493-511). Philadelphia. Elsevier Saunders.
2. Guyton AC. (1986). Hemostasis and blood coagulation. In Textbook of Medical Physiology 7th edition. (76-86). Philadelphia: WB Saunders.
3. Gillespie DL, Villavicencio JL, Gallagher C, Chang A, Hamelink JK, Fiala LA, O'Donnell SD, Jackson MR, Pikoulis E, Rich, NM. (1997). Presentation and management of venous aneurysms. *J Vasc Surg*. Nov;26(5):845-52.
4. Thrush A, Hartshorne T. (2005). Duplex assessment of deep venous thrombosis and upper limb venous disorders. In Peripheral Vascular Ultrasound, How Why and When, 2nd ed. (189-206). Edinburgh: Elsevier Churchill Livingstone.
5. Zwiebel, WJ (2005). Ultrasound Diagnosis of Venous Thrombosis. In Zwiebel WJ, Pellerito JS (Eds.), *Introduction to Vascular Ultrasonography 5th ed*, (449-465). Philadelphia: Elsevier Saunders.
6. Meissner MH. (2005). Venous duplex scanning. In Rutherford Vascular Surgery 6th edition. (254-270). Philadelphia. Elsevier Saunders.
7. Myers K, Clough A. (2004). Venous thrombosis in the lower limbs. In Making sense of vascular ultrasound: A hands on guide. (181-197). London: Hodder Arnold.
8. Dawson DL, Beals H. (2010). Acute lower extremity deep venous thrombosis. In Zierler RE (Ed.), Strandess's duplex scanning disorders in vascular diagnosis 4th ed. (179-198).Philadelphia Wolters Kluwer Lippincott Williams & Wilkins.
9. Sumner DS, Mattos MA. (1993). Diagnosis of deep vein thrombosis with real-time color and duplex scanning. In Vascular Diagnosis 4th edition. (785-800). St. Louis. Mosby.
10. Gloviczki P, Yao, JST (Eds.) (2001). Handbook of Venous Disorders, 2nd ed. (p. 38) London: Arnold.
11. Gloviczki P, Cho JS. (2005) Surgical treatment of chronic occlusions of the iliac veins and the superior vena cava. In Rutherford Vascular Surgery 6th edition. (2303-2320). Philadelphia. Elsevier Saunders.

8. Native IVC, Iliac and Venous Stent Duplex

Definition

The combination of real-time B-mode ultrasonography with Pulsed Wave (PW) and color Doppler used to diagnose the presence or absence of a hemodynamically significant obstruction, provide ultrasound guidance during stenting procedures, and allow for post-procedure surveillance.

Etiology [1,2,15,16]

- Thrombosis
- Tumors
  - Extrinsic compression by a cell mass or a tumor
  - Tumor invasion of the IVC
- Iliac vein obstruction
  - Thrombotic
  - Nonthrombotic iliac vein lesion (NIVL)
- Congenital anomalies

Risk Factors

- Age
- Immobilization
- Prothrombotic gene mutation (clotting disorders such as factor V Leiden)
- Postoperative phase (especially after orthopedic surgery)
- Peri pregnancy
- Previous deep vein thrombosis (DVT)
- Venous malformations (e.g., Klippel-Trenaunay)
- Mechanical compression of an iliac vein by an overlying artery
- Intraluminal obstruction (thrombosis, scarring, or mass)

Indications for Exam

- History of DVT involving the common femoral veins (CFV) or iliac veins
- History of pulmonary embolus
- Edema involving the upper thigh
- Edema/swelling, especially when unilateral
- Ulceration (especially in gaiter area)
- Discoloration in the gaiter area
- Venous claudication
  - Pain with physical exercise which increases with intensity and feels constrictive in the calf or thigh
  - Results in functional impairment
  - Symptoms only dissipate when the leg is positioned to enhance venous drainage (leg raised)
- History of inferior vena cava (IVC) filter placement
- Asymmetry of the CFV PW Doppler waveforms observed during lower extremity venous duplex
- Varicose veins, especially reoccurring post previous vein treatment
- Pallor (phlegmasia alba dolens)
- Cyanosis (phlegmasia cerulea dolens)
- Reoccurring lower extremity deep vein thrombosis
- Genital varicosities
- Lower extremity varicosities of pelvic origin (via the pelvic escape points)
- Routine stent surveillance

Contraindications/Limitations

- Morbid obesity
- Open wounds with bandaging that cannot be removed
- Patients who cannot cooperate or cannot be positioned adequately
- Excessive bowel gas
- Dense scar tissue from major abdominal surgery
- Patients with a large amount of peristaltic motion may produce major color and power Doppler artifacts obstructing the visualization of vessels
- Enlarged uterus overlying the IVC or iliac veins

This exam is operator-dependent; its accuracy and success depend upon the level of experience of the sonographer.

Mechanism of Disease

Inferior Vena Cava

Idiopathic/Primary obstruction [3]

- Propagation of thrombus from the iliac veins
- Isolated thrombus of the inferior vena cava can occur, even though the incidence is low.

Provoked/Secondary obstruction [3]

- Outflow obstruction, e.g., Budd Chiari-Syndrome (obstruction of veins of the liver)
- Extrinsic compression by a mass
- Intrinsic pathology (e.g., IVC filter occlusion or filter migration)
- Tumor invasion of the IVC

Anatomic variations causing obstruction may include: [4, 5]

- **Aplasia:** The failure of the IVC to develop or to function normally
- **Hypoplasia:** Underdevelopment of the IVC
- **Left-sided cava:** Refers to a variant course of the inferior vena cava. It is the most common anomaly of the IVC and occurs due to the persistence of the left supra cardinal vein.
- **Duplication of the IVC**

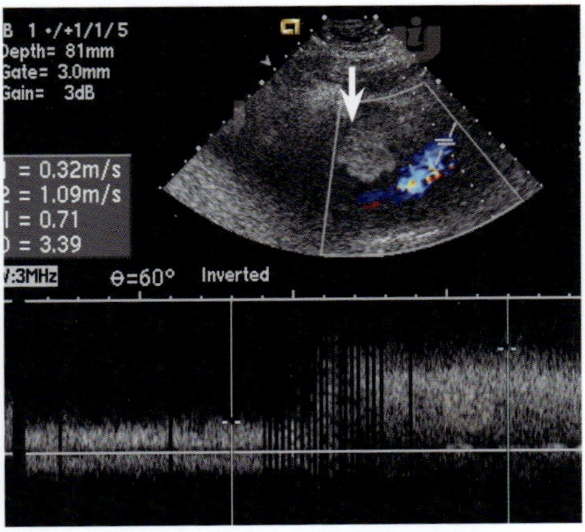

Fig. 8-1. *Color and PW Doppler tracing of extrinsically compressed IVC. A tumor is compressing the IVC narrowing the lumen. The increased velocities on the PW Doppler tracing indicate that the vein is extrinsically compressed.*

Native Common and External Iliac Veins

Iliac vein obstruction can occur due to: [2]

- Thrombotic lesions (Can occur after an incidence of DVT and cause an intrinsic obstruction).
- NIVL is the pathological compression of an iliac vein by an overlying iliac artery.
  - Extrinsic compression results if partial or complete compression of the vein lumen exists.
  - Intrinsic obstruction results in wall fibrosis and intraluminal changes caused by the pulsations of an overlying artery.
- Extrinsic compression by a cell mass or a tumor.

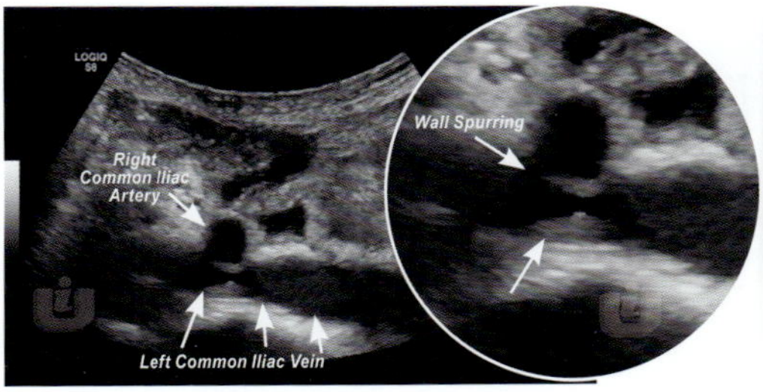

Fig. 8-2. *Longitudinal view of the left CIV with intraluminal spurring at the level of the overlying common iliac artery.*

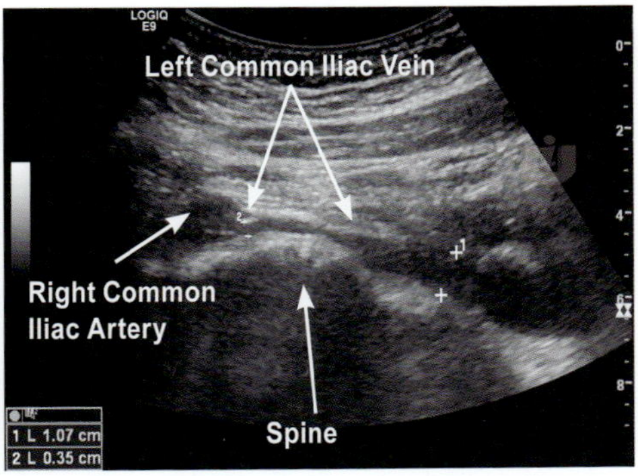

Fig. 8-3. *Longitudinal view demonstrating stenosis of the CIV due to the stretching of the vein over the spine.*

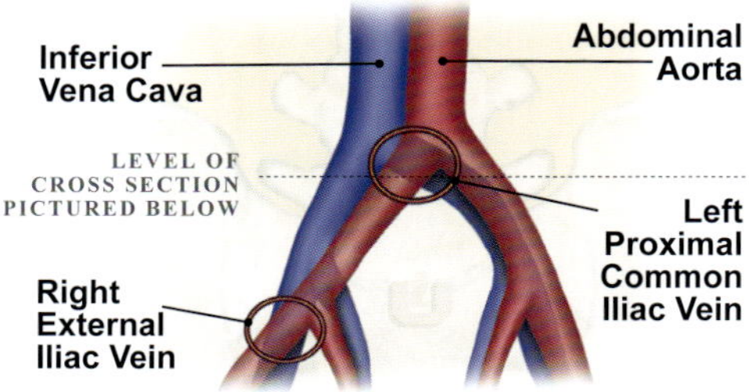

Fig. 8-4. *Most frequently occurring NIVLs*

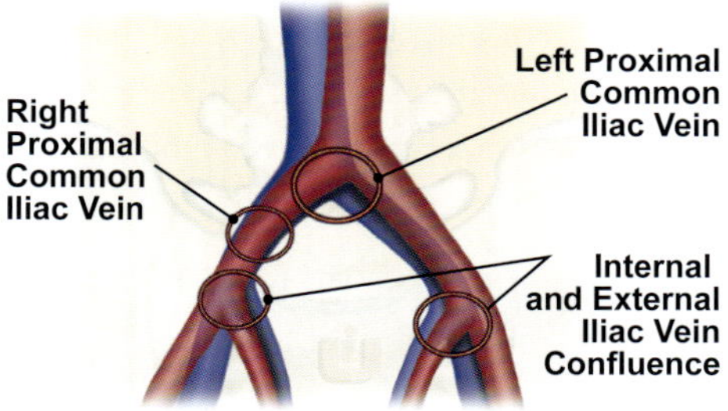

Fig. 8-5. *Less frequently occurring NIVLs*

> *Note the slight shift in the position (when comparing Figs. 8-4 and 8-5) of the aorta and the IVC creating additional sites of potential obstruction.*

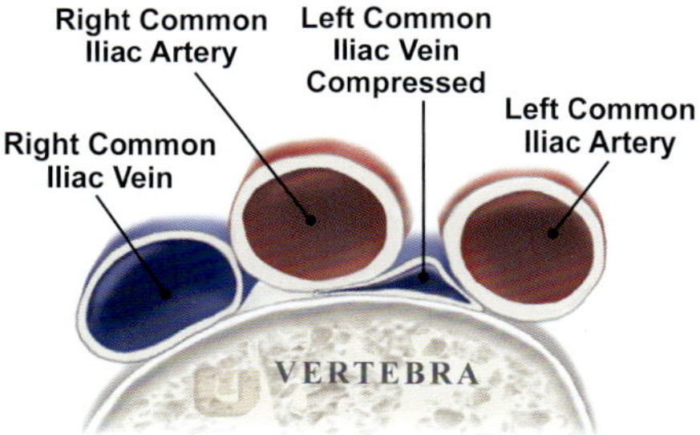

Fig. 8-6. *Cross-section view of the left CIV being compressed by the right and left CIAs.* *Adapted from www.scgvs.com*

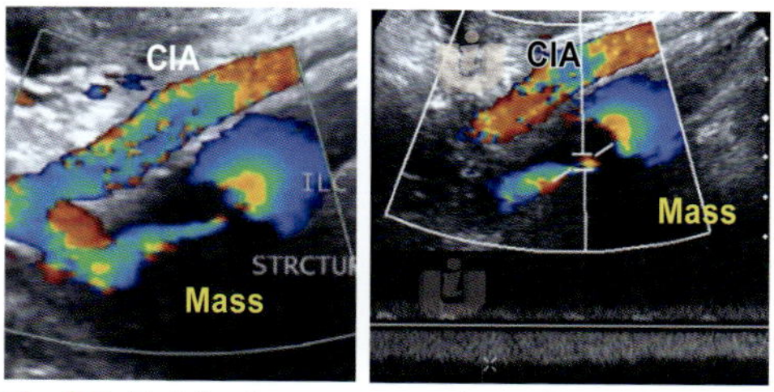

Fig. 8-7. *Extrinsic compression of the CIV by a large pelvic mass. Note the continuous PW Doppler waveform.*

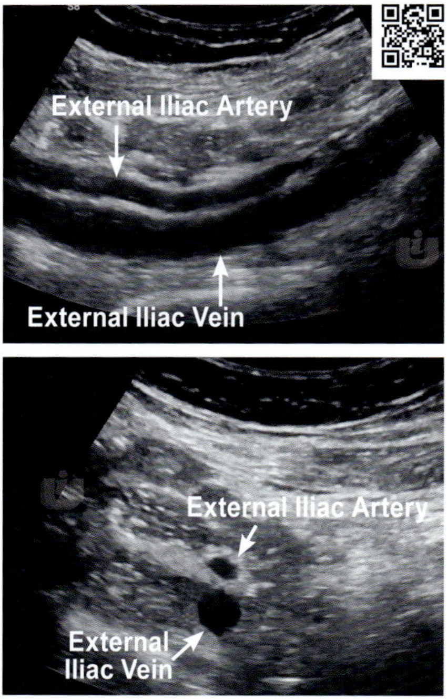

Fig. 8-8. *EIV in longitudinal and transverse views demonstrating pulsatile, repetitive compression of the EIV by the overlying EIA.*

Table 8-1. **Areas of Iliac Vein Compression***

Common Iliac Veins

- Right common iliac artery on left common iliac vein
- Right common iliac artery on right common iliac vein
- Left common iliac artery on left common iliac vein

External Iliac Veins

- Right external iliac artery on right external iliac vein
- Right internal iliac artery on right external iliac vein
- Left external iliac artery on left external iliac vein
- Left internal iliac artery on left external iliac vein
- Inguinal ligament on right external iliac vein
- Inguinal ligament on left external iliac vein

*More than one type of compression may exist.

Labropoulos Nicos, Diagnosis of Iliac Vein Obstruction With Duplex Ultrasound Criteria used during duplex ultrasound examination to identify iliac vein obstruction. Endovascular Today, July 2018, Vol. 17, No. 7, page 3

Internal Iliac Veins

- Primary valvular dysfunction (reflux occurs due to incompetent venous valves or an absence of venous valves)
- Secondary valvular dysfunction (reflux occurs due to a more central obstruction. e.g., the CIV)

> *Internal iliac vein (IIV) insufficiency is covered extensively in the Pelvic Duplex Ultrasound chapter.*

Patient History

- Acute onset of leg pain
- Acute onset of swelling
- Persistent leg/calf swelling (usually unilateral, but can be bilateral)
- Symptoms of PE (e.g., shortness of breath, chest pain, hemoptysis)
- Previous DVT
- Clotting issues (e.g., problems with anticoagulation therapy, cancer)
- Recent periods of immobilization (e.g., bed rest, long plane or car ride)
- Postoperativeve (e.g., orthopedic or neurosurgery; can occur anytime during surgery or the six months thereafter)
- Venous claudication
- Iliac vein compression
- History of endovascular treatment (angioplasty and/or stent)
- Additional history for patients being considered for stents: A combination of signs and symptoms that have been unresponsive to conservative measures may be a candidate for stenting

Family History

- DVT
- Congenital abnormalities (e.g., Klippel-Trenaunay)
- Iliac vein compression
- Anatomic variations

Physical Examination

- Edema or swelling
- Varicose veins (particularly reoccurring)
- Edema
- Venous origin changes in skin and subcutaneous tissue
- Corona Phlebectatica
- Venous ulcer

Location of Disease

- Inferior Vena Cava (IVC)
- The left Common Iliac Vein (CIV) is the most common to have obstructive pathology
- Compression of the right CIV and bilateral EIVs have been documented

Patient Preparation

If possible, the patients should be fasting for 6 - 12 hours to minimize the presence of air/bowel gas in the abdomen for better visualization. However, the iliac veins can often be visualized without a fasting preparation.

Patient Position

- The patient is in a supine position with the head of the bed slightly raised, arms by their side, or resting on their chest.
- The patient should breathe normally and not talk when PW Doppler waveforms are obtained (Valsalva should not be used when testing for phasicity).

Scanning Protocol

B-mode imaging and transverse transducer compression maneuvers are often ineffective when evaluating abdominal or pelvic veins. Therefore, color, power Doppler, and PW Doppler will be the primary modalities for evaluation. Gain settings for color or power Doppler should be adjusted for low flow states; persistence increased, sensitivity set high, velocity scale decreased, filter set low and smooth settings increased.

Inferior Vena Cava

- Locate the IVC in the upper abdomen just below the xiphoid process in the transverse view. Follow the IVC from the xiphoid process to the distal abdomen (the level of the confluence of the right and left iliac veins, record diameters at proximal, mid, and distal abdomen.
- In a transverse view, the IVC should appear as an oval; if it is seen nearly round, it may be indicative of right heart congestion or fluid overload.
- Turn the transducer to a longitudinal view and obtain PW Doppler waveforms.

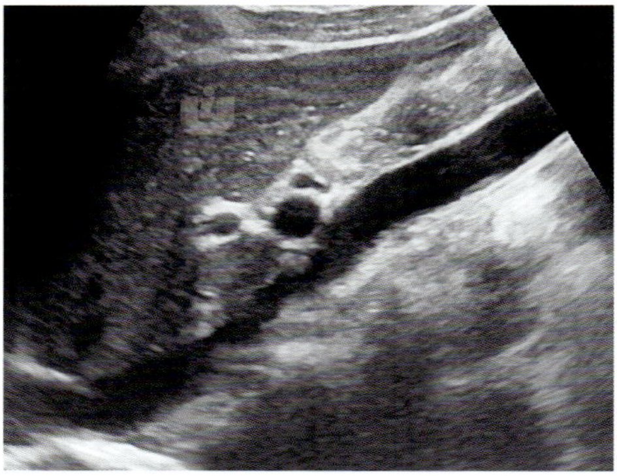

Fig. 8-9. *Longitudinal view of the IVC.*

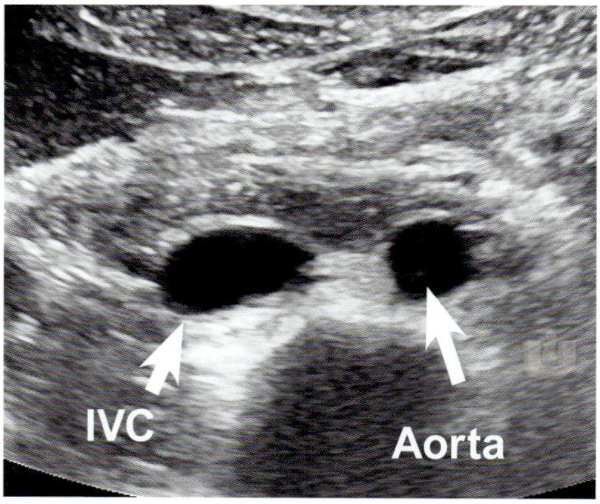

Fig. 8-10. *Transverse view of the IVC and the aorta.*

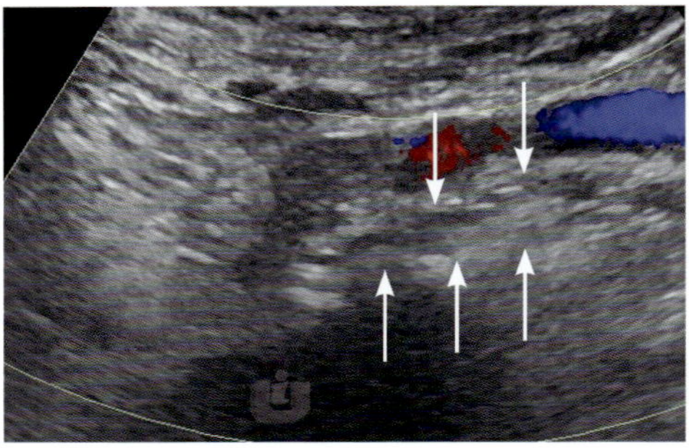

Fig. 8-11. *Occluded IVC with chronic luminal changes in a patient with an IVC filter. The narrow diameter and lack of thrombus indicate that this is a chronically occluded vein.*

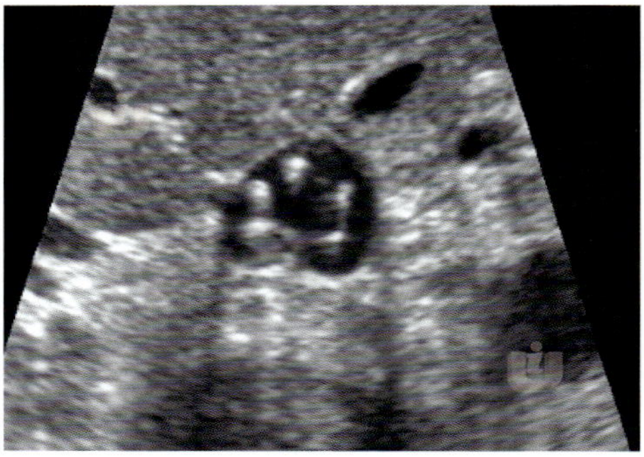

Fig. 8-12. *Transverse view of an IVC with a Greenfield filter.* *Image courtesy of Philips Healthcare*

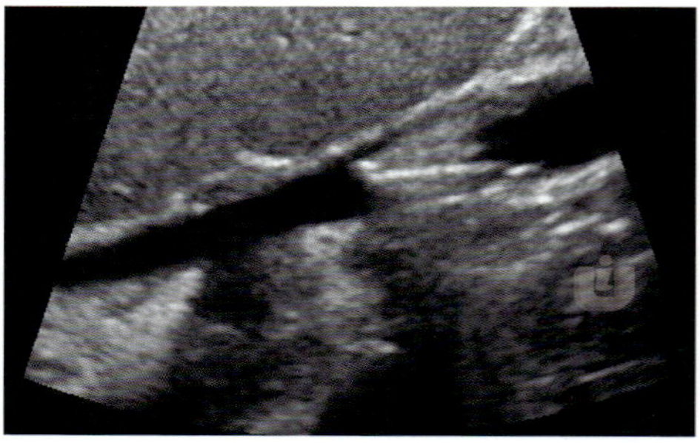

Fig. 8-13. *Longitudinal view of an IVC with a Greenfield filter.*

Images courtesy of Philips Healthcare

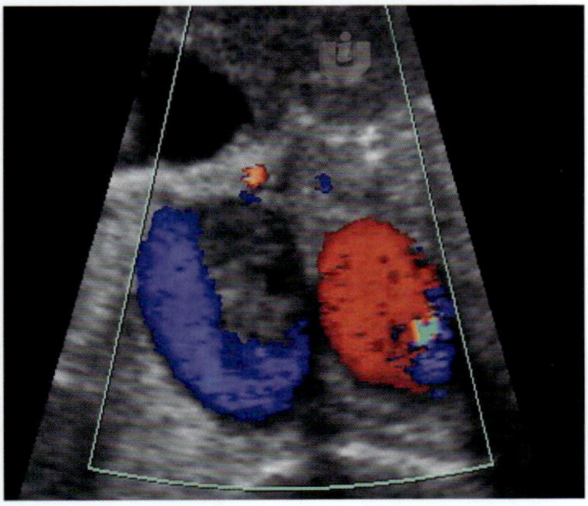

Fig. 8-14. *Partial thrombosis of the IVC in the transverse view.*

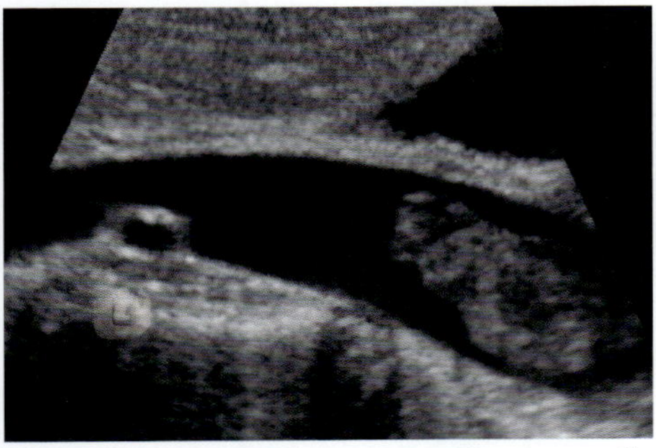

Fig. 8-15. *Acute IVC thrombus with poor wall attachment.* *Image courtesy of Philips Healthcare*

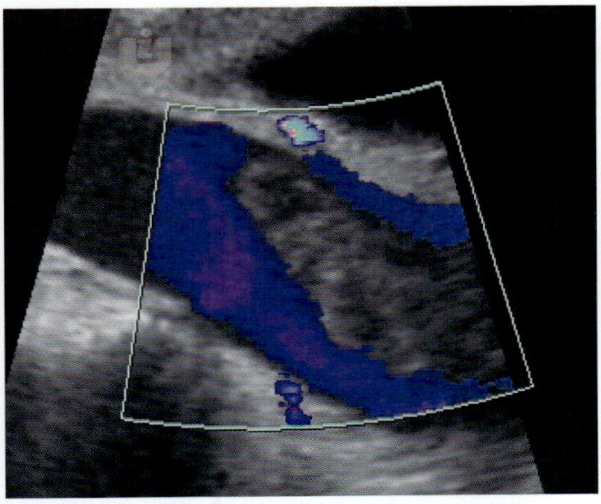

Fig. 8-16. *Partial thrombosis of the IVC in a longitudinal view.* *Image courtesy of Philips Healthcare*

Iliac Veins [5,6,7]

Indirect testing of the iliac veins should be included in all lower extremity venous duplex testing via comparison of the bilateral CFV PW Doppler waveforms. They should demonstrate phasic symmetrical flow.

When indirect signs are detected, they always indicate some form of obstruction. However, they cannot differentiate between stenosis and occlusion, extrinsic compression, or luminal changes. Therefore, direct imaging of the affected veins is important. The presence of phasic flow and good augmentation cannot exclude obstruction.

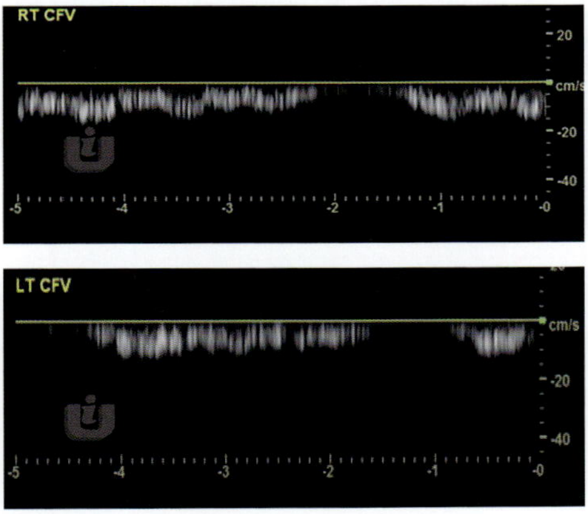

Fig. 8-17. *PW Doppler demonstrating symmetrical phasicity when comparing the right and left common femoral veins.*

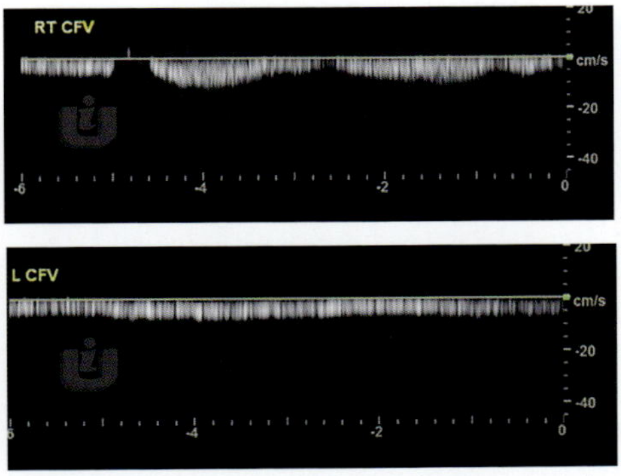

Fig. 8-18. *PW Doppler demonstrates a total lack of phasicity (aka continuous flow) in the left CFV when compared to the right CFV. This is an indirect indication of a more central obstruction.*

Native IVC, Iliac and Venous Stent Duplex

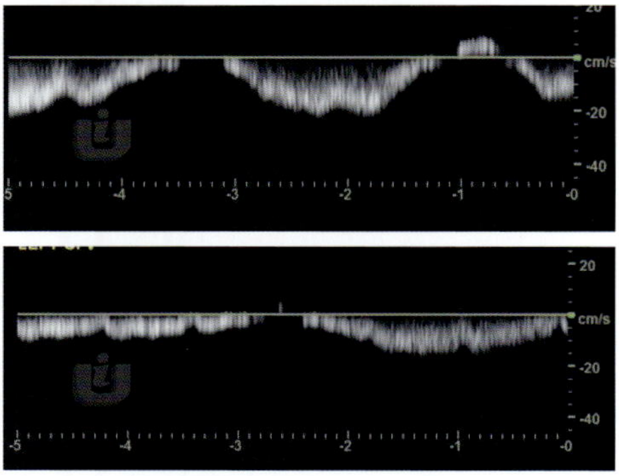

Fig. 8-19. *Asymmetry (not just an absence of phasicity) indicates a more central obstruction when comparing the common femoral Doppler waveforms.*

> *The pelvis has a robust collateral venous system which may result in the findings of phasic, symmetrical waveforms (false negative) in the CFVs. If there is a high suspicion of proximal obstruction, the iliac veins should be evaluated.*

- The confluence of the right and left CIV is identified by moving the transducer in transverse orientation caudally to the distal IVC at the level of the umbilicus.
- Because the right CIV has a fairly straight course to the IVC, a long view can be obtained by placing the transducer longitudinally just to the right of the umbilicus.
- To establish the long view of the left CIV, the transducer is positioned obliquely.
- The entire length of the iliac veins from the IVC to the inguinal ligament is imaged.

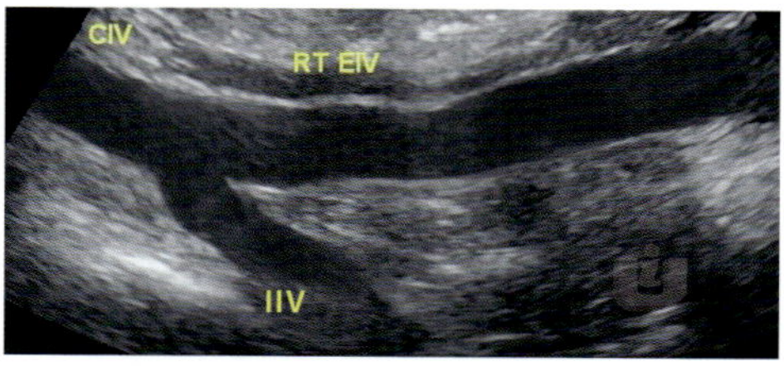

Fig. 8-20. *The confluence of the IIV and EIV forms the CIV.*

Duplex ultrasound can detect the following to aid in diagnosing significant stenosis:[7]

- Iliac vein luminal reduction
- Pre-stenotic dilation
- Increased velocity ratio
- Slow or absent venous flow
- Presence of collateral veins
- Fibrotic changes of the vein walls caused by the repetitive motion of an overlying artery

Native Iliac Veins [7,8,9]

- The exam starts at the confluence of the femoral and deep femoral veins and finishes at the inferior vena cava.
- Care should be taken to avoid heavy manual compression; this can create false positive results.
- The majority of the evaluation of the iliac system is performed in a longitudinal view.
- Transverse evaluation of the CIVs and EIVs should be included when they can be well visualized in that view.
- If a significant obstruction is present, the inflow to the iliac veins via the lower extremity and the outflow via the IVC should be imaged to:
  - Assess the veins to determine optimal stent placement from one healthy vein segment to the next
  - Ensure there is adequate inflow which allows for long-term patency of the stent
- B-mode imaging should be used to assess for:
  - Vein diameter
  - Intraluminal changes
    - » Spurring/fibrotic changes to the walls
  - Thrombosis (occlusive or nonocclusive)
    - » Chronic changes from previous thrombosis (e.g., synechiae, wall thickening)
    - » Occlusion
- Color Doppler scale should be adjusted to allow for slow venous flow and is used to assess for:
  - A color jet at the level of stenosis
  - Mosaic color flow pattern due to post stenotic turbulence
  - Direction of flow; particularly in the IIV
    - » Retrograde flow in the IIV is often seen in patients with a significant CIV compression

- PW Doppler using an angle of 60° or less is used to assess for:
  - Side-to-side (right-to-left) variability in PW Doppler waveforms
  - Peak vein velocities when a stenosis is suspected. Velocities are obtained peripheral to and at the level of the stenosis to obtain a velocity ratio.
- Grayscale, color, and PW Doppler image documentation in the longitudinal view should include:
  - The deep femoral and femoral veins just peripheral to their confluence
  - CFV
  - Peripheral EIV
  - Mid EIV
  - Central EIV
  - EIV and IIV confluence
  - Peripheral CIV
  - Mid CIV
  - Central CIV
  - IIV
  - If external compression or luminal changes are present, diameters (anterior to posterior wall) and PW Doppler peak vein velocity should be documented:
    - » Peripheral to the obstruction (pre-stenosis)
    - » At the level of obstruction
    - » Central to the obstruction (post-stenosis)

> *The terms peripheral to and central to refer to the anatomical location in reference to the IVC (e.g., the CIV is "peripheral" to the IVC and the EIV is "central to" the CFV.*

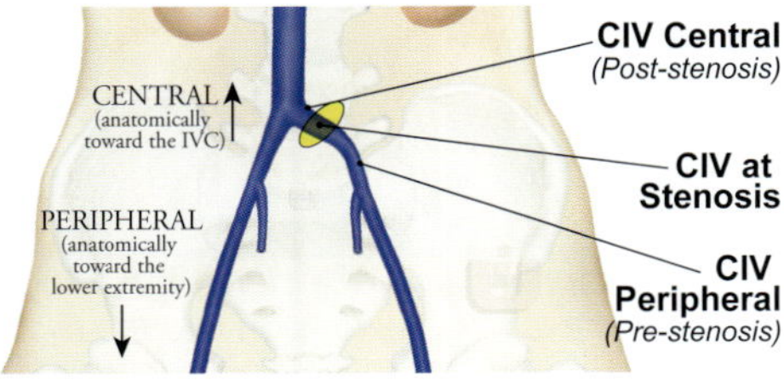

Fig. 8-21. *Diameters and PW Doppler waveforms are obtained at the level of, peripheral to, and central to the stenosis.*

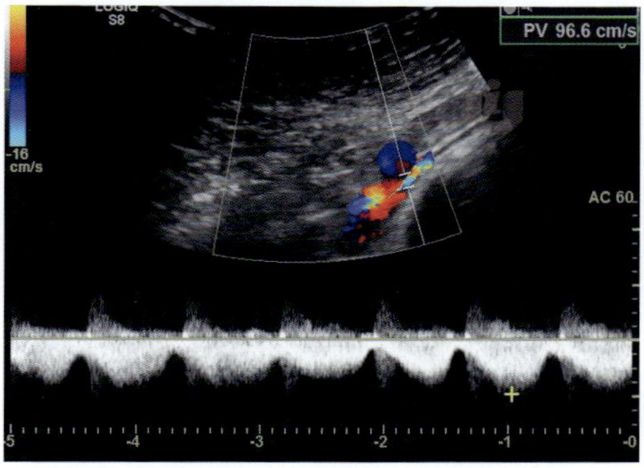

Fig. 8-22. *PW Doppler of the CIV at the level of compression.*

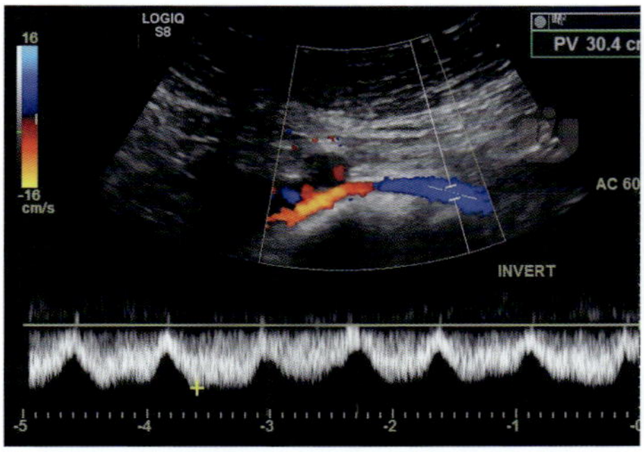

Fig. 8-23. *PW Doppler of the left CIV within the peripheral segment. These velocities are used to calculate a ratio to determine if there is a significant stenosis. Note that a ≤60° angle is used to obtain accurate velocities. 96.6cm/s (Fig. 8-22) ÷ 30.4cm/s (Fig. 8-23) = ratio of 3.18*

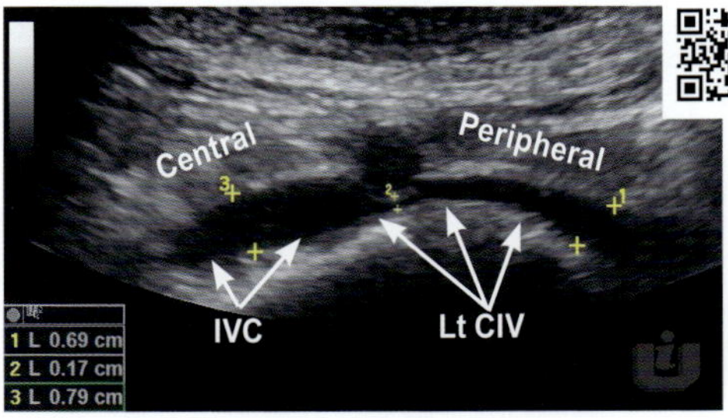

Fig. 8-24. *For accurate measurements, diameters are obtained in B-mode to ensure good visualization of the anterior and posterior wall measurements.*

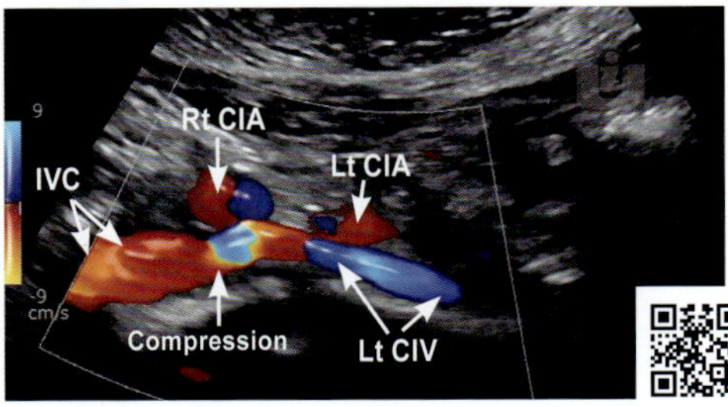

Fig. 8-25. *Left CIV as it courses posterior to the right CIA, the point of compression is demonstrated by the decreased diameter in the vein along with color flow aliasing.*

When obtaining velocities, ideally, a 60° Doppler angle should be used. A Doppler angle of >60° may be used. However, these velocities measurements should be obtained using the same angle throughout to calculate an accurate velocity ratio. The peripheral velocity will be compared with the point of compression velocity to obtain a ratio to determine if there is significant compression.

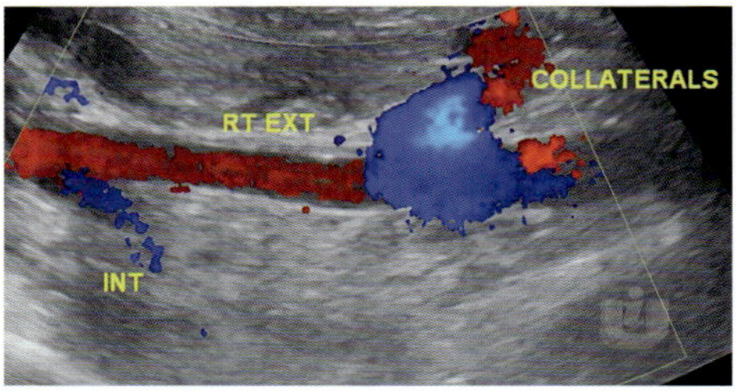

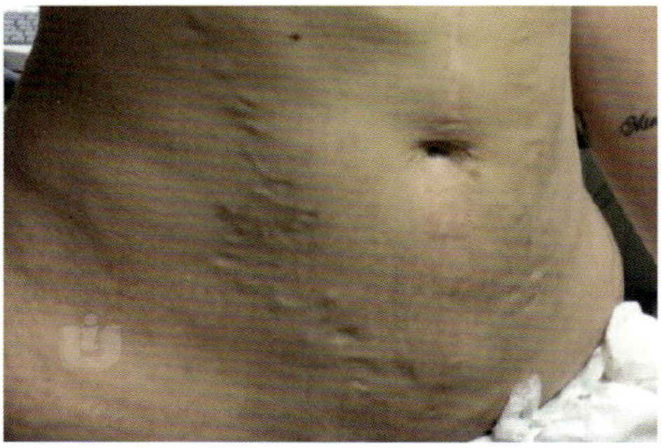

Fig. 8-26. *Patients with an IVC and CIV occlusion present with extensive abdominal varices, which are visualized as tributaries of the external iliac vein using duplex ultrasound.*

Care should be taken with transducer pressure on the abdomen to not extrinsically compress the CIVs, creating false positives. This most commonly occurs on the left side; however, this should apply to a visibly narrowed right CIV.

Internal Iliac Vein

- The bilateral IIVs should be evaluated with color and PW Doppler for flow direction and phasicity
- Spontaneous, continuous reflux within the IIV indicates a significant, more central stenosis.[7]

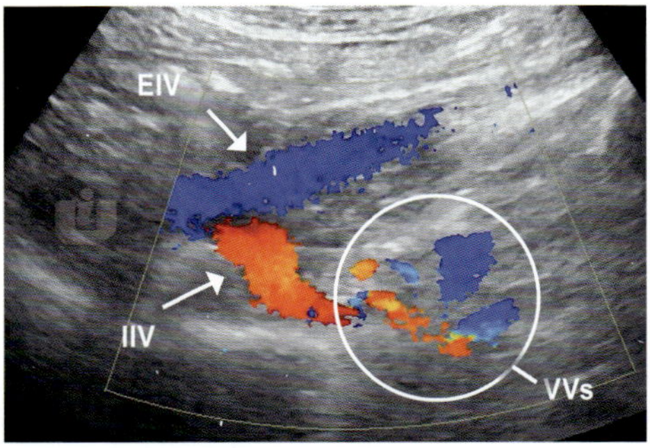

Fig. 8-27. *Transabdominal color flow demonstrating varicose veins of the IIV.*

Post-Stenting Ultrasound [9, 10, 11]

- Placement and length of a venous stent is based upon provider preference and could be:
  - Limited to the location of the lesion (typically the CIV)
  - Extending along the CIV into the EIV

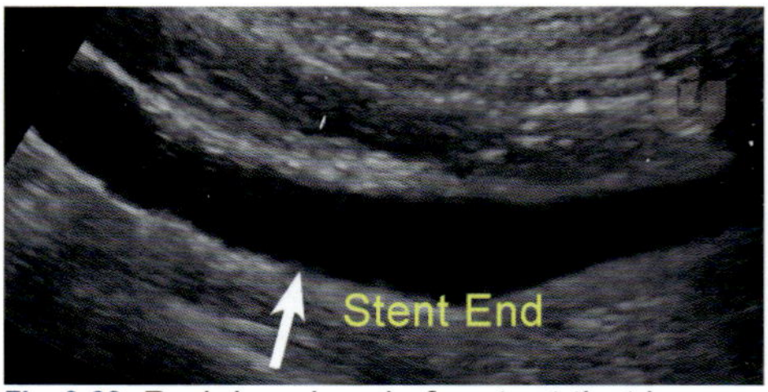

Fig. 8-28. *Peripheral end of a stent that is limited to the CIV, no extension into the EIV.*

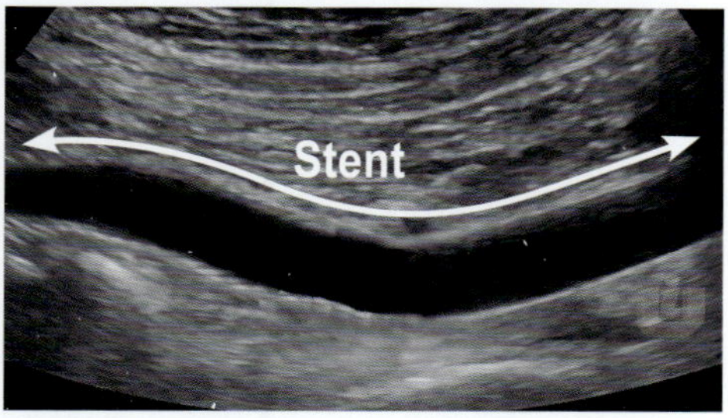

Fig. 8-29. *Left iliac vein stent extending from the IVC into the external iliac vein.*

- Follow the native iliac ultrasound protocol for the post-stenting duplex with the addition of the stent-specific measurements.
- Using B-mode, the stent is assessed along its length in longitudinal and transverse views to evaluate for any mural thrombus, visual narrowing, and intraluminal changes with particular attention paid to:
  - The region of prior compression
  - The peripheral and central ends of the stent.
- Use color Doppler, with a low scale setting for venous flow in a longitudinal view to assess the length of the stent and its inflow (native vein peripheral to the stent) and outflow (native vein central to the stent) for:
  - A color jet indicating a stenosis
  - A mosaic color flow pattern due to post stenotic turbulence at the following levels.
  - The absence of color flow indicating an occlusion
- Obtain PW Doppler waveforms in a longitudinal view using a ≤60° angle to evaluate for spontaneous flow in the following areas:
  - Inflow-to-the-stent (peripheral-to-the-stent)
  - Peripheral end-of-the-stent
  - Mid stent
  - Central end-of-the-stent
  - Outflow-of-the-stent (central-to-the-stent)
  - Additionally, peak vein velocities should be obtained at the level of a suspected stenosis, peripheral to the stenosis, and central to the stenosis

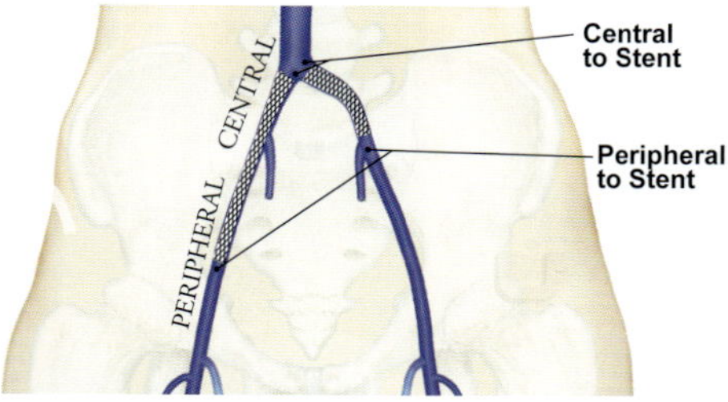

Fig. 8-30. *PW Doppler waveforms are obtained within the stent, peripheral and central to the stent. Note that two different lengths of stents are depicted. Stent length is provider-dependent.*

If a significant stenosis is suspected, the patient may have a repeat venogram and IVUS to determine the severity of stenosis, and treat it if needed.

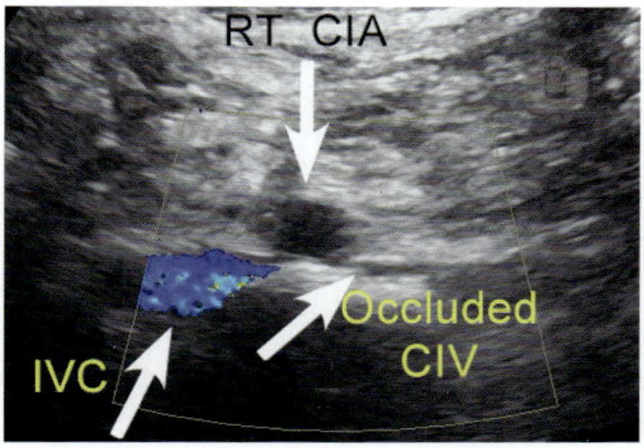

Fig. 8-31. *Near occlusion of the left CIV pre-stenting.*

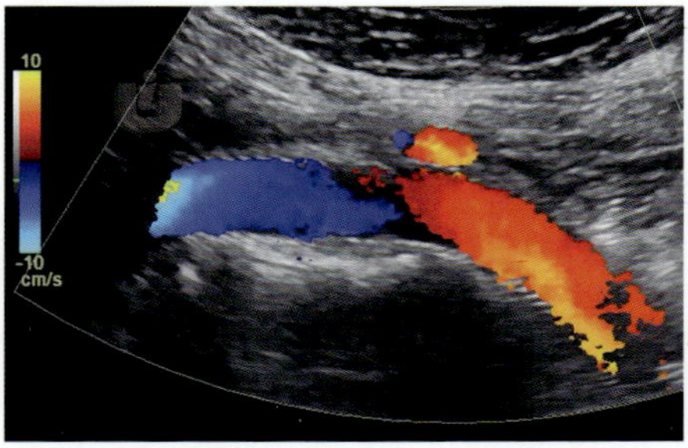

Fig. 8-32. *Resolution of the near occlusion of the left CIV post stenting.*

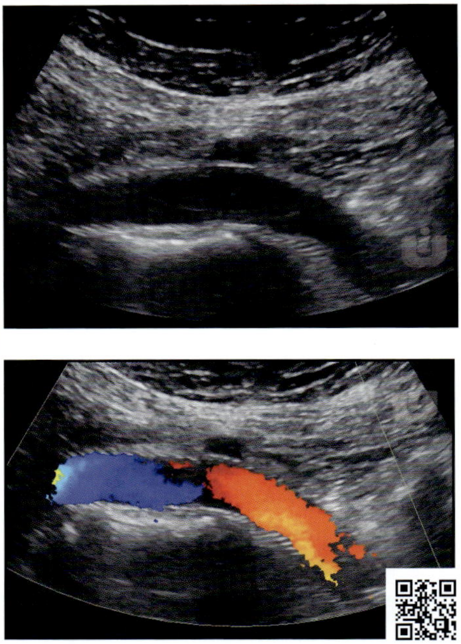

Fig. 8-33. *Cine loop of left CIV stent at the level of the right CIA.*

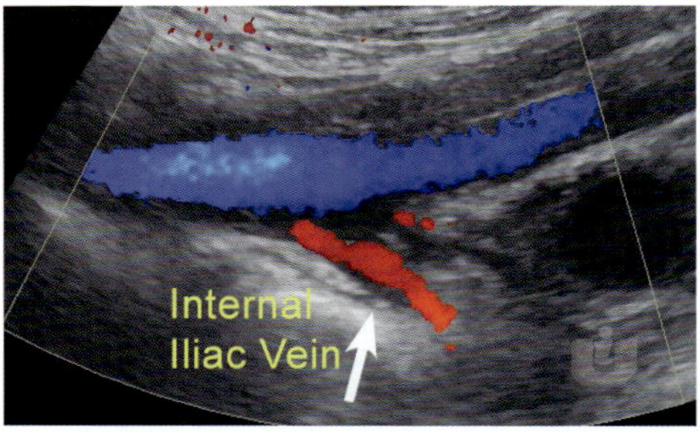

Fig. 8-34. *Patent left iliac vein stent extending into the EIV.*

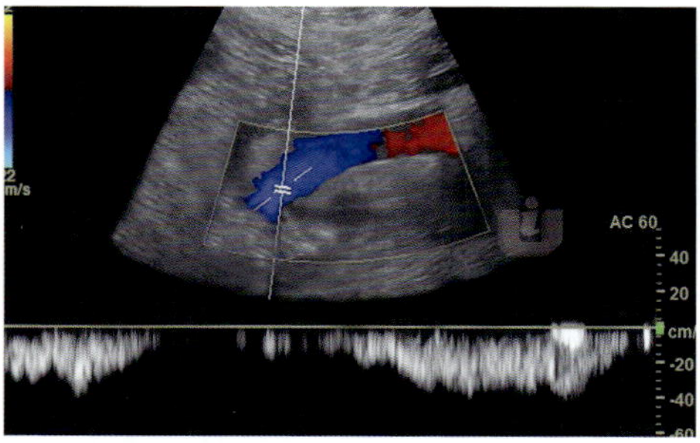

Fig. 8-35. *Spontaneous flow and respiratory variation within a CIV stent.*

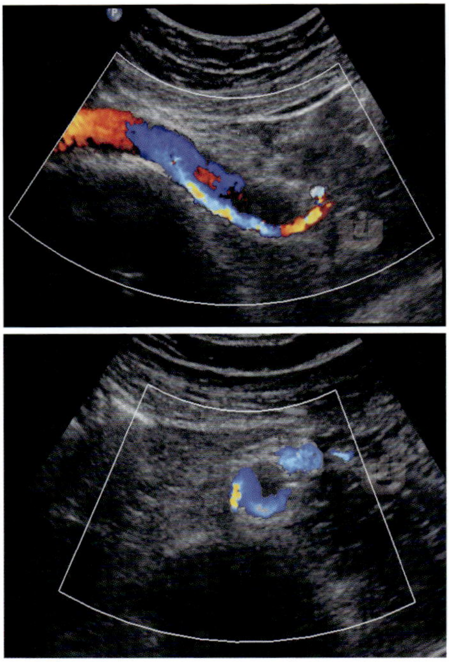

Fig. 8-36. *Longitudinal and transverse views of a partially thrombosed iliac vein stent demonstrating a lack of wall-to-wall color filling with visualization of the thrombus.*

Images courtesy of Aleta Rigsby RVT, RPhS VeinCare Centers of Tennessee

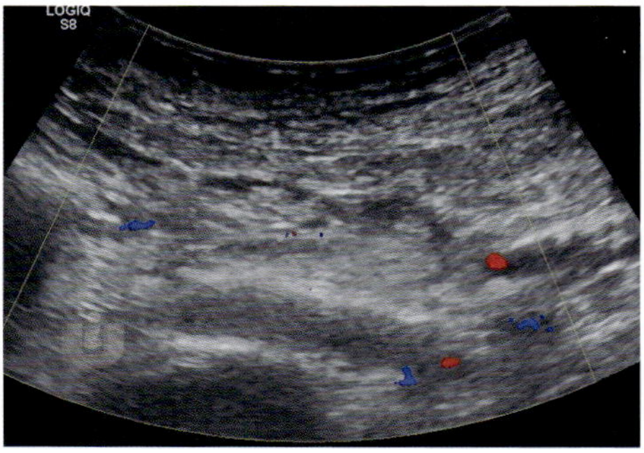

Fig. 8-37. *Longitudinal view demonstrating the absence of color flow in an occluded CIV stent.*

Iliac Venous Duplex Worksheet

Date ______________________ History ______________________

Name ______________________

DOB ______________________

MRN ______________________

Significant details are added to the diagram at the level of the anatomy that is being referred to. Including: Pathology, velocities, diameters and stents

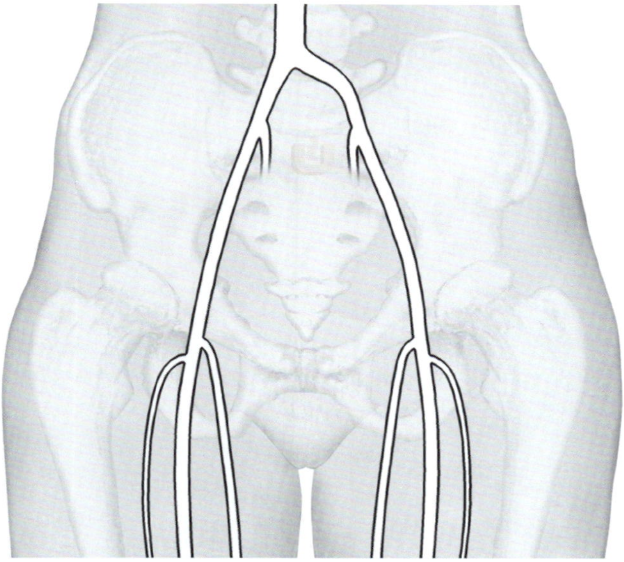

PW Doppler waveforms right to left comparison *Circle all that apply*

External iliac veins phasic aphasic symmetrical asymmetrical

Common iliac veins phasic aphasic symmetrical asymmetrical

Fig. 8-38. *Iliac vein worksheet. A PDF can be downloaded by scanning the QR code.*

Protocol: Venous Stenting

Stent deployment requires the support of multiple imaging modalities to locate diseased vessels and choose stent type and size to ensure proper deployment. Common imaging modalities include venography and IntraVascular Ultrasound (IVUS). Local anesthetic or mild IV sedation is administered.

- Venous access is obtained using a needle with ultrasound guidance.
- A guidewire is inserted into the vein via the needle's hub.
- The guidewire is advanced through the lesion.
- A venogram is performed to confirm the placement of the wire.
- The wire is advanced through to the IVC.

- A flash venogram is performed to confirm that the wire is in the IVC and has not extended into any collateral veins.
- A sheath is inserted into the vein over the guidewire to access the IVUS catheter and stent delivery system.
- The IVUS is inserted and positioned at the uppermost portion of the disease.
- Digital documentation of the IVUS is taken to demonstrate the full extent of the disease while confirming the severity of the stenosis.
- The IVUS catheter is moved centrally to a normal vein segment.
- Measurements are taken at the normal vein segment; the stent size is selected based on an average of the minimum and maximum diameter measurements.
  - Proper sizing of a stent is imperative to avoid stent migration.
  - Stent size is typically 2mm larger than the surrounding normal vein.
- A high-pressure non-compliant balloon catheter is inserted and inflated along the length of the lesion to disrupt any abnormal fibrotic tissue
- IVUS is used to identify the central stent location. It is recommended to start the stent at least 5mm central to the lesion and 5mm peripheral to the lesion.
- The stent device is inserted through the sheath, advanced through the lesion to 5mm beyond the lesion, and deployed.
  - For the successful landing of the stent, it must extend from one healthy vein segment to another.
  - Due to the curved nature of the iliac veins within the pelvis, a flexible stent system is ideal.
- The IVUS catheter is reintroduced to measure for the next stent deployment.
  - The ideal stent offers a wide range of sizes and lengths; the lesion's length will dictate the length and number of stents used.
- It is recommended that there is at least 1cm of overlap when multiple stents are needed to cover the length of a lesion.
  - The entire length of the stent system is re-dilated using the balloon catheter.
  - Self-expanding stents are used with post-placement balloon dilation to ensure that the stent is fully expanded.
- IVUS is used to confirm that the stent system is fully expanded along its length and confirms the location of the peripheral end of the stent.
- A final venogram is performed to confirm flow and absence of collateral vessels seen before the procedure.

Ideal vein stents have an increased wall strength to resist compression and can withstand repetitive motion.

There are two types of vein stents currently in use:

- **Wall stent:** *Braided, closed-cell design made with an elgiloy (a metallic wire)*
- **Nitinol stent:** *The majority have a non-braided, open-cell design made with a nickel-titanium metal*

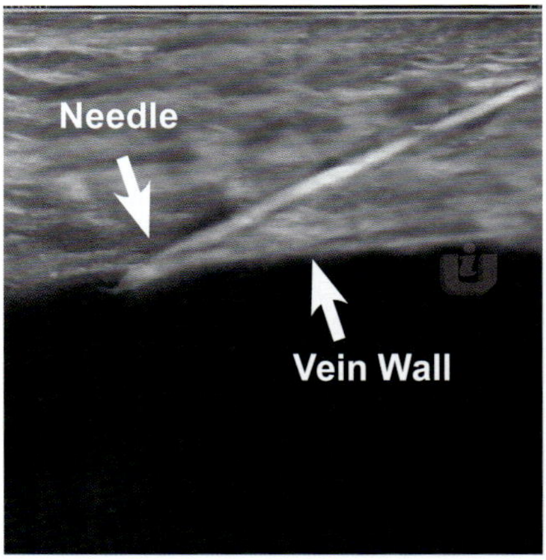

Fig. 8-39. *Ultrasound-guided venous access.*

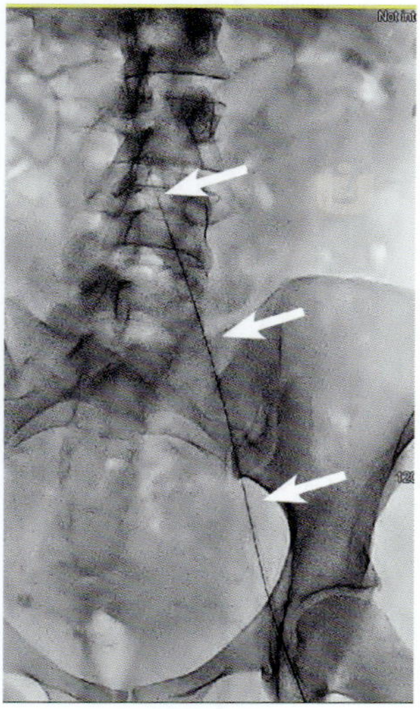

Fig. 8-40. *Visualization of the guidewire*

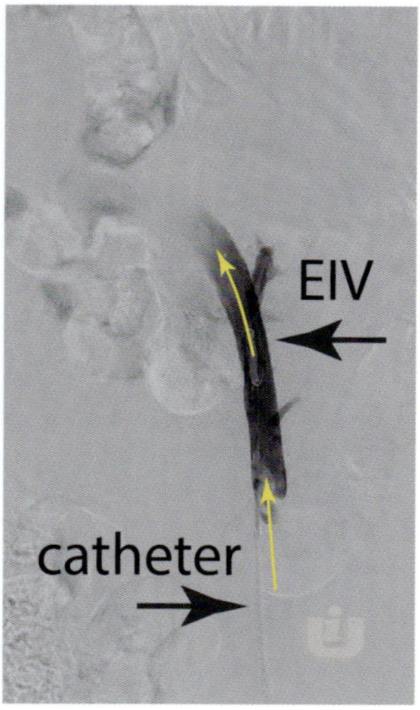

Fig. 8-41. *Injection of contrast is visualized using fluoroscopy as it moves centrally into the EIV.*

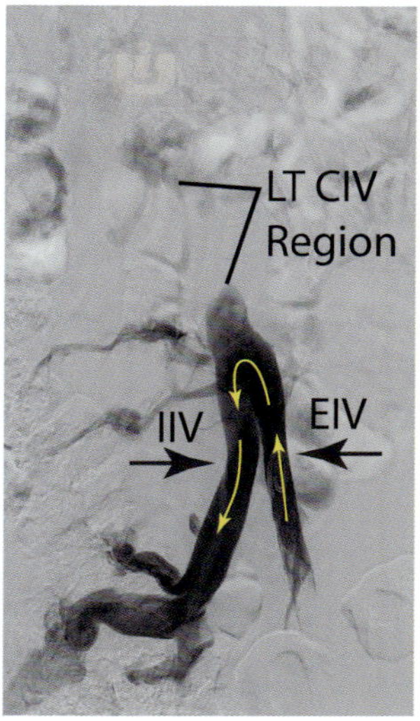

Fig. 8-42. *Contrast is visualized as it moves toward the EIV and IIV confluence. Note the absence of flow centrally toward the IVC, instead, it fills the left IIV. This is indicative of a near or complete occlusion of the CIV.*

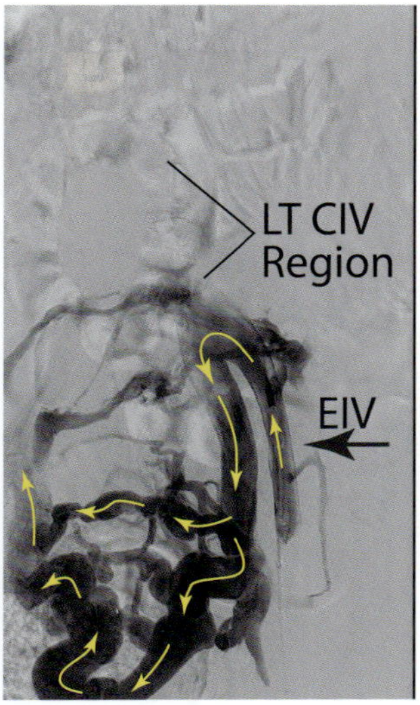

Fig. 8-43. *Contrast fills the contralateral IIV via pelvic collaterals.*

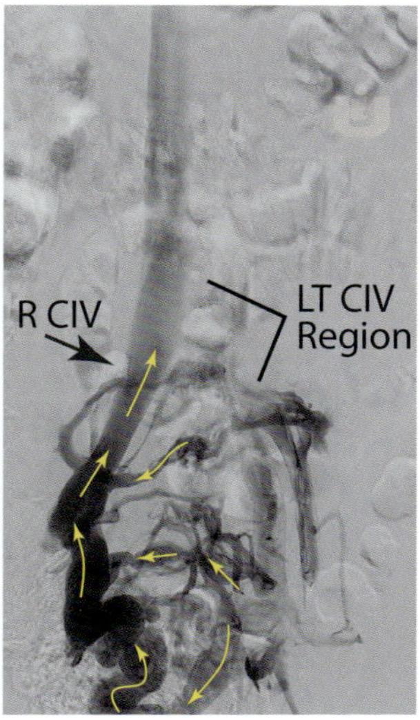

Fig. 8-44. *Contrast demonstrates the return of venous flow to the IVC via the contralateral CIV.*

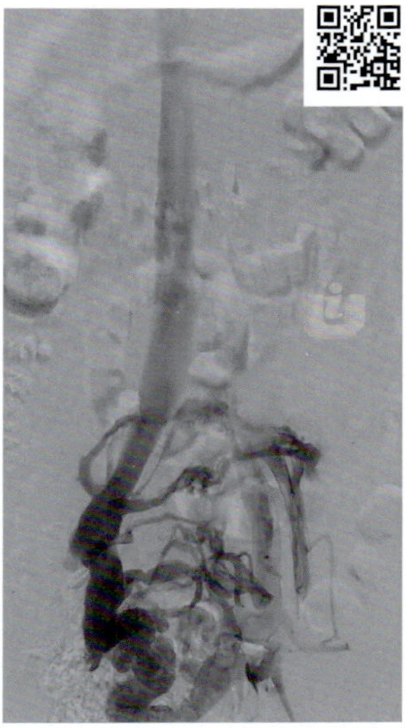

Fig. 8-45. *Cine loop using fluoroscopy with contrast demonstrates the absence of filling of the left CIV with cross pelvic collaterals allowing for venous outflow of the left lower extremity via the right CIV.*

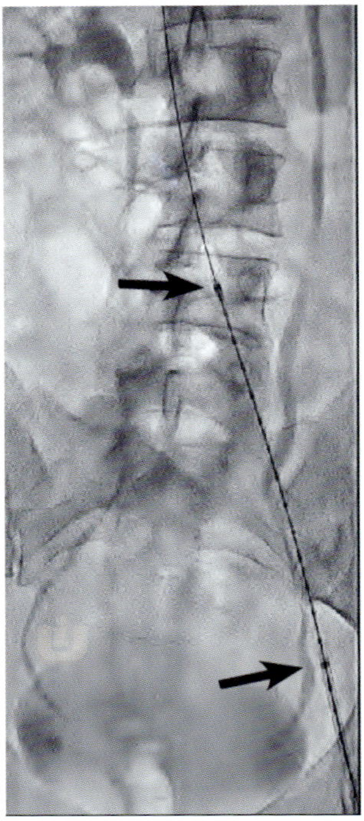

Fig. 8-46. *IVUS catheter.* *Note the markings on the catheter to aid in measuring the vessels.*

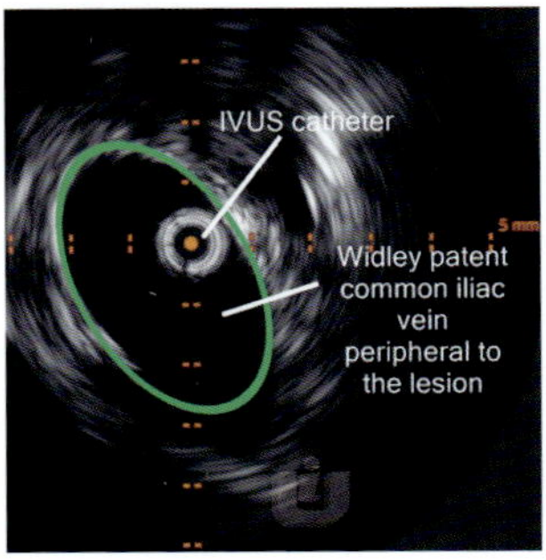

Fig. 8-47. *Visualization of the widely patent lumen of the peripheral left CIV.*

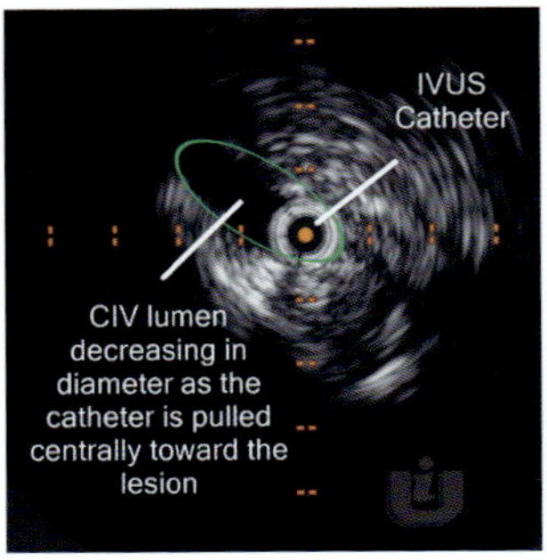

Fig. 8-48. *Visibly narrowed left CIV lumen as the catheter is moved centrally toward the lesion.*

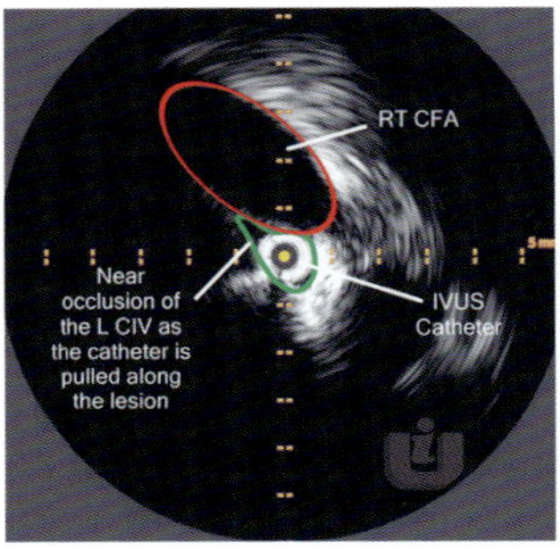

Fig. 8-49. *Near occlusion of the left CIV as the right CIA crosses anterior to it.*

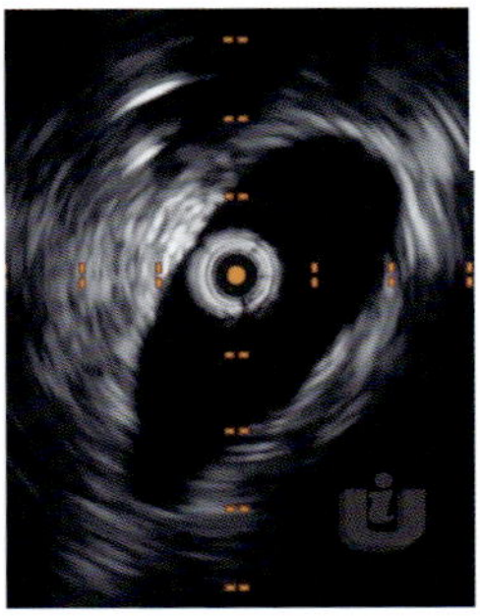

Fig. 8-50. *Cine loop of the IVUS catheter coursing from the peripheral CIV to the IVC. At the .08-second mark, note that the CIV lumen is beginning to narrow. At the .10-second mark, the Rt CIA courses anterior to the CIV, causing near occlusion, and at the .12 sec mark, the vein dilates as the catheter moves beyond the lesion.*

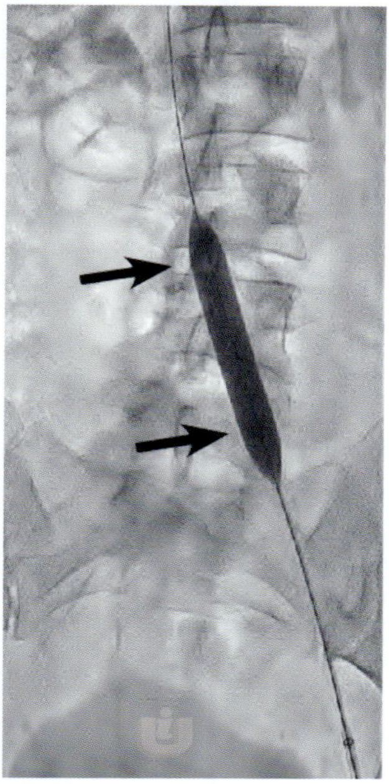

Fig. 8-51. *Balloon angioplasty pre-stent placement.*

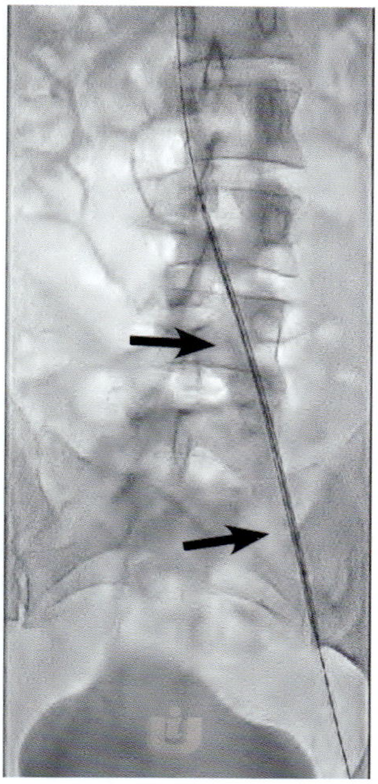

Fig. 8-52. *The venous stent is contained in an over-the-wire stent delivery catheter.*

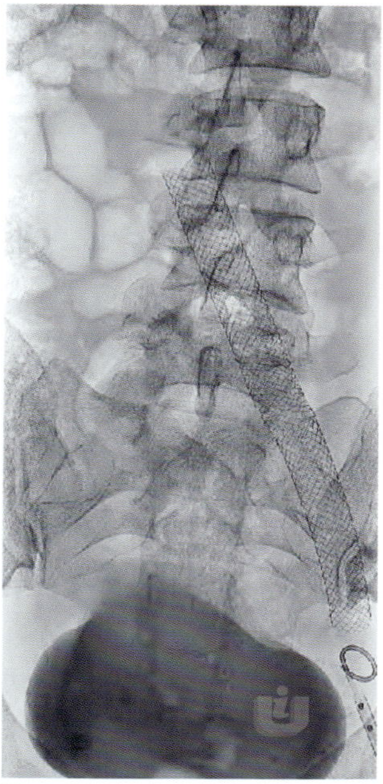

Fig. 8-53. *Fully deployed stent extending from the peripheral EIV to the IVC.*

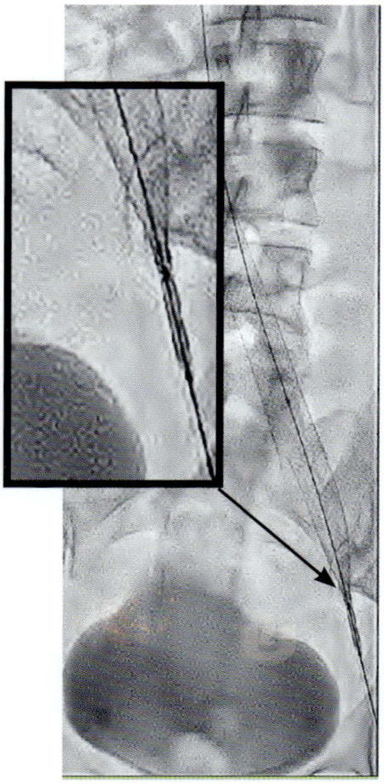

Fig. 8-54. *The stent is deployed and expands as the delivery system is withdrawn.*

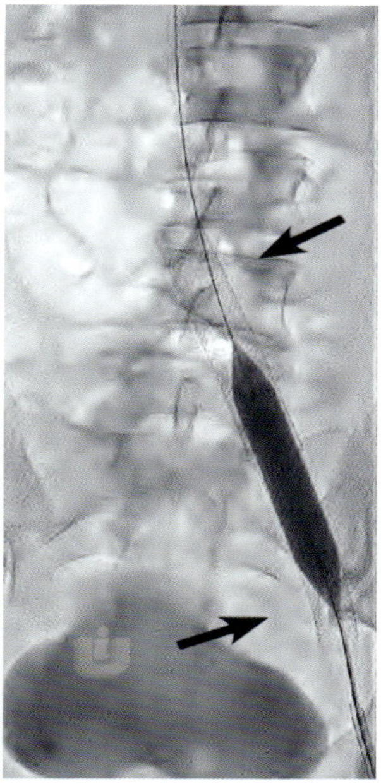

Fig. 8-55. *Balloon angioplasty is repeated in stent to ensure complete dilation of the stent.*

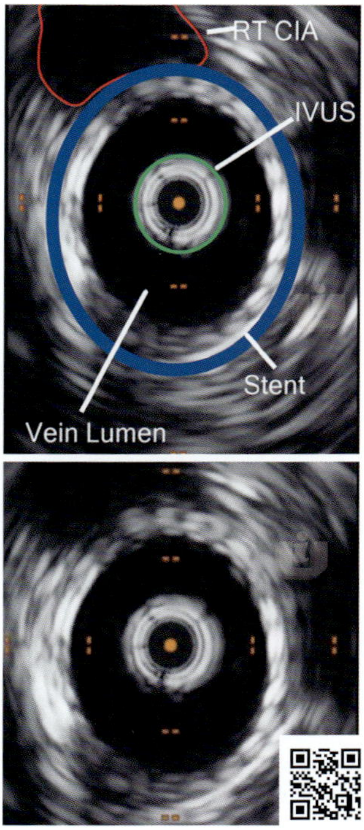

Fig. 8-56. *IVUS demonstrating widely patent stent at the level of the pre-stent lesion.*

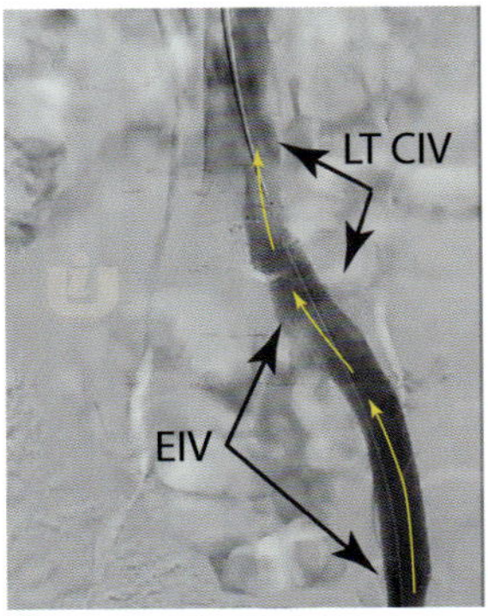

Fig. 8-57. *Cine of post-stenting fluoroscopy demonstrates decreased cross pelvic collaterals with left lower extremity outflow via the now widely patent left CIV.*

Interpretation-Diagnostic Criteria

Normal

Native IVC Illiac and Stent

B-mode Imaging

- The vein/stent is free of echogenic material
- **IVC/Native Iliac:** Variation of diameter is visualized in response to breathing
- **Stent:** No variation of diameter is visualized in response to breathing

Color Doppler

Spontaneous, antegrade color filling of the vein/stent with respiration

PW Doppler

- **Spontaneity:** The vein demonstrates spontaneous flow and symmetrical PW Doppler waveform compared to the contralateral vein.
- **Phasicity:** Venous flow varies with the respiratory and cardiac cycles. Phasicity is symmetrical when compared with the contralateral side.
- In stents, the symmetry from side to side may be slightly decreased due to the rigidity of the stent.

Abnormal [8,9,12,13,6,7,14]

B-mode Imaging

- Indirect signs of proximal obstruction/ occlusion
  - Difficulty in compressing the CFV
  - Presence of collateral veins
- Direct signs of iliac/stent obstruction or occlusion
  - Intraluminal changes, which may include thrombus, webbing, and fibrotic changes to the vein wall
  - Visible narrowing on grayscale, measure the pre-stenotic segment and the stenotic segment with calipers

Color Doppler

Color Doppler scale should be adjusted to allow for slow venous flow.

- Indirect signs
  - Reversal of flow in the ipsilateral IIV
  - Reversal of flow in the deep external pudendal vein
  - Cephalad flow in the inferior epigastric
- Direct signs
  - Absence of color flow
  - Presence of a color jet at the level of a suspected stenosis
  - Mosaic color flow pattern due to post stenotic turbulence

PW Doppler

PW Doppler scale should be adjusted to allow for slow venous flow.

- Indirect signs
  - Non-phasic flow in the proximal CFV
  - Asymmetrical flow pattern in the CFVs
  - Non-phasic flow during Valsalva maneuver
  - Low or no velocity augmentation in CFV during thigh compression or dorsi/ plantar flexion
- Direct signs
  - **Native iliac:** Peak vein velocity ratio of >2.5 when comparing the peak vein velocity of the pre- stenotic (peripheral) segment to the peak vein velocity at the stenosis
  - **Stented iliac:** Localized increase in peak vein velocity indicates an in-stent stenosis.

At present, there are no published validated diagnostic criteria to determine the severity of an in-stent stenosis.

Table 8-2. **Iliac Vein and Stent Obstruction Duplex Scan Diagnostic Criteria**

	B-mode	PW Doppler	Color Doppler
CIV and EIV	• Visible narrowing of the vein lumen • Presence of collateral veins	• Peak vein velocity ratio >2.5 (point of obstruction ÷ peripheral segment) • Lack of symmetrical and phasic waveforms when comparing left to right	• Absence of color flow • Presence of a color jet at the level of a suspected stenosis • Mosaic color flow pattern due to post stenotic turbulence
Stent	• Visible narrowing of the stent lumen	• Localized increase in peak vein velocity	• Same as above
IIV	• Presence of collateral veins	• Retrograde flow (spontaneous or with provocative maneuvers)	• Reversal of color flow with provocative maneuvers

References

1. Raju S. (2013). Best management options for chronic iliac vein stenosis and occlusion. *Journal of vascular surgery, 57*(4), 1163–1169.
2. Meissner, M. H., Khilnani, N. M., Labropoulos, N., Gasparis, A. P., Gibson, K., Greiner, M., Learman, L. A., Atashroo, D., Lurie, F., Passman, M. A., Basile, A., Lazarshvilli, Z., Lohr, J., Kim, M. D., Nicolini, P. H., Pabon-Ramos, W. M., & Rosenblatt, M. (2021). The Symptoms-Varices-Pathophysiology classification of pelvic venous disorders: A report of the American Vein & Lymphatic Society International Working Group on Pelvic Venous Disorders. *Journal of vascular surgery: Venous and lymphatic disorders, 9*(3), 568–584.
3. Shi, W., & Dowell, J. D. (2017). Etiology and treatment of acute inferior vena cava thrombosis. *Thrombosis research, 149*, 9–16. https://doi.org/10.1016/j.thromres.2016.07.010
4. Morita, S., Higuchi, M., Saito, N., & Mitsuhashi, N. (2007). Pelvic venous variations in patients with congenital inferior vena cava anomalies: Classification with computed tomography. *Acta Radiologica, 48*(9), 974–979. https://doi.org/10.1080/02841850701499409
5. Labropoulos, N., Jasinski, P. T., Adrahtas, D., Gasparis, A. P., & Meissner, M. H. (2017). A standardized ultrasound approach to pelvic congestion syndrome. *Phlebology, 32*(9), 608–619. https://doi.org/10.1177/0268355516677135
6. Kayılıoğlu, S. I., Köksoy, C., & Alaçayır, İ. (2016). Diagnostic value of the femoral vein flow pattern for detecting an iliocaval venous obstruction. *Journal of vascular surgery: Venous and lymphatic disorders, 4*(1), 2–8. https://doi.org/10.1016/j.jvsv.2015.08.002
7. Labropoulos N. (2018). Diagnosis of iliac vein obstruction with duplex ultrasound: Criteria used during duplex ultrasound examination to identify iliac vein obstruction. *Endovascular Today, 17*(7), 50–52.
8. O'Sullivan, G.J. (2020). What is the best method of imaging in iliofemoral venous obstruction? *Phlebolymphology, 27*(2). 61-69.
9. Labropoulos, N., Borge, M., Pierce, K., & Pappas, P. J. (2007). Criteria for defining significant central vein stenosis with duplex ultrasound. *Journal of Vascular Surgery, 46*(1), 101–107. https://doi.org/10.1016/j.jvs.2007.02.062
10. Raju, S., Tackett, P., Jr, & Neglen, P. (2009). Reinterventions for nonocclusive iliofemoral venous stent malfunctions. *Journal of Vascular Surgery, 49*(2), 511–518. https://doi.org/10.1016/j.jvs.2008.08.003
11. Gibson, K. (July 2021). Iliac Vein Stenting: Best Practices for Patient Safety and Successful Outcomes. Endovascular Today. https://evtoday.com/articles/2021-july/iliac-vein-stenting-best-practices-for-patient-safety-and-successful-outcomes
12. Mousa, A. Y., Broce, M., Yacoub, M., & AbuRahma, A. F. (2016). Iliac Vein Interrogation Augments Venous Ulcer Healing in Patients Who Have Failed Standard Compression Therapy along with Pathological Venous Closure. *Annals of Vascular Surgery, 34*, 144–151.
13. Metzger, P. B., Rossi, F. H., Kambara, A. M., Izukawa, N. M., Saleh, M. H., Pinto, I. M., Amorim, J. E., & Thorpe, P. E. (2016). Criteria for detecting significant chronic iliac venous obstructions with duplex ultrasound. *Journal of vascular surgery: Venous and lymphatic disorders, 4*(1), 18–27.
14. MayR., & Thurner, J. (1957). The cause of the predominantly sinistral occurrence of thrombosis of the pelvic veins. *Angiology, 8*(5), 419–427.
15. Dawson, D.L., Beals, H. (2010). Acute lower extremity deep venous thrombosis. In R.E. Zierler (Ed.), Strandess's duplex scanning disorders in vascular diagnosis (4th ed., pp. 179-198). Philadelphia Wolters Kluwer Lippincott Williams & Wilkins.
16. Zwiebel, W.J. (2005). Ultrasound assessment of the aorta, iliac arteries and inferior vena cava. In W.J. Zwiebel & J.S. Pellerito (Eds.), Introduction to vascular ultrasonography (5th ed., pp. 530-552). Philadelphia: Elsevier Saunders.

Pelvic Venous System

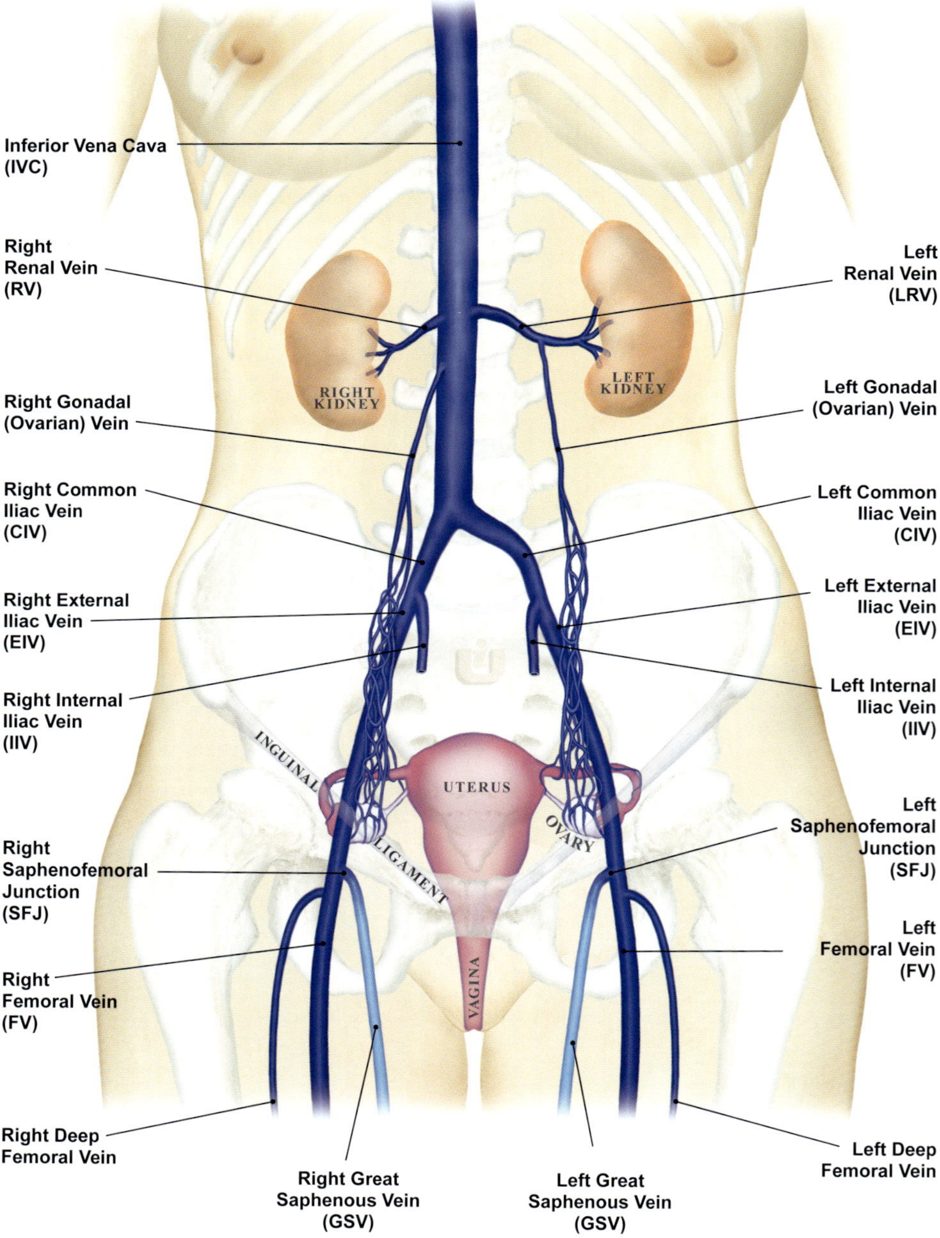

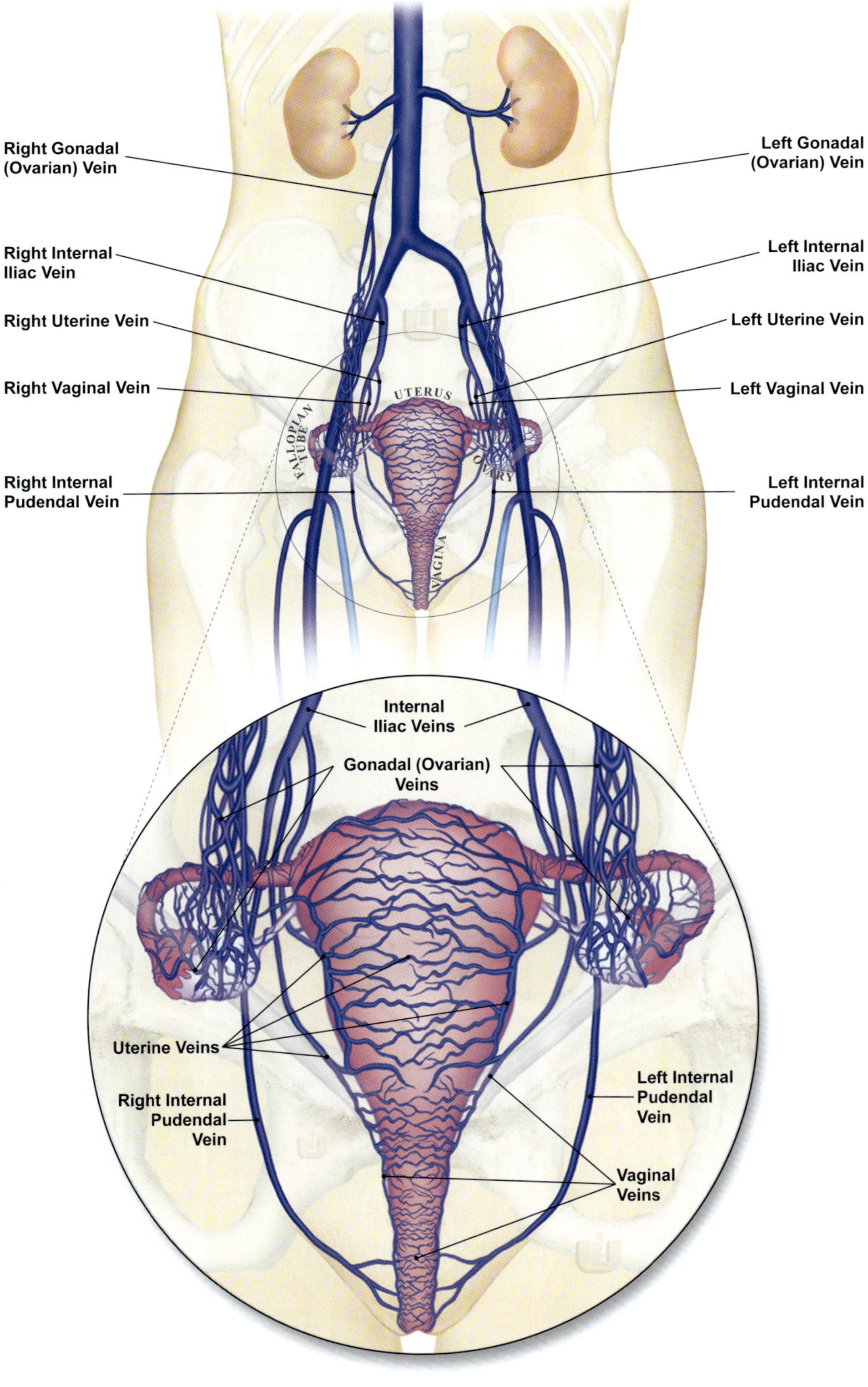
Right Gonadal (Ovarian) Vein
Left Gonadal (Ovarian) Vein
Right Internal Iliac Vein
Left Internal Iliac Vein
Right Uterine Vein
Left Uterine Vein
Right Vaginal Vein
Left Vaginal Vein
UTERUS
FALLOPIAN TUBE
OVARY
VAGINA
Right Internal Pudendal Vein
Left Internal Pudendal Vein
Internal Iliac Veins
Gonadal (Ovarian) Veins
Uterine Veins
Right Internal Pudendal Vein
Left Internal Pudendal Vein
Vaginal Veins

Definition

The combination of real-time B-mode ultrasonography with Pulsed Wave (PW) Doppler and color flow to evaluate the veins of the abdomen and pelvis for evidence of anatomical and/or flow abnormalities, valvular incompetence, and obstruction.

Etiology [1,2]

- **Thrombotic**
  - Reflux arising from a previous DVT
  - Obstruction arising from a previous DVT
- **Nonthrombotic**
  - Reflux arising from a degenerative process of the vein wall
  - Reflux arising from a proximal obstruction due to an extrinsic compression
- **Congenital**
  - Venous malformation
  - Mixed vascular malformation

Risk Factors

- Pre-menopausal, re-menopausal
- Pregnancy, especially multigravida and multiparous (more than one child at birth)
- Chronic pelvic pain
- Low BMI
- Previous DVT (particularly in the iliocaval system)
- Family history of venous insufficiency
- Varicose veins

> *During pregnancy, there is a significant increase in intravascular volume (up to 60%). Blood pooling or engorgement of the uterine or pelvic veins may have a mass effect on nearby nerves and be a source of pelvic pain. In multiparous patients this recurring distention of the veins may render the valves incompetent.*

Indications for Exam

Pelvic Symptoms

- Chronic pelvic pain present for more than 6 months [8]
- Pressure or heaviness deep within the pelvis
- Dyspareunia (pain during and after intercourse)
- Pelvic or genital pain when sitting or standing for long periods of time

Renal Symptoms

- Left flank pain
- Hematuria

Lower extremity symptoms

- Varicose veins of upper thigh, buttocks, and genitals [23]
- Lower extremity edema/swelling, especially when unilateral
- Recurring lower extremity varicose veins post previous procedures, such as stripping and ligation, endovenous ablation (thermal or chemical), cyanoacrylate (glue), or phlebectomy
- Venous claudication [25]
  - Deep pain with physical exercise increases with intensity and feels constrictive in the calf or thigh.
  - Culminates in function impairment
  - Symptoms only dissipate when the leg is positioned to enhance venous drainage (leg raised)
- Sciatic nerve pain

Contraindications/Limitations

- Pregnancy
- Poor visualization due to vessel depth, obesity, and bowel gas
- Recent pelvic surgery within 2 months; surgical scarring

Mechanism of Disease [1, 2, 3]

- The venous system of the pelvis can be considered to consist of 3 reservoirs where varices may develop.
  - The renal hilum
  - The venous plexuses of the pelvis

- The pelvic origin extrapelvic veins (tributaries of the internal iliac vein that arise in the pelvis but drain structures outside of the pelvis, e.g., genitals and buttocks)
- The lower extremity veins comprise a fourth reservoir, which may communicate with pelvic origin extrapelvic varices.
  - This reservoir differs from the other three because, although it often communicates with the pelvic origin extrapelvic veins, the severity of the lower extremity venous disease should be determined using the lower extremity classification scale known as CEAP.
    - » The CEAP scale is well defined in the *Vascular Diseases* and *Venous Insufficiency* chapters.
    - » The severity of the pelvic venous disease is determined using the SVP scale, which is defined later in this chapter.
- Increased venous pressures arising from proximal reflux or obstruction are transmitted to these reservoirs, where symptoms related to either varices or increased venous pressure may develop.
- Increased central venous pressure of the pelvic veins leads to the development of peri-uterine and trans-uterine varicosities.
  - This increased pressure occurs due to a more central obstruction and/or reflux. These may occur concurrently or independently.

Obstruction

Obstruction is most likely to occur in the Left Renal Vein (LRV)and left Common Iliac Vein (CIV)

- Extrinsic pathology
  - Mechanical (extrinsic) compression of a vein due to an overlying artery or other anatomic structure, which results in obstruction.
  - These types of compression are known as Nonthrombotic Iliac Vein Lesions (NIVLs).
- Intrinsic pathology
  - Development of an obstruction within the vein.
    - » Chronic pulsatile compression of an iliac vein by an overlying iliac artery stimulates the formation of fibrotic adhesions that can cause partial or complete iliac vein obstruction over time. This finding is associated with NIVLs.
    - » Changes associated with previous DVT

The left CIV is the most likely to have obstructive pathology. Compression of the right CIV and bilateral external iliac veins have been documented.

Reflux

Reflux is most likely to occur in the:
- Gonadal veins
- Internal iliac veins and their tributaries

Reflux within the pelvic veins has been described as uncompensated or compensated based on the anatomy and patient symptoms.

- Uncompensated reflux
  - Venous pressure is transmitted directly to the peripheral venous reservoirs (renal hilum, venous plexuses of the pelvis)
  - Will result in the development of symptoms at the location of the involved vein.
- Compensated reflux
  - Venous pressure is decompressed via collaterals into the more peripheral venous reservoirs. (Venous plexuses of the pelvis, pelvic origin extrapelvic veins, lower extremities)
  - Resulting in the development of symptoms in the peripheral venous reservoir not at the direct site of the obstruction.

Peri-uterine/Trans-uterine Veins

The peri- and trans-uterine veins are a venous reservoir that is affected by the majority of the more central obstruction and/or refluxing veins. [3]

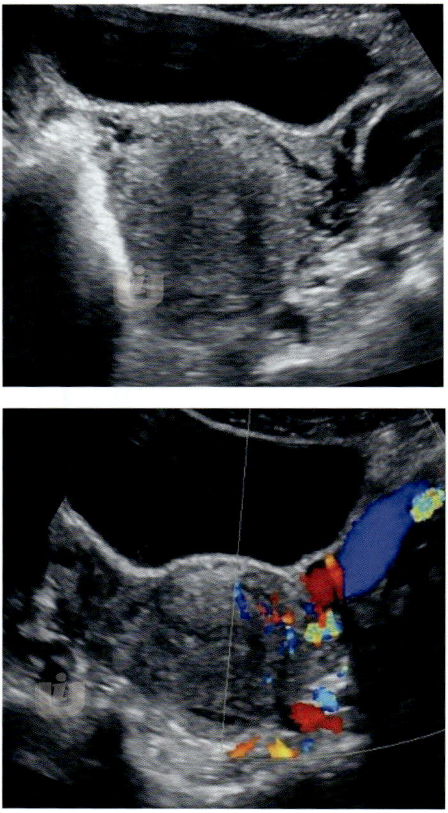

Fig. 9-1. *Transabdominal approach demonstrating the peripheral portion of the left gonadal vein in a transverse view. (with and without color flow)*

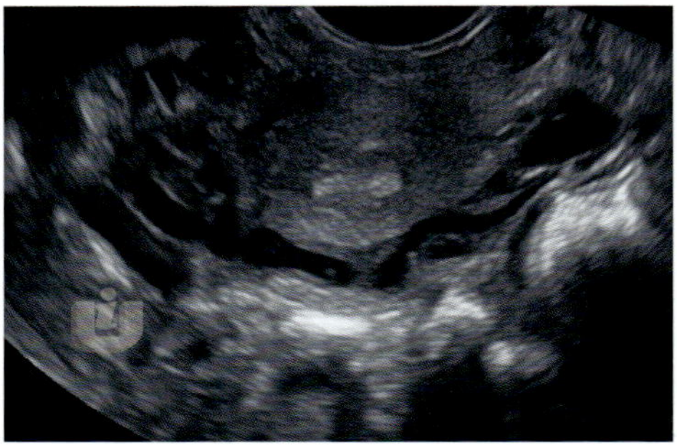

Fig. 9-2. *Endovaginal approach demonstrating peri- and trans-uterine varicose veins.*

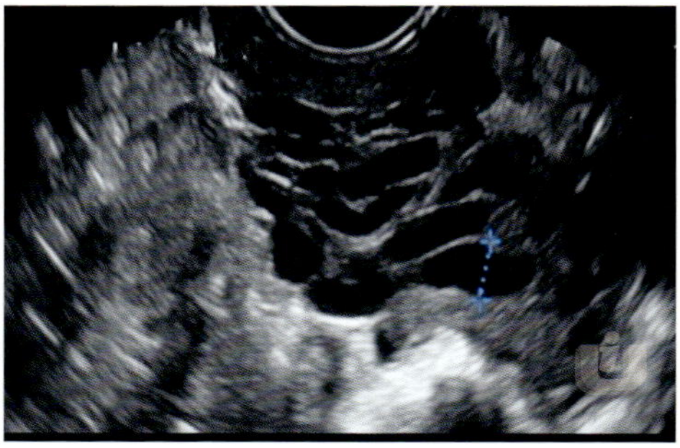

Fig. 9-3. *Endovaginal approach demonstrating peri-uterine varicose veins in a longitudinal view.*

Reflux

- Uncompensated
  - Results in an increase in the number of varicose veins present in the pelvis
  - Will most likely present with pelvic pain.
  - Could present with antegrade flow within the contralateral gonadal vein
- Compensated
  - Results in genital varicosities and sometimes, lower extremity varicose veins via the pelvic escape points (the connections between the pelvis and the lower extremities)
  - Most likely present with pelvic and genital symptoms and sometimes lower extremity venous symptoms.

Common Iliac Veins

The left Common Iliac Vein (CIV) is the most likely to have obstructive pathology. Compression of the right CIV and bilateral External Iliac Veins (EIV) have been documented.

Obstruction

- May occur due to extrinsic compression by the overlying Common Iliac Artery (CIA)
  - Fibrotic changes to the walls of the vein occur due to the repetitive pulsations of the overlying artery
- Due to the development of an obstruction within the vein lumen
  - Post-thrombotic changes occur, such as synechia (a fibrous membrane that remains in the vein)
- A stretching of the CIV over the spine

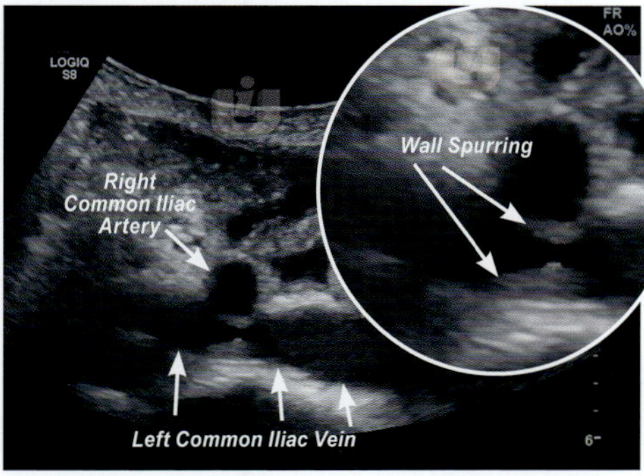

Fig. 9-4. *Compression of the left CIV causing fibrotic changes in the vein walls.*

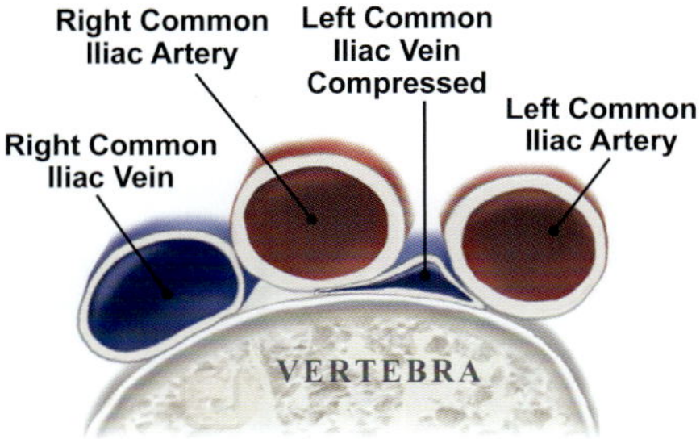

Fig. 9-5. *Transverse view of the left CIV being compressed between the vertebra and the right and left common iliac arteries.*

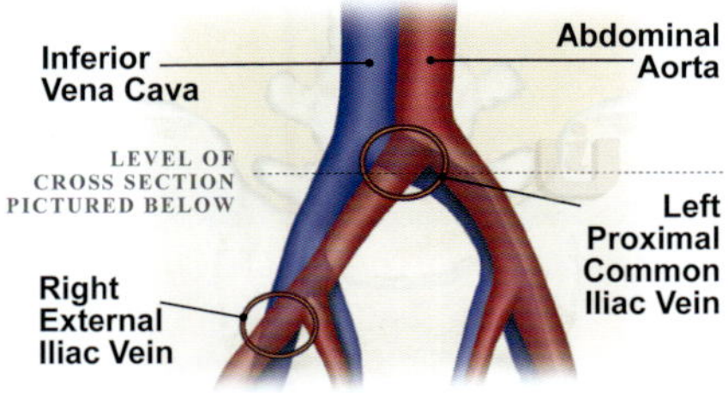

Fig. 9-6. *Most frequently occurring NIVLs.*

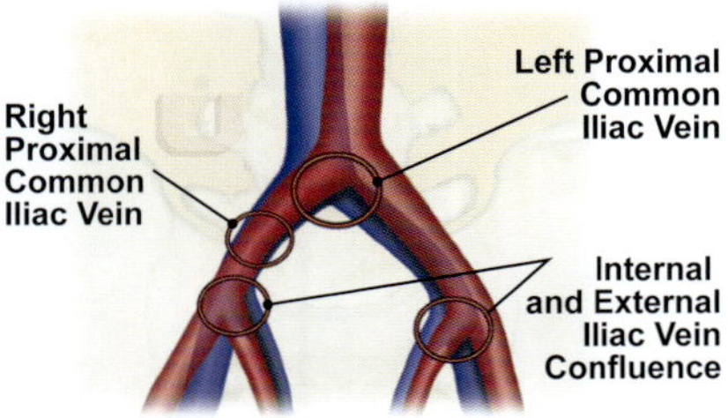

Fig. 9-7. *Less frequently occurring NIVLs.*

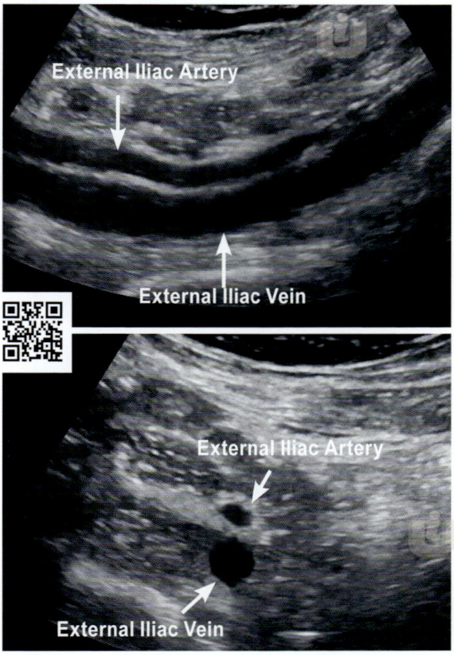

Fig. 9-8. *EIV in longitudinal and transverse views demonstrating pulsatile, repetitive compression of the EIV by the overlying external iliac artery (EIA). This repetitive compression can cause damage to the walls of the vein, which can disrupt flow.*

Reflux

- Uncompensated *(Fig. 9-22)*
  - Venous pressure is transmitted directly to the lower extremity veins resulting in lower extremity venous hypertension.
  - Most likely presents with lower extremity swelling, fullness, and pain
  - In more severe cases, patients may present with venous claudication (deep pain with physical exercise increases with intensity and feels constrictive in the calf or thigh)
- Compensated *(Fig. 9-23)*
  - Venous pressure is transmitted to the peripheral venous reservoirs resulting in hypertension of the left internal iliac vein and its branches. *(Fig. 9-9)*
  - Resulting in the formation of pelvic varicosities with or without the development of pelvic origin genital varicosities and/or lower extremity varicosities.
  - Most likely presents with chronic pelvic pain

Internal Iliac Veins

Reflux

- Primary valvular dysfunction
- Uncompensated *(Fig. 9-24)*
  - Venous pressure is transmitted directly to the peripheral venous reservoirs resulting in peri- and trans-uterine varicosities.
- Most likely presents with chronic pelvic pain
- Compensated *(Fig. 9-25)*
  - Venous pressure is transmitted to the extrapelvic tributaries, resulting in genital varicosities without or with lower extremity varicose veins.
  - Chronic pelvic pain and genital and/or lower extremity venous symptoms are most likely present.

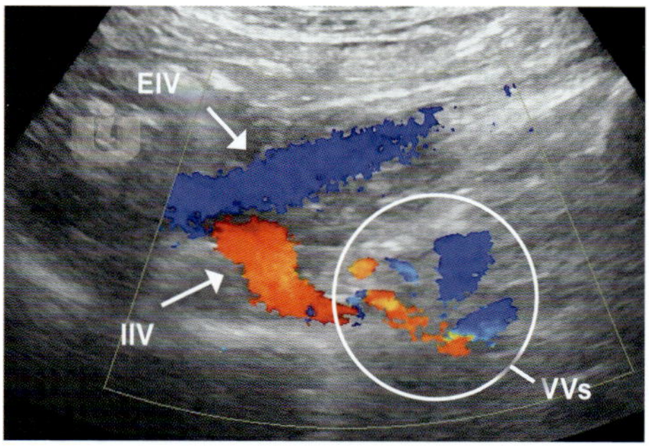

Fig. 9-9. *Transabdominal color flow demonstrating varicose veins of the IIV.*

Left Renal Vein

Obstruction

- Extrinsic compression by surrounding anatomy, such as the superior mesenteric artery (SMA), aorta, and spine.
- A secondary stretching of the vein over the aorta caused by an anatomical variant, renal ptosis or floating kidney. The kidney descends more than 2 vertebral bodies (or >5cm) during a position change.[4]

Reflux

- Uncompensated *(Fig. 9-20)*
  - Venous pressure is transmitted directly to the renal hilum resulting in renal hilar varicosities.
  - Most likely presents with left flank pain and hematuria
- Compensated *(Fig. 9-21)*
  - Venous pressure is transmitted to the peri- and trans-uterine veins via the left gonadal vein without or with genital/lower extremity varicosities.
  - Most likely presents with chronic pelvic pain without or with lower extremity symptoms.

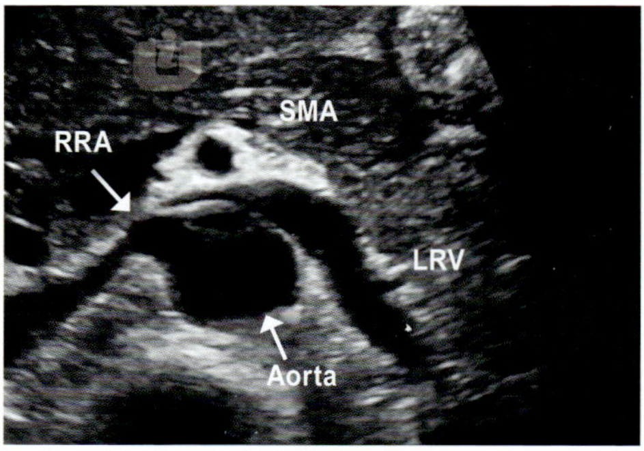

Fig. 9-10. *Stretching of the LRV over the right renal artery (RRA).*

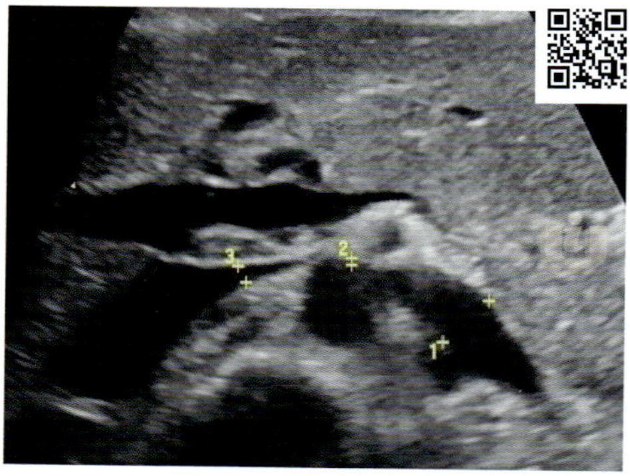

Fig. 9-11. *Compression of the LRV by the overlying SMA in the longitudinal view.*

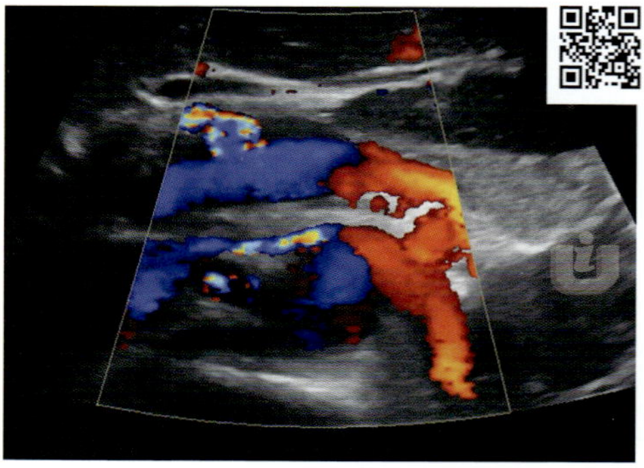

Fig. 9-12. *Color flow aliasing demonstrates a velocity increase as the LRV stretches over the aorta.*

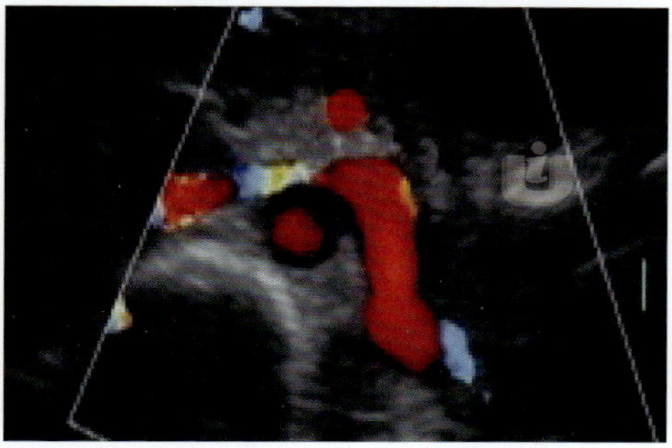

Fig. 9-13. *LRV stenosis caused by the stretching of the renal vein over the aorta.*

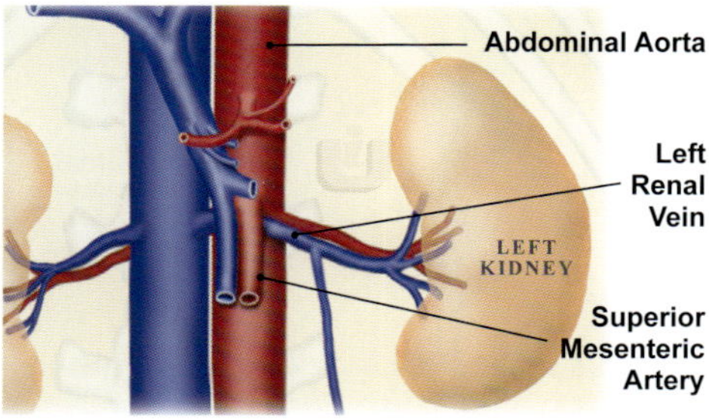

Fig. 9-14. *Mid-visceral anatomy. Note how the LRV courses between the aorta and SMA.*

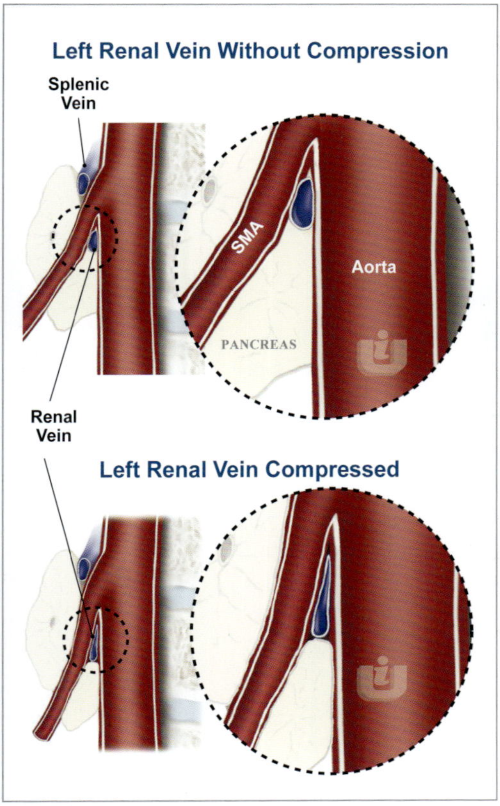

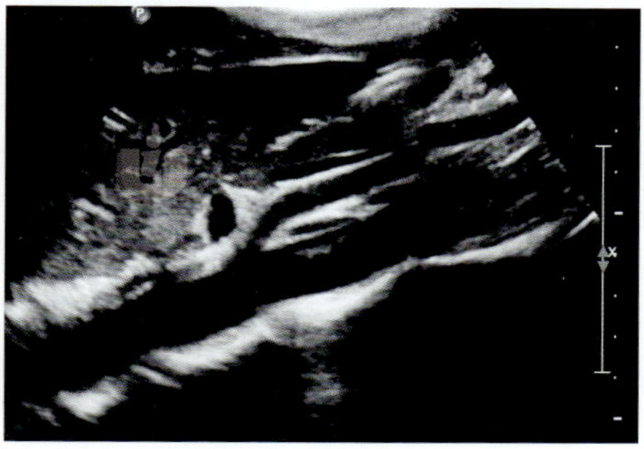

Fig. 9-15. *Longitudinal view of the LRV coursing between the aorta and SMA.*

Image courtesy of Diana Neuhardt, RPhS, RVT

Gonadal Veins

Reflux

- Gonadal vein reflux, uncompensated or compensated results in the formation of pelvic varicosities.
- Compensatory left gonadal vein reflux is due to LRV compression.
- Gonadal vein reflux can contribute to pelvic varicosities, which, if compensated, results in lower extremity and/or genital varicose veins via the pelvic escape points.
  - Uncompensated pelvic varicosities most likely present with chronic pelvic pain.
  - Compensated pelvic varicosities present with chronic pelvic pain, genital, and/or lower extremity venous symptoms.
- Right gonadal vein reflux may be considered a rarer source of pelvic varicose veins and should not be overlooked.

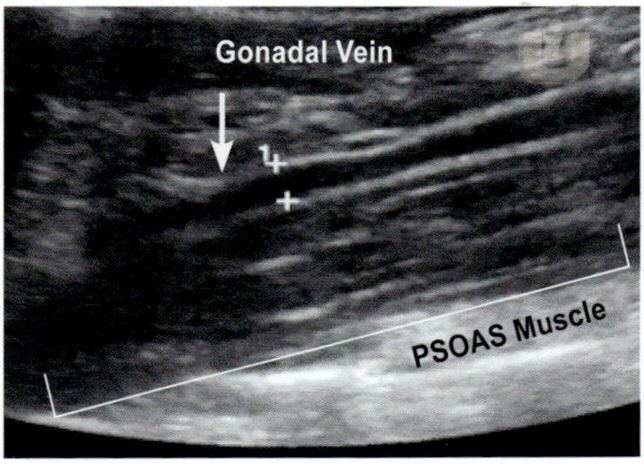

Fig. 9-16. *Image demonstrating a dilated left gonadal vein coursing along the anterior wall of the psoas muscle in a longitudinal view.*

Bilaterally, primary valvular dysfunction, can occur due to increased pressure over time due to multiple pregnancies versus genetic valvular disease.

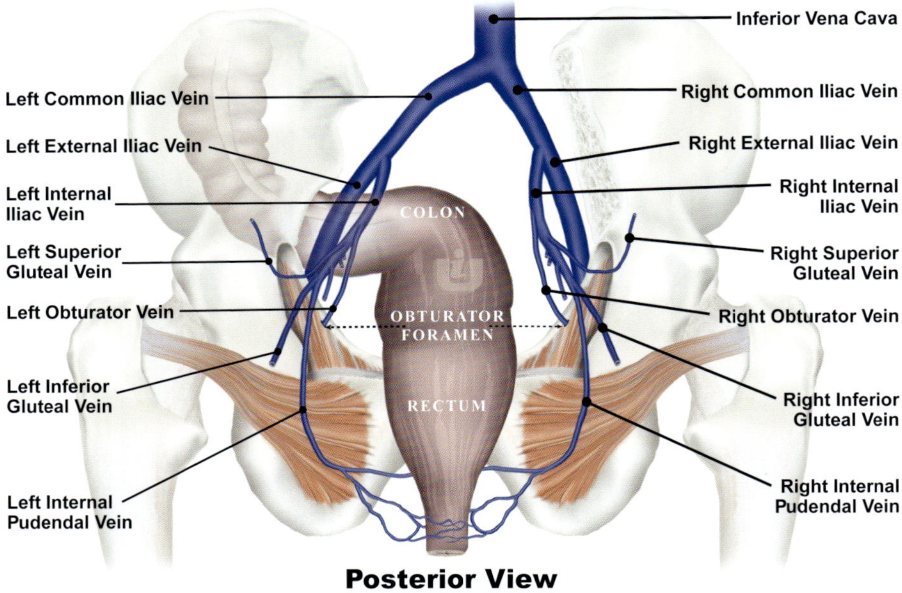

Fig. 9-17. *Posterior view of the internal iliac vein branches that act as a connection between the pelvis and the lower extremity in the setting of pelvic venous disorders. These are known as pelvic escape points.*

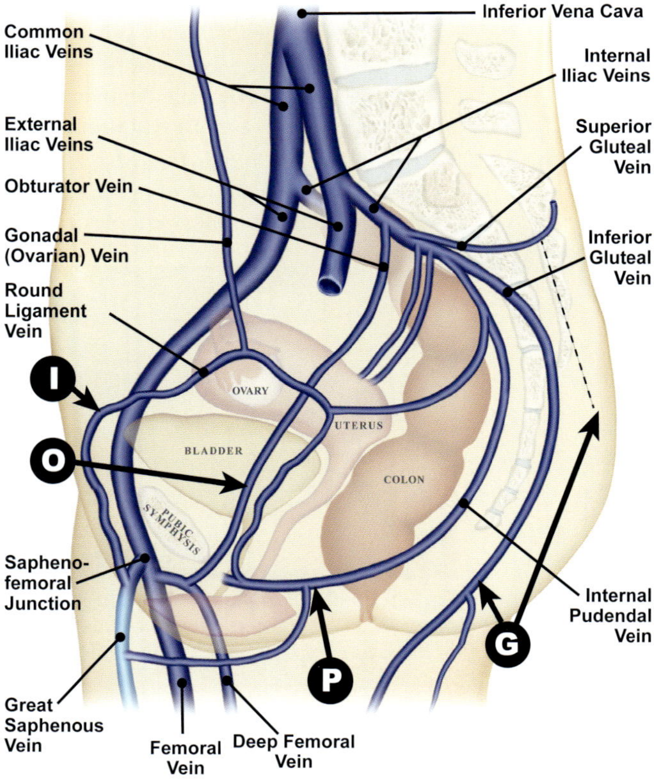

Fig. 9-18.

I = inguinal escape point

O = obturator escape point,

P= perineal escape point

G = gluteal escape point(s)

Pelvic Escape Points

- More central venous obstruction or primary valvular dysfunction results in venous hypertension within the pelvis veins.
- Retrograde (refluxing) flow in the extrapelvic veins exit the pelvis via their associated pelvic escape points.
- The pelvic escape points allow for compensation of flow for pelvic varicosities.
- The pelvic escape points and their associated IIV tributaries are:
  - Inguinal escape point, round ligament vein
  - Obturator escape point, obturator vein
  - Perineal escape point, pudendal veins
  - Gluteal (Superior and Inferior) escape points, gluteal veins

Symptoms, Varices and Pathophysiology (SVP) of Pelvic Venous Disorders [1]

Due to the complex nature of pelvic venous disorders, the American Vein and Lymphatic Society convened an international, multidisciplinary panel to develop a classification instrument for pelvic venous disorders. The varying patterns of reflux based on the path that the refluxing blood takes are depicted in Fig. 9-20 through 9-25.

The classification instrument contains three categories:

- Symptoms (S) (*Table 9-1)*
- Varices (V) *(Table 9-2)*
- Pathophysiology (P). The pathophysiology category includes the following features of the patient's disease:
  - Anatomic (*Table 9-3)*
  - Hemodynamic (*Table 9-3)*
  - Etiologic (*Table 9-3)*

Location

- The SVP classification system was designed to identify the location of the patient's symptoms (S) and their varices (V).
- To define the location, the pelvic venous system is broken into 4 anatomic zones, denoted as a subscript when reporting the symptoms (S) and the varices (V) portions of the classification. *(Fig. 9-19)*

Patients with PeVD often have symptoms and varices in more than one zone with more than one of the pathophysiological categories, all of which will be reported in the patient's SVP classification. For examples see the following figures and tables

Fig. 9-19. Pelvic Venous System (4 Anatomic Zones)

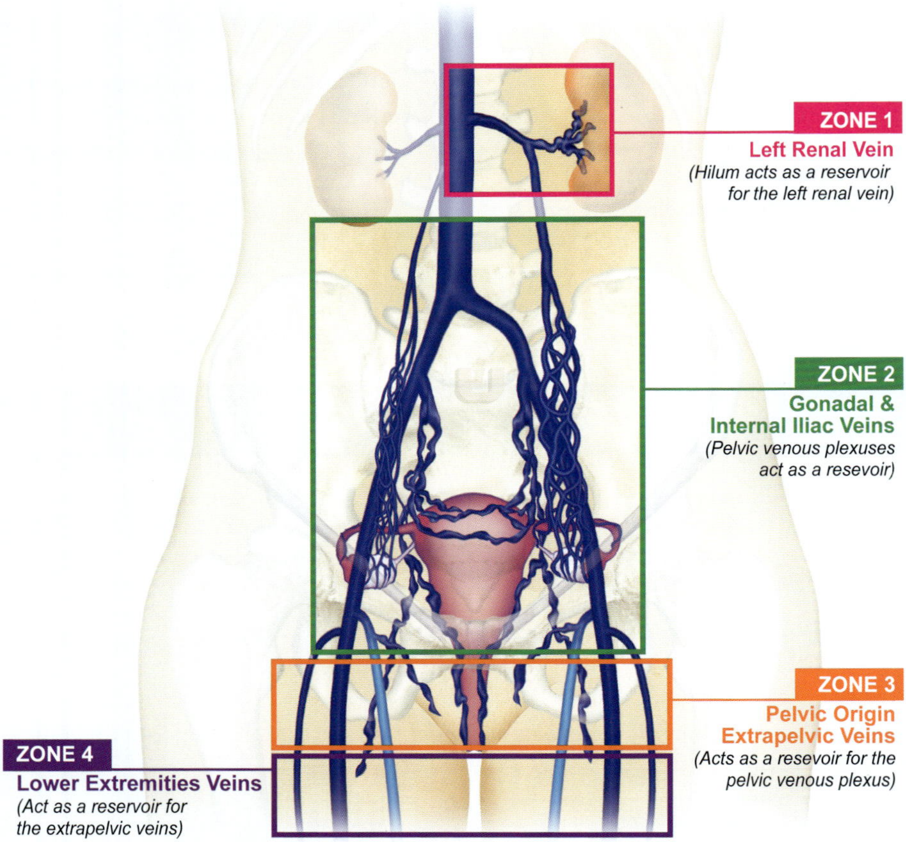

Table 9-1. SVP: Symptoms (S)

S_0	No symptoms of a PeVD (no renal, pelvic, or extrapelvic symptoms
S_1	Renal symptoms of venous origin
S_2	Chronic pelvic pain of venous origin
S_3	Extrapelvic symptoms of venous origin **a** Localized symptoms (pain, discomfort, tenderness, itching, bleeding, and superficial venous thrombosis) associated with veins of the external genitalia (vulva and scrotum) **b** Localized symptoms associated with pelvic origin nonsaphenous veins of the leg. These include those related to pelvic origin varices of the posteromedial thigh (pain, discomfort, tenderness, itching, superficial venous thrombosis) as well as those related to sciatic/tibial nerve varices (pain, paresthesia). More generalized lower extremity symptoms and signs, such as heaviness and swelling, are classified with CEAP, not SVP* **c** Venous claudication* ** Must include CEAP for full characterization of lower extremity symptoms*

PeVD Pelvic Venous Disorder; **SVP** Symptoms-Varices-Pathophysiology

Table 9-2. SVP: Varices (V)

V_0	No abdominal, pelvic, or pelvic origin extrapelvic varices on clinical or imaging examination
V_1	Renal hilar varices
V_2	Pelvic varices
V_3	Pelvic origin extrapelvic varices **a** Genital varices (vulvar varices and varicocele) **b** Pelvic origin lower extremity varicose veins arising from the pelvic escape points and extending into the posteromedial thigh, sciatic varices, and other refluxing veins transitioning through the pelvic floor.*

**Must include CEAP classification for full characterization of lower extremity varices.*

Table 9-3. SVP: Pathophysiology (P)

Hemodynamics	
Obstruction **(O)**	Thrombotic or nonthrombotic (venous compression) venous obstruction
Reflux **(R)**	Thrombotic or nonthrombotic reflux
Anatomy (Abbreviation Expansions)	
IVC	Inferior Vena Cava
LRV	Left Renal Vein
GV	Gonadal (testicular, ovarian) veins **LGV** Left gonadal vein **RGV** Right gonadal vein **BGV** Bilateral gonadal vein
CIV	Common Iliac Veins **LCIV** Left common iliac vein **RCIV** Right common iliac vein **BCIV** Bilateral common iliac veins
EIV	External Iliac Veins **LEIV** Left external iliac vein **REIV** Right external iliac vein **BEIV** Bilateral external iliac veins
IIV	Internal Iliac Veins **LIIV** Left internal iliac vein and tributaries **RIIV** Right internal iliac vein and tributaries **BIIV** Bilateral internal iliac veins and tributaries
PELV	Pelvic escape veins ("escape points"); inguinal, obturator, pudendal, and/or gluteal
Etiologic	
Thrombotic **(T)**	Venous reflux or obstruction arising from a previous episode of DVT
Nonthrombotic **(NT)**	Reflux arising from a degenerative process of the vein wall or proximal obstruction: Obstruction arising from extrinsic compression
Congenital **(C)**	Congenital venous or mixed vascular malformations

Fig. 9-20. Left Renal Vein Obstruction Uncompensated

The left renal vein is obstructed and there is no decompression (no compensation) and venous hypertension is transmitted to:

ZONE 1

- The renal hilum creating hilar varicosities
  - Renal symptoms of venous origin, including flank pain and hematuria

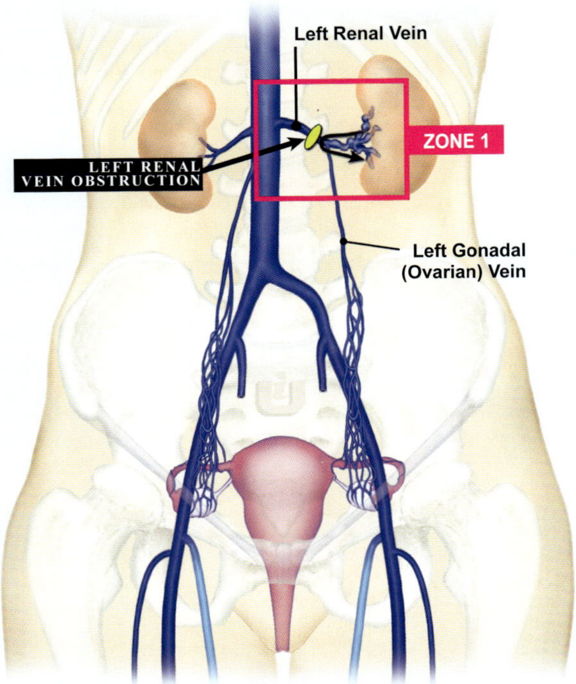

Table 9-4. SVP: Left Renal Vein Obstruction Uncompensated	
Symptoms (ZONE 1)	**1**
S_1 Renal symptoms of venous origin	
Varices (ZONE 1)	**1**
V_1 Renal hilar varices	
Pathophysiology	
Anatomic	Left Renal Vein $_{(LRV)}$
Hemodynamic	Obstruction $_{(O)}$
Etiologic	Nonthrombotic $_{(NT)}$
SVP Classification	
$S_1V_1P_{LRV,\,O,\,NT}$	

Fig. 9-21. Left Renal Vein Obstruction Compensated

The left renal vein is obstructed, and there is decompression (compensation) via the left gonadal vein. Venous hypertension is transmitted to:

ZONE 2

- Pelvic Varices
  - Chronic pelvic pain

or ZONE 2-3

- Pelvic Varices and genitalia
  - Chronic pelvic pain, genital pain, discomfort, tenderness, and itching

or ZONE 2-3-4

- Pelvic Varices, genitalia, and non-saphenous lower extremity veins
  - Chronic pelvic pain
  - Genital pain, discomfort tenderness and itching
  - Lower extremity symptoms that arise from reflux through the pelvic escape points

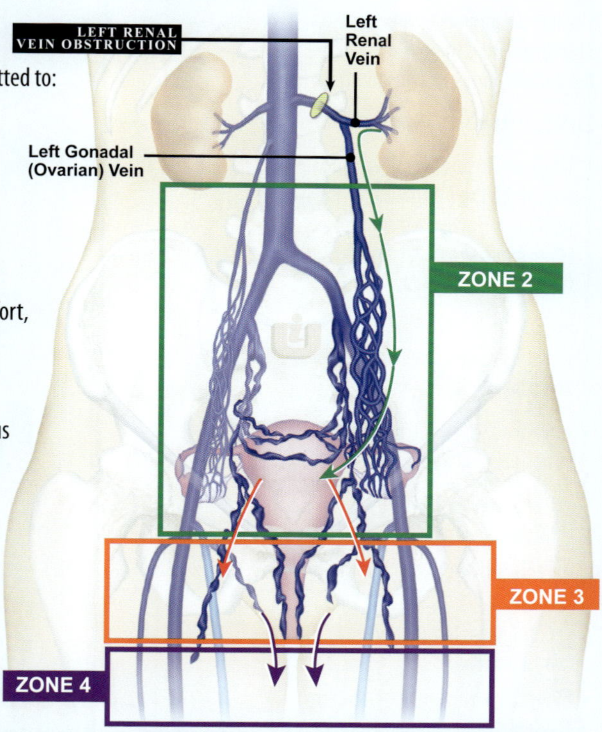

Table 9-5. SVP: Left Renal Vein Obstruction Compensated

Symptoms (ZONE 2 or 2-3 or 2-3-4)	2 3 4
S_2 Chronic pelvic pain of venous origin	
S_3 Extrapelvic symptoms of venous origin a Localized symptoms associated with veins of the external genitalia (vulva and scrotum) b Localized symptoms associated with pelvic origin nonsaphenous veins of the leg* c Venous claudication* ** Must include CEAP when the lower extremities are involved.*	
Varices (ZONE 2 or 2-3 or 2-3-4)	2 3 4
V_2 Pelvic varices	
V_3 Pelvic origin extrapelvic varices a Genital varices b Pelvic origin lower extremity veins arising from the pelvic escape points extending into the thigh	
Pathophysiology	
Anatomic	Left Renal Vein $_{(LRV)}$
Hemodynamic	Obstruction$_{(O)}$
Etiologic	Nonthrombotic $_{(NT)}$
SVP Classification Examples	
$S_2V_2P_{LRV,O,NT}$ $S_{2,3a}V_{2,3a}P_{LRV,O,NT}$	$S_{2,3a,b}V_{2,3a,b}P_{LRV,O,NT}$

Fig. 9-22. Left Common Iliac Vein Obstruction Uncompensated

The left common iliac vein is obstructed, and there is no decompression (compensation):

ZONE 4

- Venous pressure is transmitted directly to the peripheral venous reservoirs (lower extremity), resulting in lower extremity venous hypertension.
- Most likely presents with left lower extremity swelling, fullness, and pain.
- Advanced cases will present with venous claudication
  - Deep pain with physical exercise increases with intensity and
  - Feels constrictive in the calf or thigh
  - Culminates in function impairment
- Symptoms only dissipate when the leg is positioned to enhance venous drainage (leg raised)

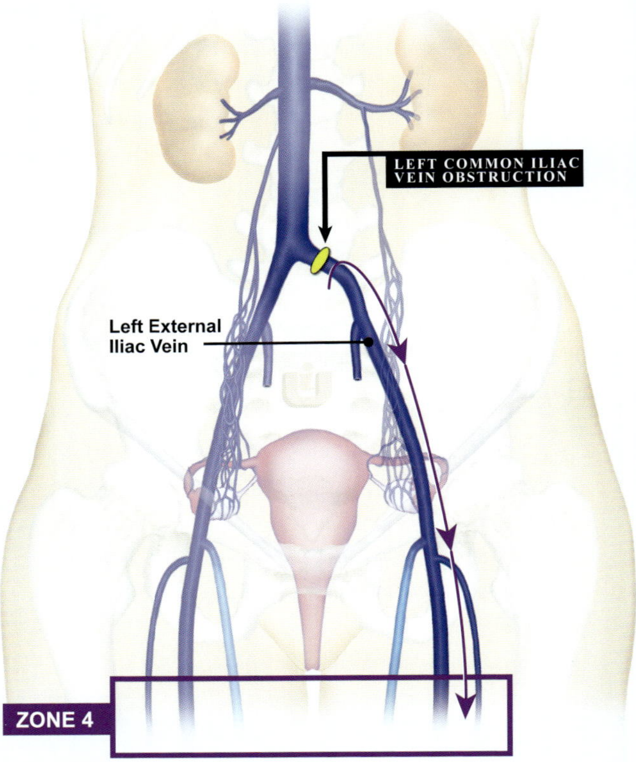

Table 9-6. SVP: Iliac Vein Compression Uncompensated

Symptoms (ZONE 4)	**4**
S_{3c}	Venous claudication (must include CEAP classification for lower ext symptoms)
Varices	
V_0	No Visible varices
Pathophysiology	
Anatomic	Left Common Iliac Vein $_{(LCIV)}$
Hemodynamic	Obstruction $_{(O)}$
Etiologic	Nonthrombotic $_{(NT)}$
SVP Classification Examples	
$S_1V_1P_{LRV,\,O,\,NT}$	$S_{3c}V_0P_{LCIV,O,T:\,LEIV,O,T}$

Fig. 9-23. Left Common Iliac Vein Obstruction Compensated

The left common iliac vein is obstructed, and there is decompression (compensation) via the internal iliac vein. Venous hypertension is transmitted to:

ZONE 2

- Pelvic varices
  - Chronic pelvic pain

or ZONE 2-3

- Pelvic varices and genitalia
  - Chronic pelvic pain, genital pain, discomfort, tenderness, and itching

or ZONE 2-3-4

- Pelvic varices, genitalia, and non-saphenous lower extremity veins
  - Chronic pelvic pain
  - Genital pain, discomfort tenderness and itching
  - Lower extremity symptoms that arise from reflux through the pelvic escape points

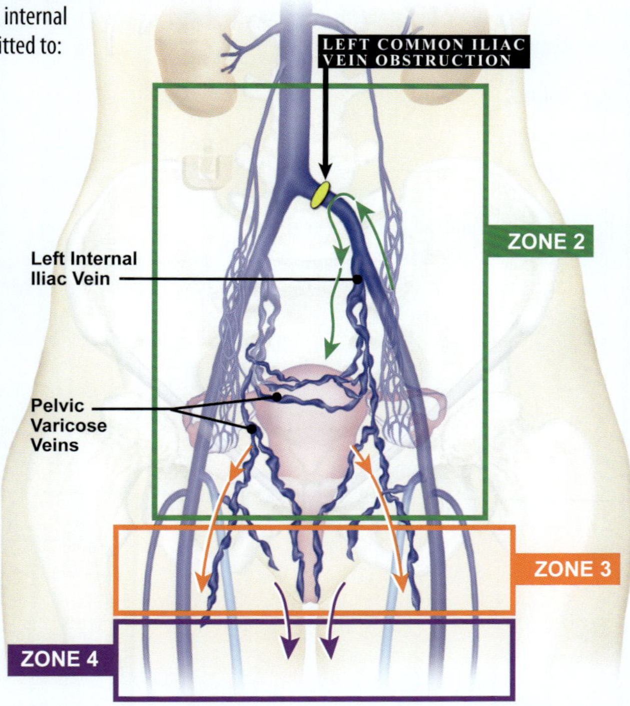

Table 9-7. **SVP: Iliac Vein Compression Compensated**				
Symptoms (ZONE 2 or 2-3 or 2-3-4)		2	3	4
S_2	Chronic pelvic pain of venous origin			
S_3	Extrapelvic symptoms of venous origin **a** Localized symptoms associated with veins of the external genitalia (vulva and scrotum) **b** Localized symptoms associated with pelvic origin nonsaphenous veins of the leg* **c** Venous claudication* ** Must include CEAP when the lower extremities are involved.*			
Varices (ZONE 2 or 2-3 or 2-3-4)		2	3	4
V_2	Pelvic varices			
V_3	Pelvic origin extrapelvic varices **a** Genital varices **b** Pelvic origin lower extremity veins arising from the pelvic escape points extending into the thigh			
Pathophysiology				
Anatomic	Left Common Iliac Vein $_{(LCIV)}$			
Hemodynamic	Obstruction$_{(O)}$			
Etiologic	Nonthrombotic $_{(NT)}$			
SVP Classification Examples				
$S_2V_2P_{LCIV,O,NT}$	$S_{2,3a}V_{2,3a}P_{LCIV,O,NT}$	$S_{2,3a,b}V_{2,3a,b}P_{LCIV,O,NT}$	$S_2V_2P_{LCIV,O,NT;LEIV,O,NT}$	

Fig. 9-24. Gonadal and/or Internal Iliac Vein Reflux Uncompensated

Gonadal vein and/or internal iliac vein(s) reflux without decompression (no compensation). Venous hypertension is transmitted to:

ZONE 2

- Pelvic varices
  - Chronic pelvic pain
- In some cases of unilateral gonadal vein insufficiency, spontaneous, antegrade flow can be seen in the contralateral GV.

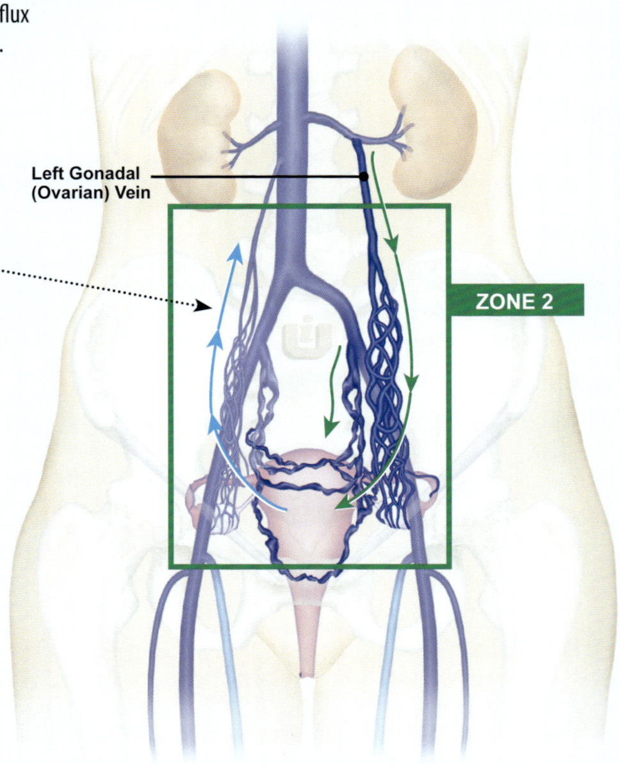

Table 9-8. SVP: Gonadal and/or Internal Iliac Vein Reflux Uncompensated	
Symptoms (ZONE 2)	**2**
S_2 Chronic pelvic pain of venous origin	
Varices (ZONE 2)	**2**
V_2 Pelvic varices	
Pathophysiology	
Anatomic	Gonadal Vein $_{(GV)}$ and /or Internal iliac vein $_{(IIV)}$
Hemodynamic	Reflux$_{(R)}$
Etiologic	Nonthrombotic $_{(NT)}$
SVP Classification Examples	
$S_2V_2P_{LGV,R,NT}$	$S_2V_2P_{BIIV,R,NT}$
An example of a combination of GV & IIV:	$S_2V_2P_{LGV,R,NT;LIIV,R,NT}$

Fig. 9-25. Gonadal and/or Internal Iliac Vein Reflux Compensated

Reflux in the gonadal and/or internal iliac vein is transmitted to:

ZONE 2

- Pelvic varices
  - Chronic pelvic pain

or ZONE 2-3

- Pelvic varices and genitalia
  - Chronic pelvic pain, genital pain, discomfort, tenderness, and itching

or ZONE 2-3-4

- Pelvic varices, genitalia, and non-saphenous lower extremity veins
  - Chronic pelvic pain
  - Genital pain, discomfort, tenderness, and itching
  - Lower extremity symptoms that arise from reflux through the pelvic escape points

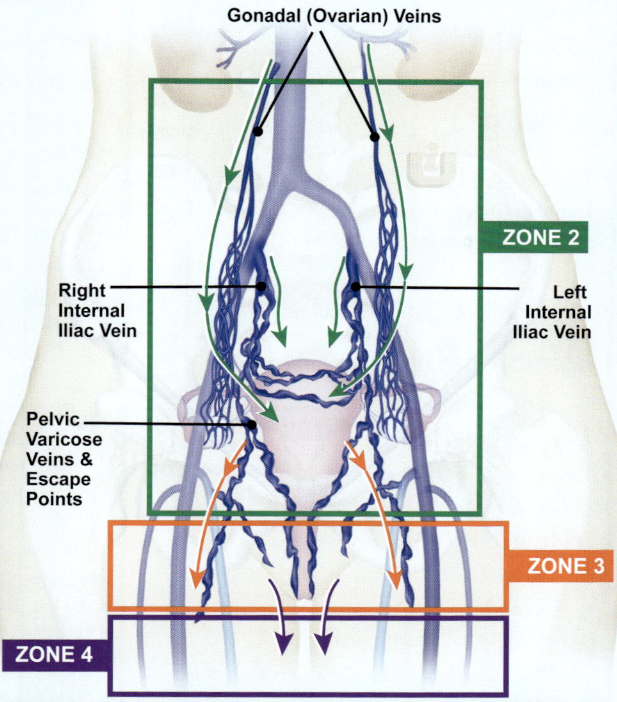

Table 9-9. SVP: Gonadal and/or internal Iliac Vein Reflux Compensated

Symptoms (ZONE 2 or 2-3 or 2-3-4)	2 3 4
S_2 Chronic pelvic pain of venous origin	
S_3 Extrapelvic symptoms of venous origin a Localized symptoms associated with veins of the external genitalia (vulva and scrotum) b Localized symptoms associated with pelvic origin nonsaphenous veins of the leg* c Venous claudication* ** Must include CEAP when the lower extremities are involved.*	
Varices (ZONE 2 or 2-3 or 2-3-4)	2 3 4
V_2 Pelvic varices	
V_3 Pelvic origin extrapelvic varices a Genital varices b Pelvic origin lower extremity veins arising from the pelvic escape points extending into the thigh	
Pathophysiology	
Anatomic	Gonadal Vein (GV) and /or Internal iliac vein (IIV)
Hemodynamic	Reflux$_{(R)}$
Etiologic	Nonthrombotic $_{(NT)}$
SVP Classification Examples	
$S_2V_2P_{LGV,R,NT}$ $S_{2,3a}V_{2,3a}P_{LGV,R,NT}$ $S_{2,3a,b}V_{2,3a,b}P_{LGV,R,N}$	
An example of a combination of BGV & BIIV:	$S_2V_2P_{BGV,R,NT;BIIV,R,NT}$

Physical Examination

- Varicose veins
  - Buttocks
  - Anterior abdominal and pelvic wall
  - Genitals
  - Posterior and medial thigh
- Lower extremity skin changes, e.g., hyperpigmentation, lipodermatosclerosis, venous ulceration (open or healed)
- Edema
- Male varicocele or hydrocele

Location of Disease

- Gonadal vein (left more often than right)
- Left renal vein
- Iliocaval
- Pelvic venous plexus (peri-uterine and/or trans-uterine)
- Extrapelvic tributaries of the IIVs
  - Round ligament vein refluxing through the inguinal escape points.
  - Obturator vein refluxing through the obturator escape points.
  - Pudendal veins refluxing through the perineal escape points.
  - Gluteal (superior and inferior) veins refluxing through the gluteal escape points.
- Scrotal pampiniform plexus reflux

Patient History

Female

- Varicose veins
- Pregnancies
- Genital varicose veins current or during pregnancy
- Pelvic heaviness
- Increasing bladder incontinency and urgency
- Increased irritable bowel
- Increased pelvic pain while standing or sitting
- Dyspareunia
- Chronic pelvic pain
  - Pain symptoms perceived to originate from pelvic organs/structures, typically lasting more than 6 months.
- History of DVT
- Long-standing history of microhematuria

Male

- Scrotal enlargement
- Scrotal pain
- Male infertility
- Scrotal varicocele

Although chronic pelvic pain also occurs in males, currently little evidence suggests that pelvic venous disease is an important contributing factor. This is likely due to both differences in venous anatomy and the role of pregnancy in PeVDs in women. The gonadal veins follow an extrapelvic course in males and the arrangement of the visceral pelvic venous plexuses are substantially different.

Pelvic Vein Disorders Duplex Protocol

Patient Preparation

- Evaluate the veins of the pelvis and the abdomen
  - Use a combination of routine pelvic and abdominal ultrasound preparations
  - Fasting for 6-8 hours helps reduce bowel gas which assists in visualization of the abdominal level veins.
- Transabdominal pelvic vein evaluation
  - Full bladder (to provide a window for peri- and trans-uterine vein, female patients only). Instruct the patient to drink 32oz of water 1/2 hour before their appointment time.
- Endovaginal peri- and trans-uterine vein evaluation
  - Empty bladder for patient comfort

Patient Position

Patient position will vary throughout the exam depending on the vein(s) being evaluated. Evaluating for pelvic venous disease can be challenging secondary to dense overlying bowel gas or difficult body habitus. A complete examination may require the sonographer to be adaptable and obtain images from protocols in a variable order.

Peri-uterine and trans-uterine Veins

- **Transabdominal**
  - Supine on a tilt table for appropriate visualization and patient comfort
  - Reverse Trendelenburg >20° (head higher than feet)
- **Endovaginal**
  - If a gynecological table is not available, place the patient in the supine position with the knees bent and the feet flat on the table, approximately shoulder width apart. The patient's hips can be elevated with a foam pad or pillow.
  - If possible, reverse Trendelenburg >20° (head higher than feet)
  - To maintain patient dignity, the patient is always covered with a sheet.

Scrotal Veins

- Supine with a rolled towel under the scrotum
- Standing

Left Renal Vein, Gonadal Vein, Iliac Veins

- Supine on a tilt table for appropriate visualization and patient comfort
- Reverse Trendelenburg ranging >20°-90° (if footboard is available)
- The gonadal veins can also be assessed in the standing position.
- Use the decubitus position if needed to avoid or change bowel gas patterns

Pelvic Escape Points

- Standing position
- Perineal escape point standing with the ipsilateral foot placed on a step stool and the leg externally rotated for easy access.

Scanning Protocol [5-13]

- Ultrasound for pelvic venous disorders involves the evaluation of multiple veins extending from the proximal abdomen to the distal pelvis/proximal lower extremity.
- Due to the complex nature of pelvic venous disorders, the protocol for scanning consists of individual protocols for each of the veins evaluated.
- Flexibility in the order in which the veins are scanned is important due to changing bowel gas patterns and the need for a full bladder.

Peri-uterine and Trans-uterine Veins

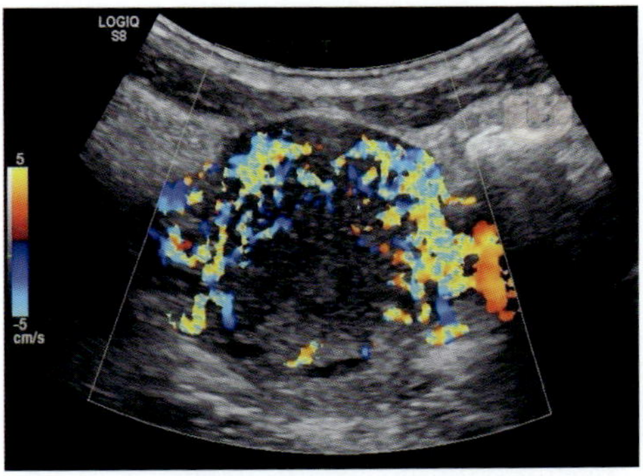

Fig. 9-26. *Transverse image of the fundus of the uterus demonstrating peri- and trans-uterine varicosities using the Valsalva maneuver. *Note the color flow scale is very low due to the slow flow within these veins.*

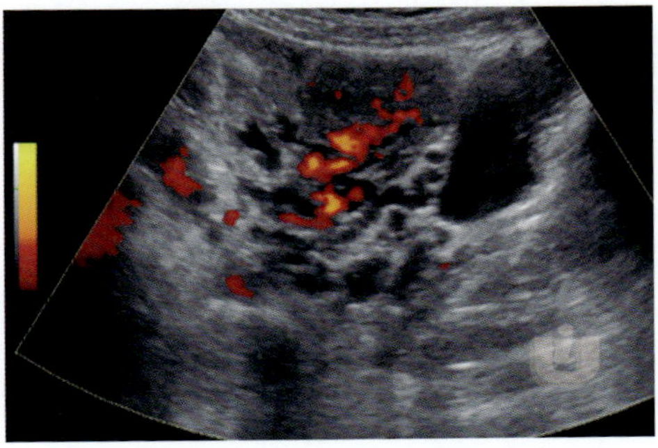

Fig. 9-27. *Longitudinal image of the left adnexa demonstrating the use of power Doppler to identify the veins.*

Duplex ultrasound can detect the following to aid in diagnosing peri-uterine and trans-uterine varicose veins:

- Increased vein diameters
- Increased number of veins
- Dilated veins traversing the uterus
- Reflux within the veins of the pelvis

Transabdominal Approach

- A curvilinear array transducer 2-5MHz is placed in a longitudinal plane just above the symphysis pubis.
- If the bladder is sufficiently full, it will provide an optimal acoustic window to the uterus.
  - If the bladder is not full, perform the next portion of the exam, returning to intermittently check for a full bladder.
- Perform longitudinal sweeps of the pelvis through the uterus, looking for dilated peri-uterine and/or trans-uterine varicosities.
- Repeat sweeps of the pelvis in the transverse plane as done in the longitudinal plane.
- Use color flow, spectral, and power Doppler to differentiate the veins from the other cystic structures present within the pelvis.
- Color and PW Doppler scales should be set low to accommodate for the slow velocities within the pelvic veins.
- Use the Valsalva maneuver to increase intra-abdominal pressure to elicit reflux.
- Obtain vein measurements from the anterior wall to the posterior wall
- Allow the patient to empty their bladder

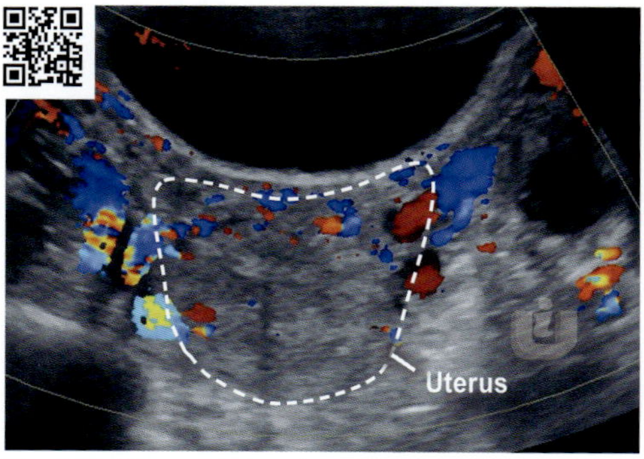

Fig. 9-28. *Transabdominal image of the fundus of the uterus with peri- and trans-uterine veins.*

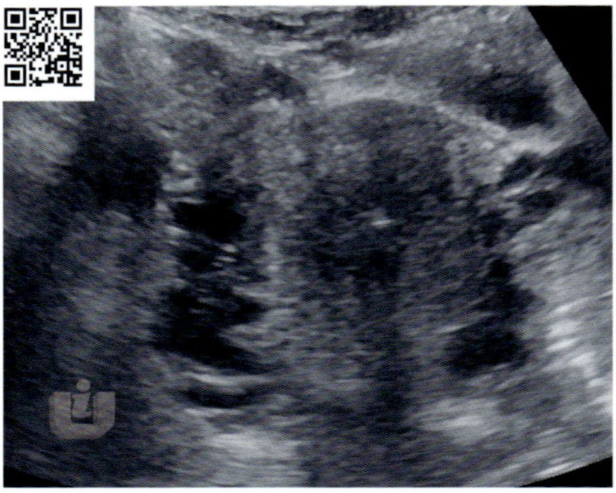

Fig. 9-29. *Transabdominal approach of a sweep of the fundus of the uterus demonstrating peri-uterine varicosities.*

Endovaginal Approach

- The 9-4 MHz transducer is inserted into the vagina
- Perform longitudinal sweeps of the pelvis through the uterus, looking for dilated peri- and/or trans-uterine varicosities.
- Repeat sweeps of the pelvis in the transverse plane as done in the longitudinal plane.
- Use color flow and PW Doppler to differentiate the veins from the other cystic structures present within the pelvis.
- Color and PW Doppler scales should be set low to accommodate for the slow velocities within the pelvic veins.
- Use the Valsalva maneuver to increase intra-abdominal pressure to elicit reflux.

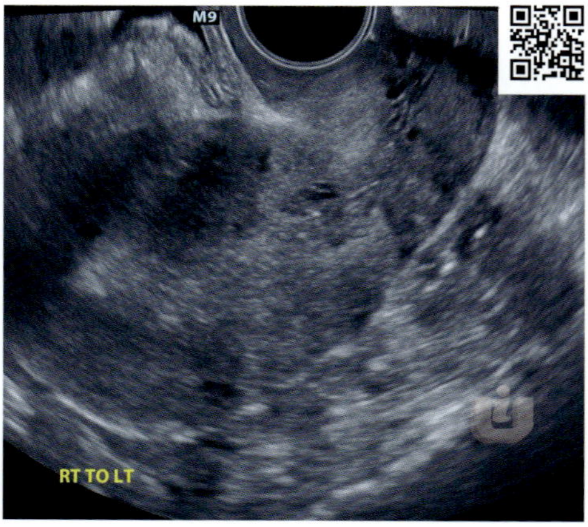

Fig. 9-30. *Longitudinal endovaginal sweep from right to left through the uterus.*

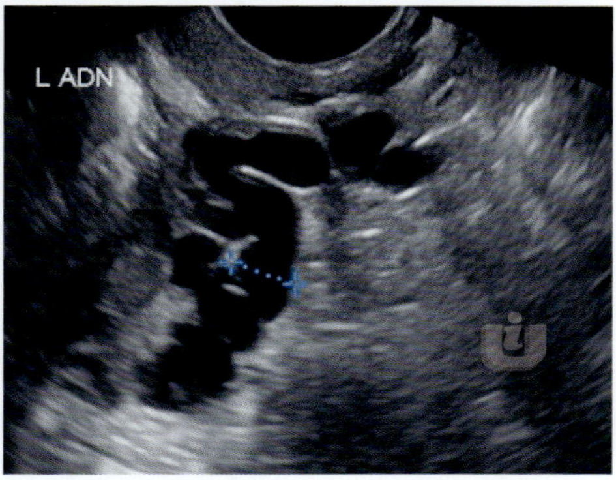

Fig. 9-31. *Endovaginal image of a pelvic adnexa varicose vein.*

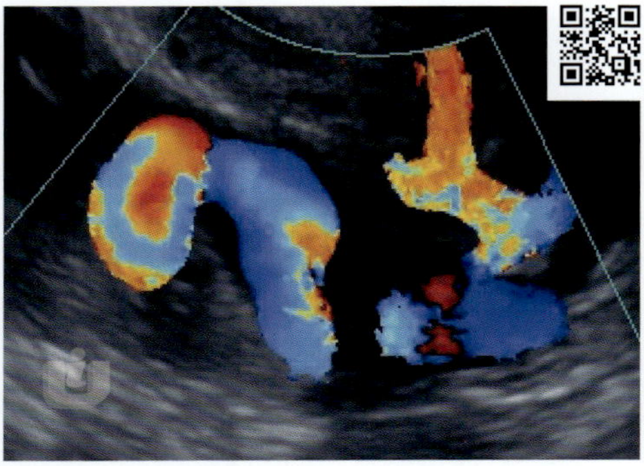

Fig. 9-32. *Endovaginal approach demonstrating reflux using the Valsalva maneuver.*

- Proceed to assess the internal iliac veins for reflux. Using a longitudinal approach, sweep through the uterus to either pelvic wall. The internal iliac vein will be found adjacent to the wall, posterior to the ipsilateral ovary. The Valsalva maneuver can be used to assess for reflux in the IIVs.
- Remove the endovaginal transducer and switch to the curvilinear transducer for the remainder of the exam.

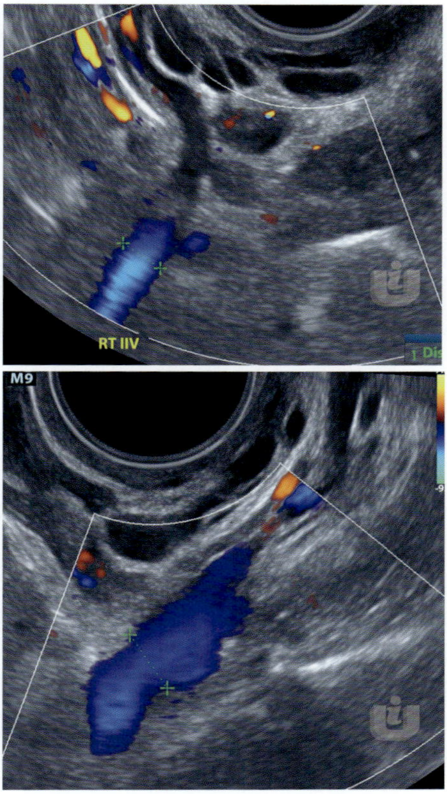

Fig. 9-33. *Endovaginal approach visualizing the left IIVs which course along the lateral walls of the pelvis. Courtesy of Aleata Rigsby RVT, RPhS. VeinCare Centers of Tennessee.*

Scrotal Veins

There is limited data on the duplex evaluation of the scrotal veins for varicocele.

The following steps should be repeated in both the supine and standing positions, at rest, and with Valsalva maneuvers.

- Bilateral grayscale imaging identifies and measures varicose veins within the scrotum.
- Flow direction assessment is performed using color and PW Doppler. Changing the patient's position and using the Valsalva maneuver will help to elicit reflux. [14]

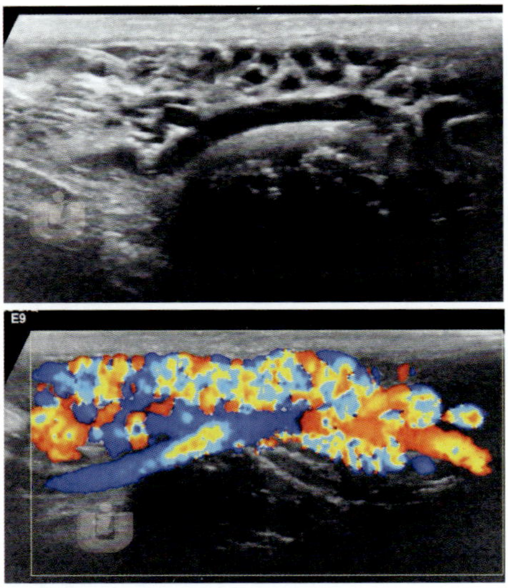

Fig. 9-34. *Scrotal varicose veins (varicocele) grayscale and color flow with Valsalva*

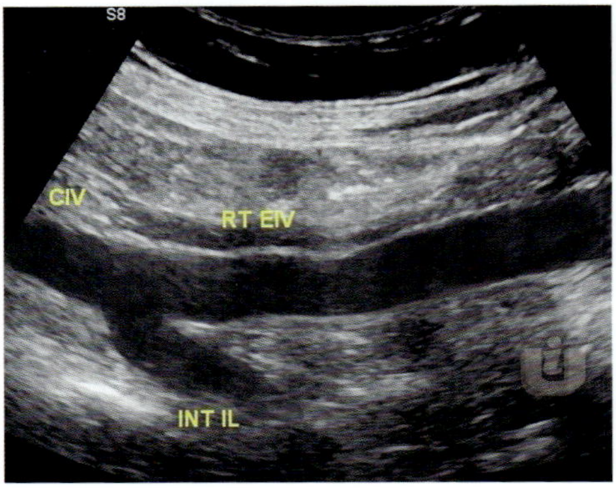

Fig. 9-35. *Longitudinal view of the confluence of the EIV and IIV to form the CIV.*

Iliac Veins [5,15,16]

Indirect testing of the iliac veins should be included in all lower extremity venous duplex testing via comparison of the PW Doppler waveforms within the bilateral CFVs. The veins should demonstrate phasic symmetrical flow.

> *The pelvis is a great "collateralizer," which may result in the findings of phasic, symmetrical waveforms in the CFVs. If there is a high suspicion of proximal obstruction, the iliac veins should be evaluated.*

- The confluence of right and left CIVs is identified by moving the transducer in transverse orientation caudally to the distal IVC at the level of the umbilicus.
- The longitudinal view of the right CIV can be visualized by placing the transducer longitudinally just to the right of the umbilicus due to a straighter course of the vessel coming to the IVC.
- To establish the longitudinal view of the left CIV, the transducer is positioned in an oblique fashion.
- The entire length of the iliac veins from the IVC to the inguinal ligament is imaged both in the longitudinal and transverse views.

Duplex ultrasound can detect the following to aid in diagnosing significant stenosis:

- Iliac vein luminal reduction
- Pre-stenotic dilation
- Increased peak vein velocity
- Increased velocity ratio
- Slow or absence of flow
- Presence of collateral veins
- Spurring of the vein walls caused by the repetitive motion of an overlying artery

Common Iliac and External Iliac Veins [10,13,16,17]

- Obtain PW Doppler waveforms in longitudinal view to evaluate for phasicity and spontaneity. When evaluating the iliac veins for phasicity and spontaneity, they should always be obtained from the right and left sides and compared for symmetry.

- Grayscale evaluation should be performed with special attention paid to areas of the vein that are in close proximity to an overlying artery.
  - The repetitive motion of the pulsatile artery on the vein can cause fibrotic changes within the vein walls.
  - Chronic changes due to the previous thrombus may also be present.
- Within the CIVs, obtain diameter measurements in B-mode and PW Doppler peak vein velocities in the longitudinal plane at the following levels:
  - Peripheral to the point of compression
  - At the suspected point of compression
  - Central to the point of compression

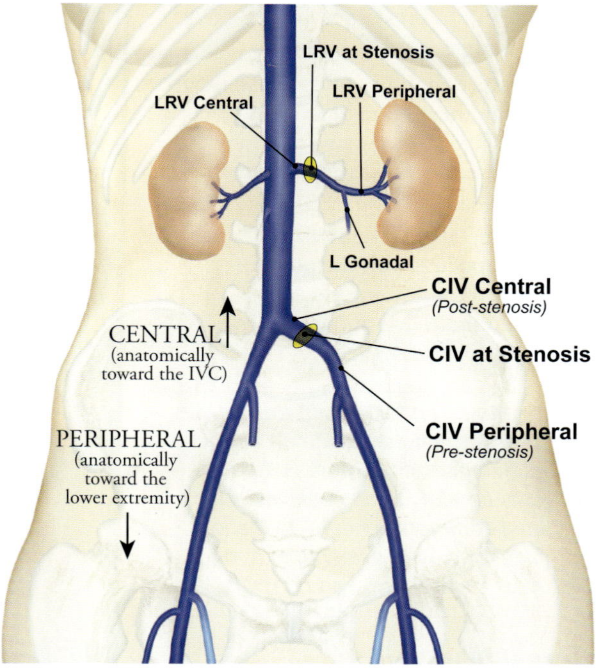

Fig. 9-36. *Diameters and PW Doppler waveforms are obtained peripheral-to, central-to, and at the stenosis.*

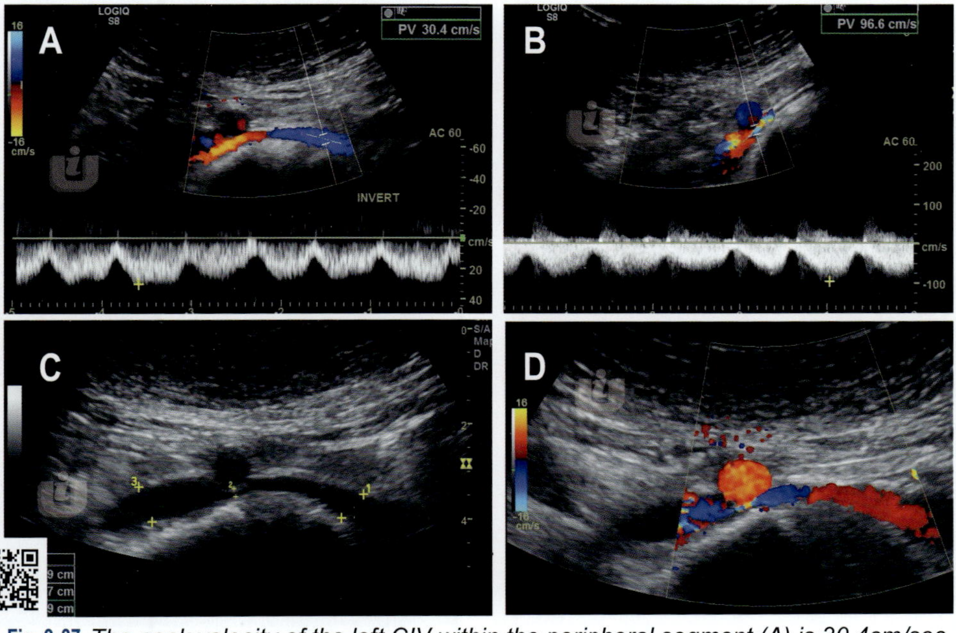

Fig. 9-37. *The peak velocity of the left CIV within the peripheral segment (A) is 30.4cm/sec and at the level of compression (B) is 96.6 cm/sec yielding a ratio of 3.2. The diameter of the peripheral portion is 6.9mm, and the stenotic portion is 1.7mm (C), yielding a ratio of 4.1, demonstrating positive findings for iliac vein compression. There is visual narrowing of the CIV (D) with color aliasing at the level of CIA.*

- When obtaining velocities, ideally a 60° Doppler angle should be used.
  - A Doppler angle of <60° may be used; however, these velocities measurements should be obtained using the same angle throughout to calculate an accurate peak systolic velocity ratio.
- The peripheral peak vein velocity will be compared with the point of compression peak vein velocity to obtain a ratio to determine if there is significant compression.

Care should be taken with transducer pressure on the abdomen as to not extrinsically compress the iliac veins creating false positives. This most commonly occurs on the left side; however, this should apply to a visibly narrowed right CIV.

Internal Iliac Vein

- The bilateral internal iliac veins should be evaluated with color and PW Doppler for flow direction and phasicity.
- Spontaneous, continuous reflux within the IIV indicates a significant, more central stenosis. [16]

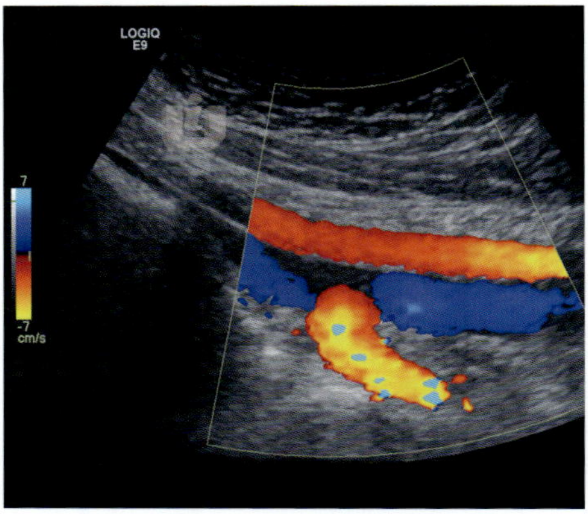

Fig. 9-38. *Spontaneous reflux within the IIV at rest.*

Left Renal Vein(s)

The LRV is evaluated for possible obstruction due to its surrounding anatomy.

The LRV is identified by imaging the IVC and aorta in transverse view just below the takeoff of the SMA.

Within the LRV, duplex ultrasound can detect the following:

- Renal vein luminal reduction
- Pre-stenotic dilation
- Increased velocity ratio
- Slow or absence of flow
- Presence of collateral veins
- Presence of a renal vein variant
  - Retroaortic renal vein
  - Circumferential renal vein

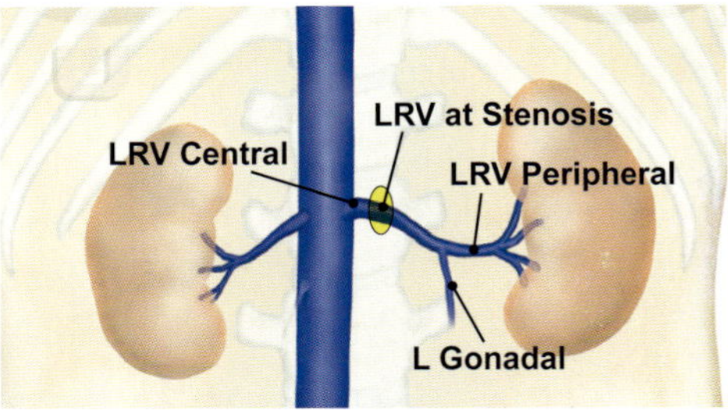

Fig. 9-39. *Diameters and PW Doppler waveforms are obtained peripheral to, central to, and at the stenosis.*

Within the veins, obtain diameter measurements in B-mode and PW Doppler peak vein velocities in the longitudinal view at the following levels:

- Peripheral to the point of compression
- At the suspected point of compression
- Central to the point of compression

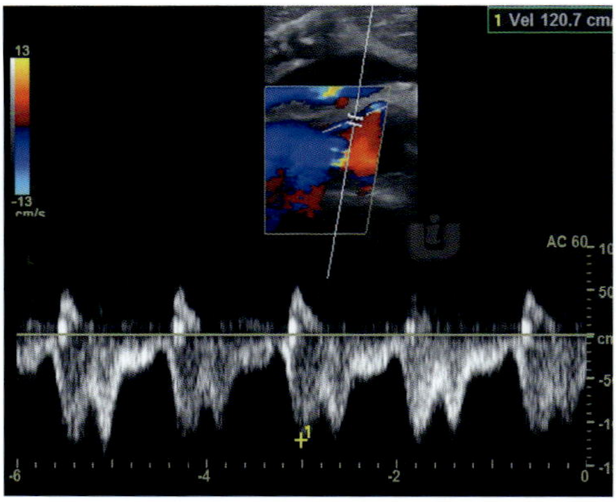

Fig. 9-40. *PW Doppler of the central segment of the LRV with a velocity of 121cm/sec.*

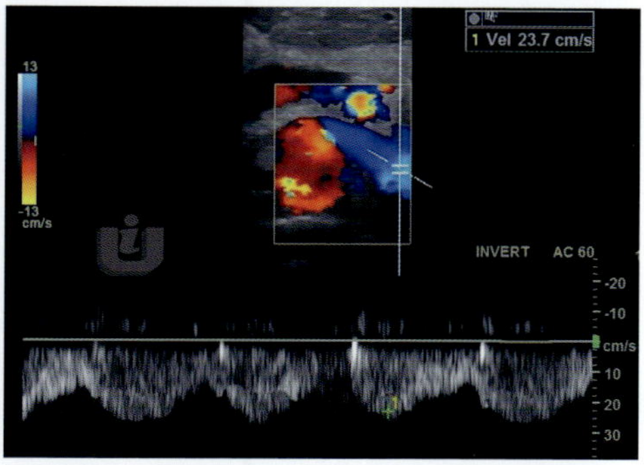

Fig. 9-41. *In the same patient, a peak velocity of 24cm/sec is obtained in the peripheral segment of the LRV. Yielding a central / peripheral renal venous ratio of 5.0.*

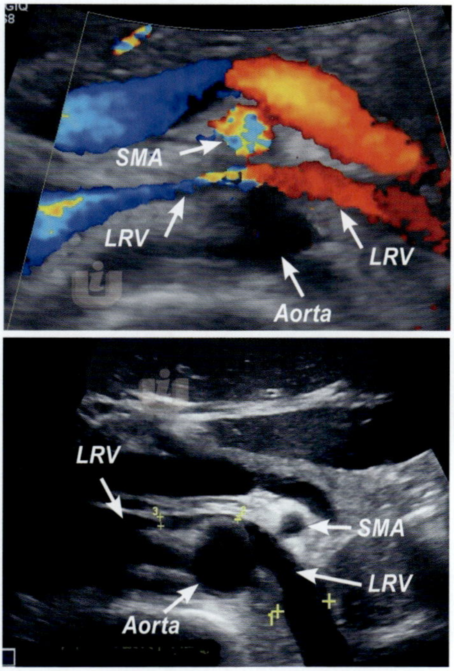

Fig. 9-42. *LRV coursing between the aorta and SMA with stenosis.*

- When obtaining velocities, ideally a 60º Doppler angle should be used.
  - A Doppler angle of <60º may be used; however, these velocities measurements should be obtained using the same angle throughout to calculate an accurate velocity ratio.

- The peripheral velocity will be compared with the point of compression velocity to obtain a ratio to determine if there is significant compression.

Stenosis can also be caused by the stretching of the vein due to anatomical variants vs. an extrinsic compression.

Gonadal Veins

Duplex ultrasound can detect the following to aid in diagnosing gonadal vein reflux:

- Increased vein diameter
- Provoked reflux
- Spontaneous reflux
- Spontaneous antegrade flow in the contralateral gonadal vein

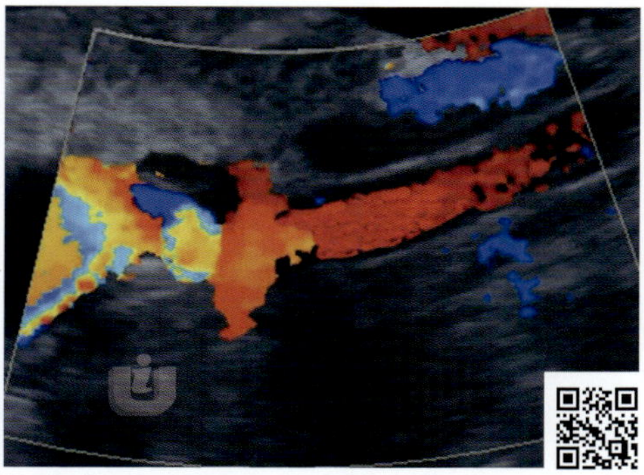

Fig. 9-43. *Confluence of the left gonadal vein with the LRV.*

Left Gonadal Vein

- To detect the left gonadal vein, the transducer is placed transversally to the left of the aorta in the mid-abdomen.
  - The gonadal vein lies anterior to the psoas muscle at this location.
- After identifying the left gonadal vein, the transducer is placed longitudinally and moved upward to visualize the communication between the left gonadal vein and the LRV.

Right Gonadal Vein

- The transducer is placed slightly to the right of the IVC, in a longitudinal plane, identifying the gonadal vein as it courses along the anterior aspect of the psoas muscle.

- A transverse view can be used to course along the IVC caudally to identify the connection with the gonadal vein.
- Obtain diameter measurements in a transverse or longitudinal plane from the following segments of the bilateral gonadal veins:
  - Proximal (central)
  - Mid
  - Distal (peripheral)

PW Doppler signals should be obtained in a longitudinal plane from the above segments of the bilateral gonadal veins to evaluate flow direction and phasicity.

If spontaneous reflux is not present, the following methods can be used to provoke reflux:

- Controlled Valsalva (minimize the motion of the abdominal wall while performing the Valsalva)
- Distal augmentation near the iliac fossa
- Reassess the veins with the patient in the standing position

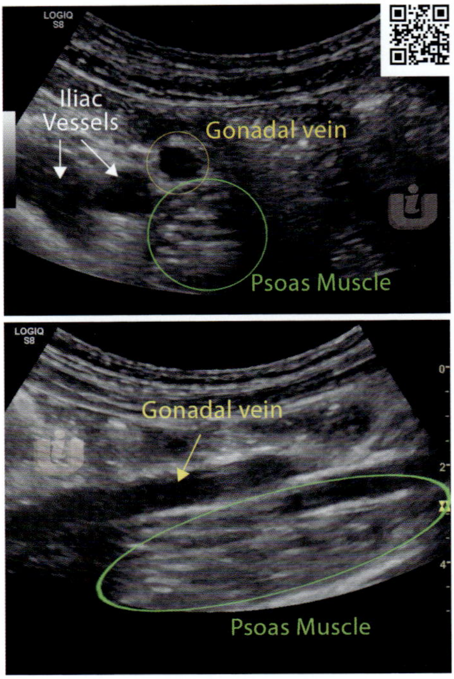

Fig. 9-45. *cine loop demonstrating the anatomical landmarks for identifying the gonadal veins.*

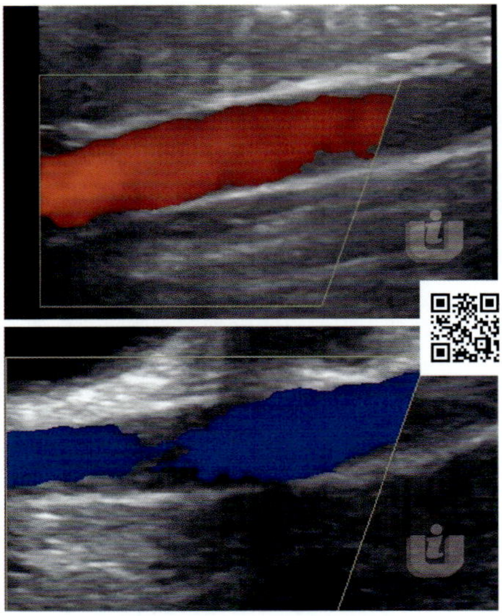

Fig. 9-44. *Color Doppler demonstrating spontaneous and continuous retrograde flow in the left gonadal vein and spontaneous, continuous antegrade flow in the right gonadal vein in the same patient.*

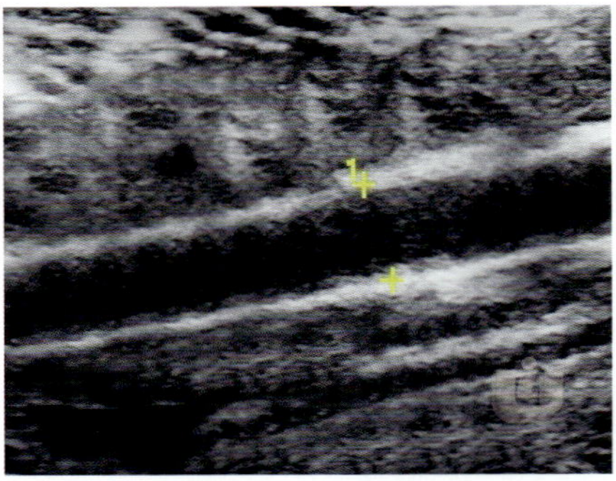

Fig. 9-46. *Longitudinal image measuring the gonadal vein.*

Pelvic Venous Disorders Duplex Worksheet

Date ______________________ **History** ______________________

Name ______________________

DOB ______________________

MRN ______________________

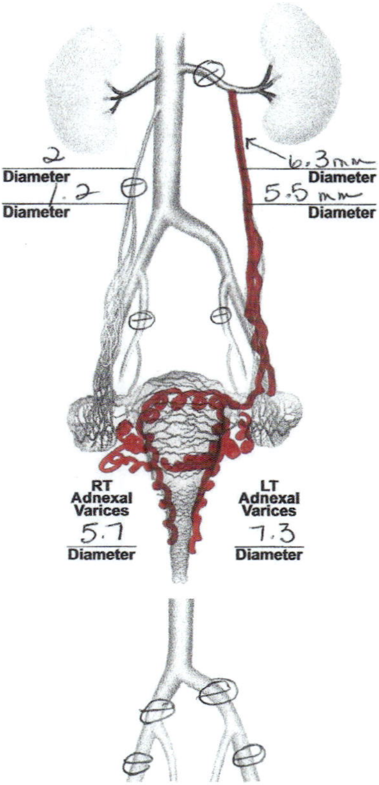

Left Renal Vein

PVV cm/sec Peripheral 18 At obstruction 80

Diam. mm Peripheral 7.5 At obstruction 2.2

Velocity Ratio 4 Diameter Ratio 3.4

Gonadal/IIV Reflux

Left gonadal vein reflux	☑ Yes	☐ No
Right gonadal vein reflux	☐ Yes	☑ No
Left internal iliac vein reflux	☐ Yes	☑ No
Right internal iliac vein reflux	☐ Yes	☑ No

Pelvic Varices

Right Adnexa	☑ Yes	☐ No
Left Adnexa	☑ Yes	☐ No
Transuterine	☑ Yes	☐ No

Left Common Iliac Vein

PVV cm/sec Peripheral 25 At obstruction 42

Diam. mm Peripheral 8.3 At obstruction 2.1

Velocity Ratio 1.6 Diameter Ratio 3.9

Other site of compression: **Rt CIV, Rt EIV, Lt EIV** N/A

PVV cm/sec Peripheral ______ At obstruction ______

Diam. mm Peripheral ______ At obstruction ______

Velocity Ratio ______ Diameter Ratio ______

⊕ Spontaneous + continuous Ⓛ gonadal vein reflux

⊕ Peri + transuterine Varices

⊖ iliac vein compression

⊖ Ⓛ renal vein compression

Fig. 9-47. *Due to the complex nature of pelvic venous disorders, it is helpful to create a map depicting any positive findings. This form can be downloaded by scanning the QR code.*

Fig. 9-48. Transducer Placement for Pelvic Imaging and DUF Images

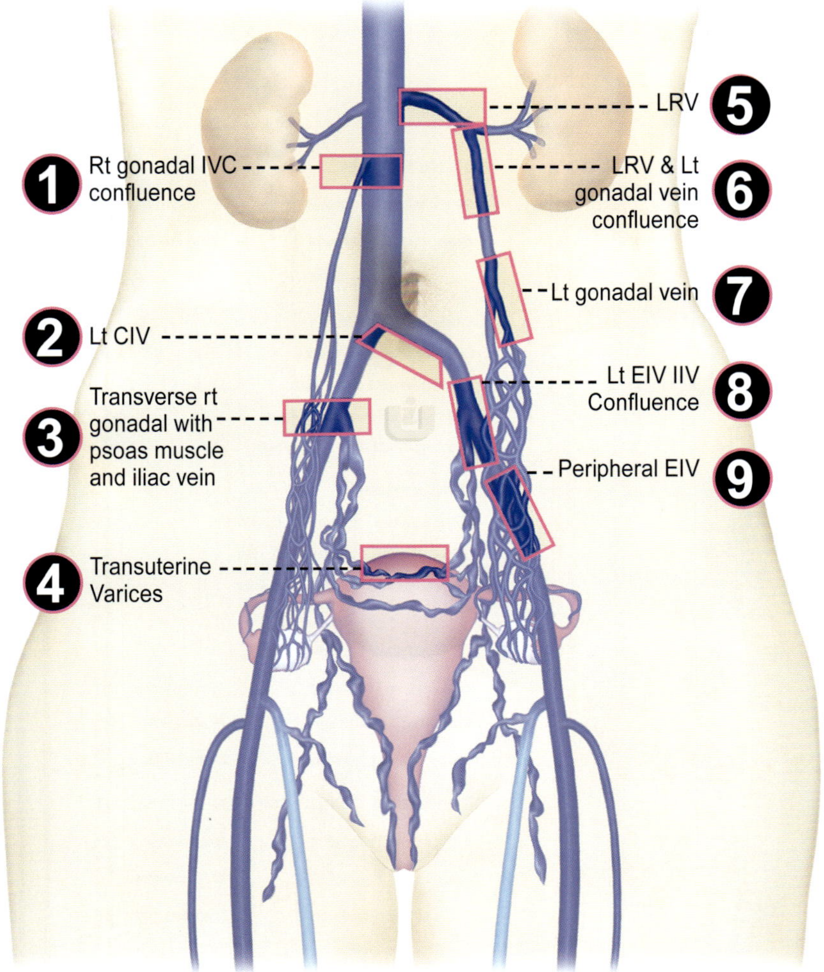

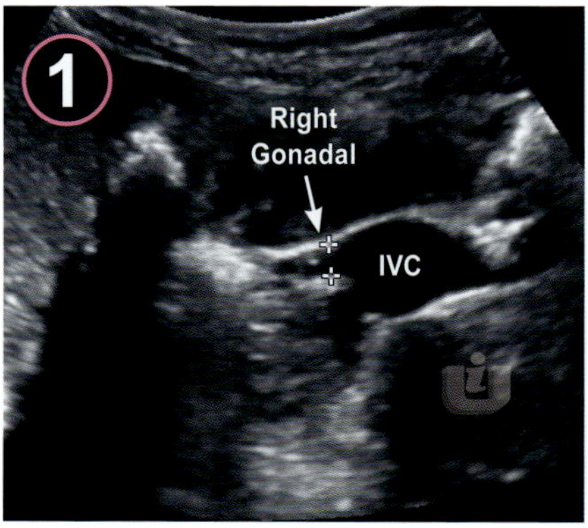

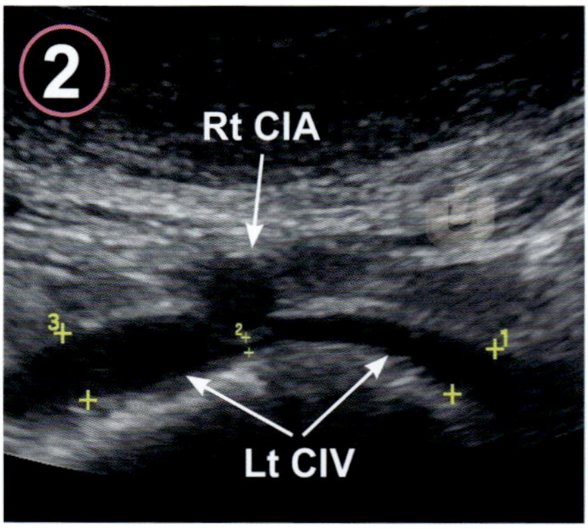

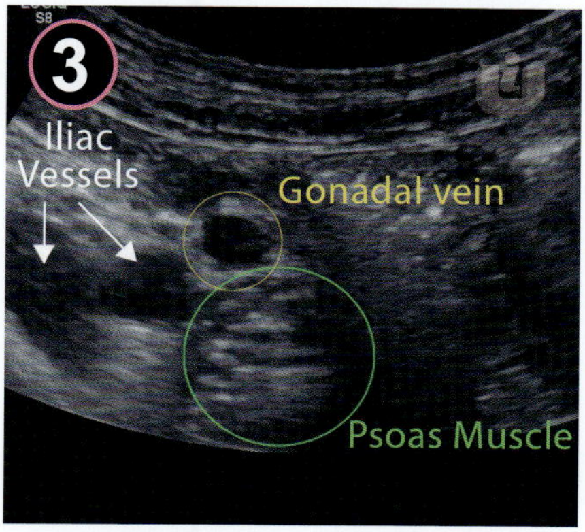

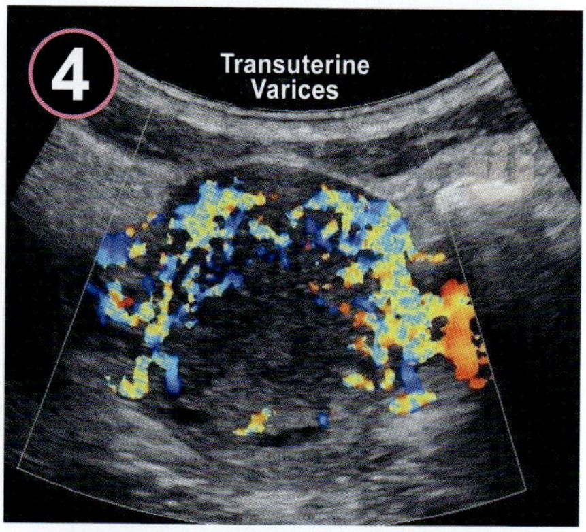

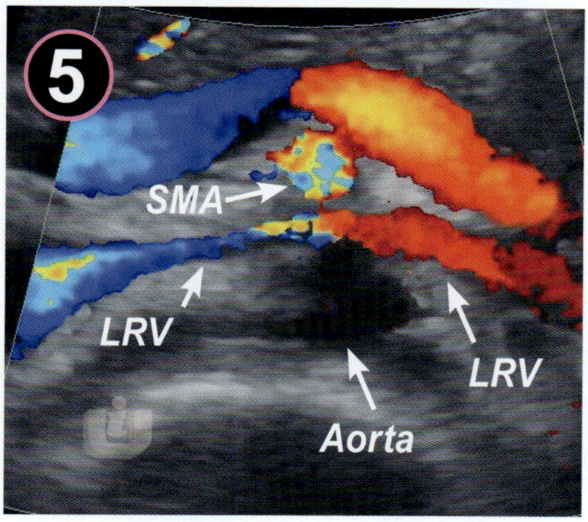

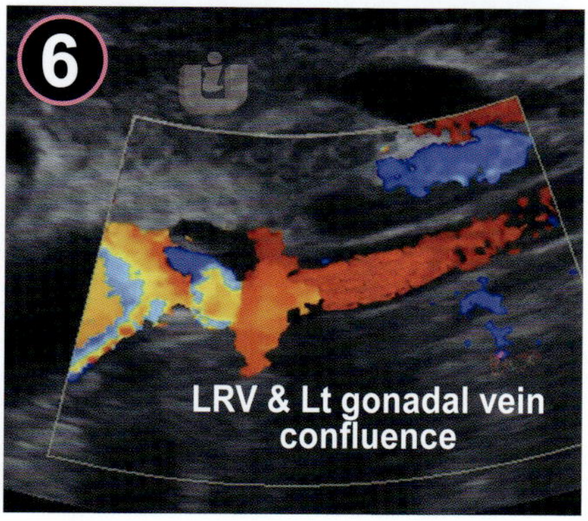

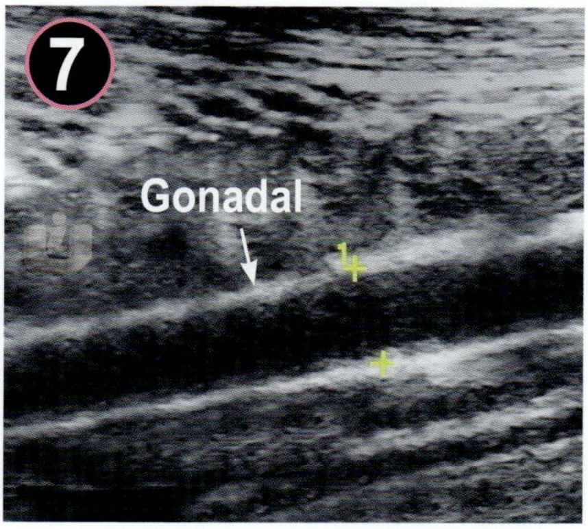

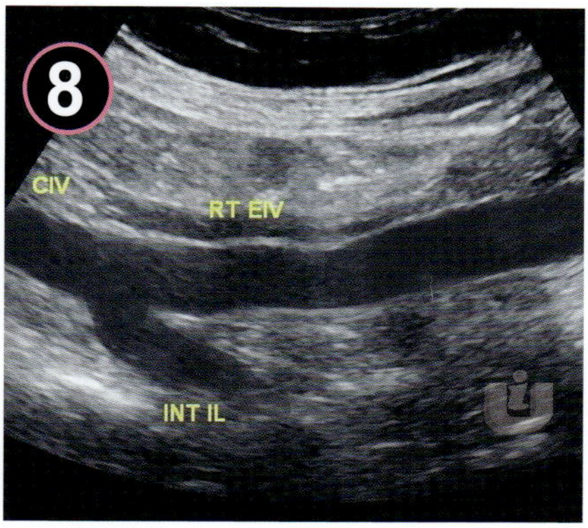

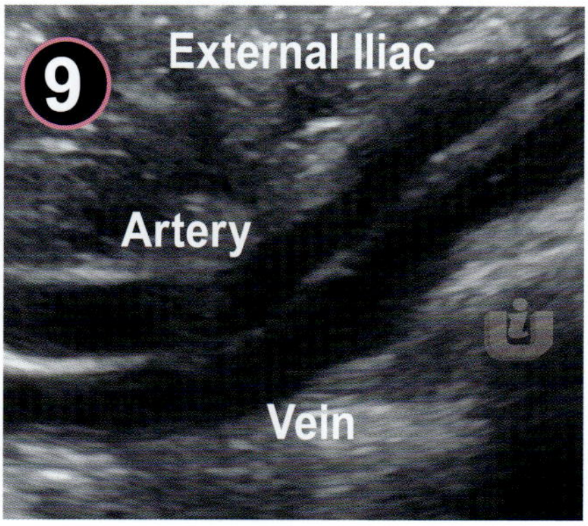

Duplex Ultrasound for Pelvic Venous Disorders

Pelvic Escape Points

If indicated, additional images of groin varicosities or genital varicosities may be obtained.

Document:

- The location of the genital and/or lower extremity varices and the associated escape point.
- Diameter measurement of varicosities
- The presence of reflux through the pelvic escape point using PW Doppler with Valsalva maneuver or distal augmentation

The following escape points should be examined (if indicated)

I point

- Inguinal point located at the superficial inguinal orifice
  - Fed by the round ligament vein
  - Can link veins of the abdominal wall and saphenous arch.
- Place the transducer in a transverse plane at groin level.
  - Identify the saphenofemoral junction.
  - Angle the transducer in a superior motion to identify the I point above the inguinal ligament.

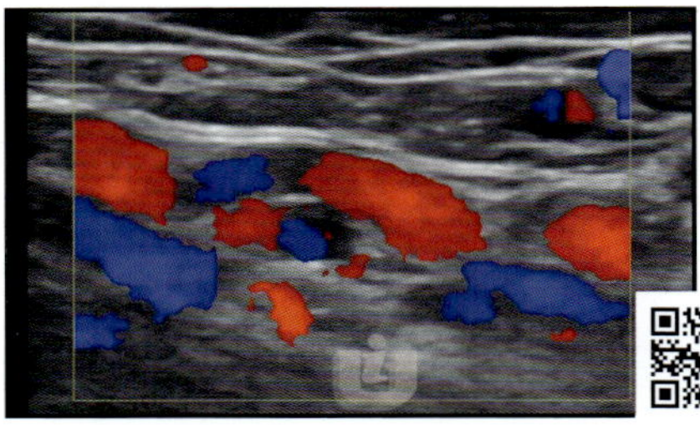

Fig. 9-49. *Inguinal escape point varices with Valsalva.*

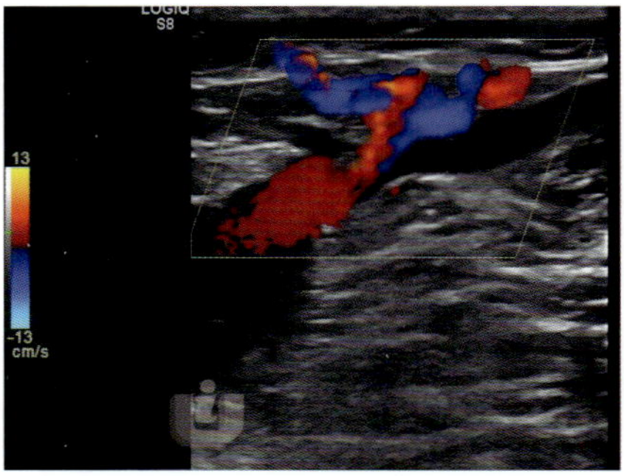

Fig. 9-50. *Inguinal escape point varices as they join the SFJ.*

P point

- Perineal escape point located at the perineal membrane
  - Fed by the pudendal vein
  - Can be the source of perineal, vulvar, and scrotal varicosities
- The perineal escape point is identified by placing the transducer in a longitudinal orientation on the perineal space on the very medial thigh and angling the transducer superiorly.

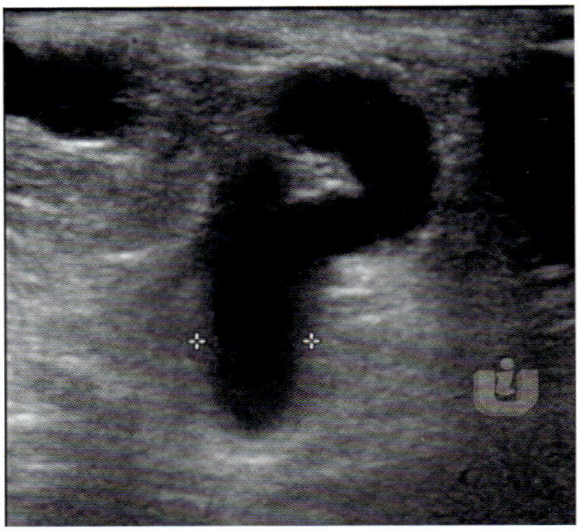

Fig. 9-51. *Varix from the pelvis escaping through the perineal escape point.*

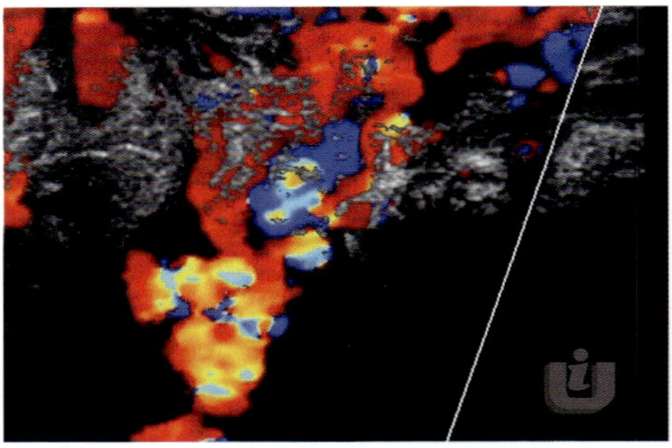

Fig. 9-52. *Labial varicosities fed by the pudendal vein through the perineal escape point with Valsalva.*

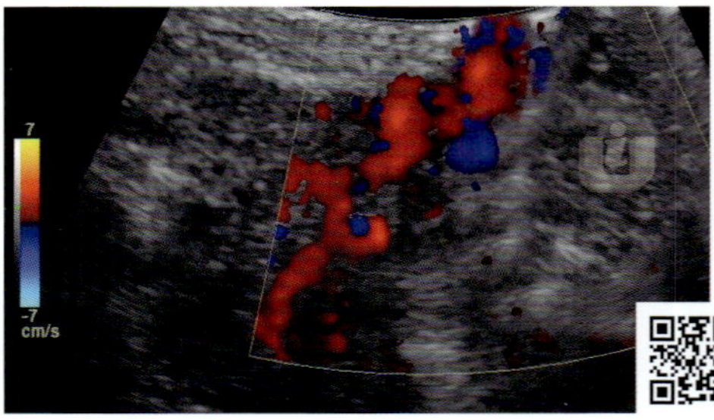

Fig. 9-53. *Color Doppler demonstrating refluxing pudendal varices through the perineal escape point.*

O escape point

- Is located in the thigh
- Fed by the obturator vein
- Usually connecting with the deep system or saphenous arch
- Is identified by angling the transducer, slightly inferior to the saphenofemoral junction and looking for a connection to the deep system.

G escape points

- The superior gluteal escape point is located at the mid portion of the buttock and linked to varicose veins involving the small saphenous vein.
- The inferior gluteal escape point is located at the infragluteal fold region, and can feed varicose veins of the sciatic nerve or posterior thigh.
- The gluteal escape points can be identified by placing a transverse transducer on the posterior thigh to follow a superficial varicosity, or varicosity within a fascial plane, proximally toward:
  - The buttocks crease to identify the inferior gluteal escape point
  - The mid buttocks to identify the superior gluteal escape point

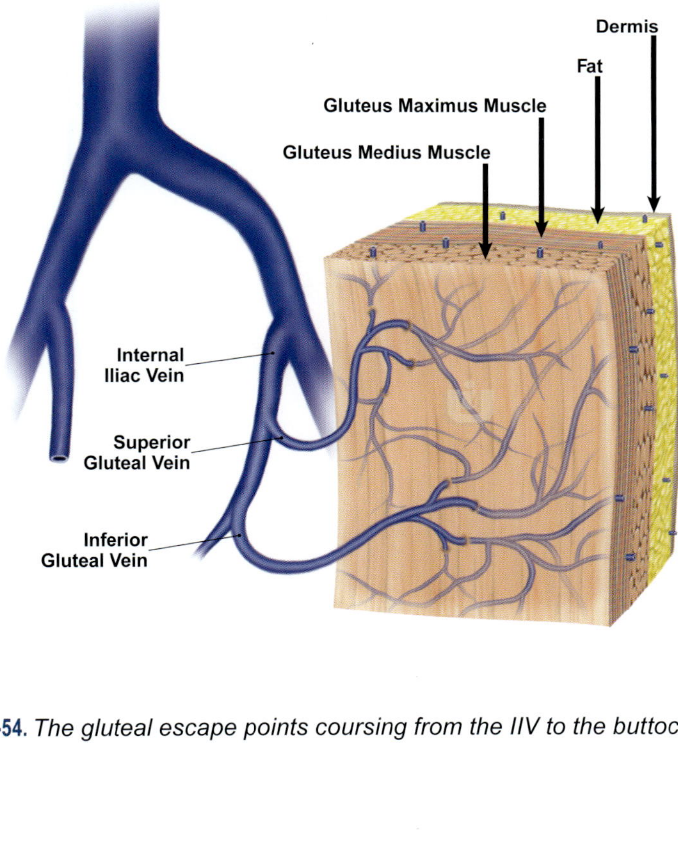

Fig. 9-54. *The gluteal escape points coursing from the IIV to the buttocks*

Transducer Placement for Pelvic Escape Points

The Inferior gluteal escape point is located at the buttocks crease and is associated with varicose veins of the sciatic nerve. These veins course along the sciatic nerve which is surrounded by a fatty sheath that is located between the muscles of the thigh.

The superior gluteal escape point is located mid buttocks and is linked with varicose veins of the small saphenous veins.

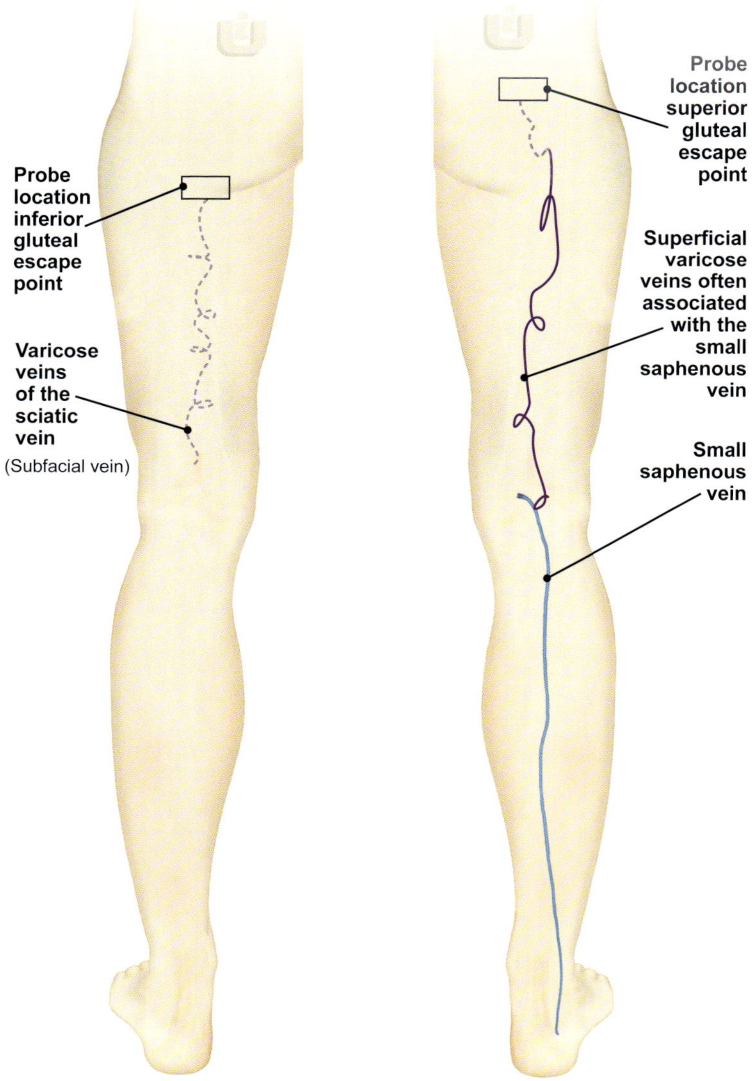

Fig. 9-55. *Transducer placement for evaluation of the gluteal leak points and the veins they are associated with.*

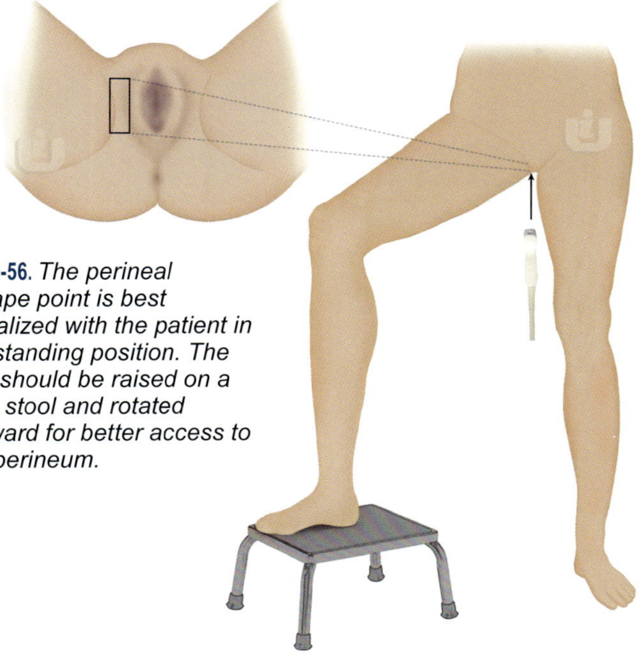

Fig. 9-56. *The perineal escape point is best visualized with the patient in the standing position. The foot should be raised on a step stool and rotated outward for better access to the perineum.*

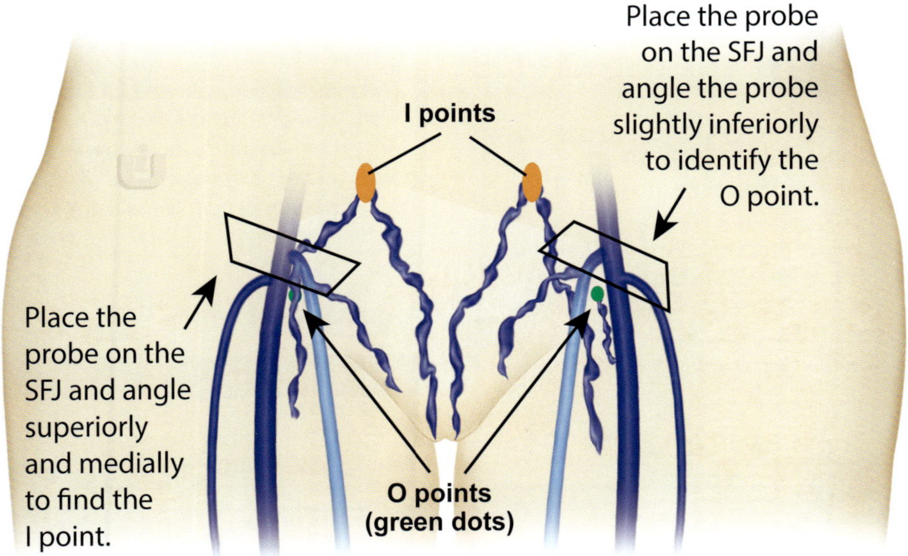

Fig. 9-57. *Transducer placement for identifying the I and O points. Note that the varices associated with the I point often join the SFJ. The varices associated with the O point join the deep system.*

Interpretation-Diagnostic Criteria

Peri-uterine and Trans-uterine Varicose Veins [6,18]

Normal

Pelvic veins measuring <5mm.

Abnormal

- Dilated and tortuous varicose veins around the uterus and ovaries measuring >5mm

> *The diagnostic criteria for defining peri-uterine varicose veins is limited to one literature source, which defines it as a vein measuring >5 mm in diameter.*

- The presence of reflux with Valsalva is considered a positive finding.

Left Renal Vein

Normal

Diameter of < 5mm and velocity ratio of <5.

Abnormal

- Diameter and velocity ratio of >5 [11]

> *Diameter and velocity ratios may not always be obtained together. The robust collateral pathways within the pelvis may alter Doppler velocities, resulting in a velocity ratio of <5.*

Left Common Iliac Vein [13,19,20,21,22,16]

Normal

- No visible narrowing on the B-mode image.
- Velocity ratio <2.5 when comparing the site of possible compression with a peripheral segment.

Abnormal

- Visible narrowing on B-mode image, which may include intraluminal scarring
- Increase in velocity >2.5 times compared to the peripheral segment
- Presence of collateral veins
- Side-to-side variability in PW Doppler waveform phasicity.

Internal Iliac Vein

Normal

Absence of reflux in the IIVs

Abnormal

- Reflux within the main trunk or its tributaries:
  - Spontaneous
  - Occur with provocative maneuvers

> *The internal iliac vein and its branches may be difficult to fully appreciate on transabdominal ultrasound; Endovaginal or transperineal ultrasound techniques may help visualize refluxing tributaries of the internal iliac vein.* [1]

Gonadal Vein [1,6,7,23,24]

Normal

- Absence of reflux
- Diameter of <6mm

Abnormal

- Reflux within the gonadal vein
  - Spontaneous
  - Occurs with provocative maneuver
  - Has been defined as >1 second in duration; however variable flow patterns have been noted in pathologic gonadal veins.
- Gonadal vein diameter of >6mm

- The diameter does not always predict disease, and veins that do not fit the size criteria should not be ruled out based on size alone.

- The right gonadal vein is often dilated due to compensatory flow, acting as the outflow pathway for a large reservoir of pelvic varicosities while remaining competent.

Pelvic Escape Points

At present time there are no published criteria for diagnosing pelvic escape points. The presence of the following findings is indicative of a positive study:

- Varicose veins in the lower extremity, particularly the medial and posterior thigh, along with varicose veins of the genitalia that can be traced to a pelvic escape point.
- Reflux with Valsalva maneuver within varicosities associated with one or more escape points.

References

1. Meissner, M. Khilnani, N. M., Labropoulos, N., Gasparis, A. P., Gibson, K., Greiner, M., Learman, L. A., Atashroo, D., Lurie, F., Passman, M. A., Basile, A., Lazarshvilli, Z., Lohr, J., Kim, M.-D., Nicolini, P. H., Pabon-Ramos, W. M., & Rosenblatt, M. (2021). The Symptoms-Varices-Pathophysiology classification of pelvic venous disorders: A report of the American Vein & Lymphatic Society International Working Group on Pelvic Venous Disorders. *Journal of vascular surgery. Venous and lymphatic disorders, 9*(3), 568–584.
2. Khilnani, Neil M., Winokur, R. S., Scherer, K. L., & Meissner, M. H. (2021). Clinical Presentation and Evaluation of Pelvic Venous Disorders in Women. *Techniques in Vascular and Interventional Radiology, 24*(1), p.100730., https://doi.org/10.1016/j.tvir.2021.100730.
3. Meissner MH, Gloviczki, P. (2019). Pelvic venous disorders. In: Almeida JI, editor. Atlas of endovascular venous surgery. 2nd ed. Philadelphia (PA): Elsevier; p. 567-99.
4. Ahmed, K., Sampath, R., & Khan, M. S. (2006). Current Trends in the Diagnosis and Management of Renal Nutcracker Syndrome: A Review. *European Journal of Vascular and Endovascular Surgery, 31*(4), pp. 410–416., https://doi.org/10.1016/j.ejvs.2005.05.045.
5. Labropoulos, N, Jasinski, P. T., Adrahtas, D., Gasparis, A. P., & Meissner, M. H. (2017). A standardized ultrasound approach to pelvic congestion syndrome. *Phlebology, 32*(9), 608–619. https://doi.org/10.1177/0268355516677135
6. Park, Seong Jin, et al. (2004). Diagnosis of Pelvic Congestion Syndrome Using Transabdominal and Transvaginal Sonography. *American Journal of Roentgenology, 182(3*), pp. 683–688., https://doi.org/10.2214/ajr.182.3.1820683.
7. Malgor R, Spentzouris, G., Adrahtas, D., Gasparis, A. P., Tassiopoulos, A. K., & Labropoulos, N. (2014). The role of duplex ultrasound in the pelvic congestion syndrome workup. *Journal of Vascular Surgery Venous lymphatic Disorders 2*(1):34-38.
8. Whiteley, M, Dos Santos, S. J., Harrison, C. C., Holdstock, J. M., & Lopez, A. J. (2015). Transvaginal duplex ultrasonography appears to be The gold standard investigation for the haemodynamic evaluation of pelvic venous reflux in the ovarian and internal iliac veins in women. *Phlebology: The Journal of Venous Disease, 30*(10), 706–713. doi: 10.1177/0268355514554638
9. Greiner, M., Gilling-Smith, G. L. (2007). Leg Varices Originating from the Pelvis: Diagnosis and Treatment. *Vascular, 15*(2), 70–78. Doi:10.2310/6670.2006.00030
10. Arnoldussen, C., de Wolf, M., Wittens, C. (2015). Diagnostic imaging of pelvic congestive syndrome. Phlebology, 30(1S), 67–72.
11. Kim SH. (1996). Nutcracker syndrome: Diagnosis with Doppler US. Radiology.1:93-97.
12. Kurklinsky A, Rooke, T. (2010). Nutcracker Phenomenon and Nutcracker Syndrome. *Mayo Clinic Procedures, 85*(6):552- 559.
13. Labropoulos, N, Borge, M., Pierce, K., & Pappas, P. J. (2007). Criteria for defining significant central vein stenosis with duplex ultrasound. *Journal of vascular surgery, 46*(1), 101–107. https://doi.org/10.1016/j.jvs.2007.02.062
14. Freeman S, Bertolotto, M., Richenberg, J., Belfield, J., Dogra, V., Huang, D. Y., Lotti, F., Markiet, K., Nikolic, O., Ramanathan, S., Ramchandani, P., Rocher, L., Secil, M., Sidhu, P. S., Skrobisz, K., Studniarek, M., Tsili, A., Tuncay Turgut, A., Pavlica, P., & Derchi, L. E. (2019). Ultrasound evaluation of varicoceles: guidelines and recommendations of the European Society of Urogenital Radiology Scrotal and Penile Imaging Working Group (ESUR-SPIWG) for detection, classification, and grading. *European Radiology.30*(1), pp. 11-25. doi:10.1007/s00330-019-06280-y
15. Kayılıoğlu, S. I, Köksoy, C., & Alaçayır, İ. (2016). Diagnostic value of the femoral vein flow pattern for the detection of an iliocaval venous obstruction. Journal of vascular surgery. *Venous and lymphatic disorders, 4*(1), 2–8. https://doi.org/10.1016/j.jvsv.2015.08.002
16. Labropoulos N. (2018). Diagnosis of iliac vein obstruction with duplex ultrasound: Criteria used during duplex ultrasound examination to identify iliac vein obstruction. *Endovascular Today, 17*(7), 50–52.
17. O'Sullivan, G.J. (2020). What is the best method of imaging in iliofemoral venous obstruction? *Phlebolymphology, 27*(2). 61-69.
18. Publishing, Licorn. (2016). Instrumental Diagnosis of Pelvic Congestion Syndrome -Servier." Phlebolymphology, https://www.phlebolymphology.org/instrumental-diagnosis-pelvic-congestion-syndrome/.
19. Mousa AY, Broce, M., Yacoub, M., & AbuRahma, A. F. (2016). Iliac vein interrogation augments venous ulcer healing in patients who have failed standard compression therapy along with pathological vein closure, *Annals of Vascular Surgery,34*,144-51.
20. Metzger PB, Rossi, F. H., Kambara, A. M., Izukawa, N. M., Saleh, M. H., Pinto, I. M. F., Amorim, J. E., & Thorpe, P. E. (2016). Criteria for Detecting Significant Chronic Venous Obstructions with Duplex Ultrasound. *Journal of Vascular Surgery Venous Lymphatic Disorders, 4*(1):18-27.
21. Kayilioglu SI. (2016). Diagnostic value of the femoral vein flow pattern for the detection of an iliocaval venous obstruction. *Journal of Vascular Surgery Venous Lymphatic Disorders, 4*, 2-8.
22. May R, Thurner J. (1957). The cause of the predominantly sinistral occurrence of thrombosis of the pelvic veins. *Angiology, 8*(5), 419-427.
23. Hansrani V, Dhorat, Z., & McCollum, C. N. (2016) Diagnosis of pelvic vein incompetence using minimally invasive ultrasound techniques. *Vascular 25*(3), 253-259. https://doi.org/10.1177/1708538116670499
24. Dos Santos SJ, S. J., Holdstock, J. M., Harrison, C. C., Lopez, A. J., & Whiteley, M. S. (2015). Ovarian vein diameter cannot be used as an indicator of ovarian venous reflux. *European Journal of Vascular and Endovascular Surgery. 49*(1):90-94.
25. Béliard, S., Feuvrier, D., Ducroux, E., & Salomon du Mont, L. (2018). May Thurner Syndrome Revealed by Left calf venous claudication during running, a case report. *BMC Sports Science, Medicine and Rehabilitation, 10*(1). https://doi.org/10.1186/s13102-018-0092-6

Definition

A combination of real time B-mode ultrasonography, with Pulsed Wave (PW) Doppler, and color Doppler imaging, to evaluate the lower extremity veins for evidence of valvular incompetence. Chronic venous disease (CVD) is caused by reflux, obstruction or a combination of both.

Rationale

Venous duplex ultrasound is the primary diagnostic imaging modality utilized for identifying patients with chronic venous disease. Duplex ultrasound can identify the presence, exact location, and extent of venous reflux and obstruction in the deep and superficial venous systems.

Etiology

Primary

The most common causes of venous insufficiency are often under-recognized or poorly defined. [1] The pathogenesis remains unclear. [5] Initially, it was thought that varicose veins were due to valvular incompetence. However, a current hypothesis states the structural changes which take place in the vein wall as they become varicose cause valvular dysfunction. [2, 51]

Secondary

DVT is the most common cause leading to chronic deep venous obstruction or valvular insufficiency. [51] Post-thrombotic valvular damage may result from initial thrombus adherence to the valve cusp or trauma to the vein wall. [44, 45]

Valvular insufficiency may develop following venous recanalization or pregnancy and progesterone-induced venous wall and valve weakness. [51]

Congenital

Congenital causes include any venous malformations. Examples include Klippel-Trenaunay variants and avalvulia. [53]

Risk Factors

- Age (greater with advanced age)
- Previous deep vein thrombosis (DVT)
- Female
- Pregnancy
- Obesity
- Family history
- Occupations requiring long periods of standing or sitting
- Congenital abnormalities (e.g., Klippel-Trenaunay)

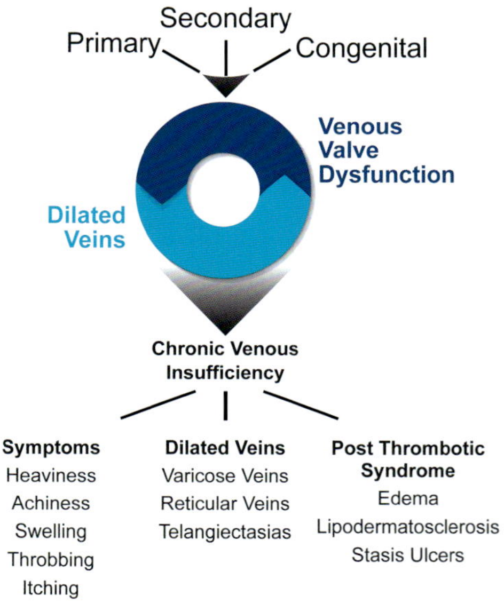

Fig. 10-1. *Pathway leading to varicose veins and other clinical manifestations of venous disease.*

Modified from Varicose Vein Surgery, Updated: Aug 19, 2021, Author: Wesley K Lew, MD; https://emedicine.medscape.com/article/462579-overview [47]

> *Symptoms may increase for women around menstruation.*
>
> *Symptoms may vary with time of day.*
>
> *Patients may present with signs without symptoms or symptoms without signs.*

The American Venous Forum's Revision of the CEAP CVD Classification
(www.veinforum.org)

CEAP Classification

C: Clinical Signs **E**: Etiologic Classification **A**: Anatomical Distribution **P**: Pathophysiologic Dysfunction

The "C" of CEAP: Clinical Signs

C0: No visible or palpable signs of venous disease

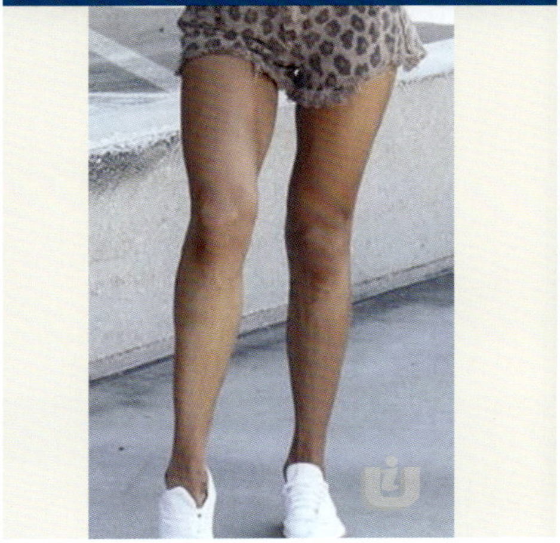

C1: Telangiectasias or reticular veins

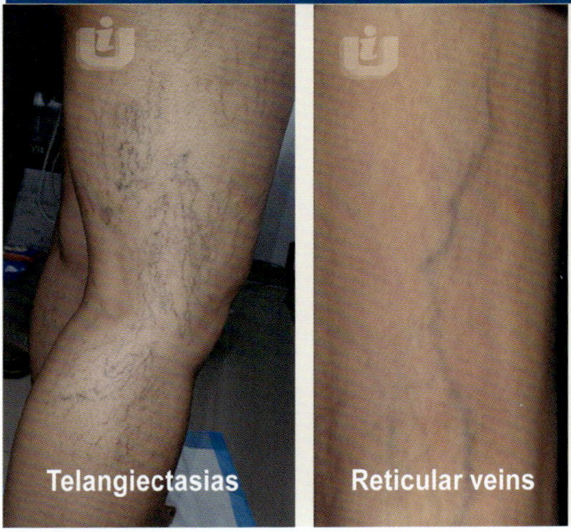

C2: Varicose veins

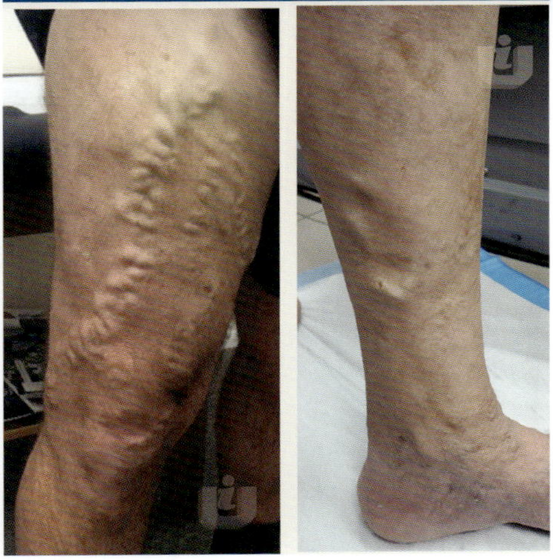

C2r: Recurrent varicose veins

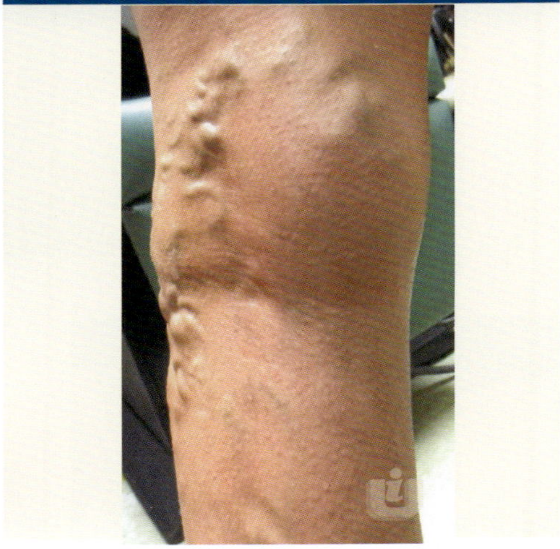

C3 Edema: When evaluating edema, compare side to side from a posterior perspective. Swelling associated with superficial venous disease is best evaluated at the ankle level.

C4: Changes in skin and subcutaneous tissue secondary to CVD

C3: Edema

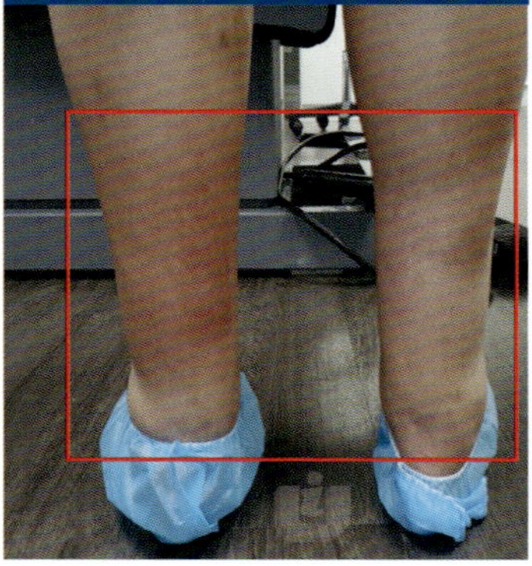

C4a: Pigmentation or eczema

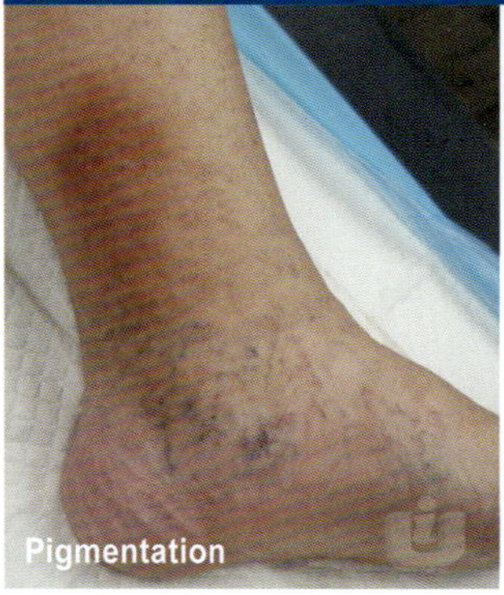

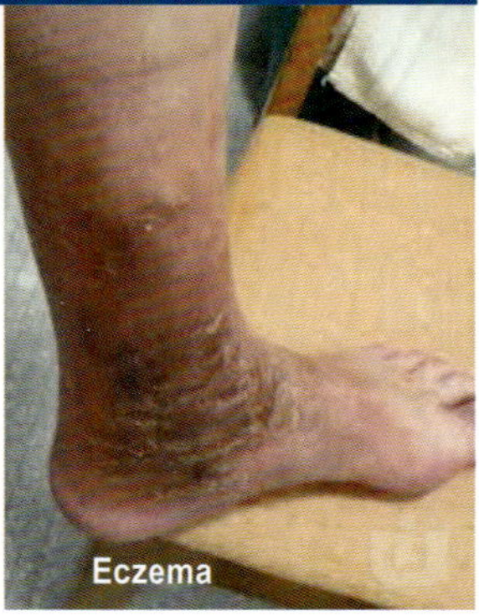

C4b: Lipodermatosclerosis or atrophie blanche

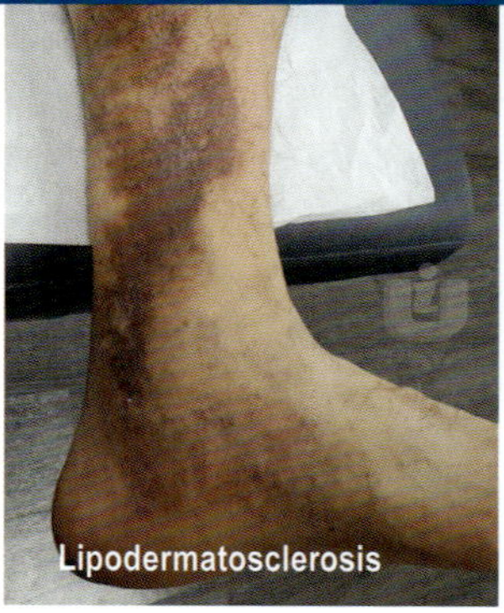

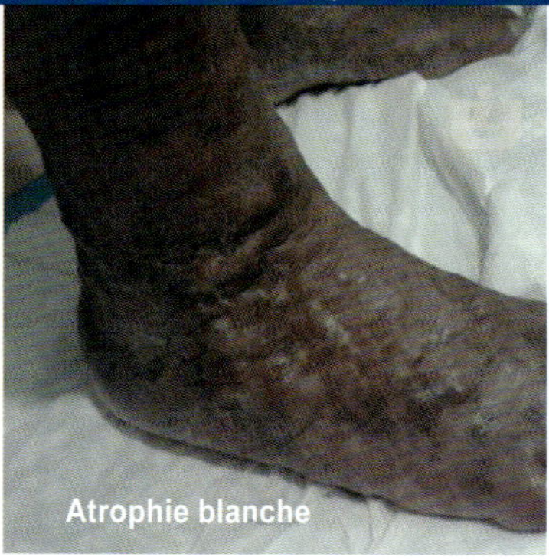

C4c Corona phlebectatica

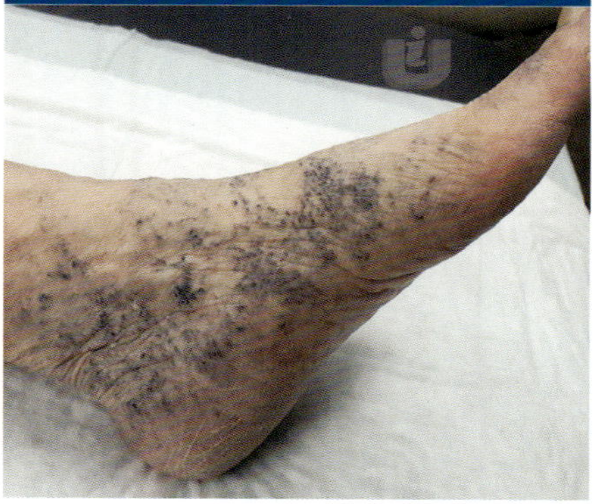

C5: Healed venous ulcer

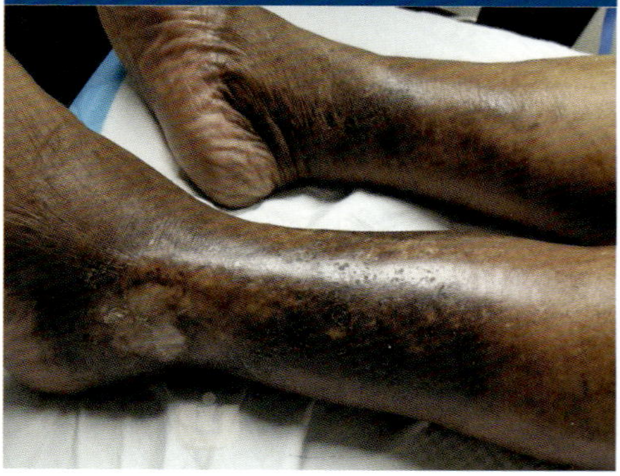

C6: Active venous ulcer

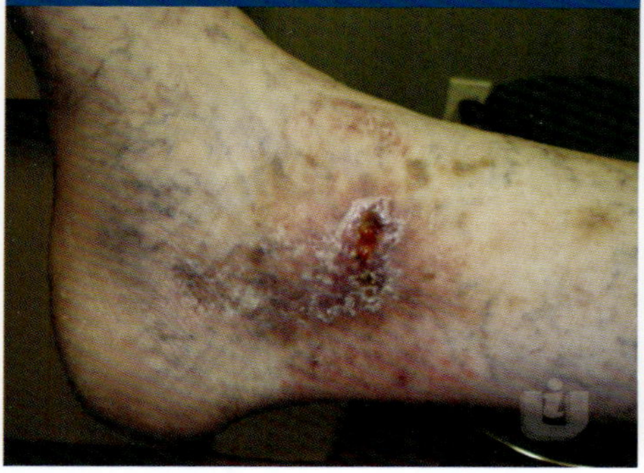

C6r: Recurrent venous ulcer

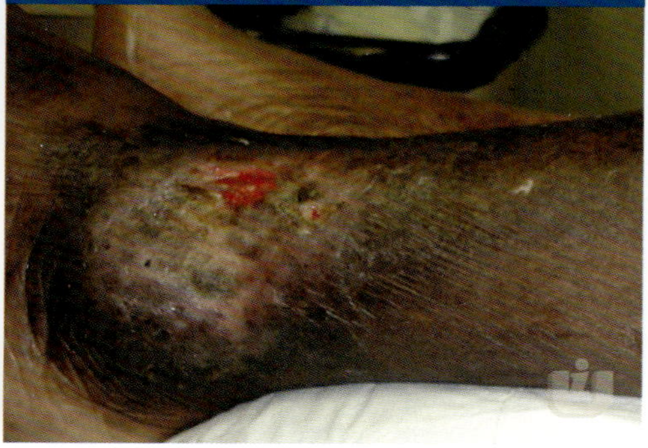

Each clinical class is further characterized by a subscript for the presence of symptoms (s, symptomatic) or absence of symptoms (a, asymptomatic), for example, C2a or C5s. Symptoms include aching, pain, tightness, skin irritation, heaviness, muscle cramps, and other complaints attributable to venous dysfunction.

s: symptomatic – the presence of symptoms attributable to venous disease

a: asymptomatic – the absence of symptoms attributable to venous disease

Taken from The American Venous Forum's Revision of the CEAP CVI Classification (www.veinforum.org)

Indications for Exam

Common indications for the performance of lower extremity venous duplex imaging for insufficiency exams include, but are not limited to:

- Pain, which may be localized to a specific varix or described as a "dull ache"
- Swelling that worsens at the end of the day
- Palpable cord or localized tenderness
- Skin changes in the gaiter region *(Fig. 10-5)*
- Active or healed ulcer
- Prior endovenous intervention (thermal, chemical or adhesive)
- Assessment of calf muscle pump or valvular incompetence
- Visible varicose vein(s)
- Venous claudication (often described as bursting pain upon walking, which is relieved with leg elevation)

Contraindications/Limitations

- Non-removable casts or tractions
- Morbid obesity or severe edema
- Patients who are unable to cooperate due to mental or physical status.
- The inability of a patient to stand, or to stand for an extended period of time.
- The inability to place the patient in an extreme reverse Trendelenburg position due to equipment limitations.

Mechanism of Disease

Normal Venous Valve Function

- Venous blood normally flows toward the heart and from the superficial venous system to the deep venous system. [3]
- In the perforating veins, blood flows from the superficial veins to the deep veins. [7]
- When standing still, with the calf muscle relaxed, the veins in the calf fill with blood. Pressure on the valves from retrograde flow force the valves to close, preventing blood from flowing toward the feet. [7]
- While walking, muscle contractions squeeze the veins initiating venous blood flow. Venous flow opens the venous valves allowing the blood to flow towards the heart. As the muscle relaxes, the valves close to prevent backflow of blood (reflux). [3]

- There are multiple components that facilitate effective venous return from the lower extremities.
  - **Cardiac pump:** During cardiac contraction and relaxation, there is a passive push from the arterial system and a mild suction from the cardiac valves that assist venous blood flow. [42]
  - **Respiratory pump:** During the inspiration and expiration process, pressure changes occur in the thoracic and abdominal cavities. These pressure changes compress the nearby veins and assist blood return to the heart. [42]
  - **Peripheral muscle pumps:**
    - » **Foot:** during flexion the plantar venous plexus is compressed and it primes the calf muscle pump [4, 5]
    - » **Calf:** gastrocnemius and soleus muscles eject 40-60% of venous volume with a single contraction [4]
    - » **Thigh:** although the thigh level veins are surrounded by muscle the contribution to venous return is less when compared to the calf [4]

> *Of the three lower extremity muscle pumps, the calf muscle pump is the most important. It is highly efficient, has the largest capacitance and generates the highest pressures (200mmHg during muscular contraction).* [4, 7, 8]

- **Pressure gradient and muscle pumps:** the muscle pumps drive blood into the popliteal and femoral veins.
  - » The valves prevent retrograde flow (reflux) during relaxation, generating negative pressure and drawing blood from the superficial to the deep system through perforating veins. [7]
  - » Venous pressure is lowered until arterial inflow equals venous outflow. [7]
  - » When exercise ceases, the veins slowly fill from the capillary bed, causing a slow return to the resting venous pressure. [7]
- **Competent venous valves:**
  - » Allow unidirectional flow
  - » Function to divide the hydrostatic column of blood into segments [7, 9]
  - » Prevent retrograde venous flow [7, 9]

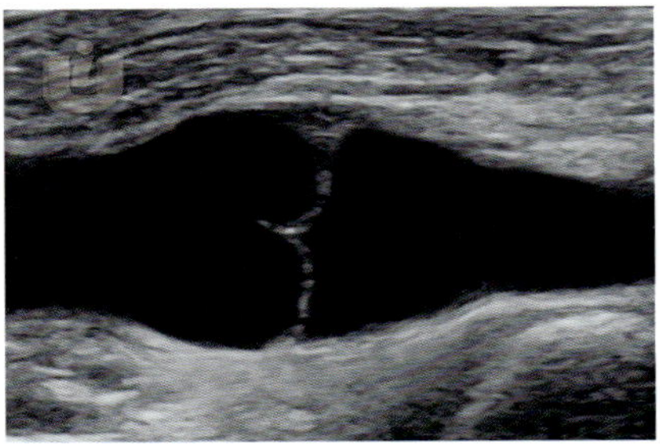

Fig. 10-2. *Longitudinal view of the right popliteal vein: standing, non-weight bearing.*

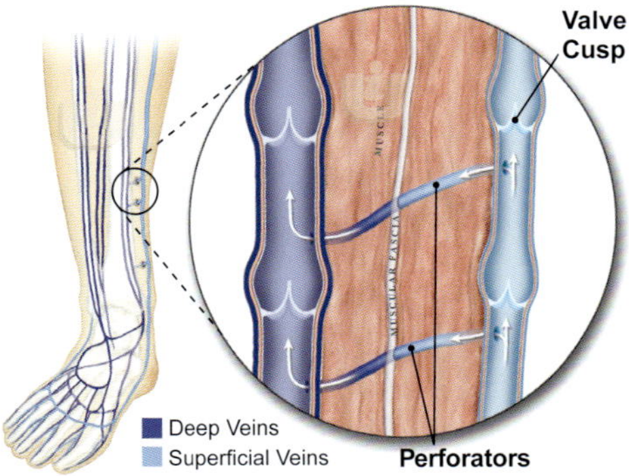

Fig. 10-3. *Perforating veins drain blood from the superficial veins to the deep veins.*

Venous Disease

- Chronic venous obstruction
- Reflux
- A combination of both obstruction and reflux
- Dysfunction of the muscular pumps
- Less common venous diseases
  - Malformations
  - Aneurysms
  - Tumors

Venous Obstruction [11, 12]

- There are three factors responsible for the formation of venous thrombosis. A combination of any of these events may result in venous thrombosis.
  - Vein wall injury
  - Hypercoagulability
  - Stasis of blood flow

- Obstruction of the iliac veins can directly affect the lower extremities and should be considered when assessing the lower extremities for venous disease; in particular, when the signs and symptoms are out of proportion with the ultrasound findings.
- Compression, although most often found in the left common iliac vein, may be observed in the right common iliac and both external iliac veins.

Venous Reflux

- Reflux is defined as retrograde flow of blood caused by incompetent valves and in rare cases, absent valves.
- Reflux or pathologic retrograde flow occurs when the valves are absent or rendered incompetent either by degenerative processes (primary venous disease) or by an episode of DVT (secondary venous disease). [2]

Dysfunction of the Muscular Pump

- Retrograde flow during calf muscle relaxation prevents the usual reduction in pressure and rapid venous refilling occurs from the retrograde flow of blood, as well as slow capillary inflow. [2]
  - When walking (contracting and relaxing the calf muscles), the calf muscle pump is activated, which propels blood upwards toward the heart, reducing blood volume and venous pressure.
  - When venous valves are incompetent, blood flows backwards during calf muscle relaxation, which can cause a significant increase in venous pressure.
- Increased venous pressure may also be transmitted from the deep to the superficial veins through incompetent perforators. [2]

The function of the calf muscle pump may be impaired in patients with chronic venous disease, an observation that is at least partially related to a reduced ankle range of motion. [2]

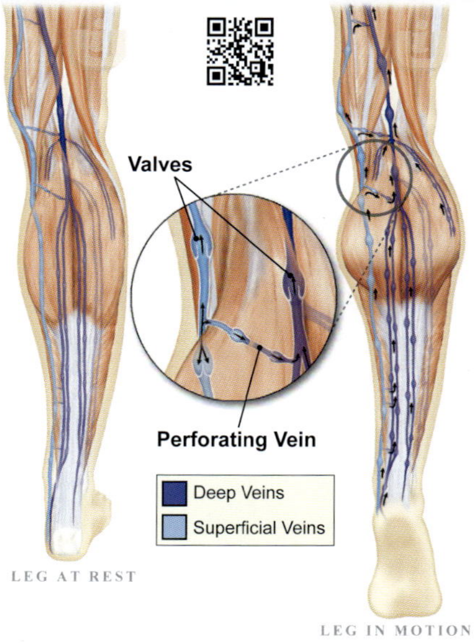

Fig. 10-4. *The calf muscle pump drives venous flow. While walking, muscle contractions squeeze the veins initiating venous blood flow. Venous flow opens the venous valves allowing the blood to flow towards the heart. As the muscle relaxes, valves close to prevent the backward flow of blood (reflux).*

Location of Disease

- Incompetent valves may be located anywhere within the deep, superficial or perforating venous systems, including:
  - Common femoral vein
  - Femoral vein
  - Popliteal vein
  - Saphenofemoral junction (SFJ)
  - Saphenopopliteal junction (SPJ) if present
  - Saphenous veins
  - Superficial tributaries
  - Perforating veins (most commonly those in the gaiter area)

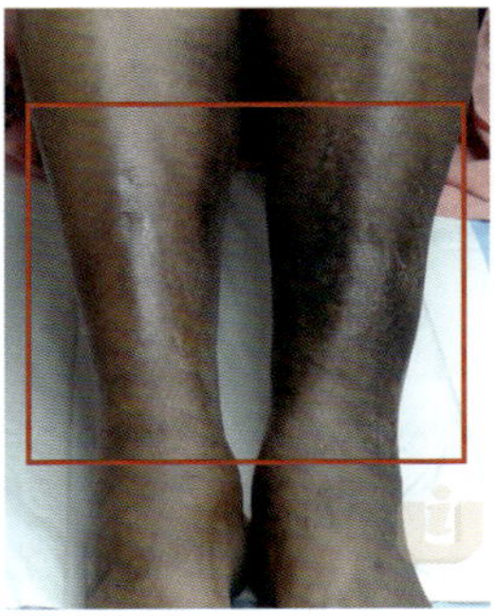

Fig. 10-5. *Located within the box is the gaiter area. Hyperpigmentation may occur in this area on the lateral or medial aspect of the leg, or both.*

Lower Extremity Venous Insufficiency Duplex

Patient History

- Family history of disease in both venous and arterial systems
  - Arterial: PAD, CAD, CVA
  - Venous: DVT, VVs, ulcers, thrombophilia
- Surgical history of the venous and arterial systems
- Prior deep or superficial vein thrombosis
- Localized pain, burning, or itching
- Tired, heavy legs after prolonged standing
- Persistent swelling (especially at the end of the day)
- Symptoms worsen at the end of the day
- Symptoms worsen at different times of the month; can be worse for women around menstruation
- Medications: blood thinners, birth control or hormone replacement
- Heavy lifting due to work or exercise regimen
- Standing or sitting for prolonged periods of time

Many times, patients will insist they had a ligation and stripping, but really only had an ambulatory phlebectomy.

Physical Examination

- Edema or irregularity in limb circumference
- Tenderness
- Warm or redness along a superficial vein or varicosity
- Varicose veins, reticular veins or telangiectasias (spider veins)
- Hyperpigmentation or skin changes associated with venous disease
- Active or healed venous ulcer
- Dermatitis
- Venous claudication
- Swelling
- Scars (possible indication of prior treatment)
- Local dilatations or blow outs (may be a perforating vein or muscle fascia hernia)

Alternate positions for calf vein evaluation Figs. 10-8 and 10-9

Patient Position

- The vein size can be affected by patient position or room temperature (a cold room may cause veins to constrict).
- To image the deep and superficial systems for thrombus and document spectral waveforms and color images, position the patient as follows:
  - Supine on a tilt table (for appropriate visualization and patient comfort)
  - Reverse Trendelenburg >20° (head higher than feet)
  - Lower extremity slightly abducted and externally rotated
  - Calf veins (alternative positions)
    - » Lateral decubitus
    - » Seated with legs dependent

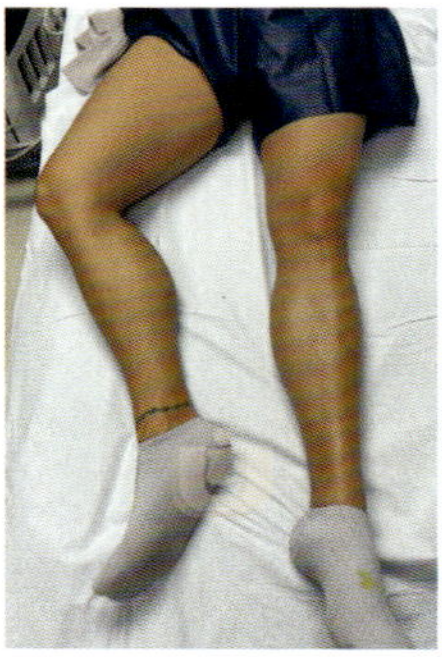

Fig. 10-6. *Position for evaluation of the deep and superficial systems for DVT, SVT and resting PW waveforms and color Doppler images of the CFV, FV, and PopV.*

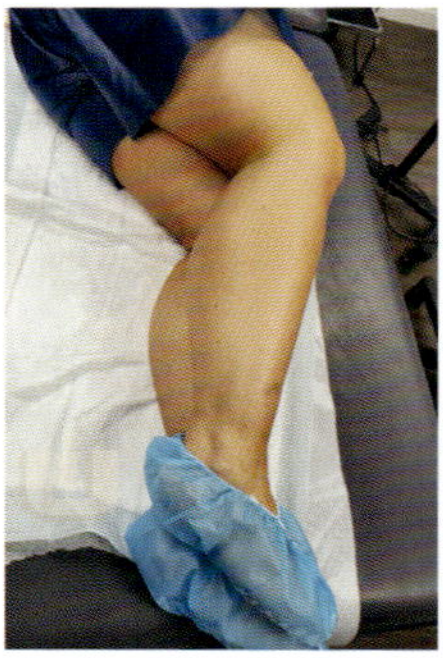

Fig. 10-7. *An alternate position for evaluation of the calf veins is the decubitus position (left decubitus position shown).*

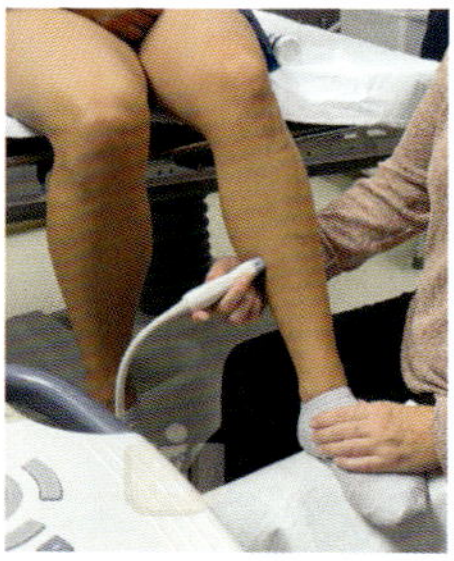

Fig. 10-8. *Evaluation of calf veins; patient is seated on the side of the bed with leg dependent and foot resting on examiner's lap or stool.*

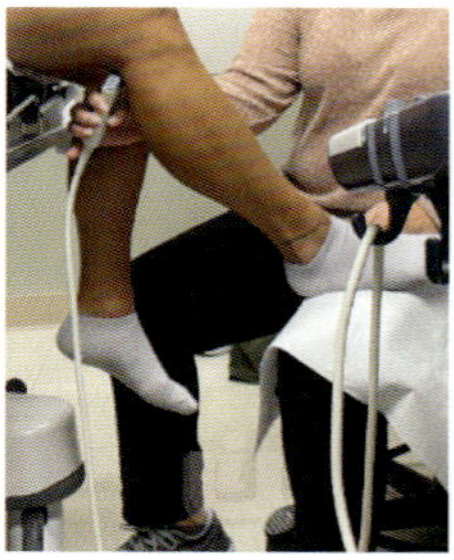

Fig. 10-9. *When using this position, be sure the back of the leg or knee is not resting against the bed.*

Deep and Superficial Systems for DVI/SVI

- Stand the patient on the floor or a platform when imaging:
  - Common Femoral, Femoral, Popliteal, Great Saphenous, and when present, other Accessory Great Saphenous and associated tributary veins
- Facing the examiner
  - Open stance with hip externally rotated
  - Knee slightly flexed—heel flat on the floor
  - Weight shifted to the contralateral limb
- Small Saphenous Vein, Thigh Extension of the SSV and associated tributaries
  - Face away from the examiner
  - Open stance with a step forward
  - Knee slightly flexed - heel flat on the floor
  - Weight shifted to the contralateral limb
- Perforating Veins (PVs)
  - Depends on topography

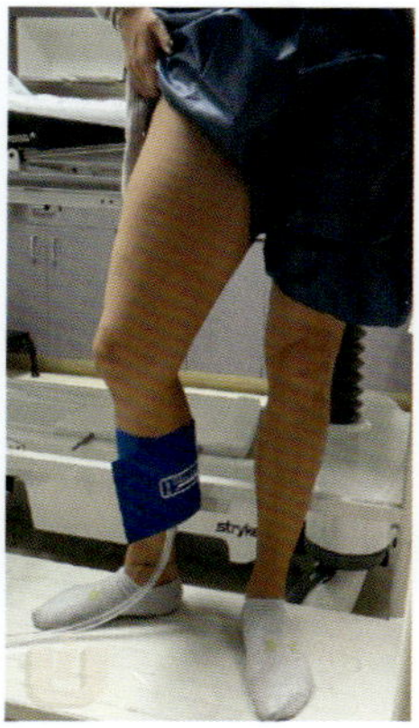

Fig. 10-10. *Position for evaluation of the CFV, SFJ, FV, GSV, AAGSV, and PAGSV.*

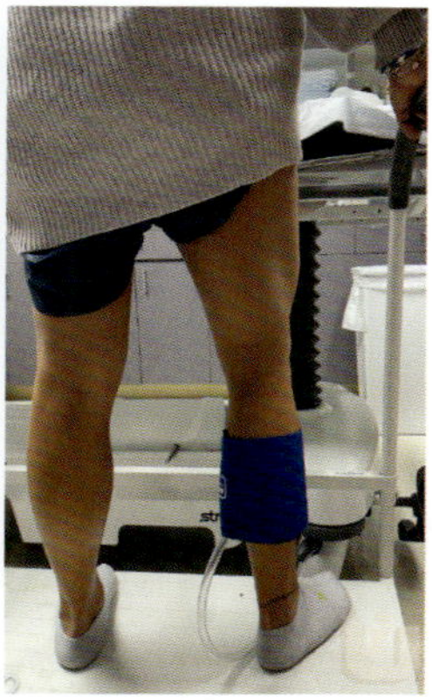

Fig. 10-11. *Position for evaluation of the PopV, SSV, and TE-SSV.*

Lower Extremity Venous Duplex Ultrasound Protocol [13-20]

B-Mode Analysis of the Deep Veins

Using the transverse view, evaluate the following vessels every 1-2cm for vein wall compressibility:

- Common Femoral Vein (CFV)
- SaphenoFemoral Junction (SFJ)
- Deep Femoral Vein (DFV)
- Femoral Vein (FV)
  - Proximal Thigh (PT)
  - Mid-Thigh (MT)
  - Distal Thigh (DT)
- Popliteal vein (PopV)
- Tibio-Peroneal Trunk (TPT)
- Posterior Tibial Veins (PTVs)
- Peroneal Veins (PerVs)
- Great Saphenous Vein (GSV)
- Small Saphenous Vein (SSV)
- Gastrocnemius Veins (GVs)
- Soleal Veins (SolVs)
- If present:
  - Sapheno Popliteal Junction (SPJ)
  - Anterior Accessory Great Saphenous Vein (AAGSV)
  - Posterior Accessory Great Saphenous Vein (PAGSV)
  - Thigh Extension of the SSV (TE-SSV)

When pathology (thrombus or intraluminal echoes) is present, document compressibility, appearance, location, and extent.

Doppler Analysis of the Deep Veins

5-7 MHz frequency transducers achieve adequate visualization of the deep, saphenous and perforating veins. If the deep veins are not easily visualized, you may need to use a lower frequency transducer. With the patient supine in the reverse Trendelenburg position, using a longitudinal view, demonstrate spontaneous venous flow, phasicity and color Doppler filling at the following levels:

- CFV
- FV
- PopV

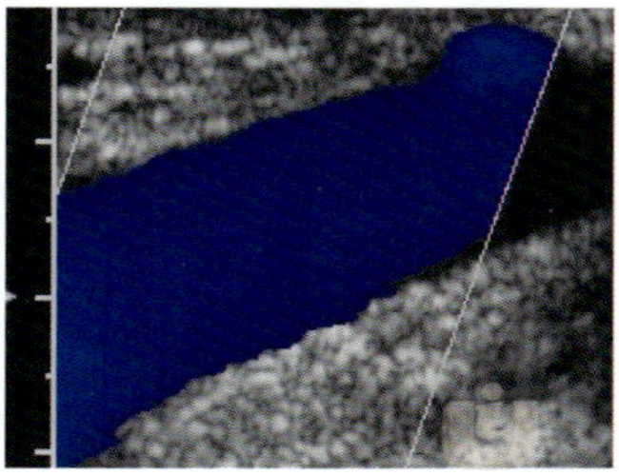

Fig. 10-12. *Color Doppler image demonstrating complete filling of the vein at rest.*

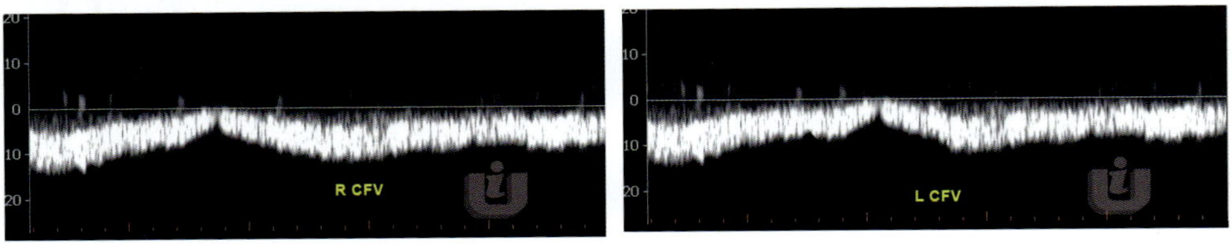

Fig. 10-13. *PW Doppler waveforms displaying symmetry between the right and left lower extremity common femoral veins.*

> *If unilateral testing is performed, Doppler waveforms must be obtained from the contralateral common femoral vein to assess for symmetrical phasicity.*

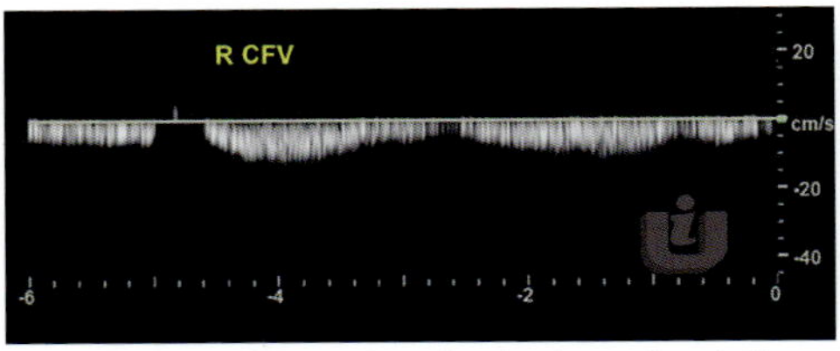

Fig. 10-14. *PW Doppler displaying phasicity in the right common femoral vein.*

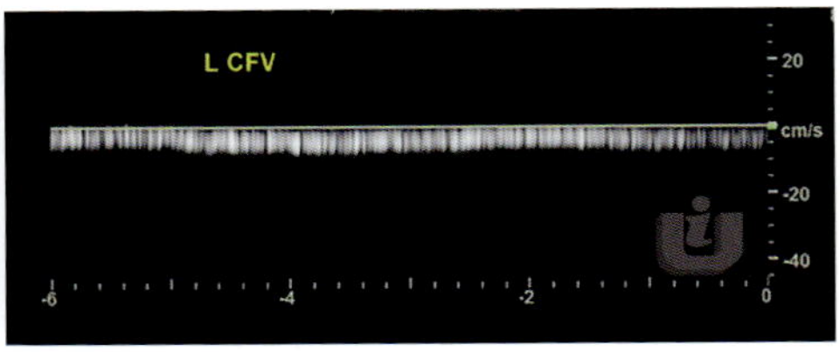

Fig. 10-15. *PW Doppler displaying a lack of phasicity in the left common femoral vein.*

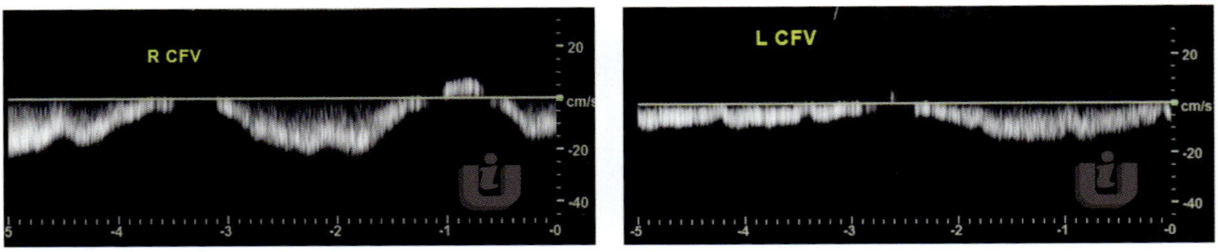

Fig. 10-16. *Asymmetry between the right and left lower extremity common femoral veins.*

> *Changes that are the result of central, systemic conditions will be seen bilaterally. Symmetry between left and right-sided waveforms is an important aspect of duplex studies requiring comparison of spontaneous signals.[21] By comparison, a lack of phasicity or asymmetry in the common femoral veins is an indirect indication of a central obstruction.*

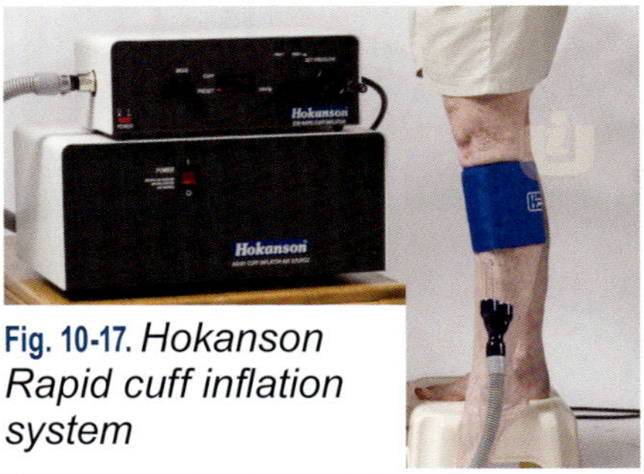

Fig. 10-17. *Hokanson Rapid cuff inflation system*

Photo courtesy of Hokanson, Bellevue, WA hokansonvascular.com

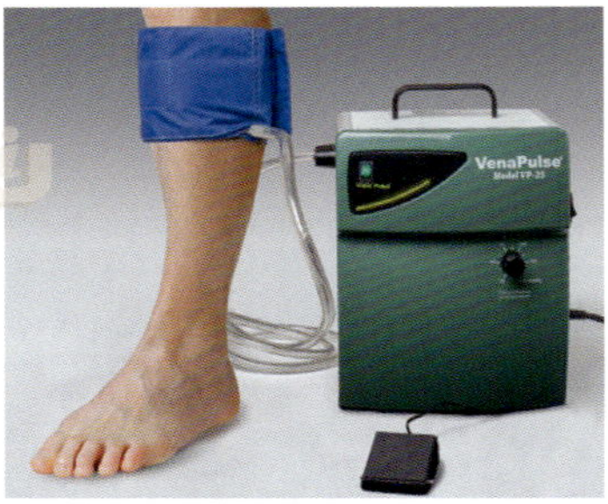

Fig. 10-18. *VenaPulse® Hands-Free Augmentation Device* *Photo courtesy of ACI Medical San Marcos, CA. acimedical.com/products/venapulse*

> *The use of a hands-free pneumatic rapid cuff inflation device is recommended to provide reproducible peripheral augmentation and reduce sonographer twisting and bending during the insufficiency examination.*

Venous Insufficiency Examination

- Higher frequency transducers achieve adequate visualization of the saphenous and superficial tributaries. If the deep veins are not easily visualized, you may need to use a lower frequency transducer.
- Evaluate all veins for the presence or absence of reflux using PW and/or color Doppler.
- Optional maneuvers mentioned earlier may be used.

Use PW Doppler without or with color Doppler to document the presence or absence of reflux in the following vessels:

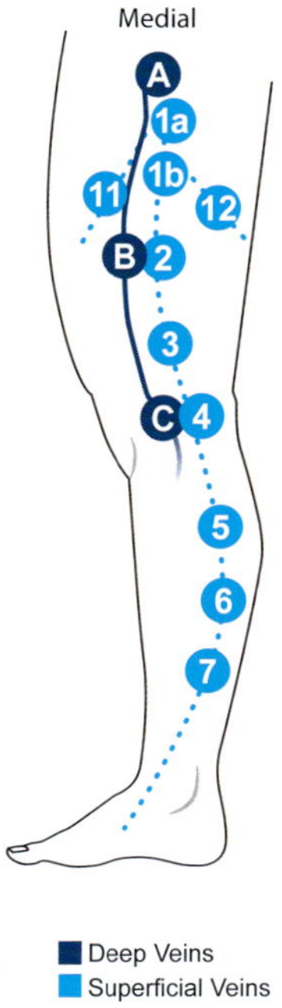

Deep Veins

A Common Femoral Vein (CFV)
B Femoral Vein (FV)
C Popliteal Vein (PopV)

Superficial Veins

Great Saphenous Vein (GSV)

1a Sapheno Femoral Junction terminal valve (SFJtv)
1b Sapheno Femoral Junction pre-terminal valve (SFJptv) and or Proximal Thigh (PT)
2 Mid Thigh (MT)
3 Distal Thigh (DT) (if vein is present at this level)
4 Knee (if vein is present at this level)
5 Proximal Calf (PC) (if vein is present at this level)
6 Mid Calf (MC) (if vein is present at this level)
7 Distal Calf (DC) (if vein is present at this level)

Small Saphenous Vein (SSV)

8 Sapheno Popliteal Junction (SPJ)
9 Mid Calf (MC)
10 Distal Calf (DC) (optional)

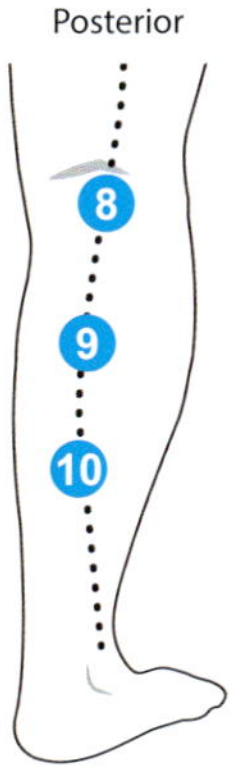

If present or relevant

11 Anterior Accessory Great Saphenous Vein (AAGSV)
12 Posterior Accessory Great Saphenous Vein (PAGSV)
- Anterior Thigh Circumflex Vein (ATCV)
- Posterior Thigh Circumflex Vein (PTCV)
- Thigh Extension of the SSV (TE-SSV)
- Associated tributaries and perforating veins

The saphenous compartment contains the saphenous veins. Saphenous tributaries lie above the saphenous fascia in the epifascial compartment.

At times the posterior thigh circumflex vein forms a connection between the great saphenous vein and the small saphenous vein.

- To record PW Doppler waveforms, place the Doppler sample gate in the center of the flow stream. Adjust the gate to 2-4mm wide depending on the diameter of the vessel.
- Perform peripheral augmentation release to assess for the presence or absence of reflux by using any of the following maneuvers:
  - Calf and thigh rapid augmentation/ release maneuver
  - Dorsiflexion
  - Valsalva maneuver

The augmentation maneuver used must be noted in the final report.

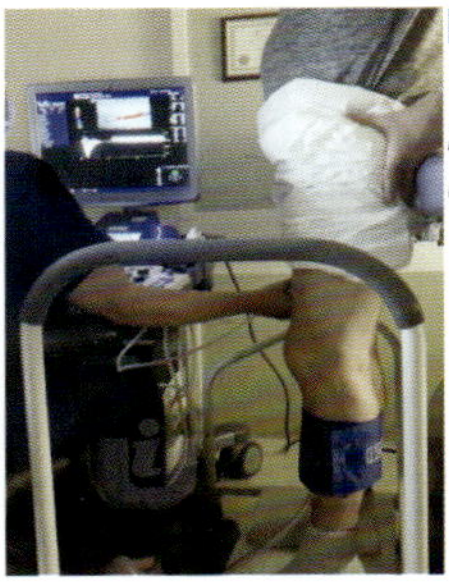

Fig. 10-19. *Venous insufficiency evaluation*

- Color Doppler may be used to demonstrate response to peripheral augmentation release maneuvers. Reversal of color signifies flow reversal and may be indicative of reflux. Color Doppler can expedite the evaluation, but is not required. PW Doppler is a more reliable and reproducible means of documenting reflux.[48]
- A unilateral examination may be performed if the patient has unilateral symptoms. If unilateral testing is performed, a Doppler waveform must be obtained from the contralateral common femoral vein and should be assessed for symmetrical phasicity.
- If DVT is present, compression maneuvers and Doppler waveforms must be obtained from the contralateral common femoral vein.
- If DVT is identified, augmentation is not performed; however, resting grayscale images in both longitudinal and transverse views along with PW waveforms and color Doppler images should be documented.

Interpretation-Diagnostic Criteria

Normal

Criteria for patency

- Absence of intraluminal thrombus on grayscale image
  - Common femoral veins
  - Femoral veins
  - Popliteal veins
  - Calf veins
  - Saphenous veins
  - Intramuscular veins
- Complete coaptation of vein walls with transducer pressure
- PW Doppler waveforms demonstrating spontaneity and phasicity
  - Common femoral veins
  - Femoral veins
  - Popliteal veins
- Visualization of color flow throughout the lumen
  - Common femoral veins
  - Femoral veins
  - Popliteal veins

Abnormal

Criteria for the presence of thrombosis

- Partial or incomplete coaptation of vein walls with transducer pressure.
- Presence of intraluminal thrombus (echogenic material) on grayscale image (in early acute stage of thrombus, the vein may be dilated with no sign of intraluminal thrombus).
- Abnormal PW Doppler waveforms: absence of phasicity, diminished or continuous flow.

Normal

Criteria for normal resting venous waveforms[50]

- **Spontaneous flow:** Blood flow is spontaneous when it is observed actively moving in a vein without any external maneuvers such as Valsalva, muscle contraction or compression peripheral to the vein being evaluated.

- **Respirophasic flow:** A cyclical increase and decrease in flow velocity, which correlates with respiratory phases.

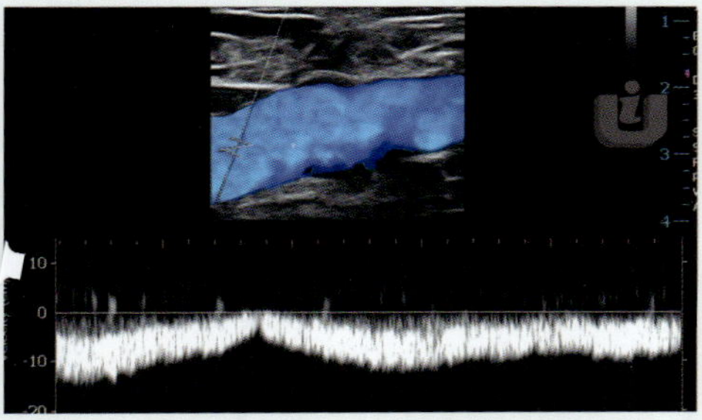

Fig. 10-20. *Spontaneous phasic flow in the femoral vein.*

Abnormal

Criteria for abnormal resting waveforms [50]

- **Pulsatile flow:** Cyclical increase and decrease, which inversely correlates with the cardiac cycle.
- **Continuous flow:** Characterized by the lack of respiratory or cardiac influence on flow velocity variation resulting in a steady and consistent Doppler signal with minimal to no variation in flow.
- **Absent flow:** No blood flow is detected with an absent PW Doppler signal.

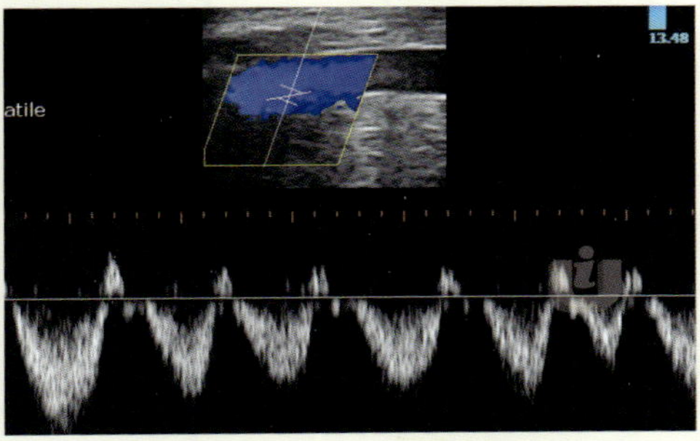

Fig. 10-21. *Pulsatile flow in the femoral vein.*

In the presence of congestive heart failure, central venous pressure increases and may be a cause of pulsatile waveforms in the lower extremities (not all pulsatile venous waveforms are caused by CHF). [10]

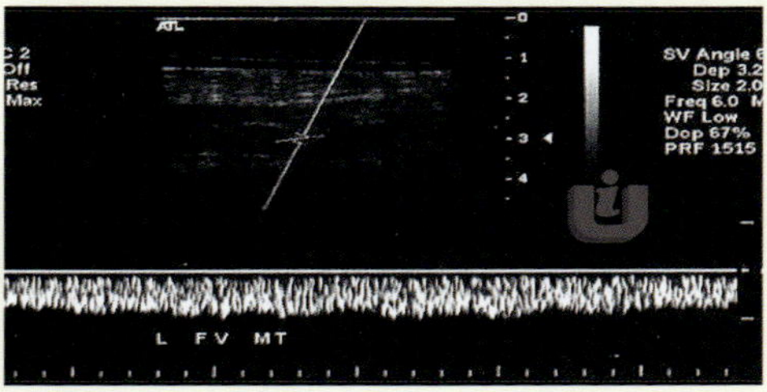

Fig. 10-22. *Continuous flow in the femoral vein.*

Table 10-1. Lower Extremity Venous DVT, SVT, DVI and SVI Examination Protocol Summary

DVT/SVT

Reverse Trendelenburg position using B-mode. Scan using the transverse view (SAX) without and with transducer compression to assess deep, superficial and intramuscular veins for thrombus.

		Superficial veins
• CFV	• PTVs	• GSV
• SFJ	• PerVs	• SSV
• FV	• GVs	• Other if present
• PopV	• SolVs	

Resting Doppler

Trendelenburg position using pulsed wave and color Doppler. Scan in longitudinal view (LAX) to assess for spontaneity, phasicity and color filling in the:

- CFV
- FV
- PopV
- Deep veins of the calf are optional
- Intramuscular calf veins are optional

Standing Position with peripheral augmentation release maneuver in longitudinal view (LAX) using PW and/or CD for present or absence of reflux:

Deep veins	Superficial veins
• CFV	• GSV
• SFJ	• SSV
• FV	• Other if present
• PopV	
• Deep veins of the calf are optional	
• Intramuscular calf veins are optional	

Provocative maneuvers and venous reflux criteria

- **Peripheral Augmentation and Release:** Normally, as the valve is closing there is a brief period of reverse flow. After the valve has closed there is no flow.
  - Reflux in the deep veins of the thigh (CFV, FV, PopV) is defined as reverse flow >1sec (>1000msec). [14, 23, 25, 26]
  - Reflux in the deep veins of the calf, superficial veins and perforating veins is defined as reverse flow >0.5sec (>500msec). [14, 23, 25, 26]
- **Valsalva:** Cessation of the PW Doppler signal (should result in flow velocity = 0). If the PW Doppler signal is augmented (flow velocity increases) there is venous reflux. Valsalva should be used only at the CFV/SFJ level. The remaining vein segments should be evaluated using peripheral augmentation and release. [14, 23, 25, 26]
- **Central Compression and Release:** Cessation of flow during central compression after a brief valve closure, with augmentation upon release, is a normal finding. Similar to the Valsalva response, augmentation during central compression proves valvular incompetence. [22]

> *Central compression is a form of augmentation where an area central to the vein segment being evaluated is compressed and released, e.g., the left lower quadrant (left side of the pelvis).*

Normal

No Venous Reflux

- Venous flow should be directed towards the heart (negative deflection of the Doppler tracing).
  - Both during and after augmentation below the probe
  - During the Valsalva maneuver
- A brief period of reflux immediately after maneuvers is most likely just the normal reverse flow that occurs during valve closure [23, 24]

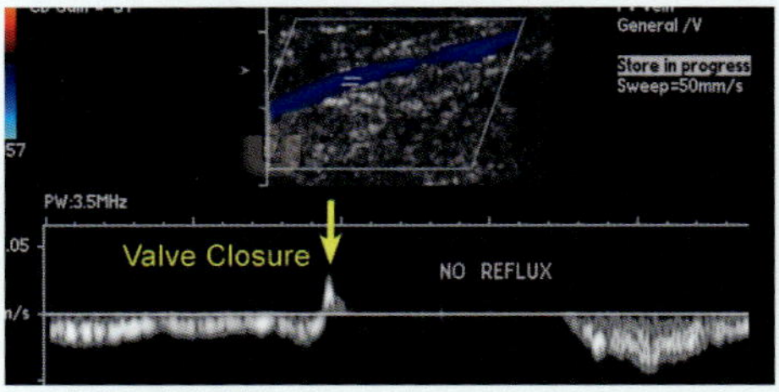

Fig. 10-23. *PW Doppler waveform displaying valve closure following peripheral augmentation release maneuver. A brief period of flow reversal may be observed during the closure of a healthy venous valve.*

Abnormal

Venous Reflux

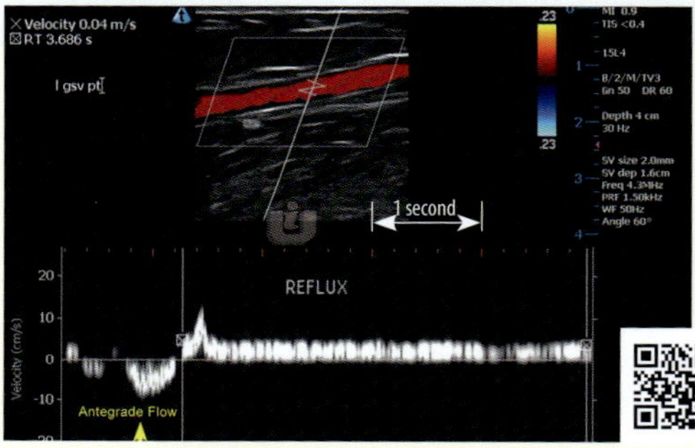

Fig. 10-24. *Waveform displaying >3500msec of reflux in the GSV. Reflux is indicated by retrograde flow above the baseline for a duration of >500msec.*

- Abnormal, incompetent valves allow both forward and reverse flow (negative and positive) deflection of the PW Doppler waveform.
- Venous reflux (reverse flow) may be seen:
  - Upon release when using peripheral augmentation release maneuver.
  - During the Valsalva maneuver while the abdomen muscles are contracted
- Reflux is considered to be clinically significant when it lasts in the: [14, 23, 25, 26]
  - **Deep veins (CFV, FV, PopV):** >1sec (>1000msec)
  - **Superficial veins:** >0.5sec (>500msec)
  - **Tibial veins:** >0.5sec (>500msec)
  - **Perforating veins:** >0.5sec (>500msec)

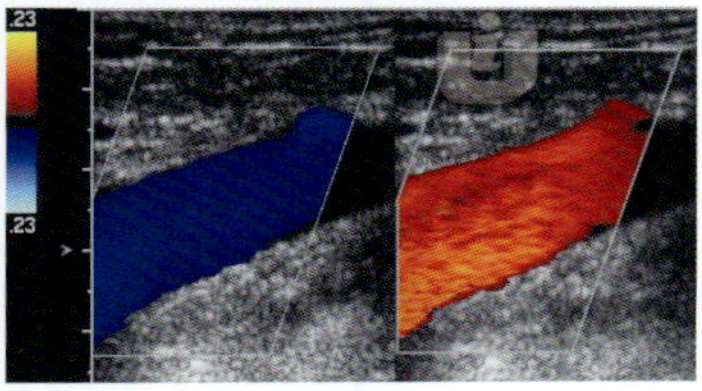

Fig. 10-25. *The image on the left displays normal (antegrade) flow in the vein. The image on the right displays abnormal (retrograde) flow in the vein during the Valsalva maneuver.*

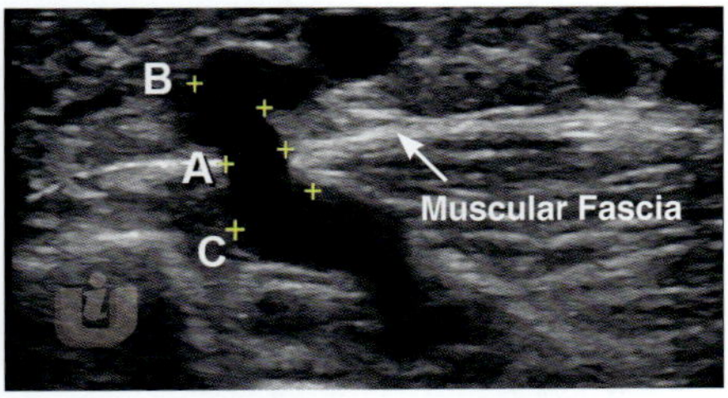

Fig. 10-26. *Pathologic perforating vein measuring 4.1mm in diameter at the level of the muscular fascia.*

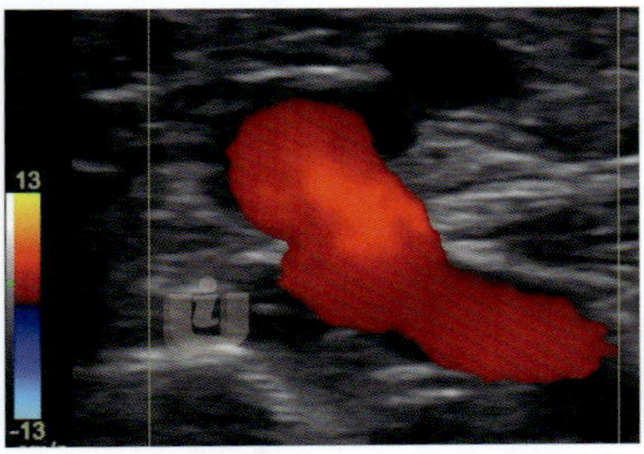

Fig. 10-27. *Color Doppler image of an incompetent perforating vein.*

Perforating Veins

- Investigate and evaluate perforating veins that connect directly to varicosities and/or are in close proximity to dermatologic changes.
- Assess perforating veins for size and competence. Perforating veins are considered incompetent if they show >0.5 seconds of reversed flow or reflux.
- Measure the diameter of the incompetent perforating vein at three levels (if possible).
  - at the location where the vein perforates the deep fascia *(Fig. 10-26 A)*
  - largest diameter above the fascia *(Fig. 10-26 B)*
  - largest diameter below the fascia *(Fig. 10-26 C)*

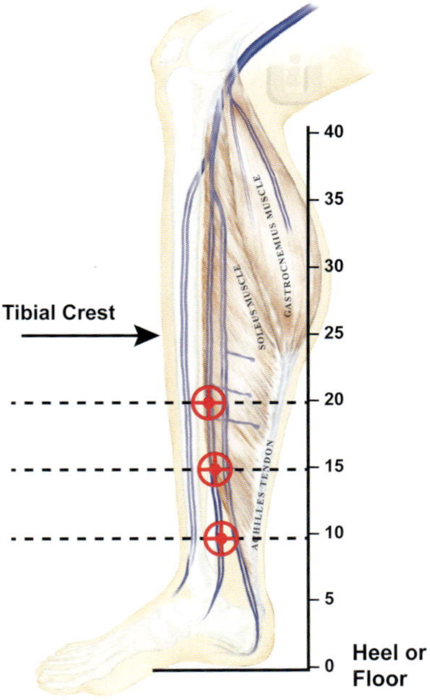

Fig. 10-28. *Measuring a pathologic perforating vein: Use the sole of the foot or the floor to generate a longitude coordinate and use the tibial crest to generate a latitude coordinate.*

Interpretation

Table 10-2. Diagnostic Criteria for Venous Reflux [14, 23, 25, 26]

	Valve Closure Time Normal	Valve Closure Time Abnormal
Common Femoral Vein (CFV)	<1sec or <1000msec	>1sec or >1000msec
Femoral Vein (FV)	<1sec or <1000msec	>1sec or >1000msec
Popliteal Vein (PopV)	<1sec or <1000msec	>1sec or >1000msec
Calf Veins	<0.5sec or <500msec	>0.5sec or >500msec
Perforating Veins [50]	<0.5sec or <500msec	>0.5sec or >500msec
Superficial Veins	<0.5sec or <500msec	>0.5sec or >500msec

There is no consensus currently for normal/abnormal vein diameters in published literature. [14]

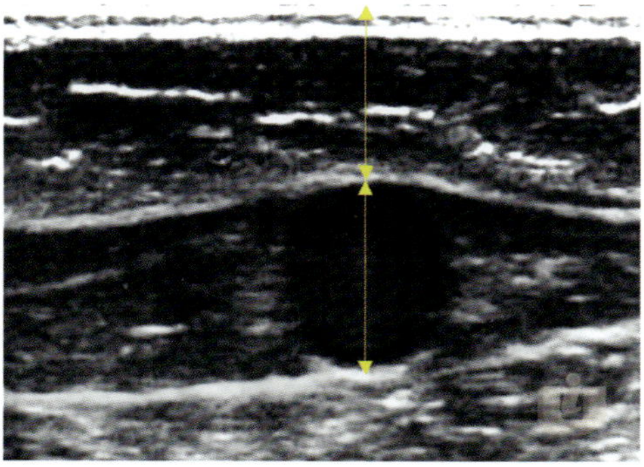

Fig. 10-29. *Diameter and depth measurements of the GSV.*

- Vein diameter should be measured, but not used as a criterion for reflux.
  - Mean diameter GSV: 5.0 ± 2.4 [46]
  - Mean diameter SSV: 3.1 ± 1.3 [46]
- Perform all measurements in the standing position.
- Using the transverse view, measure the maximum diameter from the anterior outer wall to the posterior outer wall.
- Measure the depth of the vein from the skin surface when relevant.

Many small diameter veins have reflux, and many large diameter veins do not have reflux.

Incidental Findings

- **Venous aneurysm:** A region in the vein where the lumen has become significantly larger than that of the central segment. Historically, superficial venous aneurysms were rarely identified; however, due to increased use of venous ultrasound, they are seen more frequently. Superficial venous aneurysms may be associated with thrombosis and pulmonary emboli and are found more often in females than males. [37]
- **Neovascularization:** Recurrence through the growth of new vessels. [27]
- **Revascularization:** Veins can recur in the saphenous compartment after a saphenous vein procedure. [43]
- **Recanalization:** Restoration of a lumen in a blood vessel following thrombotic occlusion by organization of the thrombus with formation of new channels. [28]
- **Popliteal cyst (e.g., Baker's cyst):** is a fluid-filled sac behind the knee. [29]
- **Enlarged lymph node:** The majority of lymph nodes are considered normal if they measure less than 1cm in short axis. There are a few exceptions, including inguinal region, where lymph nodes less than 1.5cm in short axis are considered normal. [30]
- **Edema:** A swelling caused by excess fluid trapped in your body's tissues. Although edema can affect any part of your body, you may notice it more in your hands, arms, feet, ankles and legs. [31]
- **Phlebosclerosis (chronic wall changes):** Refers to thickening and hardening of the venous wall. Phlebosclerosis creates a fibrous degeneration of the venous wall, predominantly the intima, with or without calcification. [33]
- **Synechiae (webbing):** Organization and subsequent contraction of a thrombus leading to adherence of thrombus to the vein wall and spontaneous lysis of areas within the thrombus. A fibrous membrane may remain within the lumen of the vein. [32]
- **Rouleaux flow:** A phenomenon that is slow flowing RBCs moving together producing spontaneous contrast. This should not be confused with thrombosis. It can easily be corrected with probe compression to distribute the RBCs. [34]
- **Vein wall dissection:** A dissection is a tear within the wall of a blood vessel, which allows blood to separate the wall layers. Usually, a dissection is an arterial wall dissection, but rarely it may be a vein wall dissection. [35]

A superficial venous aneurysm is a localized dilatation of a vein segment where the diameter is >50% diameter of the adjacent vein segments.

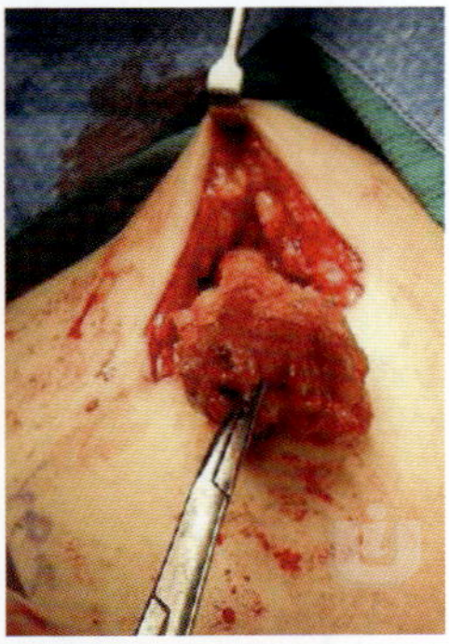

Fig. 10-30. *Surgical image of a venous aneurysm.* *Image courtesy of John Mauriello, MD*

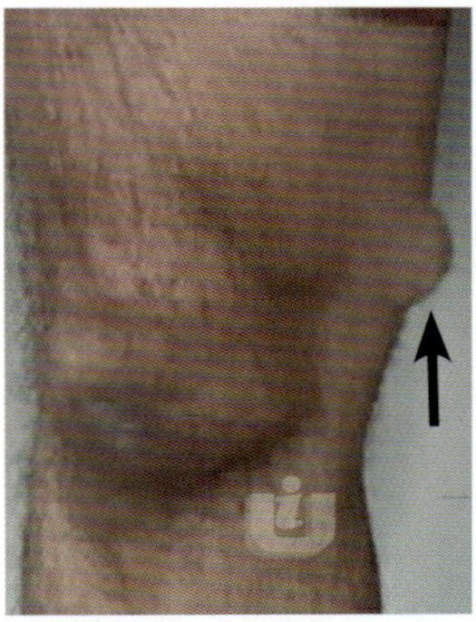

Fig. 10-31. *A venous aneurysm located on the medial aspect of the distal thigh.*

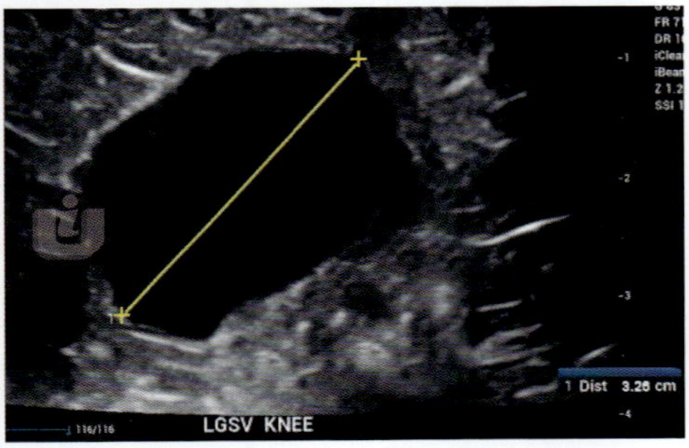

Fig. 10-32. *A venous aneurysm displayed using B-mode. The diameter is 32.6mm.*

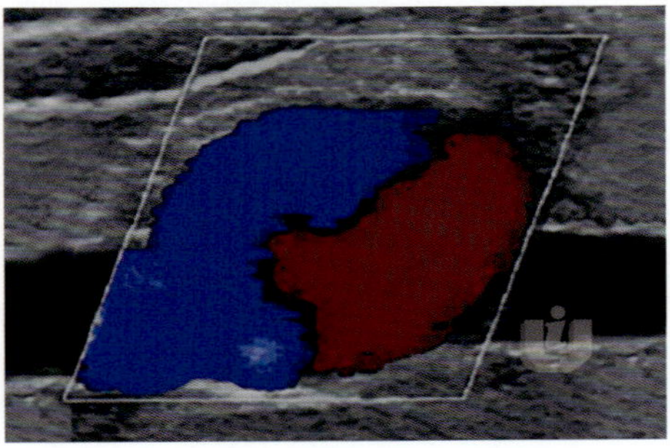

Fig. 10-33. *Color Doppler image displaying bidirectional flow within an aneurysmal segment.* *Image courtesy of Joseph Caprini MD*

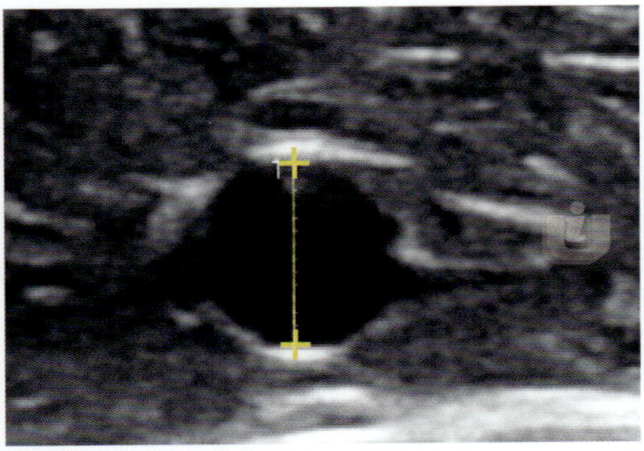

Fig. 10-34. *Diameter of the GSV is 7mm central to the aneurysmal segment in Fig. 10-35.*

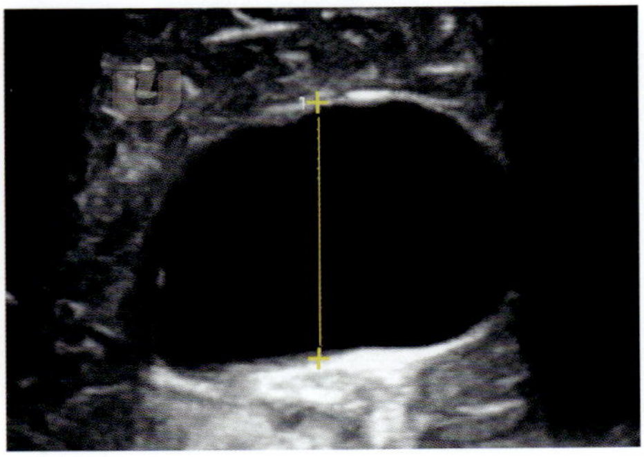

Fig. 10-35. *Great saphenous venous aneurysm measuring 20.7mm in diameter.*

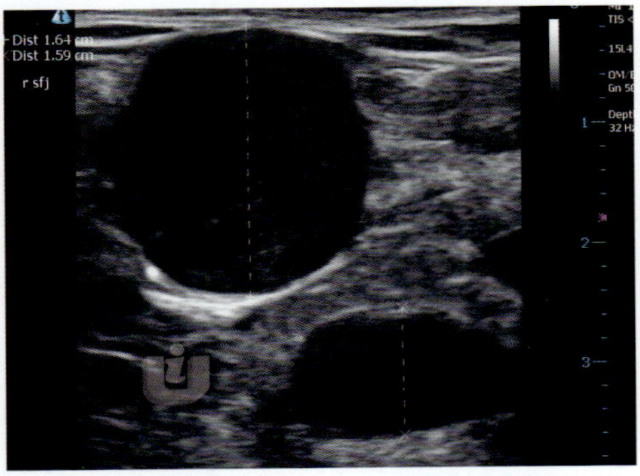

Fig. 10-36. *Venous aneurysm at the SFJ in the transverse view. The GSV diameter is 1.64mm and the CFV diameter is 1.59mm.*

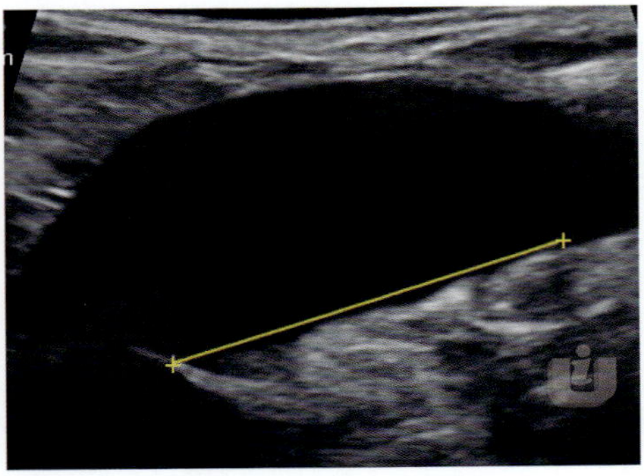

Fig. 10-37. *Venous aneurysm in the longitudinal view.*

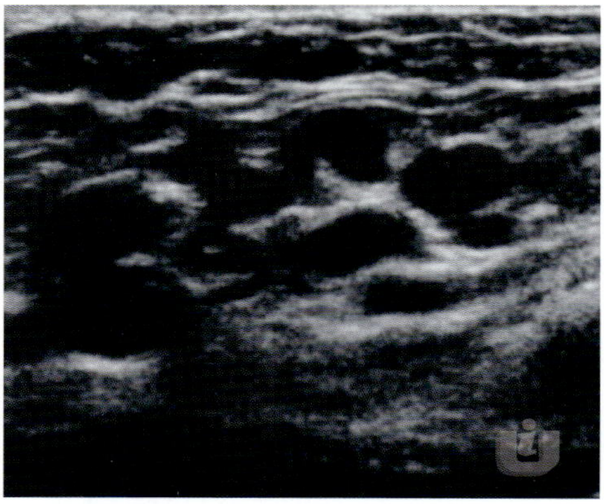

Fig. 10-38. *Inguinal neovascularization displayed in grayscale.*

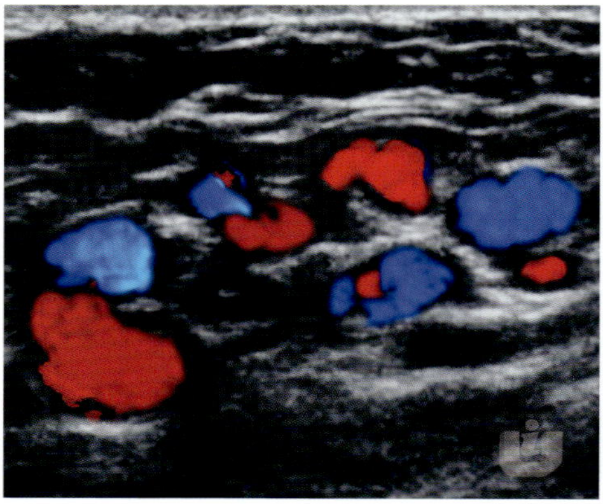

Fig. 10-39. *Inguinal neovascularization displayed using color Doppler during Valsalva maneuver.*

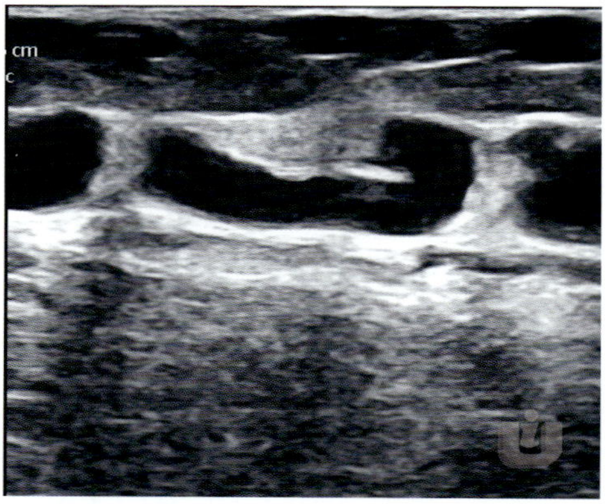

Fig. 10-40. *Revascularization within the small saphenous compartment at the mid-calf level.*

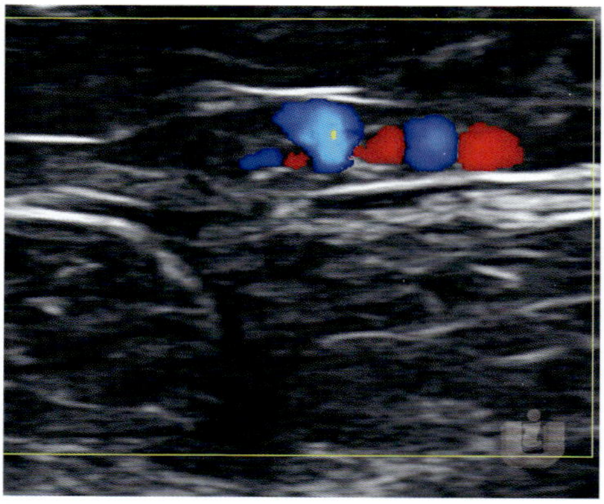

Fig. 10-41. *Revascularization within the great saphenous compartment at the mid-thigh level with color.*

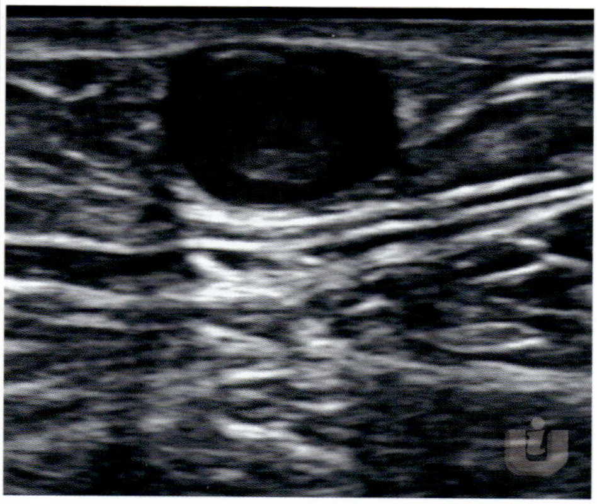

Fig. 10-42. *Recanalization displayed in the transverse view using B-mode.*

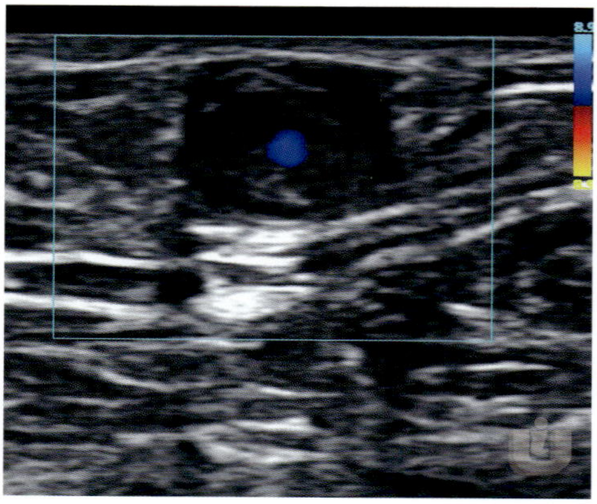

Fig. 10-43. *Recanalization displayed in the transverse view using color Doppler imaging.*

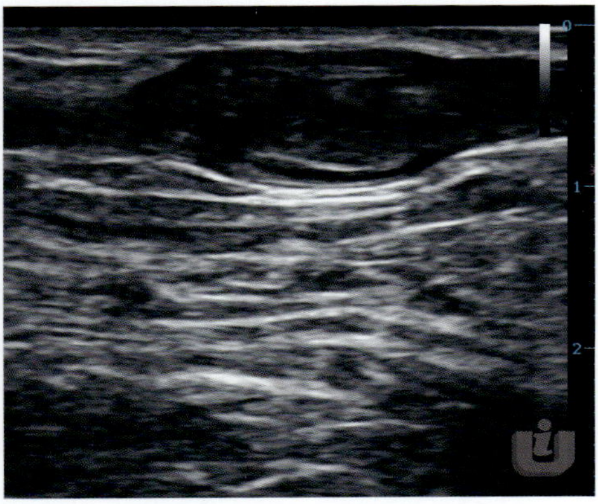

Fig. 10-44. *Recanalization displayed in the longitudinal view using B-mode.*

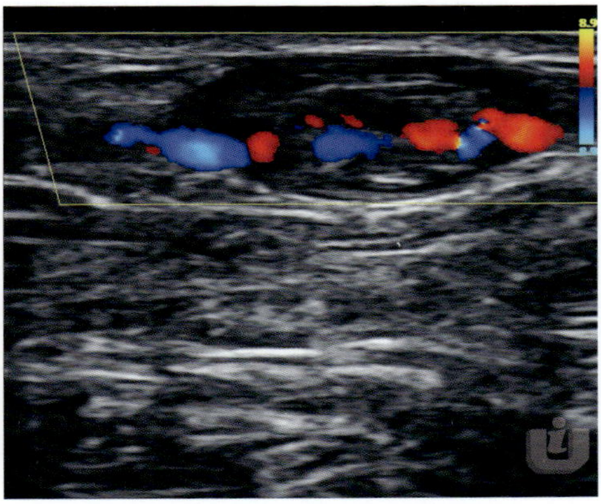

Fig. 10-45. *Recanalization displayed in the longitudinal view using color Doppler imaging.*

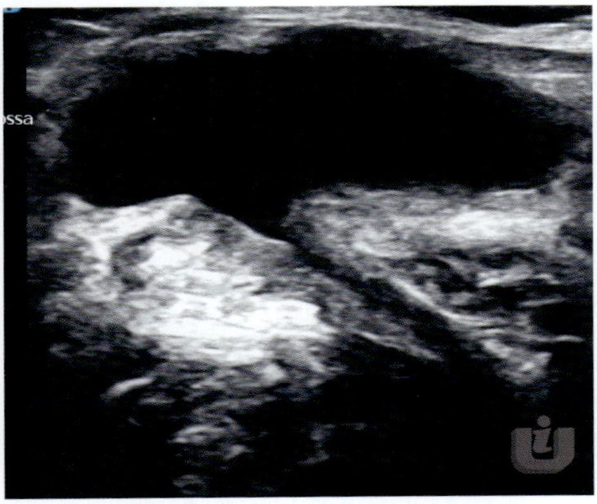

Fig. 10-46. *Simple popliteal cyst displayed using B-mode.*

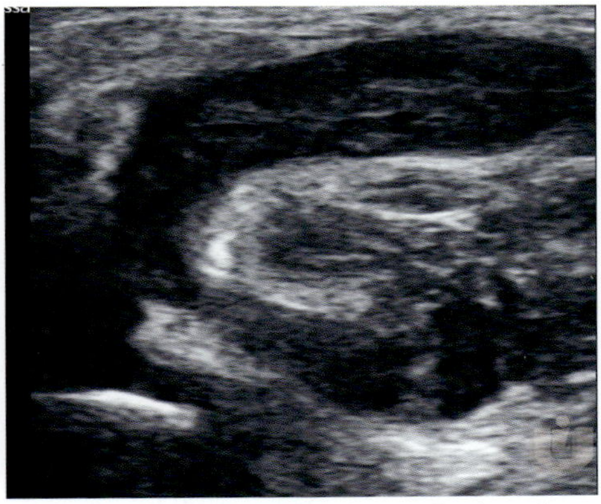

Fig. 10-47. *Complex popliteal cyst displayed using B-mode.*

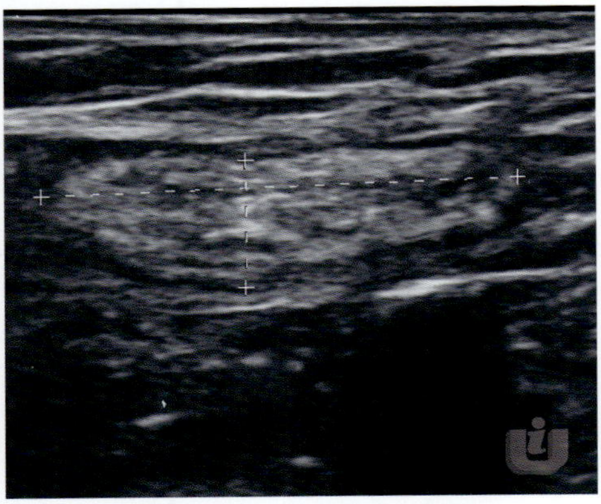

Fig. 10-48. *Inguinal lymph node displayed using B-mode.*

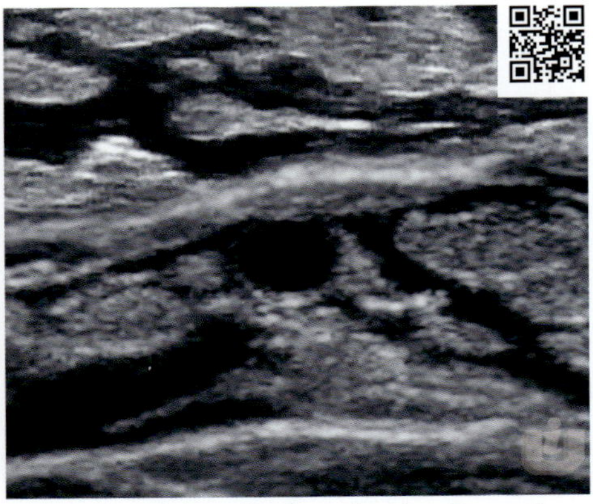

Fig. 10-49. *Edema displayed using B-mode.*

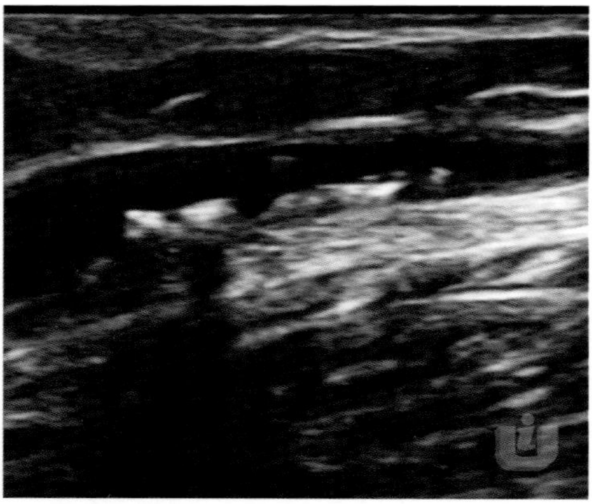

Fig. 10-50. *Phlebosclerosis displayed in the longitudinal view using B-mode.*

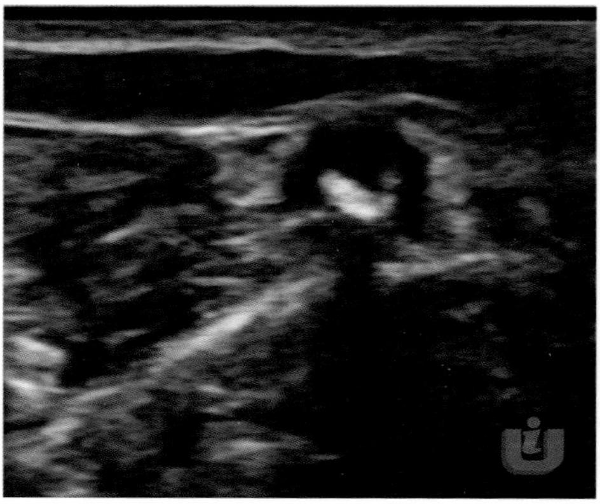

Fig. 10-51. *Phlebosclerosis displayed in the transverse view using B-mode.*

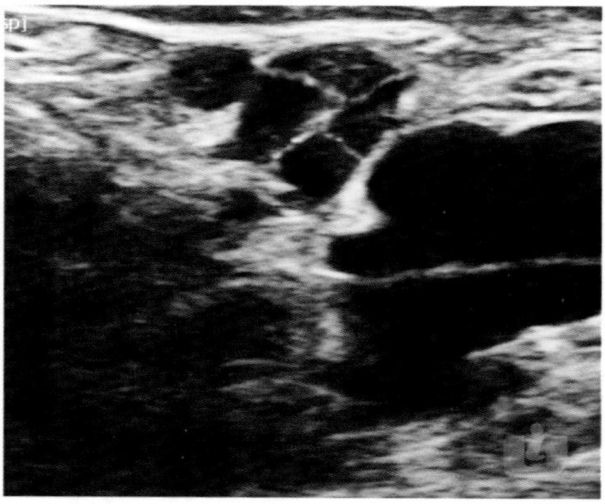

Fig. 10-52. *Webbing displayed in the transverse view using B-mode.*

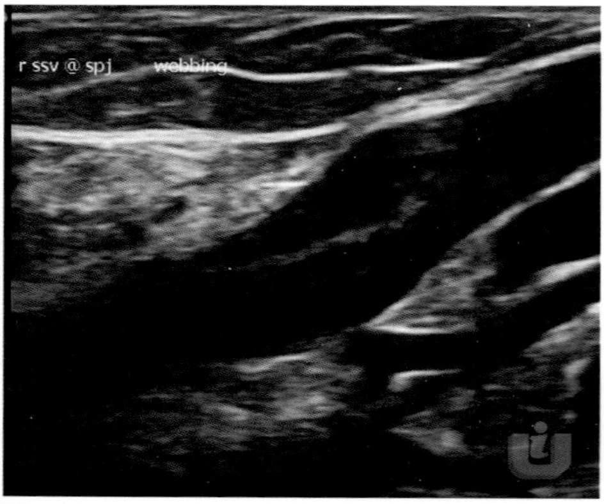

Fig. 10-53. *Webbing displayed in the longitudinal view using B-mode.*

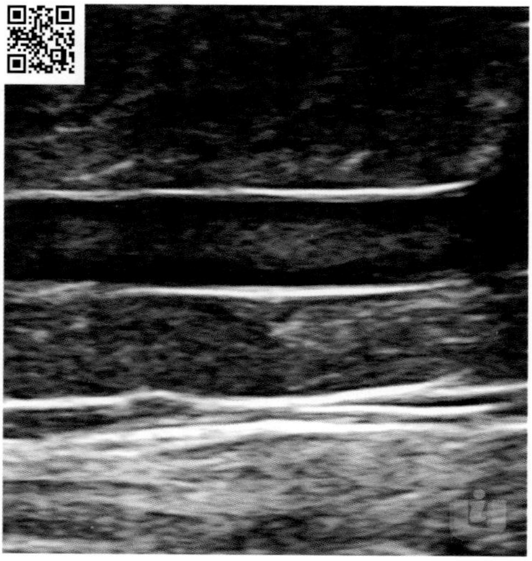

Fig. 10-54. *Rouleaux flow displayed in the longitudinal view using B-mode.*

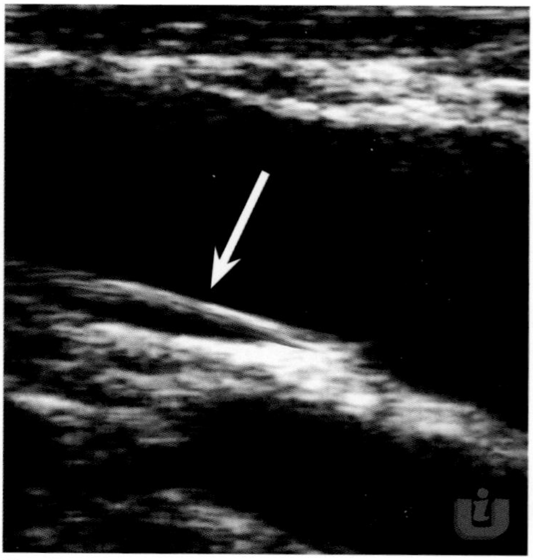

Fig. 10-55. *Vein wall dissection displayed in the longitudinal view using B-mode.*

How To Create A Lower Extremity Venous Map

A completed mapping should accompany all positive reflux studies indicating the following:

- Note patient position on the mapping form.
- Document augmentation method used.
- Draw all patterns of reflux.
- Measure diameter and depth of all incompetent veins.
- Using duplex pictures and other notes taken during the ultrasound examination, it is recommended to draw a detailed map of the superficial system, tributaries, perforating veins and any unusual anatomy or disease.
- Draw the vein course and caliber. Use the best estimation that accurately represents the venous tree.
- Use key on the map form provided to accurately code pathology.

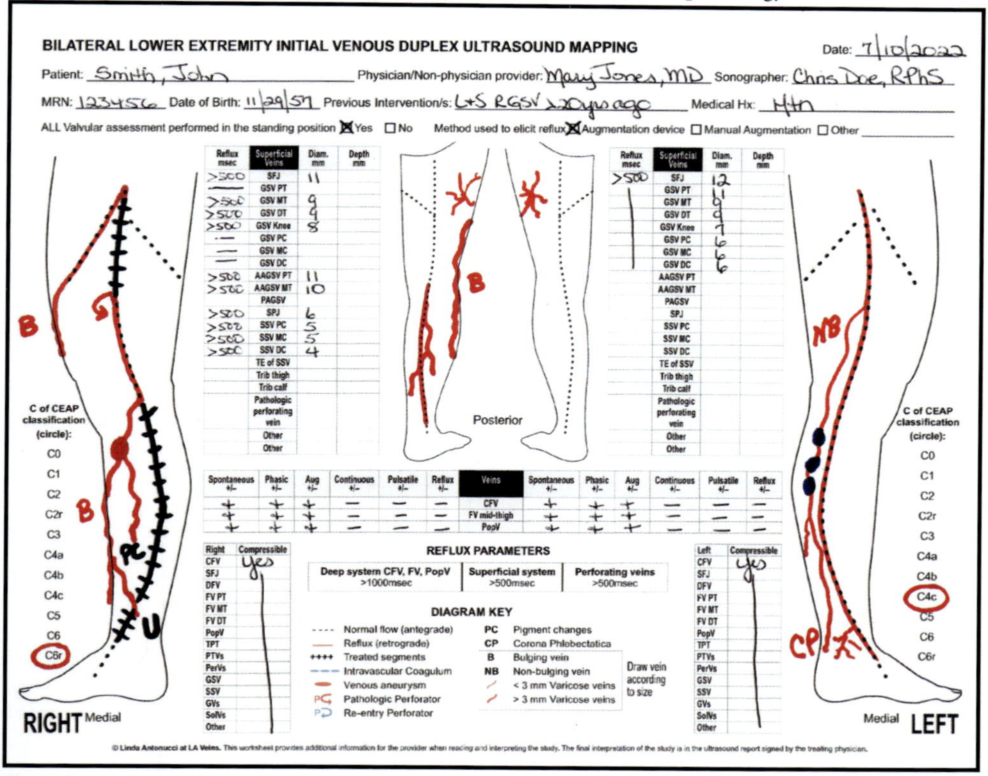

Fig. 10-56. *Venous lower extremity mapping form and example can be downloaded with the QR code.*

Points to Remember

- The superficial veins do not have a corresponding artery, which makes them easy to distinguish from deep veins.
- The femoral and popliteal veins may be duplicated.
- An estimated 40% of people in the United States have CVD. [38]
- Venous disease occurs more often in women than in men. [38]
- Venous disease occurs more frequently in people over age 50. Approximately 50% of those over 50 years of age have VVs. [38]
- The prevalence of venous ulcers in the U.S. is approximately 600,000 annually. [39]
- If both parents had VVs, it is estimated that their children have a 90% chance of developing VVs. If only one parent had VVs, the son has a 25% chance and the daughter a 62% chance of developing VVs. If neither parent had VVs, there is still a 20% chance of developing VVs. [40]

- Varicose veins can occur anywhere in the body, though they occur most often in the lower extremities.
- There are several terms used to describe venous issues which are sometimes used incorrectly. Thrombophlebitis is defined as inflammation of a vein associated with a thrombus. Phlebitis simply means venous inflammation and can occur in the absence of a thrombus.
- Superficial vein thrombosis can occur with or without inflammation.
- Studies estimate that 69% of patients with a history of DVT will develop chronic venous insufficiency within 1 year. [23]
- Dilatation of the lower extremity venous system can be due to venous or portal hypertension. [10]
- Birth control pills and hormone replacement therapy may increase the risk of varicose/spider veins and thrombosis. [41]
- The number and severity of varicose veins can increase with each pregnancy. Varicose veins can improve postpartum. [41]
- To study veins, the settings on the ultrasound machine need to be set for "low-flow" (low wall filter, low color scale and high gain), as the machine needs to be able to detect blood flow with a velocity of 5-10cm/s.
- Compression should always be performed using the transverse view to ensure full coaptation of the vein walls and to avoid missing duplicate veins and/or collaterals.
- Standing is the preferred position for reflux evaluation of both the deep and superficial veins.
- A clear understanding of the fascial boundaries and the many variations that occur within the lower extremity venous system is essential for accurate reporting.
- A strong understanding of the possible treatments will assist in performing a focused and targeted exam.
- Document all necessary information and whenever possible, identify the highest source of reflux.
- Create a lower extremity venous map to accompany the ultrasound report displaying all pertinent details.
- Measure saphenous vein diameters in the thigh and calf, along with the distance of the vein from the skin. Veins that are located less than 5mm from the skin surface are at higher risk of skin discoloration and dermal injury.
- Obtain diameter and depth measurements of insufficient superficial axial veins while the patient is standing.
- Diameter measurements of superficial veins are obtained in the transverse view and measured from the anterior outer wall to the posterior outer wall (OTO).
- Diameter measurement of pathologic perforating veins are obtained in the longitudinal view where the vein perforates the muscular facial border.
  - Use the sole of the foot or the floor to generate a longitude coordinate, and use the tibial crest to generate a latitude coordinate of the pathologic perforating vein.
  - Use the knee crease for thigh perforating vein.
- Document areas that may hinder navigation of the wire or catheter during treatment.
- In the final report, it is helpful to include incidental findings. Edema, enlarged lymph nodes, Baker's cyst and other findings may contribute to the patient's symptoms.

References

1. Eberhardt, R.T., Raffetto, J.D. (2014). Chronic venous insufficiency. Circulation, 130, 333–346. https://doi: 10.1161/CIRCULATIONAHA.113.006898
2. Meissner, M.H. Lower extremity venous anatomy. (2005). Semin Intervent Radiol, 22(3), 147-56. https://doi: 10.1055/s-2005-921948. PMID: 21326687; PMCID: PMC3036282
3. Sumner, D.S., Zierler, R.E. (2005). Vascular physiology: essential hemodynamic principles. In Rutherford Vascular Surgery (6th ed., pp. 75 - 123). Philadelphia. Elsevier Saunders.
4. Ludbrook, J. (1966). The musculovenous pumps of the human lower limb. American Heart Journal, 71(5), 635-641. https://doi.org/10.1016/0002-8703(66)90313-9
5. Meissner, M.H., Gloviczki, P., Bergan, J., Kistner, R.L., Morrison, N., Pannier, F., Pappas, P.J., Rabe, E., Raju, S., Villavicencio, J.L. (2007). Primary chronic venous disorders. J Vasc Surg. Dec 46 Suppl S, 54S-67S. https://doi: 10.1016/j.jvs.2007.08.038. PMID: 18068562
6. Uhl, J. F., Gillot, C. (2012). Anatomy of the foot venous pump: physiology and influence on chronic venous disease. Phlebology, 27(5), 219–230. https://doi.org/10.1258/phleb.2012.012b01
7. Meissner, M.H., Moneta, G., Burnand, K., Gloviczki, P., Lohr, J.M., Lurie, F., et al. (2007). The hemodynamics and diagnosis of venous disease. J Vasc Surg 46(suppl S), 4-24S.
8. Burnand, K.G. (2001). The physiology and hemodynamics of chronic venous insufficiency of the lower limb. In: P. Gloviczki & J.S.T. Yao (Eds.), Handbook of venous disorders Guidelines of the American Venous Forum. (2nd ed., pp. 49-57). London: Hodder Arnold.
9. Goldman, M.P., Fronek, A. (1989). Anatomy and pathophysiology of varicose veins. J Dermatol Surg Oncol 15, 138-45.

10. Size, G.P., Lozanski, L., Russo, T. (2013). Cardiac Effects on Spectral Doppler. In C. L. Skelly & E.F. Sherry (Eds). Inside Ultrasound Vascular Reference Guide (pp. 336-344). Inside Ultrasound Inc.
11. Kushner A., West, W.P., Pillarisetty, L.S. (2021). Virchow Triad. [Updated 2021 Sep 14]. In: StatPearls [Internet]. Treasure Island (FL): StatPearls Publishing; 2021 Jan-. Available from: https://www.ncbi.nlm.nih.gov/books/NBK539697/
12. Labropoulos, N. (2018). Diagnosis of Iliac Vein Obstruction with Duplex Ultrasound Criteria used during duplex ultrasound examination to identify iliac vein obstruction. Endovascular Today, 17 (7), 50-52.
13. Franceschi, C., Cappelli, M., Escribano, J.M., Mendoza, E. (2020). Dynamic Fractioning of the Gravitational Hydrostatic Pressure: A hemodynamic model for the venous pressure control by the valvo-muscular pump. Journal of Theoretical and Applied Vascular Research, 5(2), 1-10.
14. Coleridge-Smith, P., Labropoulos. N., Partsch, H., Myers, K., Nicolaides, A., Cavezzi, A., et al. (2006). Duplex ultrasound investigation of the veins in chronic venous disease of the lower limbs: UIP consensus document: Part I. Basic principles. Eur J Vasc Endovasc Surg, 31(1), 83-92.
15. Cavezzi A., Labropoulos, N., Partsch, H., Ricci, S., Caggiati, A., Myers, K., et al. (2006). Duplex ultrasound investigation of the veins in chronic venous disease of the lower limbs—UIP consensus document. Part II. Anatomy. Eur J Vasc Endovasc Surg, 31(3), 288-299.
16. Caggiati, A., Bergan, J.J., Gloviczki, P., Eklof, B., Allegra, C., Partsch, H., et al. (2005). Nomenclature of the veins of the lower limb: extensions, refinements, and clinical application, J Vasc Surg 41(4), 719-24.
17. Society for Vascular Ultrasound. (2019). Vascular Technology Professional Performance Guidelines: Lower Extremity Venous Duplex Evaluation for Insufficiency. Retrieved from https://www.svunet.org/practicemanagementmain/professionalperformanceguidelines
18. American Institute for Medical Ultrasound. (2015). AIUM Practice Parameter for the Performance of Peripheral Venous Ultrasound Examinations. Retrieved from https://www.aium.org/resources/guidelines/peripheralvenous.pdf
19. Intersocietal Accreditation Commission. (2019). IAC Standards and Guidelines for Vascular Testing Accreditation. Retrieved from https://www.intersocietal.org/vascular/standards/IACVascularTestingStandards2019.pdf
20. Consensus Conference on Work Related Musculoskeletal Disorders. (2016). Industry Standards for the Prevention of Work-Related Musculoskeletal Disorders in Sonography. Retrieved from https://www.sdms.org/docs/default-source/Resources/industry-standards-for-the-prevention-of-work-relatedmusculoskeletal-disorders-in-sonography.pdf
21. Kim, E.S., Sharma, A.M., Scissons, R., et al. (2020). Interpretation of peripheral arterial and venous Doppler waveforms: A consensus statement from the Society for Vascular Medicine and Society for Vascular Ultrasound. Vascular Medicine, 25(5), 484-506. doi:10.1177/1358863X20937665
22. Ermini, S., Passariello, F., Cappelli, M., Franceschi, C. (2017). Experimental validation of the Paraná maneuver compared to the squeezing test. JTAVR, Dec 31;2(2), 97–105. doi: 10.24019/ jtavr.42
23. Labropoulos, N. (2005). Evaluation of chronic venous disease. In: M.A. Mansour & N. Labropoulos (Eds.), Vascular Diagnosis (pp. 447-461). Philadelphia: Elsevier Saunders.
24. Meissner, M.H. (2005). Venous duplex scanning. In Rutherford Vascular Surgery (6th ed., pp. 254 - 270). Philadelphia. Elsevier Saunders.
25. Cina, A., Pedicelli, A., Di Stasi, C., Porcelli, A., Fiorentino, A., Cina, G., Rulli, F., Bonomo, L. (2005). Color-Doppler sonography in chronic venous insufficiency: What the radiologist should know. Current Problems in Diagnostic Radiology, 34(2), 51-62. ISSN 0363-0188, https://doi.org/10.1067/j.cpradiol.2004.12.001
26. Pascarella, L., Mekenas, L. (2006). Ultrasound examination of the patient with primary venous insufficiency. In The Vein Book (pp. 171 - 181). Philadelphia, Elsevier.
27. Mouton, W., Heim, D., Janzen, J. (2019). Neovascularization of saphenous veins. J Vasc Bras. 18, e20190030. https://doi:10.1590/1677-5449.190030
28. Proebstle, T.M., Moehler, T., Gül, D., Herdemann, S. (2005). Endovenous treatment of the great saphenous vein using a 1,320 nm Nd:YAG laser causes fewer side effects than using a 940 nm diode laser. Dermatol Surg : official publication for American Society for Dermatologic Surgery [et al.], 31(12), 1678-83.
29. Leib, A.D., Roshan, A., Foris, L.A., et al. [Updated 2022 Feb 12]. Baker's Cyst. In: StatPearls [Internet]. Treasure Island (FL): StatPearls Publishing; 2022 Jan-. Available from: https://www.ncbi.nlm.nih.gov/books/NBK430774/
30. LAVascular. (2022, March 1). Lymph-nodes and Swollen lymph nodes. LA Vascular Healthcare and Beyond. https://Lavascular.com/lymphnode
31. Mayo Clinic Staff. (2022, March 14), Edema. Mayo Clinic. https://www.mayoclinic.org/diseases-conditions/edema/symptoms-causes/syc-20366493
32. Synechiae in femoral vein. (2016, September 16). Critical Care Sonography. Retrieved January 31, 2022 from https://www.criticalcare-sonography.com/2016/09/16/synechiae-in-femoral-vein
33. Labropoulos N, Tzogias L, Malgor RD, Antoniou G, Giannoukas AD. Phlebosclerosis in lower extremities veins. Phlebology. 2014 Apr;29(3):186-90. doi: 10.1258/phleb.2012.012113. Epub 2013 May 6. PMID: 23270828.
34. Kibria, F. et al. (2016, November). Sonographic Tendencies. https://sonographictendencies.com/2016/11
35. Salgado, O.J., Chacón, R.E., Alcalá, A., Alvarez, G. (2005). Vein wall dissection: a rare puncture-related complication of brachiocephalic fistula. Gray-scale and color Doppler sonographic findings. J Clin Ultrasound, 33(9), 464-467. https://doi.org/10.1002/jcu.20171
36. Chen, S.I., Clouse, W.D., Bowser, A.N., Rasmussen, T.E. (2009). Superficial venous aneurysms of the small saphenous vein. J Vasc Surg, 50(3):644-647. https://doi.org/10.1016/j.jvs.2009.04.025
37. Pascarella, L., Al-Tuwaijri, M., Bergan, J.J., Mekenas, L.M. (2005). Lower extremity superficial venous aneurysms. Ann Vasc Surg, 19(1), 69-73. https://doi.org/10.1007/s10016-004-0135-1
38. Chronic-Venous-Insufficiency. (2019, May 14). My Cleveland Clinic. Retrieved April 29, 2022, fro my.clevelandclinic.org/health/diseases/16872-chronic-venous-insufficiency-cvi
39. Sen, C.K., Gordillo, G.M., Roy, S., et al. (2009). Human skin wounds: a major and snowballing threat to public health and the economy. Wound Repair Regen, 17(6), 763-771. https://doi.org/10.1111/j.1524-475X.2009.00543
40. Cornu-Thenard, A., Boivin, P., Baud, J.M., De Vincenzi, I., Carpentier, P.H. (1994). Importance of the familial factor in varicose disease. Clinical study of 134 families. J Dermatol Surg Oncol, 20(5), 318-326. https://doi.org/10.1111/j.1524-4725.1994.tb01631.x
41. Min, R.J., Rosenblatt, M. (2010). US Department of Health and Human Services, Office on Women's Health. Varicose Veins and Spider Veins. Retrieved July, 7 2010, from http://www.womenshealth.gov/faq/varicosespider veins.cfm
42. Pagel, P.S., Freed, J.K. (2018). Cardiac Physiology. In JA. Kaplan (Ed.), Kaplan's Essentials of Cardiac Anesthesia (2nd ed., pp. 62-79). Elsevier. ISBN 9780323497985, https://doi.org/10.1016/B978-0-323-49798-5.00004-8
43. Kostas T, Ioannou CV, Touloupakis E, Daskalaki E, Giannoukas AD, Tsetis D, Katsamouris AN. Recurrent varicose veins after surgery: a new appraisal of a common and complex problem in vascular surgery. Eur J Vasc Endovasc Surg. 2004 Mar;27(3):275-82. doi: 10.1016/j.ejvs.2003.12.006. PMID: 14760596.
44. Meissner, M.H., Eklof, B., Smith, P.C., Dalsing, M.C., DePalma, R.G., Gloviczki, P., et al. (2007). Secondary chronic venous disorders. J Vasc Surg 46 Suppl S, 68S-83S
45. Labropoulos, N., Gasparis, A. P., Pefanis, D., Leon, L. R., Jr, & Tassiopoulos, A. K. (2009). Secondary chronic venous disease progresses faster than primary. Journal of vascular surgery, 49(3), 704–710.
46. Joh, J. H., & Park, H. C. (2013). The cutoff value of saphenous vein diameter to predict reflux. Journal of the Korean Surgical Society, 85(4), 169–174. https://doi.org/10.4174/jkss.2013.85.4.169
47. Lew, W.K. (2021, August 19). Varicose Vein Surgery. Medscape. https://emedicine.medscape.com/article/462579
48. Khilnani, N.M., Min, R.J. (2005). Imaging of venous insufficiency. Semin Intervent Radiol, 22(3), 178-184. https://doi:10.1055/s-2005-921950
49. Fan, C. M. (2005). Venous pathophysiology. Seminars in interventional radiology, 22(3), 157–161. https://doi.org/10.1055/s-2005-921949
50. Kim, E. S., Sharma, A. M., Scissons, R., Dawson, D., Eberhardt, R. T., Gerhard-Herman, M., Hughes, J. P., Knight, S., Marie Kupinski, A., Mahe, G., Neumyer, M., Poe, P., Shugart, R., Wennberg, P., Williams, D. M., & Zierler, R. E. (2020). Interpretation of peripheral arterial and venous Doppler waveforms: A consensus statement from the Society for Vascular Medicine and Society for Vascular Ultrasound. Vascular medicine (London, England), 25(5), 484–506. https://doi.org/10.1177/1358863X20937665
51. Gloviczki, P., Comerota, A.J., Dalsing, M.C., Eklof, B.G., Gillespie, D.L., Gloviczki, M.L., Lohr, J.M., McLafferty, R.B., Meissner, M.H., Murad, M.H., Padberg, F.T., Pappas, P.J., Passman, M.A., Raffetto, J.D., Vasquez, M.A., Wakefield, T.W. (2011). Society for Vascular Surgery; American Venous Forum. The care of patients with varicose veins and associated chronic venous diseases: clinical practice guidelines of the Society for Vascular Surgery and the American Venous Forum. J Vasc Surg, 53(5 Suppl), 2S-48S. https://doi: 10.1016/j.jvs.2011.01.079. PMID: 21536172
52. Raffetto, J. D., & Khalil, R. A. (2021). Mechanisms of Lower Extremity Vein Dysfunction in Chronic Venous Disease and Implications in Management of Varicose Veins. Vessel plus, 5, 36. https://doi.org/10.20517/2574-1209.2021.16
53. Patel, S. K., & Surowiec, S. M. (2021). Venous Insufficiency. In StatPearls. StatPearls Publishing.
54. Allegra, Claudio & Antignani, Pier & Bergan, J.J. & Carpentier, P.H. & Coleridge-Smith, Philip & Cornu-Thénard, André. (2002). The "C" of CEAP: Suggested definitions and refinements: an International Union of Phlebology conference of experts. J Vasc Surg. 37. 129-131.
55. Lurie, Fedor & Passman, Marc & Meisner, Mark & Dalsing, Michael & Masuda, Elna & Welch, Harold & Bush, Ruth & Blebea, John & Carpentier, Patrick & Maeseneer, Marianne & Gasparis, Anthony & Labropoulos, Nicos & Marston, William & Rafetto, Joseph & Santiago, Fabricio & Shortell, Cynthia & Uhl, Jean-François & Urbanek, Tomasz & van Rij, Andre & Wakefield, Thomas. (2020). CEAP classification system and reporting standard, revision 2020. Journal of Vascular Surgery: Venous and Lymphatic Disorders. 8. 10.1016/j.jvsv.2019.12.075.

Definition

A combination of real time B-mode imaging, Pulsed Wave (PW) and color Doppler imaging utilized during ablative and surgical procedures to treat venous insufficiency in symptomatic and aesthetic patients.

Rationale

Venous duplex ultrasound is the primary diagnostic imaging modality utilized to accurately examine the anatomic characteristics and functional status of the target vein to confirm that the vein is a viable candidate for an intervention. It is also used preoperatively to precisely mark the course of the vein and all relevant anatomical characteristics. During the procedure, ultrasound is used as an assistive tool for vascular access, device placement, and administration of tumescent anesthesia. Immediately post-procedure, ultrasound will be used to assess deep system patency, as well as for all follow-up examinations.

Indications [7, 8, 18]

- Telangiectasias
- Reticular veins
- Varicose veins
- Swelling or edema (related to CVD)
- Skin changes
- Active or healed venous ulcers
- Prior endovenous intervention
- Heaviness/tiredness
- Aching, pain, cramping
- Throbbing
- Itching
- Restless legs (may be a symptom of CVD) [31]

Contraindications / Limitations [9]

- Pregnancy or breast feeding
- Obstructed deep venous system (e.g., acute thrombosis, KTS)
- Coagulopathy
- Patient immobility
- Thermal ablation
  - Allergy to anesthetic
  - Epifascial tributary veins
  - Vein is in close proximity to a nerve
  - Areas which may hinder device navigation e.g., tortuous vessel, aneurysmal segment, large valve cusp, or synechiae
- Chemical ablation
  - Allergy to sclerosing agent
  - Local infection in the area of sclerotherapy
  - Severe generalized infection
  - Long-lasting immobility and confinement to bed
- Adhesive ablation
  - Allergy to adhesive or cyanoacrylates
  - Acute superficial vein thrombosis
  - Acute sepsis

Patient History

- Family and surgical history of both venous and arterial system disease
- Prior endovenous intervention
- Prior deep or superficial vein thrombosis
- Soft tissue leg pain or tenderness
- Enlarged varicose veins or spontaneous venous hemorrhage
- Localized pain, burning or itching
- Tired, heavy legs after prolonged standing
- Persistent swelling (especially at the end of the day)
- Medications – blood thinners, birth control or hormone replacement
- Heavy lifting due to their work or exercise regimen
- Standing or sitting for prolonged periods of time
- Restless legs

Symptoms may increase for women around menstruation.

Symptoms may vary with time of day.

Patients may present with signs without symptoms or symptoms without signs.

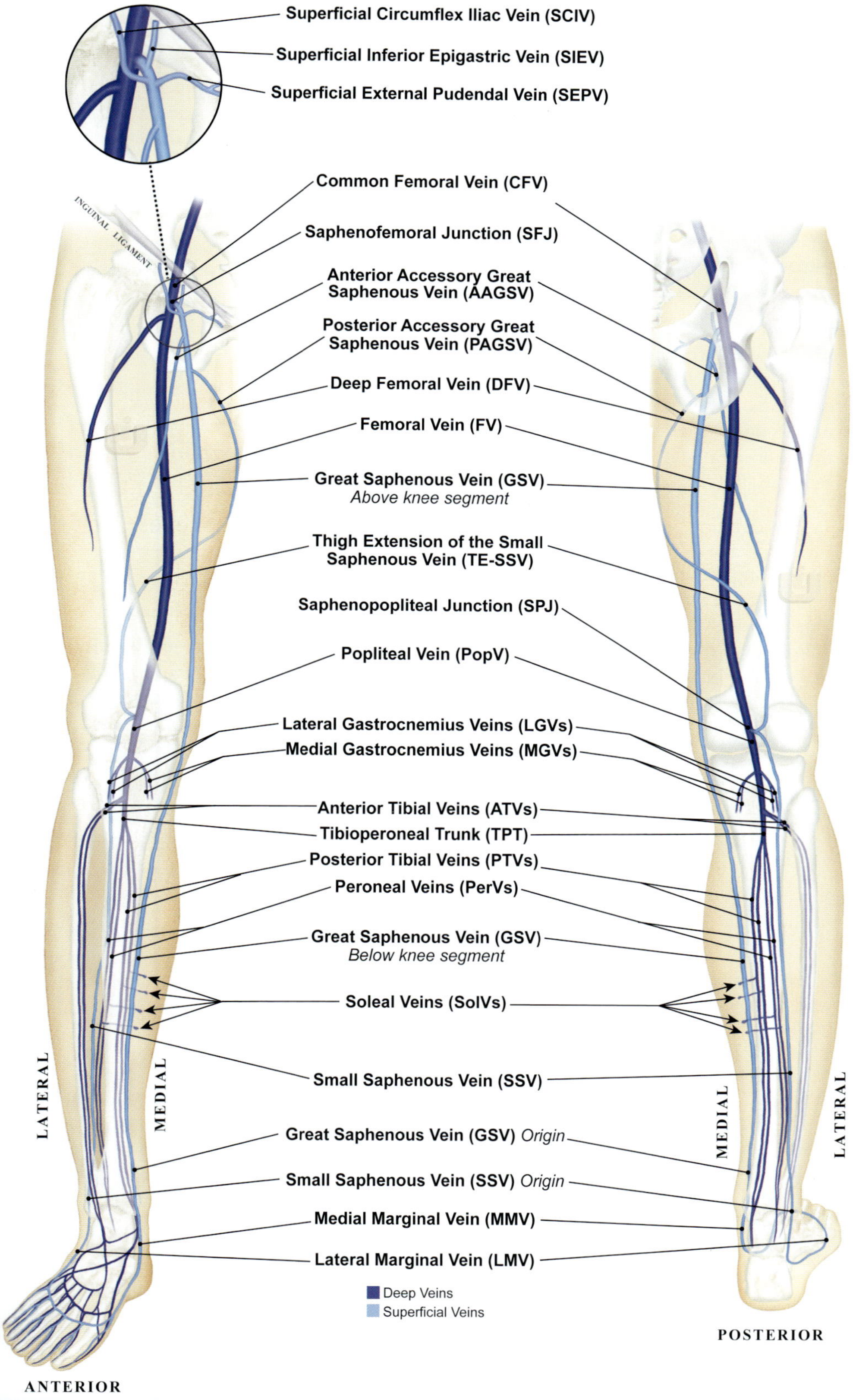
Superficial Circumflex Iliac Vein (SCIV)
Superficial Inferior Epigastric Vein (SIEV)
Superficial External Pudendal Vein (SEPV)
INGUINAL LIGAMENT
Common Femoral Vein (CFV)
Saphenofemoral Junction (SFJ)
Anterior Accessory Great Saphenous Vein (AAGSV)
Posterior Accessory Great Saphenous Vein (PAGSV)
Deep Femoral Vein (DFV)
Femoral Vein (FV)
Great Saphenous Vein (GSV) Above knee segment
Thigh Extension of the Small Saphenous Vein (TE-SSV)
Saphenopopliteal Junction (SPJ)
Popliteal Vein (PopV)
Lateral Gastrocnemius Veins (LGVs)
Medial Gastrocnemius Veins (MGVs)
Anterior Tibial Veins (ATVs)
Tibioperoneal Trunk (TPT)
Posterior Tibial Veins (PTVs)
Peroneal Veins (PerVs)
Great Saphenous Vein (GSV) Below knee segment
Soleal Veins (SolVs)
Small Saphenous Vein (SSV)
Great Saphenous Vein (GSV) Origin
Small Saphenous Vein (SSV) Origin
Medial Marginal Vein (MMV)
Lateral Marginal Vein (LMV)
Deep Veins
Superficial Veins
LATERAL
MEDIAL
MEDIAL
LATERAL
ANTERIOR
POSTERIOR

Table 11-1. **Diagnostic Criteria for Venous Reflux** [2, 10, 11, 12, 13]

Deep venous system CFV, FV, PopV	>1000ms
Deep venous system calf	>500ms
Superficial venous system	>500ms
Perforating venous system [1, 7]	>500ms

Treatment Approach

Treatment approach is best described to patients using a river system analogy. The source of reflux (the large river) is commonly treated first, which is typically the superficial truncal vein. Once the truncal vein has been successfully treated, the tributaries (smaller rivers) are addressed. Finally, the reticular veins and telangiectasias (streams and brooks) may be treated if desired.

Approaching venous disease from the source, and moving superficially, yields improved patient outcomes and minimizes the likelihood of recurrence and revascularization. [4, 33]

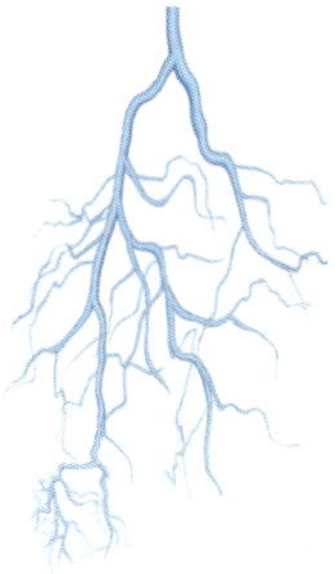

Fig. 11-1. *River system analogy for comparison to venous system drainage.*

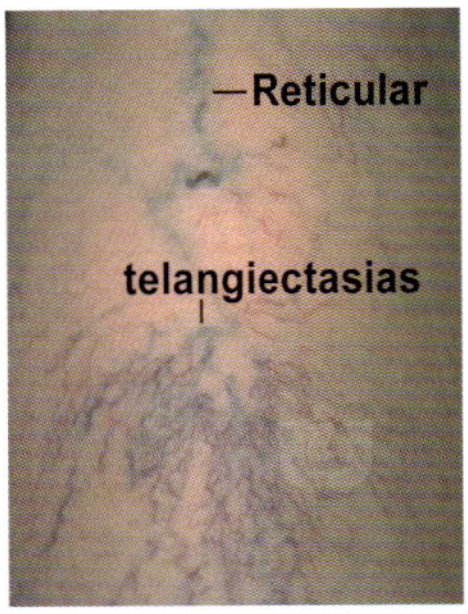

Fig. 11-2. *Reticular vein feeding a cluster of telangiectasias.*

> *The most important feature regarding venous sinuses, and veins in general, is to keep in mind that veins are like rivers. The size of any vein or sinus is determined by the sum total of the tributaries it gathers, much like a river is exactly as large as the total volume of streams which feed it. Nearly all variations in venous size can be explained by this simple and powerful analogy.* [3]

Treatment Options for Superficial Venous Insufficiency

A variety of treatment modalities are available for the treatment of chronic venous insufficiency, including surgery, thermal ablation, chemical ablation and cyanoacrylate adhesive ablation.

Surgical Options

- Ligation and Stripping
  - Ligation of the central vein segment
  - Stripping of the vein may be performed concomitantly
- Ambulatory Phlebectomy
  - Removal of large tortuous varicose veins

> *Patients may insist they had a ligation and stripping when they only had an avulsion phlebectomy.*

Thermal Ablative Options

Definition

Thermal ablation is a procedure using heat to remove tissue or destroy its function. [15]

Currently, two types of thermal ablation methods are used: endovenous LASER ablation, and radiofrequency ablation. Both methods may be used in an operating room or in an out-patient setting. [8]

Rationale

The procedure uses heat to achieve venous closure of the diseased veins, decreasing the risk of complications and symptoms from venous disease.

Thermal ablation when compared with traditional surgical techniques, is less invasive, offers the same cosmetic results with virtually no scarring, and a faster return to normal activities. [4]

Technique

The underlying goal for all thermal ablation procedures is to deliver sufficient thermal energy to the wall of an incompetent vein segment to produce irreversible occlusion, fibrosis, and ultimately disappearance of the vein. [8]

A thermal device is placed into the target vein using ultrasound guidance and positioned at the level of its junction with the deep venous system.

A local anesthetic is administered between the vein wall and soft tissue, within the saphenous compartment. Then thermal energy is delivered to the diseased vein through the device tip. As the catheter is withdrawn, heat causes the vein to collapse and eventually close.

Tumescent anesthesia involves the injection of a very dilute local anesthetic solution, into tissue until it becomes firm and engorged. The technique was initially pioneered in the 1980s for the purposes of liposuction, but its application has since expanded to cover a variety of surgeries. [14]

Tumescent anesthesia is administered by the provider and directed into the perivenous space within the superficial fascia.

The purpose of tumescent anesthesia is to: [14, 17, 27]

- Increase the depth between the skin and the target vein to avoid injuring the skin.
- Create a heat sink, protecting the soft tissue surrounding the vein from thermal injury.
- Compress and exsanguinate the vein.
- Enhance patient comfort during and after treatment.
- Push structures away from the heat source (e.g., tissue, nerves and arteries), if administered directly within the vein sheath.

Veins Treated Using Thermal Ablation

- Great Saphenous Vein (GSV)
- Anterior Accessory Great Saphenous Vein (AAGSV)
- Posterior Accessory Great Saphenous Vein (PAGSV)
- Thigh Extension of the Small Saphenous Vein (TE-SSV)
- Small Saphenous Vein (SSV)
- Anterior Circumflex Vein (ATCV)*
- Posterior Circumflex Vein (PTCV)*
- Pathologic Perforating Vein (PPV)

*If found within the saphenous compartment

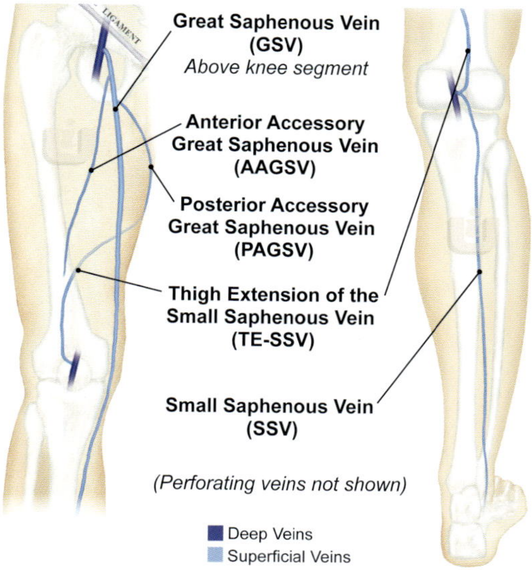

Fig. 11-3. *Veins treated using thermal ablation.*

For a comprehensive description of lower extremity superficial venous duplex exam, please refer to the Lower Extremity Venous Insufficiency Duplex exam chapter.

Ultrasound Imaging Pre, During, and Post Thermal Intervention

Ultrasound Immediately Prior to Thermal Intervention

To ensure safe, effective, and efficient outcomes, ultrasound is used immediately prior, during and post intervention.

Following your facilities protocol, perform a quick scan to identify the following:

- Proposed viable access point
  - Diameter (large enough to accept the device)
  - Depth (approximately 5mm from skin surface) [18]

Relay quick scan findings to the provider. This discussion may prevent difficulty during the procedure or lead to a different treatment approach.

Epifascial veins are not candidates for thermal ablation due to complications (Tissue and skin damage, sterile abscess) [18]

- Areas which may hinder navigation:
  - Significant tortuosity
  - Aneurysmal segments
  - Large valve cusps
  - Synechiae (webbing)
  - Hypoplastic segments
  - "Phlebosclerosis" fibrous degeneration of the venous wall, predominantly the intima, with or without calcification. [5]

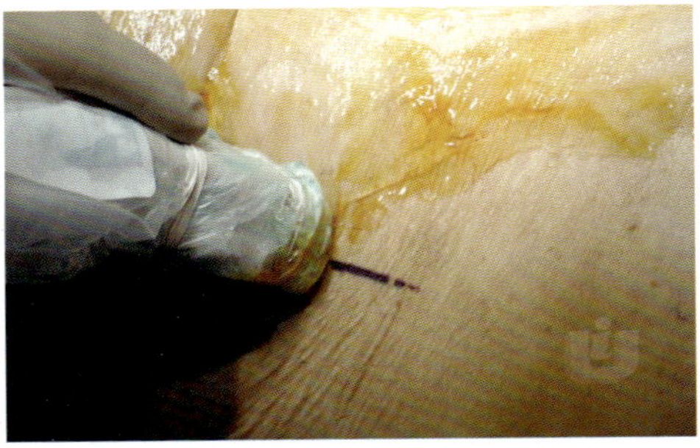

Fig. 11-4. *Mark the proposed access site.*

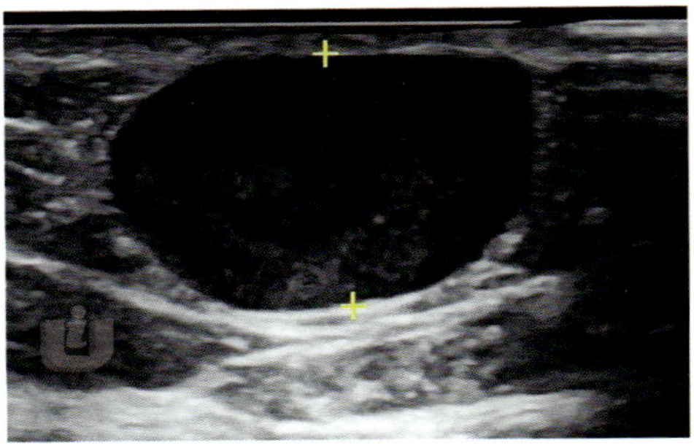

Fig. 11-5. *B-mode of an aneurysmal segment.*

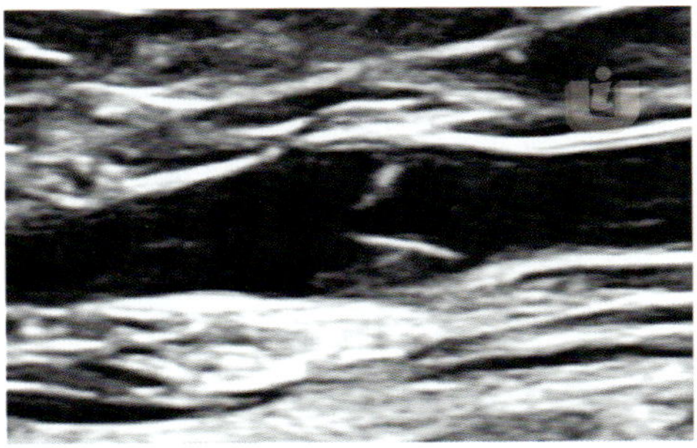

Fig. 11-6. *B-mode of valve cusps within a venous sinus.*

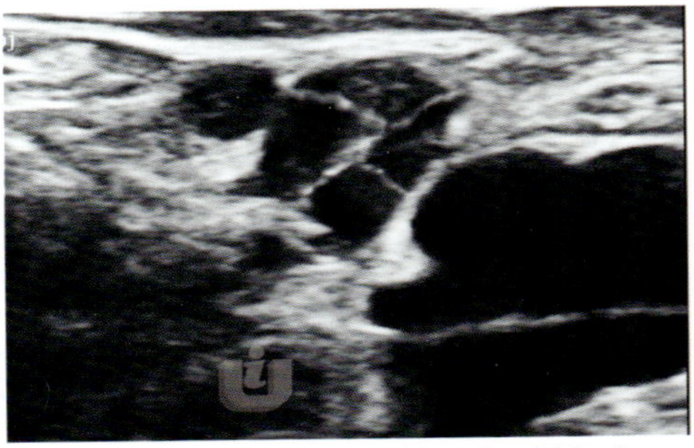

Fig. 11-7. *B-mode of Synechiae (webbing).*

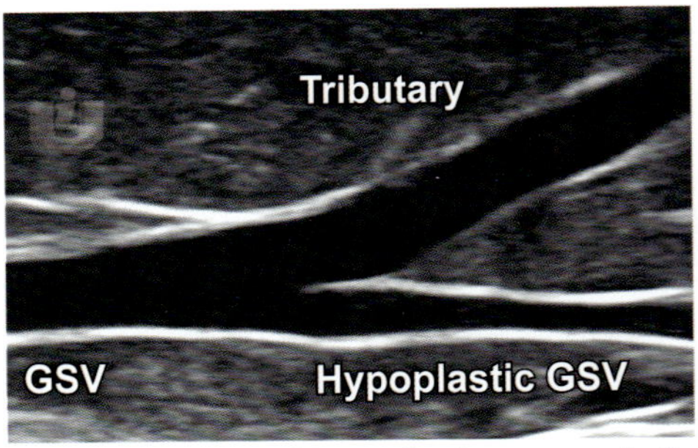

Fig. 11-8. *B-mode of hypoplastic segment of the GSV*

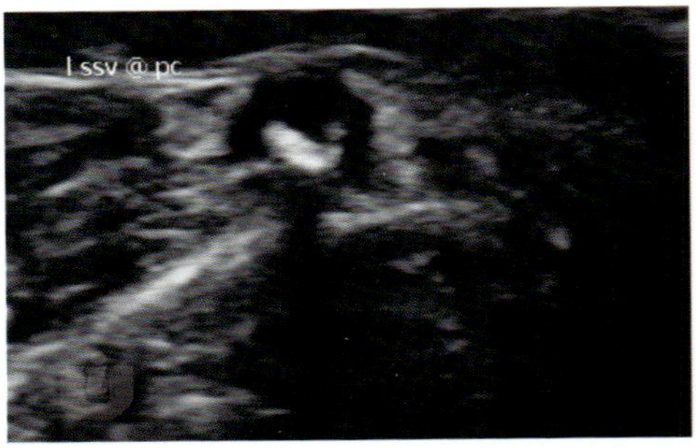

Fig. 11-9. *B-mode of chronic postphlebotic changes with acoustic shadowing demonstrating calcification.*

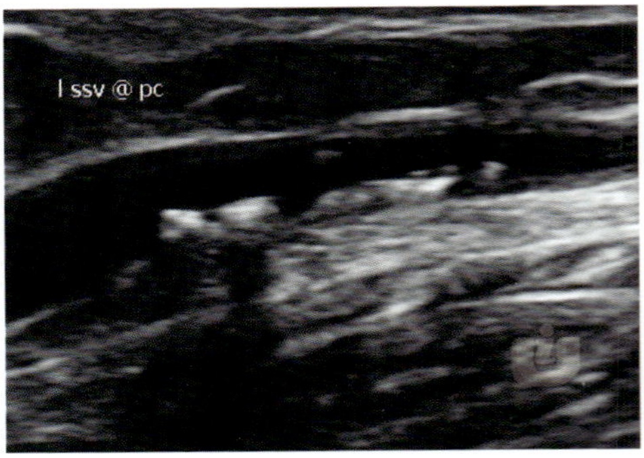

Fig. 11-10. *B-mode of phlebosclerosis displayed in the longitudinal view.*

Large tributaries and/or large perforating veins may lead to post procedure problems or treatment failure. [7, 19, 20]

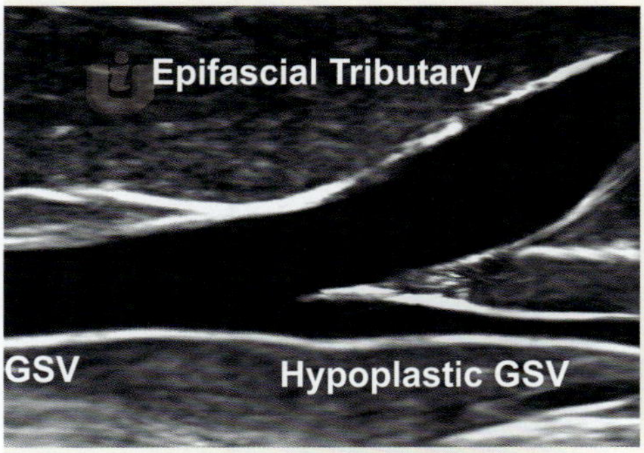

Fig. 11-11. *B-mode of large epifascial tributary joining the GSV.*

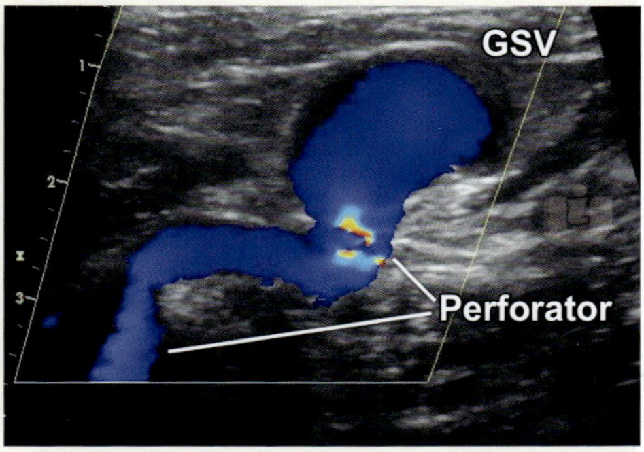

Fig. 11-12. *Color Doppler of Large perforating vein joining the GSV.*

GSV Nerve location

The great saphenous vein and great saphenous nerve merge approximately 8-10cm below the knee crease. [7]

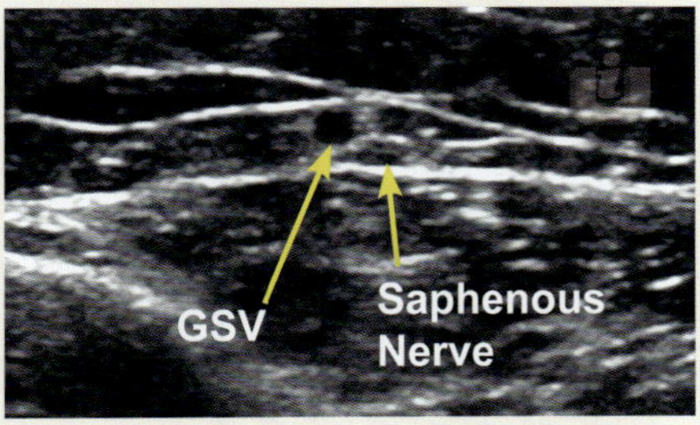

Fig. 11-13. *B-mode of GSV and saphenous nerve.*

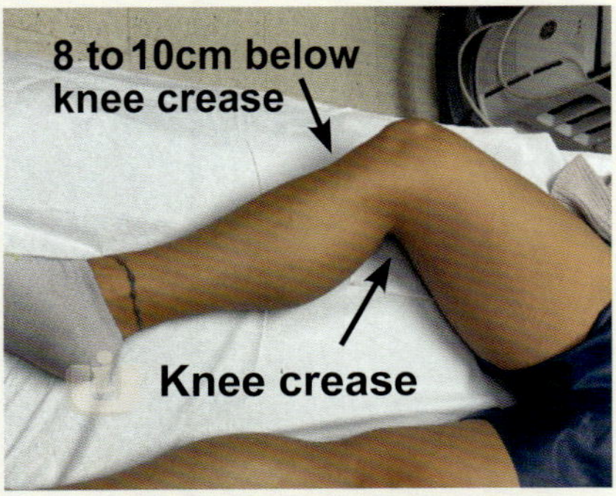

Fig. 11-14. *The great saphenous vein and saphenous nerve merge 8 to 10cm below the knee crease.*

SSV Nerve location

The small saphenous vein and the sural nerve merge at the descent of the calf (tail end of the gastrocnemius muscle). [21]

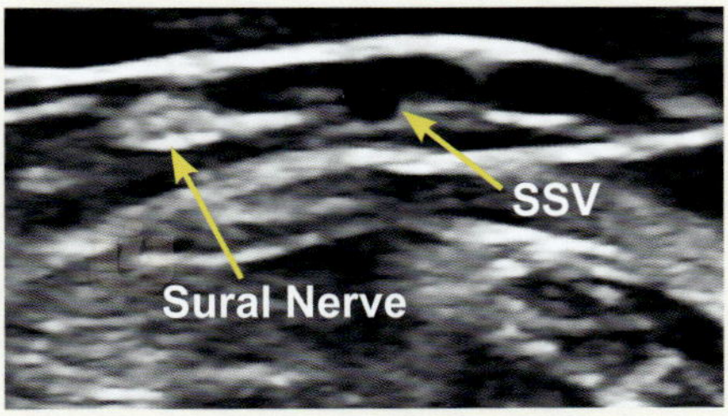

Fig. 11-15. *B-mode of SSV and sural nerve.*

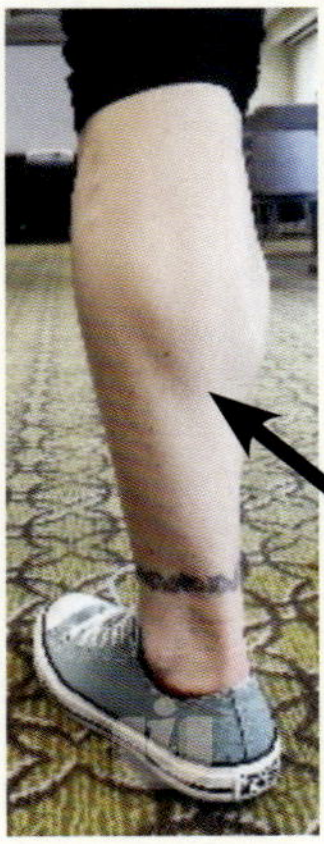

Fig. 11-16. *The small saphenous vein and sural nerve merge at the tail end of the gastrocnemius muscle.*

Tail end of the gastrocnemius muscle.

If a nerve is visualized at the level of the access the provider may choose an alternate access site.

Position for marking the GSV

Supine, >20° reverse Trendelenburg with the lower extremity externally rotated and a slight flexion of the knee joint.

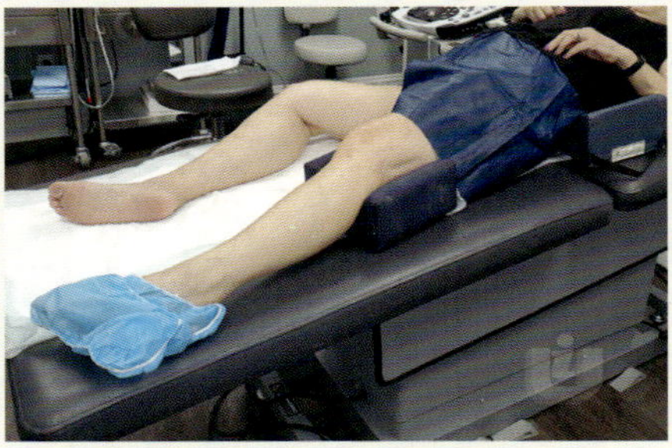

Fig. 11-17. *A cushion may be placed under the knee and lower back.*

Position for marking the SSV

Prone, >20° reverse Trendelenburg with a bolster under the ankle to flex the knee joint.

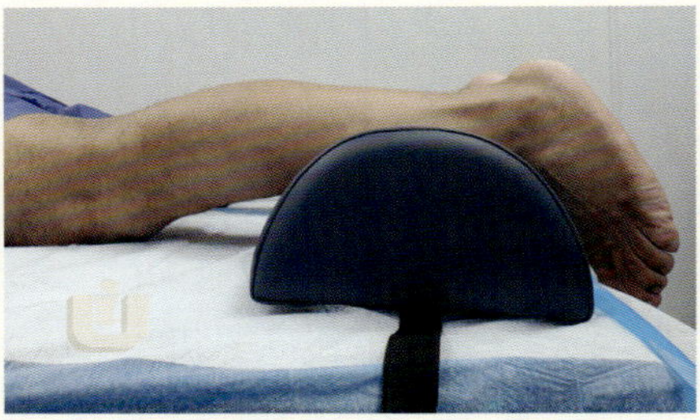

Fig. 11-18. *A bolster is placed under the ankle to flex the knee joint.*

> *When the leg is straight, it may be difficult to visualize and assess the popliteal vein.*

Comprehensive Marking

In addition to marking the access site, a provider may request a complete marking of the entire course of the vein.

- Create a reference point on the center of your transducer or transducer cover.
- Image the vein in transverse and position the vein in the center of the field of view. This should correspond with the reference point/center of the transducer.
- Use an indelible marker so the marker will remain visible despite skin preparation. Gently press for a few seconds to create and indentation or a dot on the skin.
- Move the transducer centrally from the proposed access site to the junction, making a mark every two inches.

> *Moving centrally will wipe away the gel as you go, making it easier to mark the skin.*

- After you have marked the limb, wipe off the gel, make hashmarks over the dots or completely connect the dots. Map the entire course of the vein.
- Mark any areas of concern (areas which may hinder navigation: see descriptions on pg. 176).
- Mark the diameter and depth at the access point.

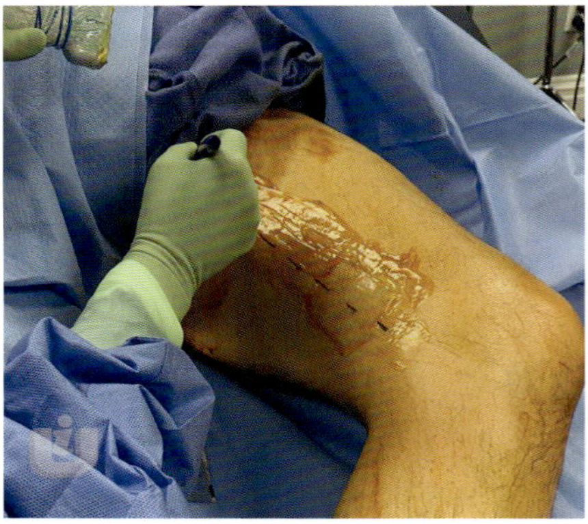

Fig. 11-19. *Marking the entire course of the vein using hash marks.*

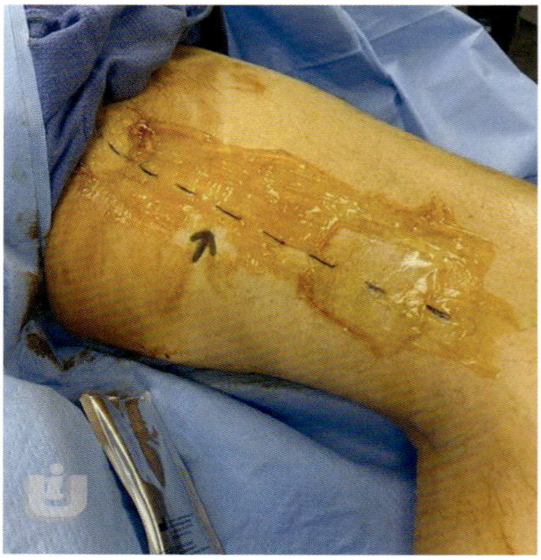

Fig. 11-20. *Area that may hinder navigation marked with an arrow on the limb.*

Ultrasound During Thermal Ablation

Position for GSV Ablation

Supine, >20° reverse Trendelenburg with the lower extremity externally rotated and a slight flexion of the knee joint.

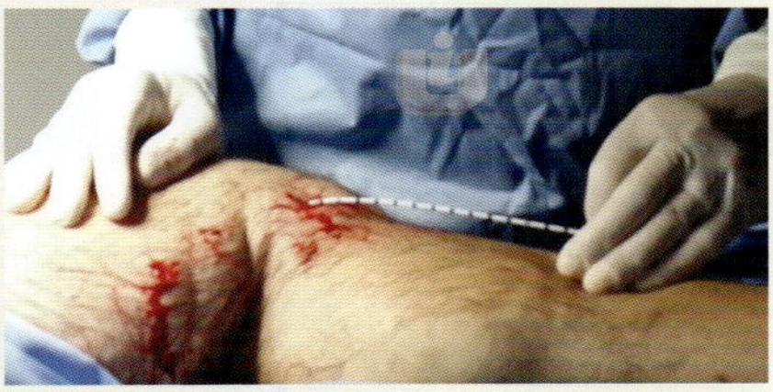

Fig. 11-21. *Provider performing a thermal ablation of the GSV. The extremity is externally rotated and there is a slight flexion of the knee joint.*

Photo courtesy of Joseph Fretta, MD

The dependent position will dilate the vein for an easier access.

Position for SSV Ablation

Prone, >20° reverse Trendelenburg with a pillow under the ankle to flex the knee joint.

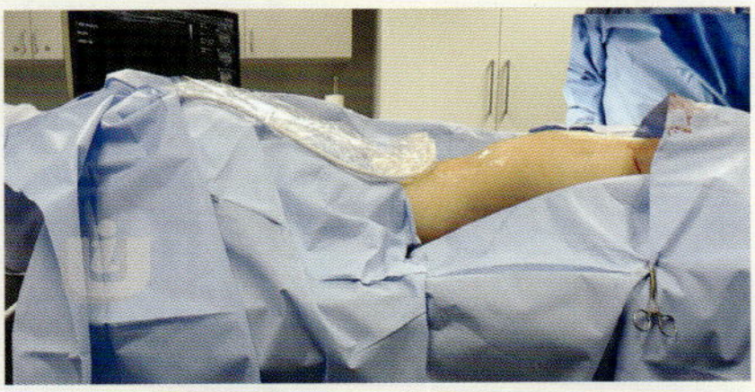

Fig. 11-22. *Provider about to perform a thermal ablation of the SSV. The patient is in the prone position with a pillow under the ankle to flex the knee joint.*

Photo courtesy of John Capitanelli, MD

Protective barriers:

- Sterile keyboard cover
- Sterile transducer cover
- Sterile single-use gel packets (used to decrease the risk of infection)
- Sterile gloves
- Sterile gown

Per your facilities protocol, surgical caps and shoe coverings may be worn.

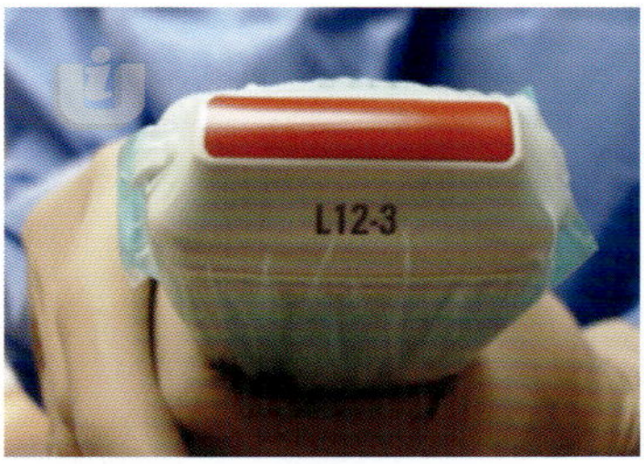

Fig. 11-23. *Be certain you have no air bubbles between the transducer and the cover. Air bubbles will obstruct your view.*

Technique

- Apply sterile gel over the proposed treatment area.
- Identify the target vein at the level of the junction. Move peripherally, evaluating the vein down to the level of the access.
- Administration of local anesthetic will be injected directly over the marked location or in real time by positioning the transducer over the access site.
- The provider determines the orientation of the transducer to gain access. The sonographer should orient the transducer accordingly.
- The transducer should remain perpendicular to the limb, allowing accuracy during access.

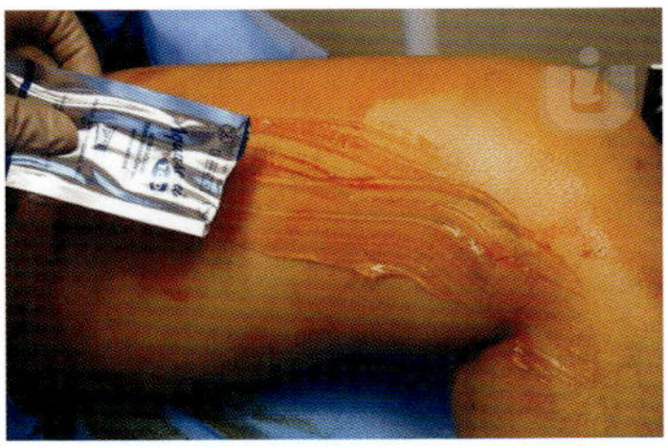

Fig. 11-24. *Application of sterile gel.*

If possible, anchor the transducer to create a stress point (an area to relieve tension from the weight of the cord) with a towel clamp or a Velcro strip.

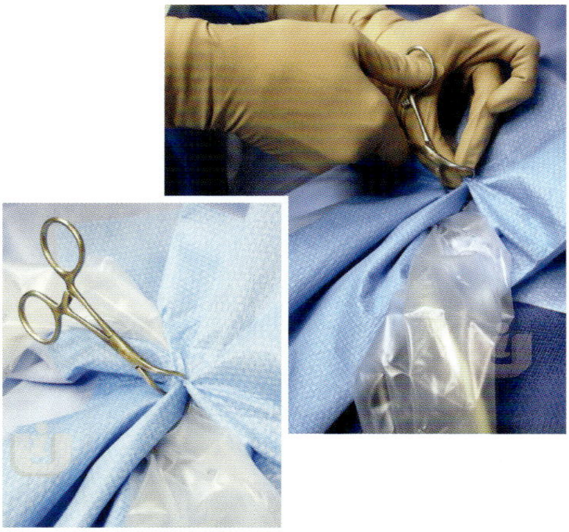

Fig. 11-25. *Creating a stress point by securing the cord to the sterile field will reduce tension on the transducer.*

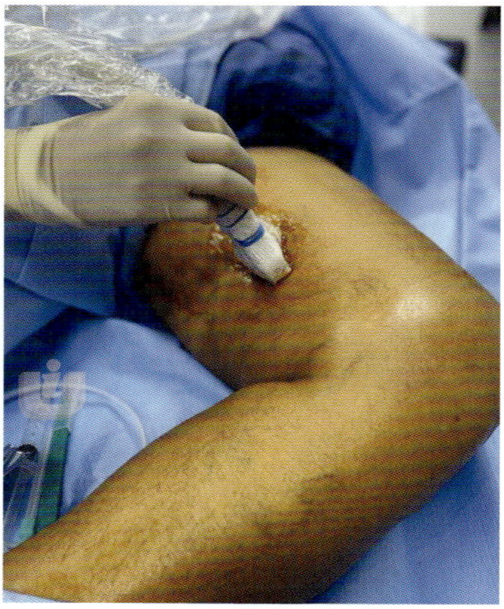

Fig. 11-26. *Transducer orientation for guidance using the longitudinal view.*

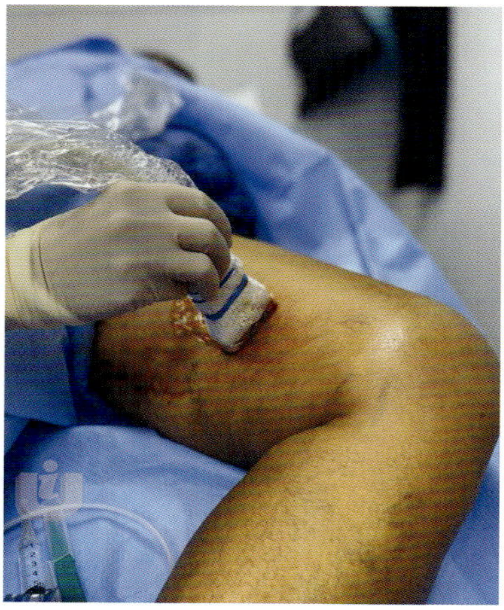

Fig. 11-27. *Transducer orientation for guidance using the transverse view.*

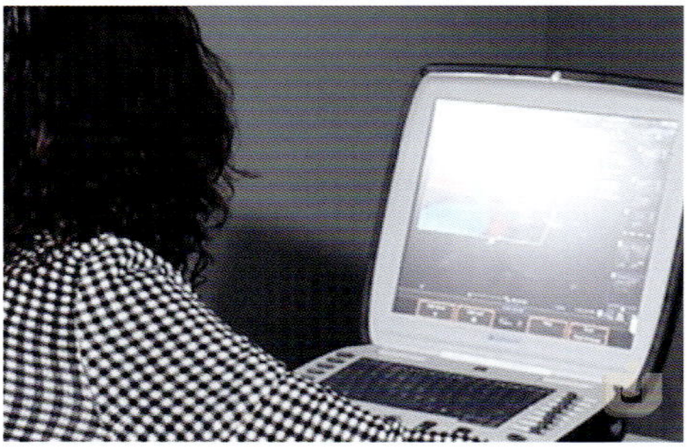

Fig. 11-28. *Keep your eyes on the monitor at all times during access. Turning your head will undoubtedly move your hand, making it more difficult to remain on your target. This may delay access, and even worse, dislodge the needle.*

During access it is important to hold the transducer properly to avoid needle sticks.

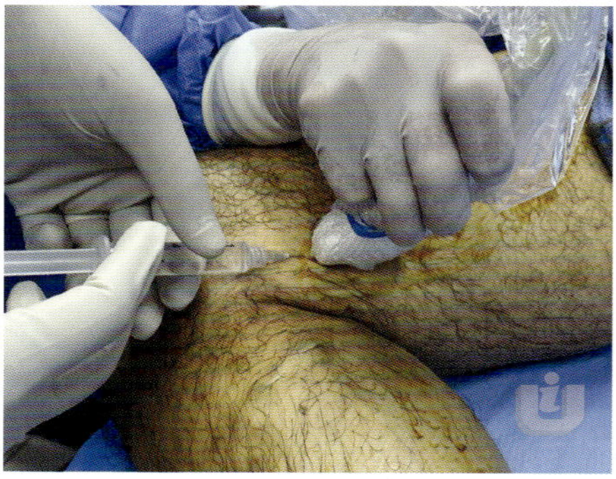

Fig. 11-29. *Administration of local anesthetic.*

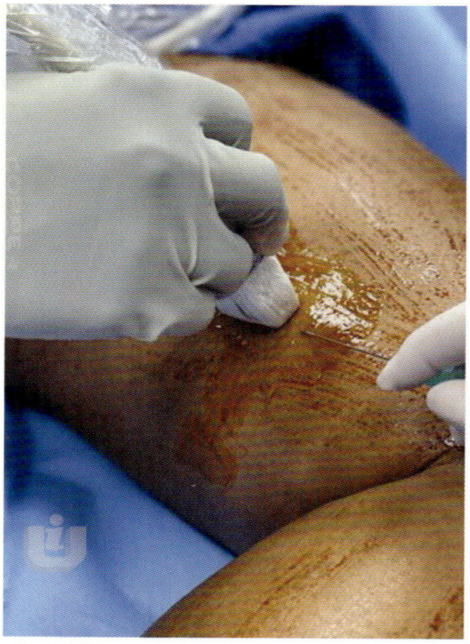

Fig. 11-30. *Gaining access for ablation procedure.*

- The vein is accessed via needle, and a guidewire is placed in the vein. Maintain a steady hand while guiding the provider into the vein.
- Confirm the entry and presence of the needle and the guidewire.
- A dilator and catheter are placed over the guidewire.
- Confirm the entry and presence of the catheter. Once placed at the desired level, the wire is removed.
- Confirm the device (LASER, RF) is inserted in the vein and positioned peripheral to the ostium.
- Using ultrasound, take a preliminary distance measurement of the location of the device tip within the superficial vein in relation to its associated deep vein. This step ensures safe, effective, and precise placement of the tip. The suggested distance for veins are: [16]
  - GSV, AAGSV (other inguinal vein) 2-3cm peripheral to the ostium. [6]
  - SSV at the descent of the small saphenous vein before it dives toward the popliteal vein.
  - Perforating vein at or just below the muscular (deep) fascia. [1]

> *During access, use a gentle touch to avoid compressing the vein. Conversely, during administration of the tumescent, use a steady hand to avoid sliding off the region of interest.*

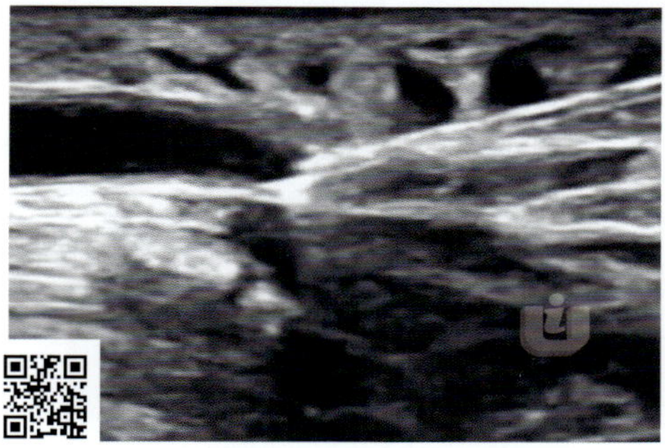

Fig. 11-31. *Access in longitudinal view.*

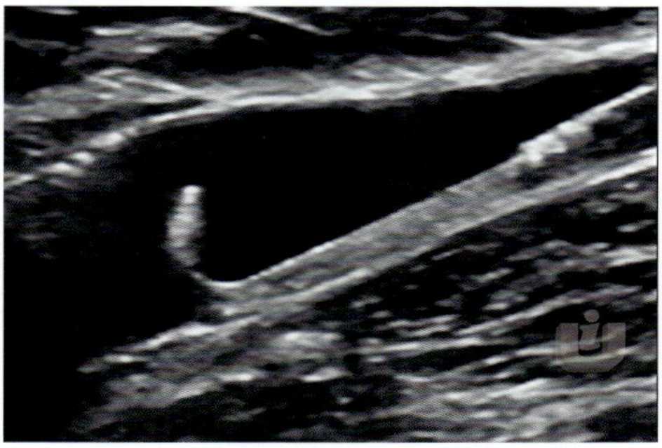

Fig. 11-32. *J-wire placed in the GSV to be treated.* Image courtesy of Patrick Washko, BS RT RDMS RVT

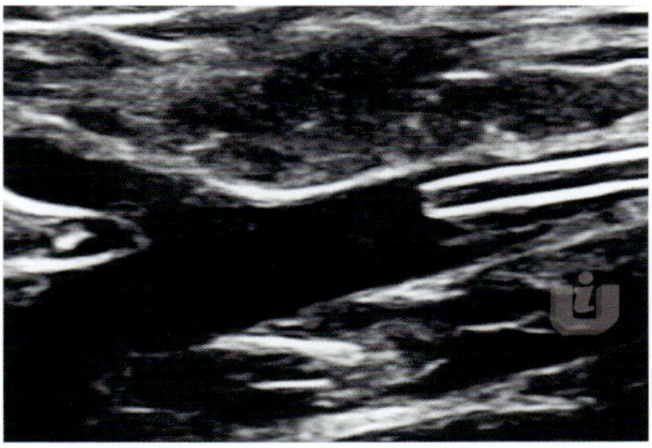

Fig. 11-33. *Catheter peripheral to the SFJ.*

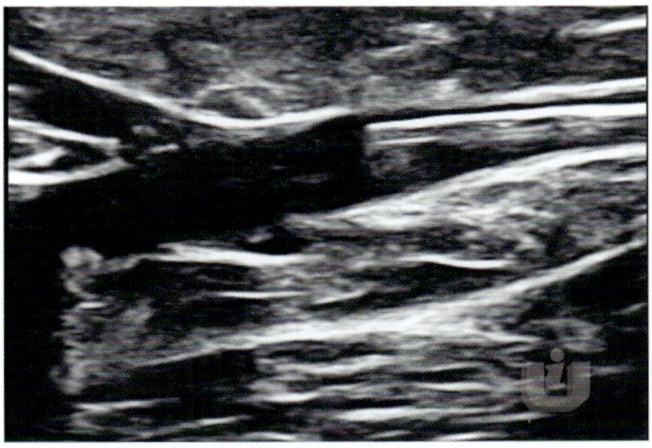

Fig. 11-34. *Device tip peripheral to the SFJ.*

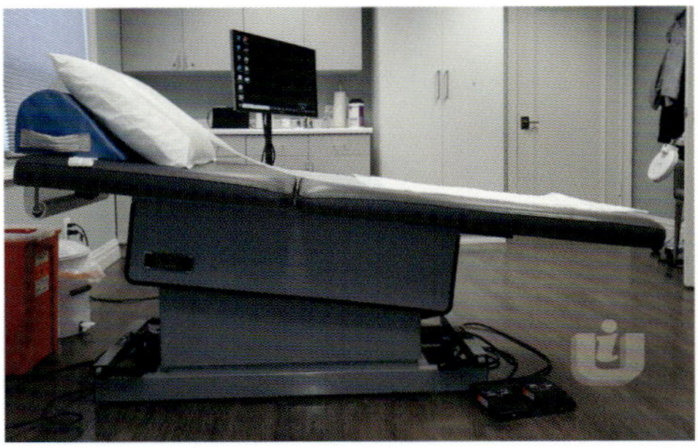

Fig. 11-35. *Reverse Trendelenburg*

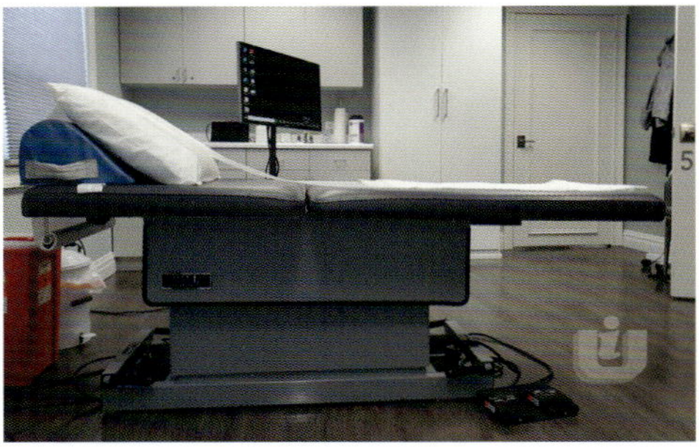

Fig. 11-36. *Flat*

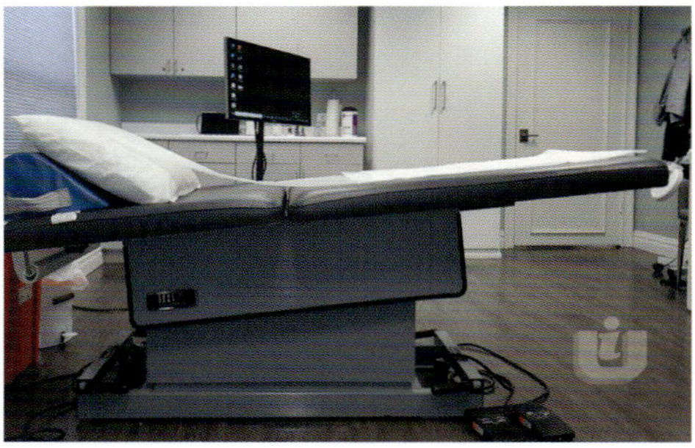

Fig. 11-37. *Trendelenburg*

- Adjust the table to 0º (flat) or mild Trendelenburg position. [28]
- As infiltration of tumescent anesthesia begins, it is essential for the sonographer to maintain a steady hand, keeping the transducer perpendicular to the limb and parallel to the catheter.
- In the transverse view, it is important to keep the vein in the center of the image.
- In the longitudinal view, it is important that the entire length of the catheter is visible on the screen.

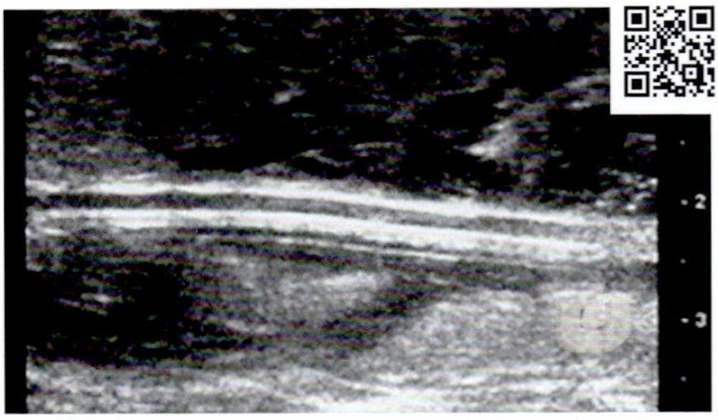

Fig. 11-38. *Tumescent displayed in the longitudinal view (fractured tissue effect).*

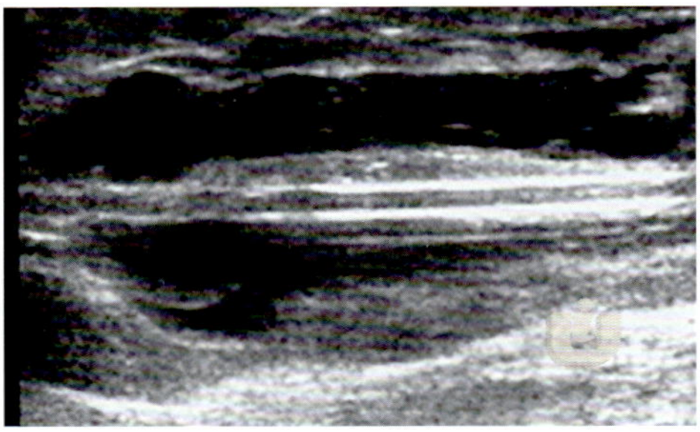

Fig. 11-39. *Tumescent displayed in the longitudinal view (banana peel effect).*

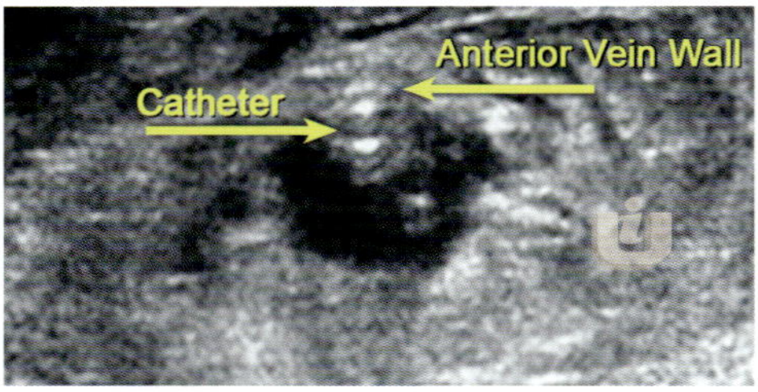

Fig. 11-40. *Transverse view displaying inadequate separation of the device and the vein wall after administration of the tumescent solution.*

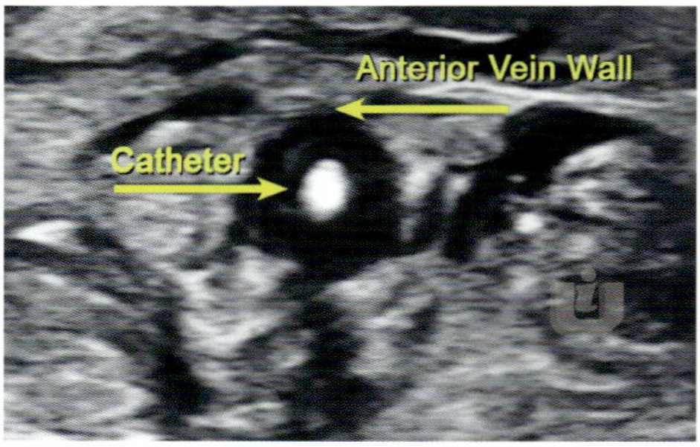

Fig. 11-41. *Transverse view displaying adequate separation of the device and the vein wall after administration of the tumescent solution. Perform a sweep of the entire length of the vein to ensure adequate tumescent anesthesia infiltration. If tip cannot be visualized look for an acoustic shadow (10sec on cine).*

- Remeasure the distance between the junction and the tip (should be approximately 4-5cm) before infiltration is complete. The device may be displaced during administration, and it will be easier to visualize the tip before infiltration is complete.

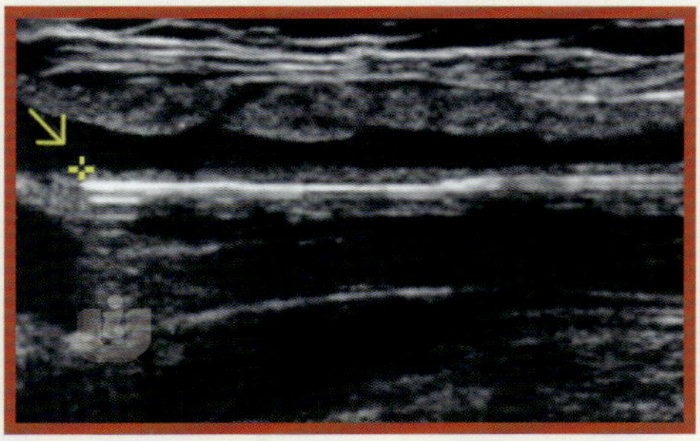

Fig. 11-42. *Tip placement is too close to the ostium.*

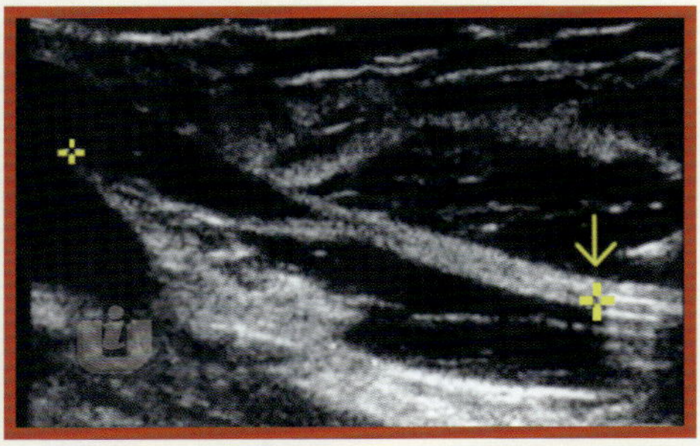

Fig. 11-43. *Tip placement is too far from the ostium.*

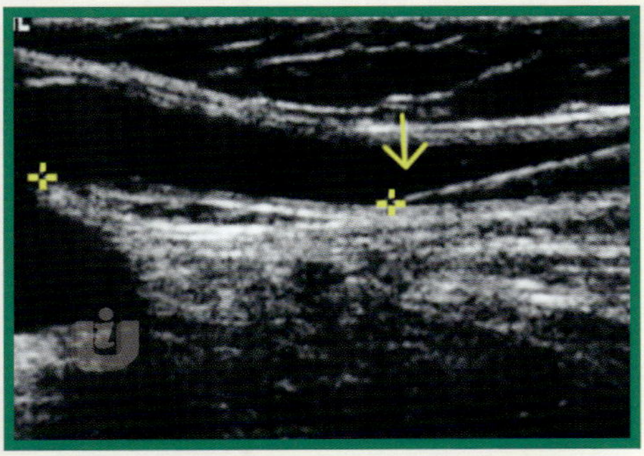

Fig. 11-44. *Tip placement is perfect. Typically, somewhere between 2-3cm peripheral to the ostium for the inguinal veins.* [6, 27]

This target measurement may vary according to your facility's protocol.

To ensure accurate tip placement double check tip in transverse view fanning centrally and peripherally to show tip presence and absence.

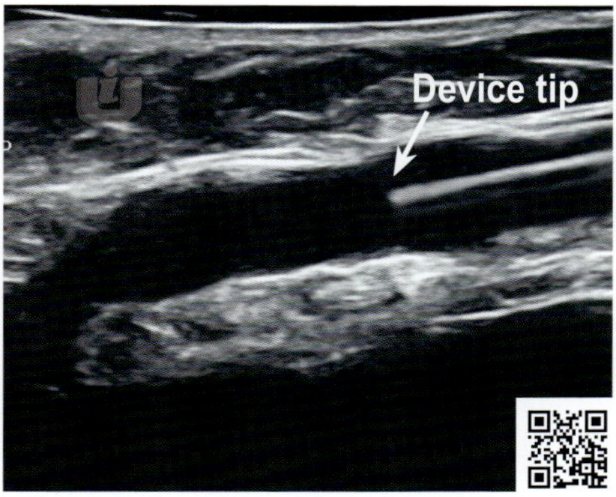

Fig. 11-45. *Device tip at the saphenofemoral junction before infiltration of tumescent anesthesia.*

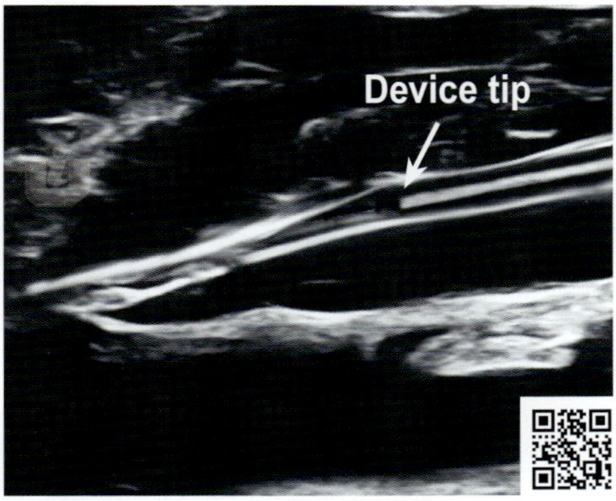

Fig. 11-46. *After infiltration of the junction.*

It is important that adequate tumescent is administered in the area of the junction, ensuring it is entirely compressed. This will help prevent heat from the device entering into the deep vein.

- Continue and complete infiltration of the junction at this time.
- Prior to activation of the device, using the transverse view, follow the entire length of the vein to ensure adequate tumescent anesthesia infiltration.

- Adequate tumescent should appear as a halo effect. The vein should lie at a depth of >10mm from the skin surface and 10mm of fluid should surround the device. [14, 37]

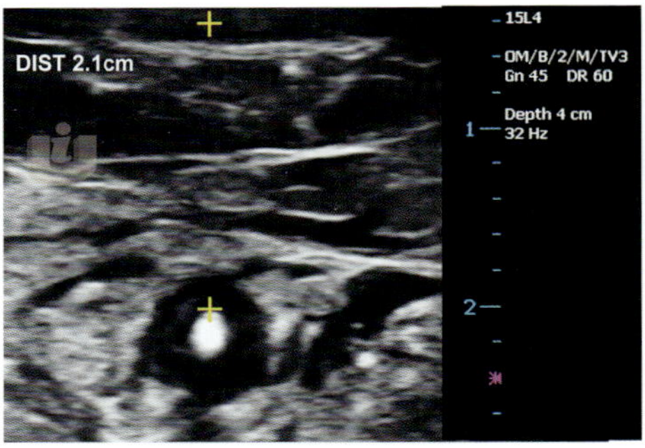

Fig. 11-47. *Tumescent anesthesia demonstrating the "Halo effect". The device is >20mm from the skin surface with >10mm of fluid surrounding it.* [37]

> *When administered accurately, tumescent is an effective tool to minimize the risk of thermal injury to the surrounding tissue and structures.*

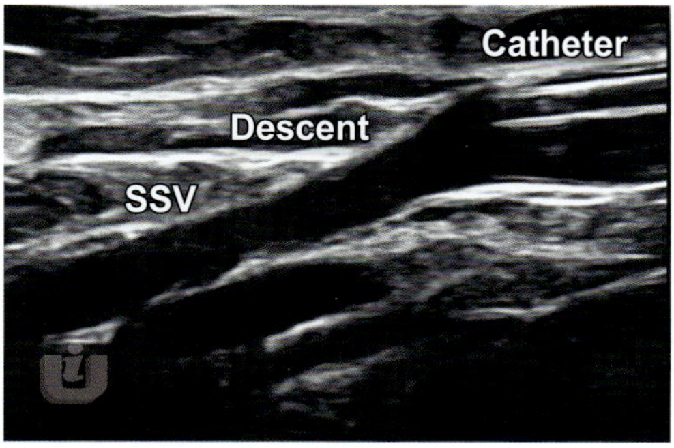

Fig. 11-48. *Catheter is positioned at the descent of the SSV.*

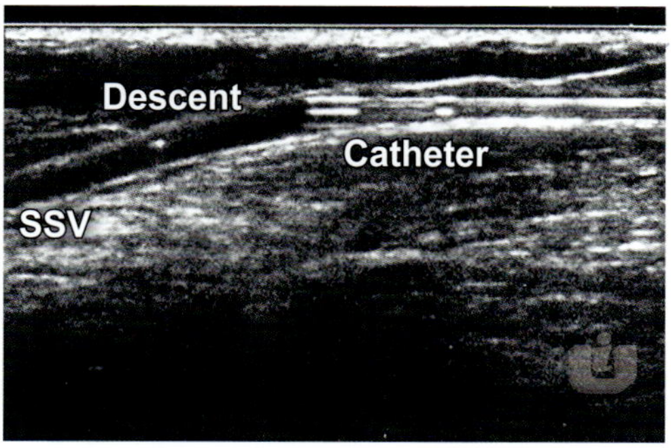

Fig. 11-49. *Device tip placement at the descent of the small saphenous vein.*

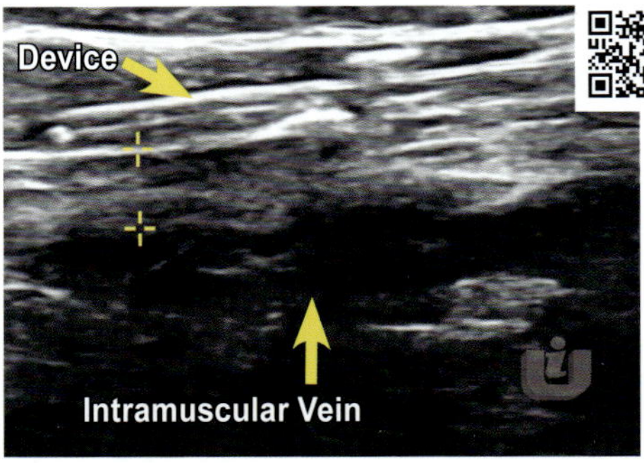

Fig. 11-50. *Due to the close proximity of the SSV and the intramuscular veins, adequate tumescent must be administered below (as well as above) the SSV to push the intramuscular vein away from the device.*

- To maintain a safe and optimal junctional distance, use transverse and longitudinal views to document a final junctional measurement before activation:
  - Typically, somewhere between 2-3cm peripheral to the ostium for the inguinal veins e.g., great saphenous, accessory great saphenous veins. [6]
  - Typically, at the descent of the small saphenous vein before it dives toward the popliteal vein. [21]
- The table is then positioned to 20-30° Trendelenburg.
- Imaging during the procedure will be defined according to the device being used.

Ultrasound Immediately Post-Thermal Ablation

- Patient position immediately post-procedure
  - GSV supine, >20° reverse Trendelenburg with the lower extremity externally rotated and a slight flexion of the knee joint.
  - SSV prone, >20° reverse Trendelenburg with a pillow under the ankle to flex the knee joint.

Remember to adjust the table from Trendelenburg back to reverse Trendelenburg. The dependent position dilates the vein, making it easier to visualize. Skipping this step will not only make it difficult to visualize the vein, it will result in poor filling of the untreated segment.

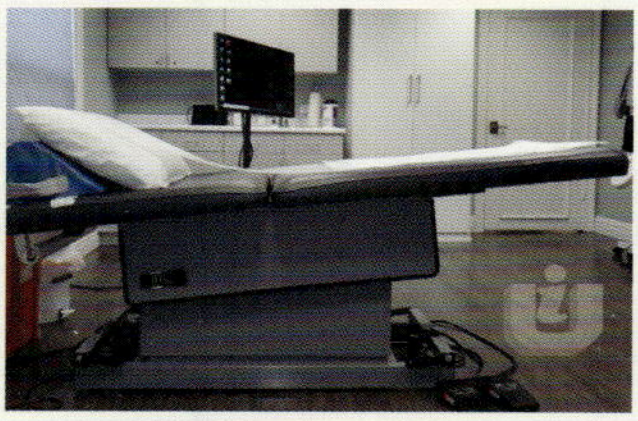

Trendelenburg

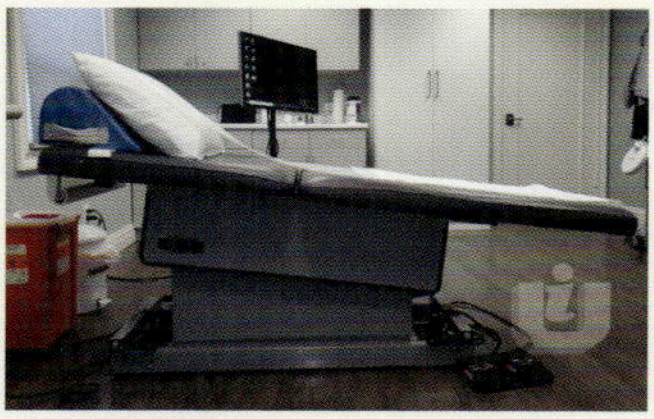

Reverse Trendelenburg

- Locate the junction using the transverse view.
- Evaluate the confluence of the treated vein and the associated deep vein using B-mode imaging without and with transducer compression.
- Turn the transducer longitudinally.
- Evaluate the junction for patency using both B-mode and color Doppler imaging.
- Demonstrate color Doppler filling of the untreated vein segment where it joins with its associated deep vein (cul-de-sac).
  - The first few centimeters of the treated vein segment should be patent, leaving a small cul-de-sac where it joins with the associated deep vein.
- Document PW Doppler of the associated deep vein.

Documentation should include at a minimum:

- Transverse split screen grayscale images of the associated deep vein/s without and with compression
- Resting PW flow pattern of the associated deep vein
- Grayscale image of the SFJ displaying a patent junction
- Color Doppler filling of the of the untreated vein segment where it joins with its associated deep vein (cul-de-sac)
- Any unusual anatomy or disease

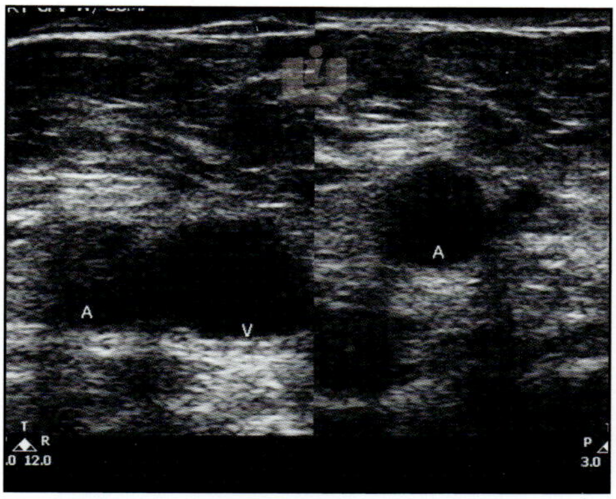

Fig. 11-51. *CFV split screen without and with compression.*

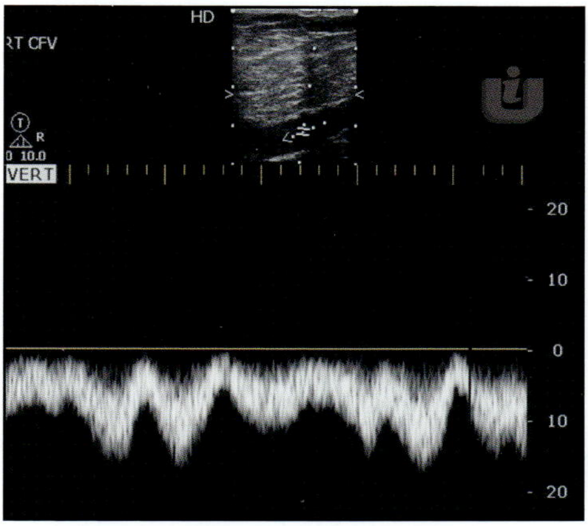

Fig. 11-52. *PW Doppler of the CFV immediately after the ablation displaying post-ablation disturbed flow.*

Image order for an immediate post intervention exam should start with the compression images first, followed by color Doppler images and spectral waveforms. Spectral waveform may appear disturbed due to increased blood temperature.

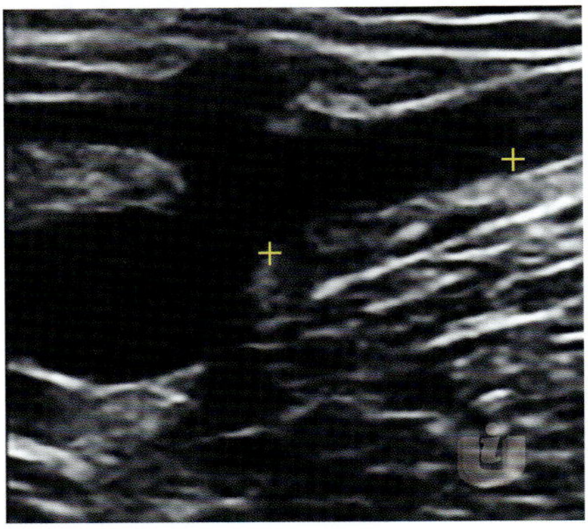

Fig. 11-53. *Grayscale image of the saphenofemoral junction displaying patency in the cul-de-sac, CFV and epigastric vein immediately post thermal ablation procedure.*

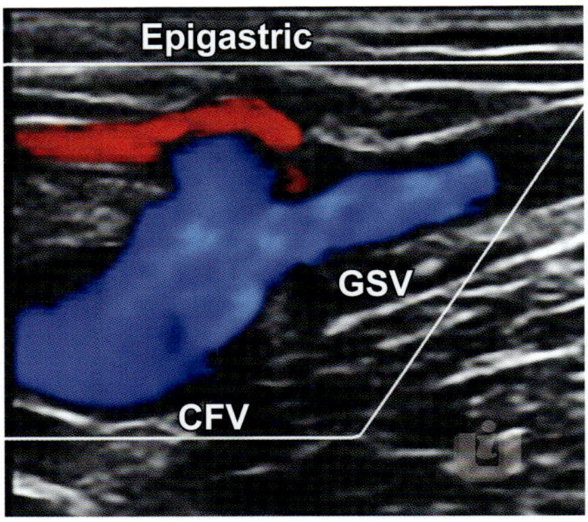

Fig. 11-54. *Color Doppler image of the saphenofemoral junction displaying adequate color filling in the cul-de-sac, CFV and epigastric vein immediately post thermal ablation procedure.*

If an inguinal vein is involved, use color Doppler imaging to assess the epigastric vein for patency.

Non-Thermal Non-Tumescent (NTNT) Ablative Options

Chemical and Adhesive

As the field of phlebology is constantly growing, additional research and treatment options to ablate superficial veins have become available. In the last decade, additional venous closure methods emerged:

1. Chemical
2. Adhesive ablation

Chemical Ablation

Definition

Chemical Ablation or Sclerotherapy: A procedure using a chemical to remove tissue or destroy its function. Sclerotherapy is the targeted chemical ablation of a varicose vein by intravenous injection of a liquid or foam sclerosant. [25]

There are various types of chemical ablation methods: mechanochemical, proprietary endovenous micro foam, physician compounded foam, and liquid. All methods can be used in an operating room or as an office-based procedure.

Rationale

The procedure uses a sclerosing agent, to achieve venous closure. Chemical ablation, also known as sclerotherapy, may be performed with or without ultrasound guidance. Sclerotherapy used to treat noticeable dermal and hypodermal veins that appear near the skins surface, known as telangiectasias and reticular veins, will not be discussed in this chapter.

Veins Treated Using Chemical Ablation

- Great Saphenous Vein (GSV)
- Anterior Accessory Great Saphenous Vein (AAGSV)
- Posterior Accessory Great Saphenous Vein (PAGSV)
- Thigh Extension of the Small Saphenous Vein (TE-SSV)
- Small Saphenous Vein (SSV)
- Anterior Circumflex Vein (ATCV)*
- Posterior Circumflex Vein (PTCV)*
- Pathologic Perforating Vein (PPV)
- Varicose tributaries
- New, remaining and recurrent varicose veins after previous procedures *(Fig. 11-87)*

* *Within or outside of the saphenous compartment*

Ultrasound is used immediately prior to, during, and post procedure to ensure safe, effective, and efficient administration.

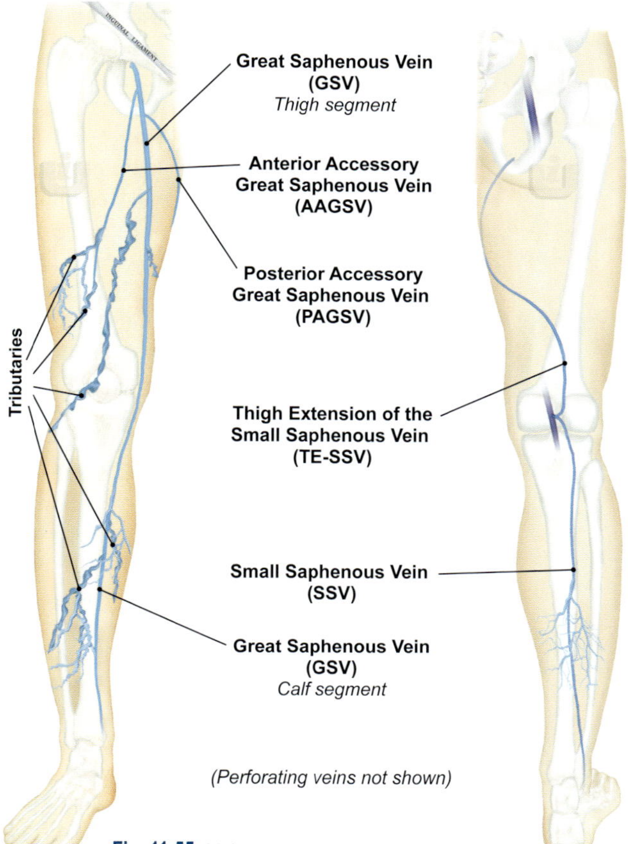

Fig. 11-55. *Veins treated using chemical ablation.*

Ultrasound Immediately Prior to Chemical Ablation

Following your facilities protocol, perform a quick scan to identify and mark the following:

- Proposed access point for catheter-based technique
- Vein segment to be injected for non-catheter/percutaneous direct needle technique
- Common causes that may lead to post procedure problems or treatment failure [7, 19, 20]
  - Large perforators
  - Large tributaries

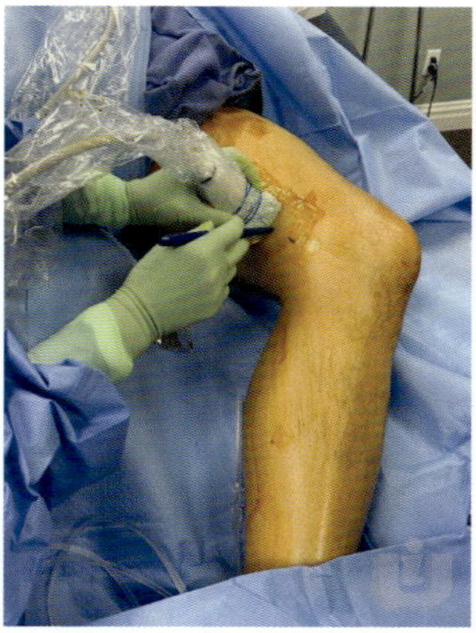

Fig. 11-56. *Target vein (GSV) marked in preparation of a catheter based sterile technique.*

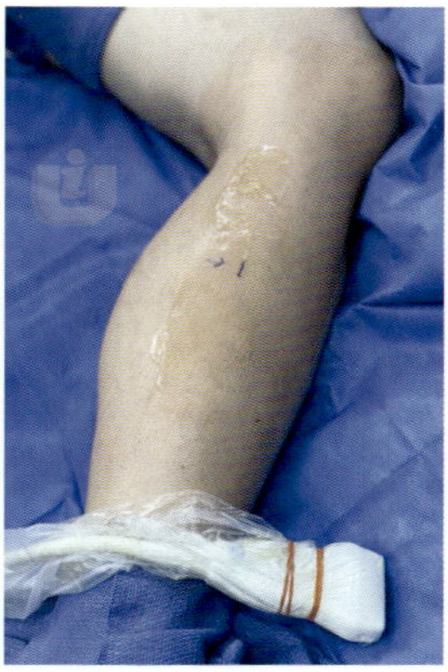

Fig. 11-57. *Target vein (GSV) marked in preparation of a direct needle stick technique.*

Relay quick scan findings to the provider. This discussion may prevent difficulty during the procedure or lead to a different treatment approach.

Marking the limb gives a visual location of the target vein/s. This allows for a systematic approach to treatment and proper positioning, reducing the need to shift position during the procedure.

Ultrasound During Chemical Ablation

Position for GSV and Accessory Great Saphenous Veins

- Supine
- 45° Trendelenburg
- Lower extremity externally rotated and a slight flexion of the knee joint

Position for GSV Below Knee

- Supine
- 45° Trendelenburg* (if administering sclerosant peripheral to central)
- >20° Reverse Trendelenburg (if administering sclerosant central to peripheral)
- Lower extremity externally rotated and a slight flexion of the knee joint

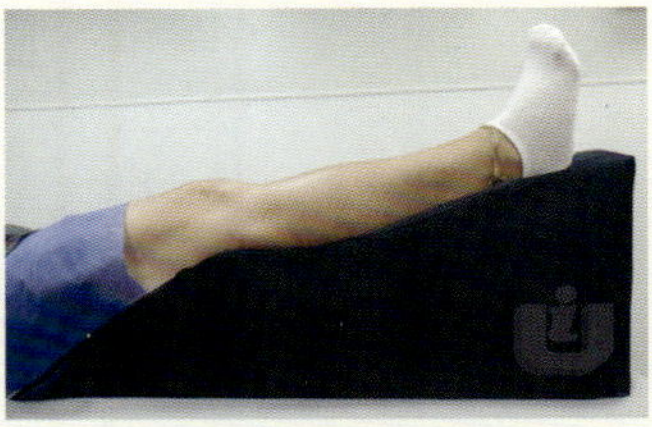

Fig. 11-58. *Position of the limb during chemical ablation of the below knee GSV segment, when using a peripheral to central approach.*

Position for SSV

- Prone
- 45° Trendelenburg (if administering sclerosant peripheral to central)
- >20° Reverse Trendelenburg (if administering sclerosant central to peripheral)

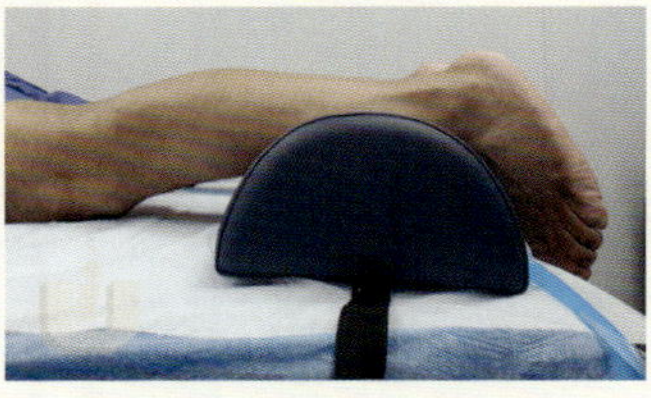

Fig. 11-59. *Position of the limb during chemical ablation of the SSV segment, when using either the central to peripheral or the peripheral to central access approach.*

Catheter-based technique

Protective barriers:

- Sterile keyboard cover
- Sterile transducer cover
- Sterile single-use gel packets (used to decrease the risk of infection)
- Sterile gloves
- Sterile gown

Per your facilities protocol, surgical caps and shoe coverings may be worn.

Technique

- Apply sterile gel over the proposed treatment area.
- Identify the target vein at the level of the junction. Move peripherally, evaluating the vein down to the level of the access.
- Administration of local anesthetic will be injected directly over the marked location or injected under ultrasound guidance in real time by positioning the transducer over the access site.
- The provider determines the orientation of the transducer to gain access. The sonographer should orient the transducer accordingly.
- The transducer should remain perpendicular to the limb, allowing accuracy during access.
- The vein is accessed via needle, and a guidewire is placed in the vein. Maintain a steady hand while guiding the provider into the vein.
- Confirm the entry and presence of the needle and the guidewire.
- A dilator and catheter are placed over the guidewire. Once placed at the desired level, the wire is removed.
- The sclerosant is then injected into the vein.

Non-catheter/percutaneous direct needle technique

Protective barriers:

- Sterile or non-sterile gloves
- Sterile or non-sterile keyboard cover
- Sterile or non-sterile transducer cover
- Sterile single-use gel packets (used to decrease the risk of infection)

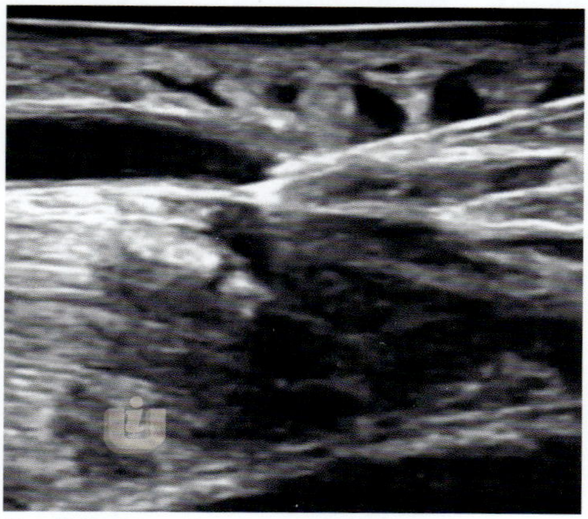

Fig. 11-60. *Needle access displayed in the longitudinal view.*

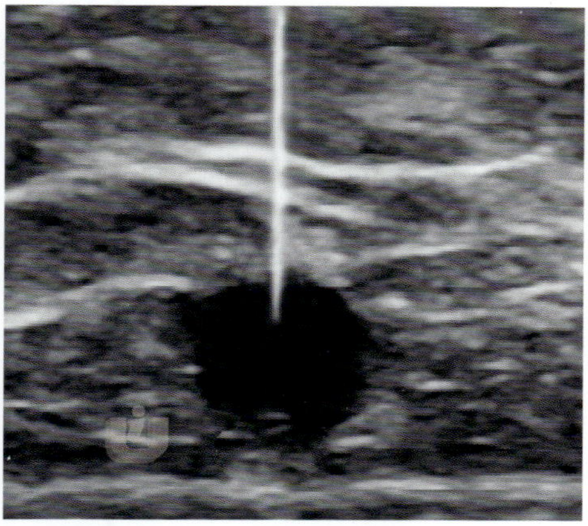

Fig. 11-61. *Needle access displayed in the transverse view.*

Technique

- Apply sterile gel over the treatment area.
- Identify the target vein.
- The vein is accessed via needle. Maintain a steady hand while guiding the provider into the vein.
- Confirm the entry and presence of the needle.
- The sclerosant is then injected into the vein.

> *During access, use a gentle touch to avoid compressing the vein.*

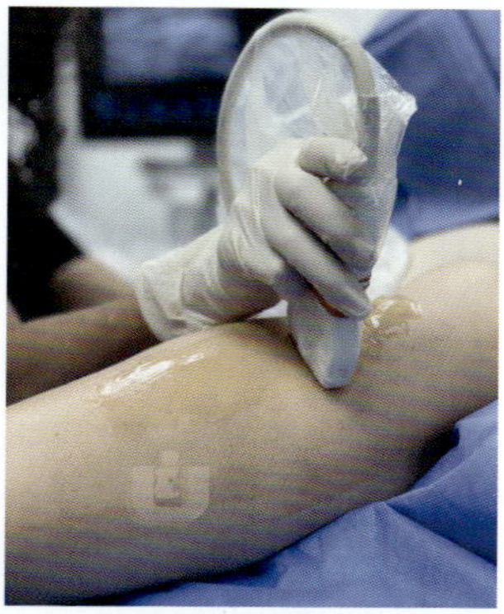

Fig. 11-62. *Hand position for guidance using transverse/ short axis.*

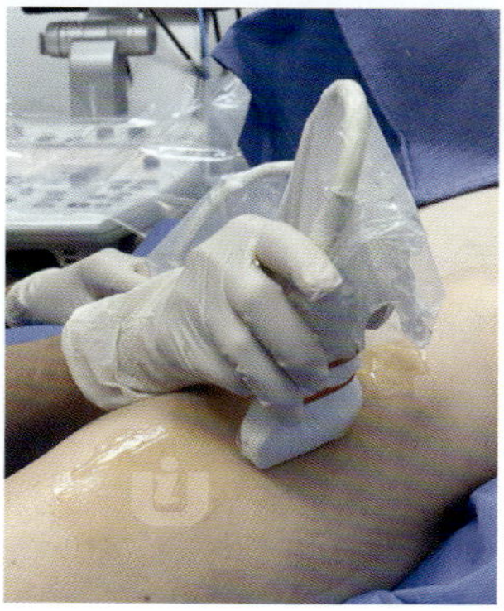

Fig. 11-63. *Hand position for guidance using longitudinal/ long axis.*

Ultrasound Immediately Post-Chemical Ablation

Patient position immediately post-procedure is dependent upon the vein/s injected.

- If possible, follow the sclerosant to ensure full coverage of target vein, and to identify areas where it may be traveling into the deep veins. If sclerosant is seen flowing into the deep system, alert the provider immediately. The provider may instruct the patient to perform dorsiflexion to flush the deep system of sclerosant.

> *During chemical ablation of the superficial truncal veins, alert the provider when the sclerosant approaches the junction. A safe, optimal distance is typically 3-5cm peripheral to the junction.*

Documentation should include at a minimum:

- Transverse split screen grayscale images of the associated deep vein/s without and with compression
- Any unusual anatomy or disease

Remember to adjust the table from Trendelenburg back to reverse Trendelenburg. The dependent position dilates the vein, making it easier to visualize. Skipping this step will not only make it difficult to visualize the vein, it will result in poor filling of the untreated segment.

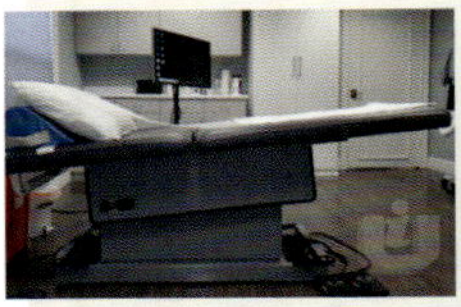

Trendelenburg

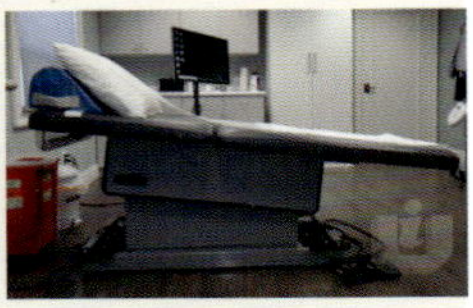

Reverse Trendelenburg

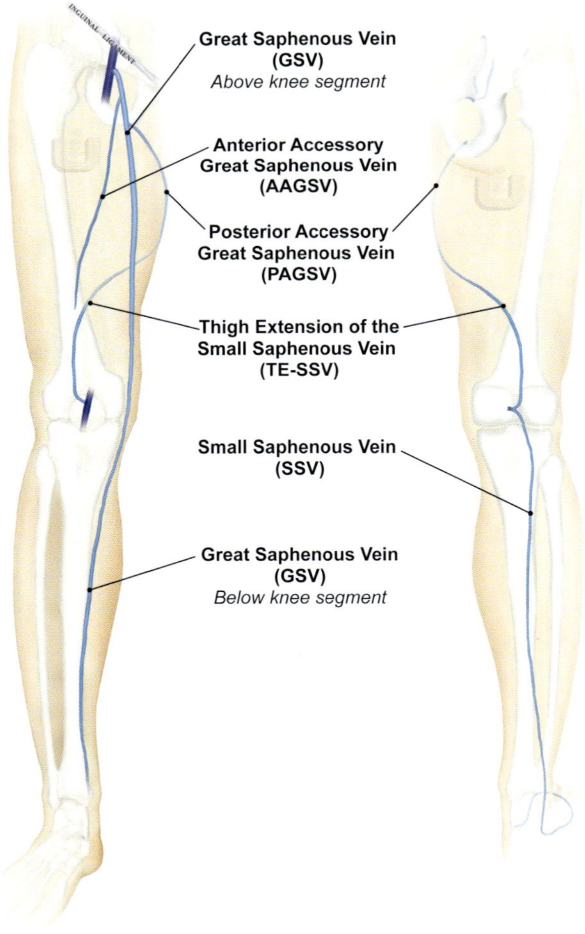

Fig. 11-64. *Veins treated using adhesive ablation.*

Adhesive Ablation

Definition

A procedure using cyanoacrylate to close a vein. Cyanoacrylate (Superglue) is a strong, biodegradable tissue adhesive that polymerizes upon contact with tissues. [30]

Rationale

The procedure uses a cyanoacrylate, also known as glue, to achieve venous closure. The procedure differs from heat and chemical ablation by leaving the glue in the vein as a medical implant. [30, 32]

Veins Treated Using Adhesive Ablation

- Great Saphenous Vein (GSV)
- Anterior Accessory Great Saphenous Vein (AAGSV)
- Posterior Accessory Great Saphenous Vein (PAGSV)
- Thigh Extension of the Small Saphenous Vein (TE-SSV)
- Small Saphenous Vein (SSV)

Ultrasound Immediately Prior to Adhesive Ablation

Perform a quick scan to identify and mark the target vein.

- Position for marking (perform pre-operative marking in the same position as the surgery):
  - GSV: Supine, >20° reverse Trendelenburg with the lower extremity externally rotated and a slight flexion of the knee joint.
  - SSV: Prone, >20° reverse Trendelenburg with a pillow under the ankle to flex the knee joint.

Ultrasound is used immediately prior to, during, and post procedure to ensure safe, effective, and efficient intervention.

Comprehensive marking

- Create a reference point on the center of your transducer or transducer cover.
- Image the vein in transverse and position the vein in the center of the field of view. This should correspond with the reference point/center of the transducer.
- Use an indelible marker so the marker will remain visible despite skin preparation. Gently press for a few seconds to create an indentation or a dot on the skin.
- Move the transducer centrally from the proposed access site to the junction, making a mark every two inches.

Moving centrally will wipe away the gel as you go, making it easier to mark the skin.

- After you have marked the limb, wipe off the gel, make hashmarks over the dots or completely connect the dots. Map the entire course of the vein.

Marking the skin improves accuracy while tracking the course of the vein.

Ultrasound During Adhesive Ablation

Position for GSV	Position for SSV
Supine, >20° reverse Trendelenburg with the lower extremity externally rotated and a slight flexion of the knee joint.	Prone, >20° reverse Trendelenburg with a pillow under the ankle to flex the knee joint.

Protective barriers:

- Sterile keyboard cover
- Sterile transducer cover
- Sterile single-use gel packets (used to decrease the risk of infection)
- Sterile gloves
- Sterile gown

Per your facilities protocol, surgical caps and shoe coverings may be worn.

Anchor the transducer to create a stress point (an area to relieve tension from the weight of the cord) with a towel clamp or a Velcro strip.

Technique

- Apply sterile gel over the proposed treatment area.
- Identify the target vein at the level of the junction. Move peripherally, evaluating the vein down to the level of the access.
- Administration of local anesthetic will be injected directly over the marked location or in real time by positioning the transducer over the access site.
- The provider determines the orientation of the transducer to gain access. The sonographer should orient the transducer accordingly.
- The transducer should remain perpendicular to the limb, allowing accurate access.
- The vein is accessed via needle, and a guidewire is placed in the vein. Maintain a steady hand while guiding the provider into the vein.
- Confirm the entry and presence of the guidewire.
- A dilator and catheter are placed over the guidewire.
- Confirm the entry and presence of the catheter. Once placed at the desired level, the wire is removed.
- Using ultrasound, take a preliminary measurement of the location of the device tip within the superficial vein in relation to its associated deep vein. This step ensures safe, effective, and precise placement of the device.
- To prevent glue from entering the deep system, apply pressure cephalad to the catheter by using the ultrasound transducer in the transverse view.
- A medical grade adhesive is then placed in the vein via a catheter.
- Subsequent placement of glue is administered as needed

Keep your eyes on the monitor at all times during access. Turning your head will undoubtedly move your hand, making it more difficult to remain on your target. This may delay access and even worse, dislodge the needle.

Occlusion rate after cyanoacrylate glue treatment is not influenced by vein length, diameter, dispensing device, or use of postoperative compression stockings. [30]

Ultrasound Immediately Post-Adhesive Ablation

- Patient position immediately post-procedure is dependent upon the vein/s injected.
- Locate the junction using the transverse view.
- Evaluate the confluence of the treated vein and the associated deep vein using B-mode without and with transducer compression.
- Turn the transducer into a longitudinal view.
- Evaluate the junction for patency using both B-mode and color Doppler imaging.
- Demonstrate color Doppler filling of the untreated vein segment where it joins with its associated deep vein. The first few centimeters of the treated vein segment should be patent, leaving a small cul-de-sac where it joins with the associated deep vein.

Documentation should include at a minimum:

- Transverse split screen grayscale images of the associated deep vein/s without and with compression
- Color Doppler filling of the of the untreated vein segment where it joins with its associated deep vein (cul-de-sac)
- Any unusual anatomy or disease

Short-term Ultrasound Post-Procedure Follow-up [29]

A post-procedure venous exam is recommended to evaluate for patency of the deep system at its confluence with the treated vein. However, an expanded post-procedure venous examination may be performed to assess the deep and superficial venous system for patency, insufficiency, and to evaluate the treated vein at its confluence with the deep vein.

Most patients resume normal activity immediately following the procedure. Graduated compression stockings that follow thermal and chemical ablation are not required. [30]

Patient Position Post-Procedure Examination

- Post-procedure examination performed with patient standing.
- Expanded post-procedure performed with patient standing and supine.

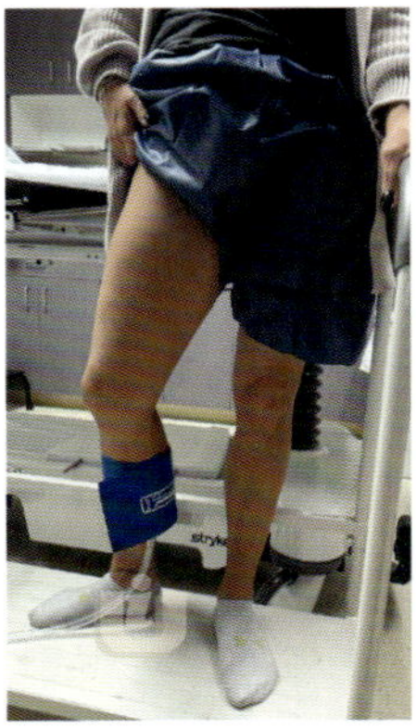

Fig. 11-65. *Position for evaluation of the CFV, SFJ, FV, GSV, AAGSV, and PAGSV.*

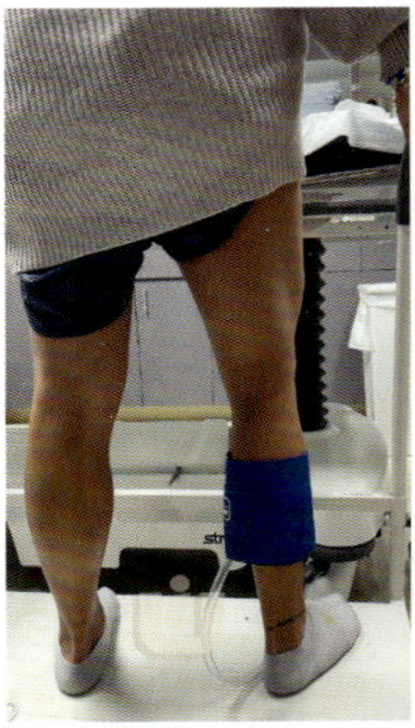

Fig. 11-66. *Position for evaluation of the PopV, SSV, and TE-SSV.*

Standing is the preferred position. Sitting or reverse Trendelenburg may be used if the patient cannot stand. Patient position must be noted in the final report.

Post-Procedure Ultrasound Examination

Position for GSV	*Position for SSV*
Facing the examiner, the lower extremity is externally rotated with a slight flexion of the knee joint.	Facing away from the examiner with a slight flexion of the knee joint.

Technique

- Evaluate the confluence of the treated vein and the associated deep vein using B-mode without and with transducer compression.
- Demonstrate color Doppler filling of the untreated vein segment where it joins with its associated deep vein (cul-de-sac).
- Measure the cul-de-sac in the longitudinal view by placing calipers on the posterior wall of the treated vein from the ostium to the beginning of the treated segment. *(Fig. 11-53)*
- The first few centimeters of the treated vein should be patent, leaving a small cul-de-sac where it joins with the associated deep vein.

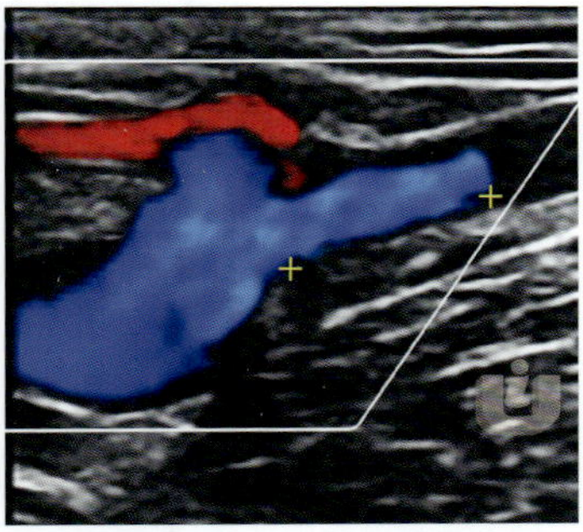

Fig. 11-67. *Color Doppler image of saphenofemoral junction displaying adequate color filling in the cul-de-sac, CFV and epigastric vein immediately post thermal ablation procedure.*

Expanded Post-Procedure

Supine

- DVT, SVT, treated segment and iatrogenic thrombus evaluation
  - >20° reverse Trendelenburg with the lower extremity externally rotated and a slight flexion of the knee joint.
  - Perform B-mode evaluation with and without transducer compressions of all deep, superficial and intramuscular calf veins to assess for thrombus.
  - Document spontaneity and phasicity of the deep veins using PW Doppler.
  - Assess for filling defects using color Doppler.
  - Using B-mode and color Doppler, demonstrate patency and adequate color Doppler filling of the untreated vein segment where it joins with its associated deep vein (cul-de-sac).
  - Measure the cul-de-sac in the longitudinal view by placing calipers on the posterior wall of the treated vein from the ostium to the beginning of the treated segment. *(Fig. 11-53)*

> *If an inguinal vein is involved, use color Doppler to assess the epigastric vein for patency.*

  - The first few centimeters of the treated vein should be patent, leaving a small cul-de-sac where it joins with the associated deep vein.

Standing

- **GSV:** Facing the examiner, the lower extremity is externally rotated with a slight flexion of the knee joint.
- **SSV:** Facing away from the examiner with a slight flexion of the knee joint.

Documentation should include at a minimum:

- Transverse split screen grayscale images of the associated deep vein/s without and with compression
- Color Doppler to demonstrate color filling
- B-mode and color Doppler imaging of the of the untreated vein segment where it joins with its associated deep vein (cul-de-sac)
- Any unusual anatomy or disease

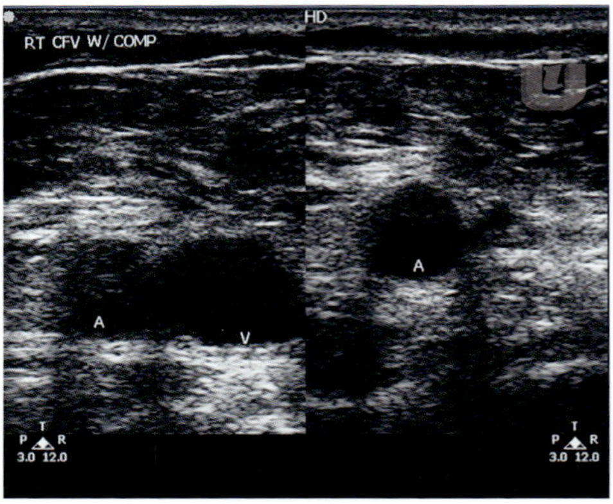

Fig. 11-68. *Transverse split screen grayscale images demonstrating venous compression.*

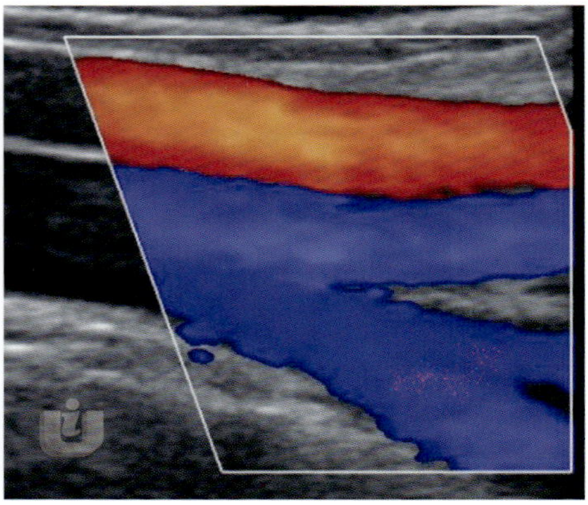

Fig. 11-69. *Color Doppler imaging to demonstrate color filling.*

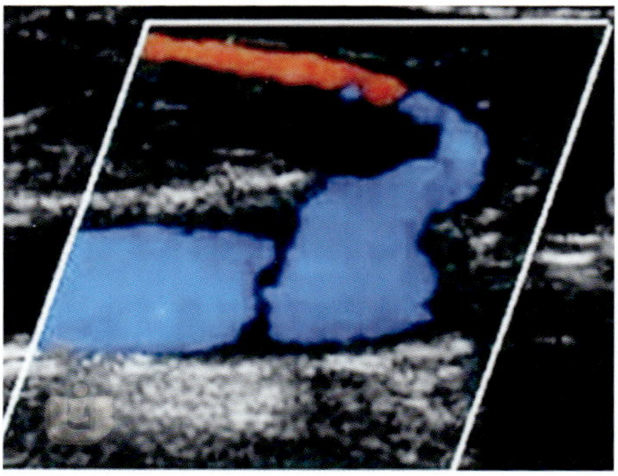

Fig. 11-70. *Color Doppler of the untreated vein segments.*

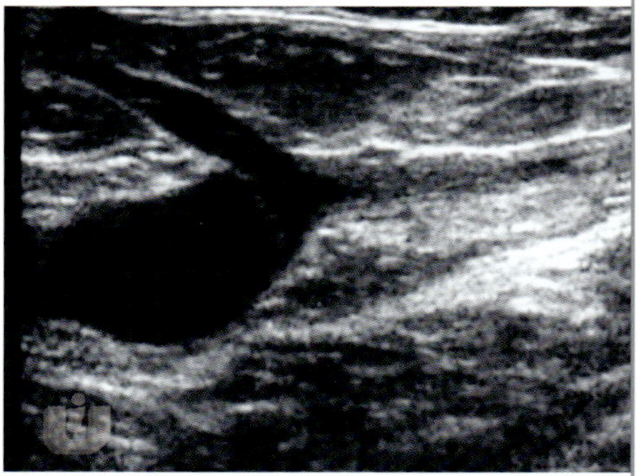

Fig. 11-71. *B-mode image displaying filling of the treated vein segments.*

There may be a difference in the closure point based on patient position.

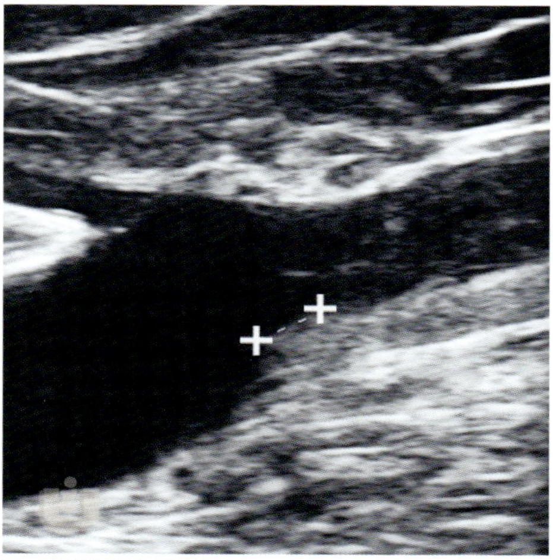

Fig. 11-72. *PASTE measuring 0.5cm from the ostium supine.*

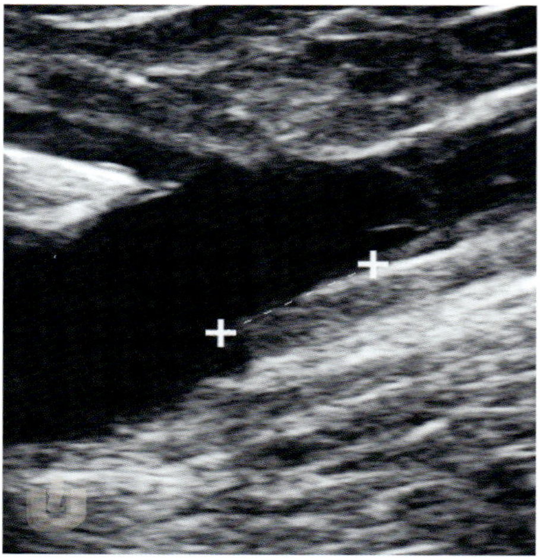

Fig. 11-73. *PASTE measuring 1.48cm from the ostium standing.*

As the field of phlebology continually grows, further research and treatment options to ablate superficial veins have become available. Additional venous closure methods have emerged in the last decade, such as Steam and Microwave Vein Sclerosis; however, these methods are not approved for use in the USA. [26]

Expected Complications

Routine follow-up scans to assess for complications should be performed 3-7 days following all procedures.

- Pain and bruising
- Hyperpigmentation
- Tenderness
  - Inflammation of the treated vein
  - Inflammation of adjacent vein segments
- PASTE [24]

Ablation procedures work in different ways. Some produce inflammation, which can lead to thrombus. Iatrogenic thrombus is defined as thrombus induced by a procedure. These thrombi are known as Post Ablation Superficial Thrombus Extension (PASTE), a general term used for all thrombus caused by ablative procedures. Thrombus extension is categorized based on the type of ablative procedure used. [24]

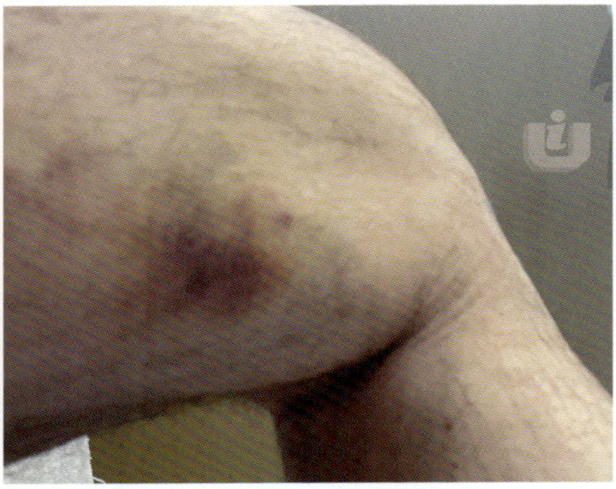

Fig. 11-74. *Post procedure bruising at access site.*

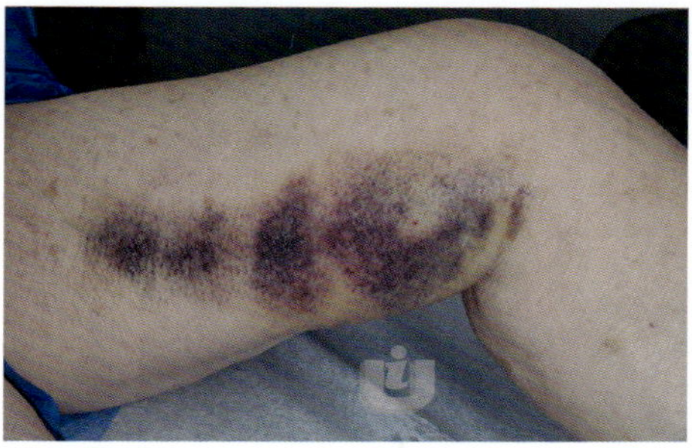

Fig. 11-75. *Post procedure bruising along vein tract as a result of tumescent administration.*

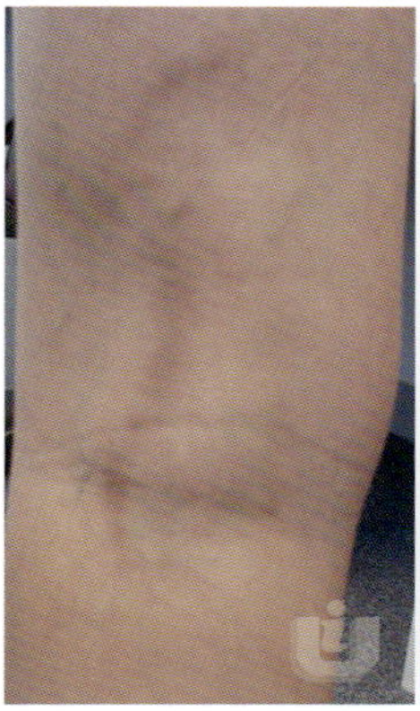

Fig. 11-76. *Staining*

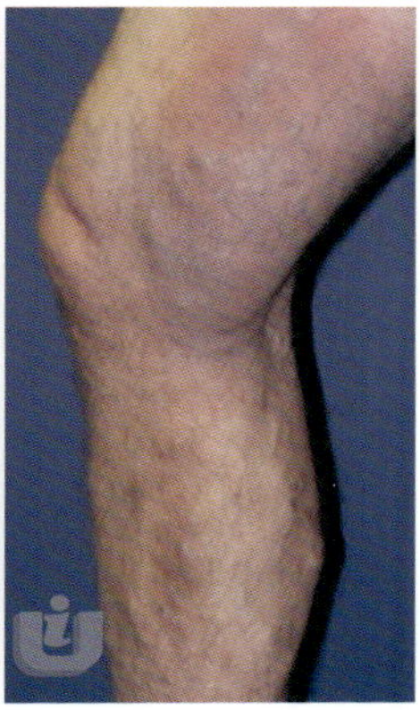

Fig. 11-77. *Phlebitis*

Photos courtesy of John Golan, MD

> *The majority of iatrogenic thrombi are asymptomatic.* [23]

Table 11-2. **Post Ablation Superficial Thrombus Extension (PASTE)** [24]

Device Used	Thrombus Extension
ETA Endovenous Thermal Ablation (ELA, EVLA, EVLT, RFA)	**EHIT** Endovenous Heat Induced Thrombus
UGFS (foam) **UGS** (liquid) **MOCA** (Mechanochemical ablation)	**EFIT** Endovenous Foam Induced Thrombus
EVAA Endovenous Adhesive Ablation	**EGIT** Endovenous Glue Induced Thrombus

If thrombus is present: [22, 23, 24, 33]

- Assess the severity and extent
- Grade if required by your facility
- Perform serial studies to assess for progression, regression, and stability

All images should be obtained in the supine and standing position.

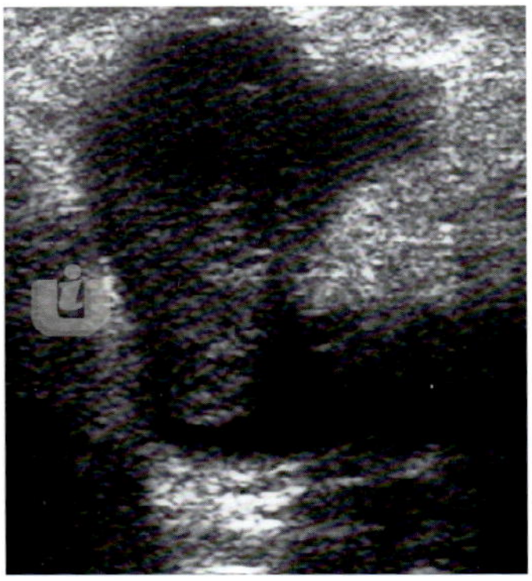

Fig. 11-78. *PASTE - Class 3 transverse view*

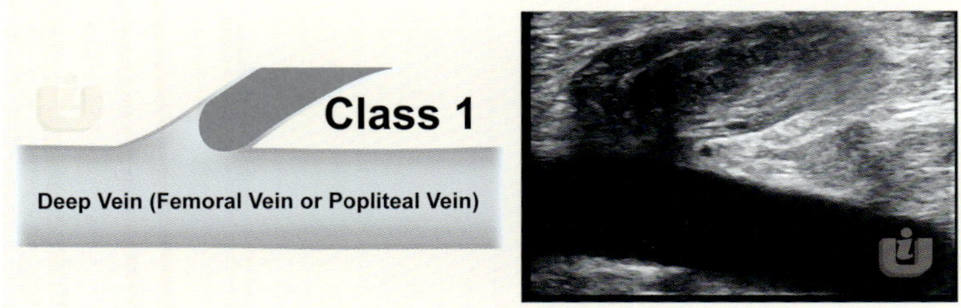

Fig. 11-79. *Venous thrombosis extending to the superficial-deep junction, but not into the deep system.*

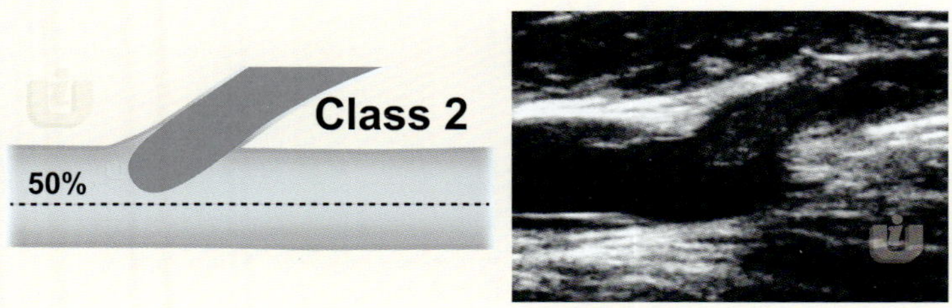

Fig. 11-80. *Non-occlusive venous thrombosis, with an extension into the deep system of a cross sectional area of <50%.*

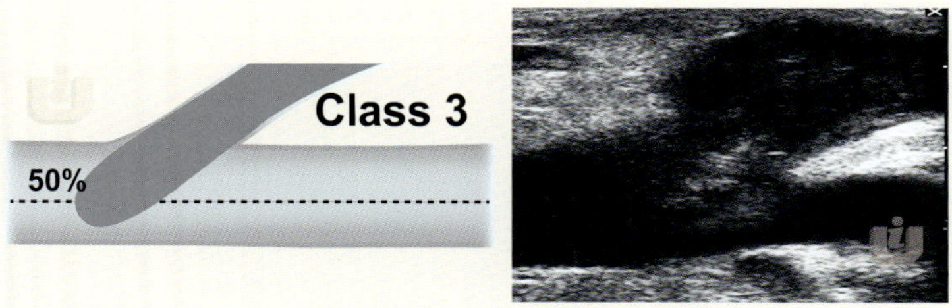

Fig. 11-81. *Non-occlusive venous thrombosis, with an extension into the deep system of a cross sectional area of >50%.*

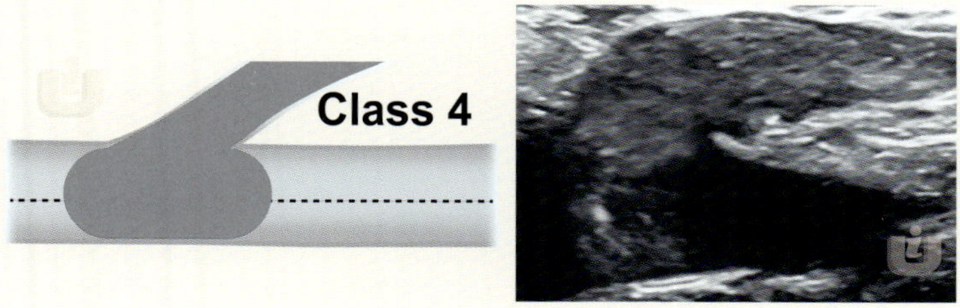

Fig. 11-82. *Occlusive deep vein thrombosis of the deep vein.*

Thrombus Extension Classification [29, 33, 34]

Some authors have introduced the broader term "post-ablation superficial thrombus extension" to indicate a thrombus extension from the superficial to the deep system after any kind of chemical or thermal endovenous ablation. [24]

Documentation should include at a minimum:

- Transverse split screen grayscale images of the associated deep vein/s without and with compression
- Longitudinal view in B-mode, demonstrating sonographic characteristics
- Longitudinal and transverse views using color Doppler imaging, demonstrating flow through or around any thrombosed segment
- Measurements of thrombus [29]
  - Length into the junction
  - Width
  - Height
  - Cross-sectional diameter
- Thrombus characteristics (obtained from B-mode images at varying angles of insonation)
- Resting PW flow pattern of the associated deep vein

Unexpected Complications

- Venous thrombosis
  - Deep
  - Superficial
- Tissue damage
  - Thermal or chemical skin burn
    - Dermal or Subdermal
  - Ulceration
- Matting
- Skin puckering/dimpling
- Nerve injury
- Sterile abscess
- Visual disturbance
- Infection (<1%)
- Treatment failure
  - Recanalization
  - Nonocclusion or reopening

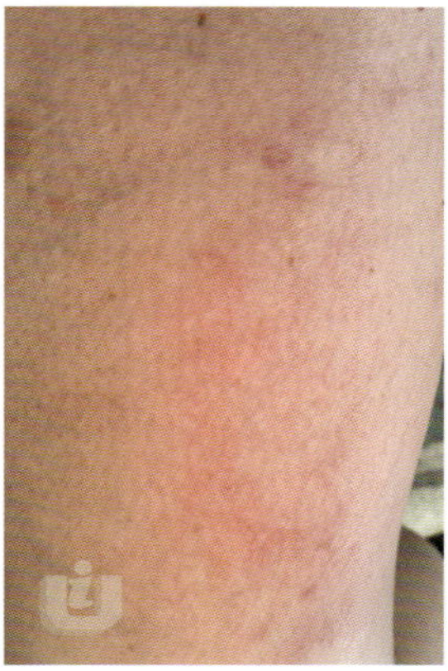

Fig. 11-83. *Matting*

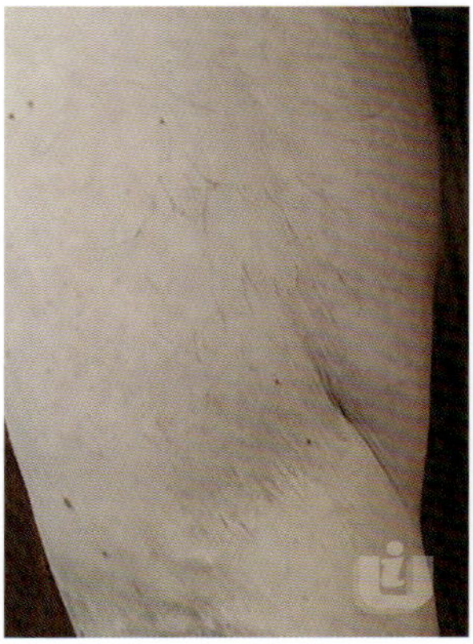

Fig. 11-84. *Skin puckering/ dimpling*

Photo courtesy of John Golan, MD

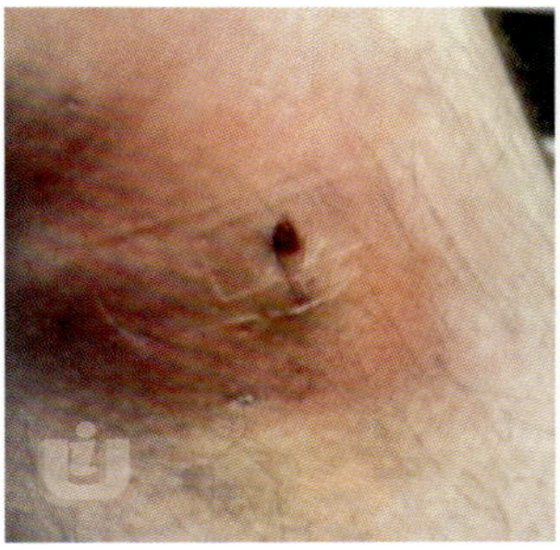

Fig. 11-85. *Tissue damage at the access area with cauterization of the access site.*

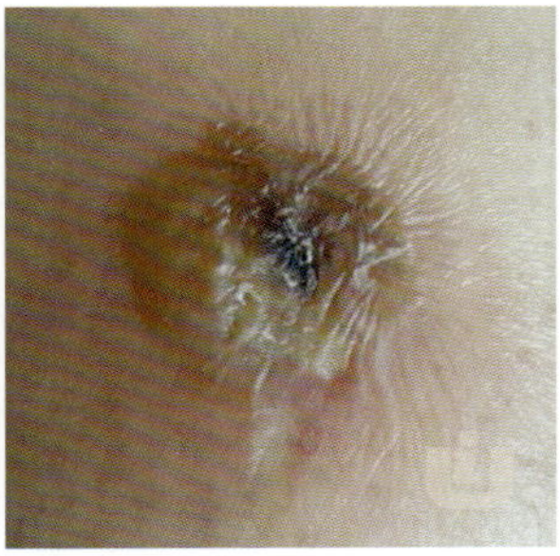

Fig. 11-86. *Chemical burn after sclerotherapy treatment.*

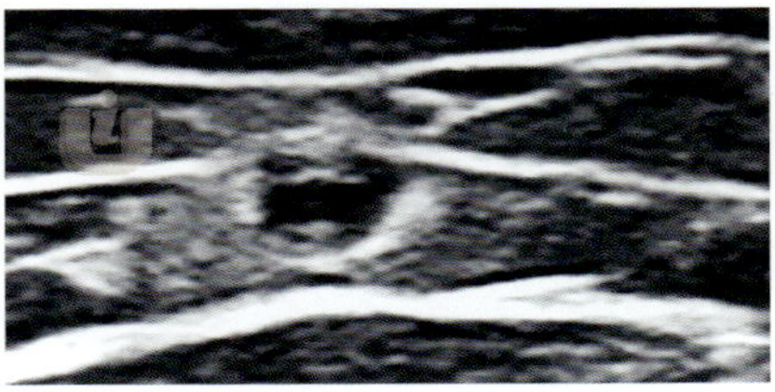

Fig. 11-87. *Treatment failure: Recanalization displayed in grayscale using the transverse view.*

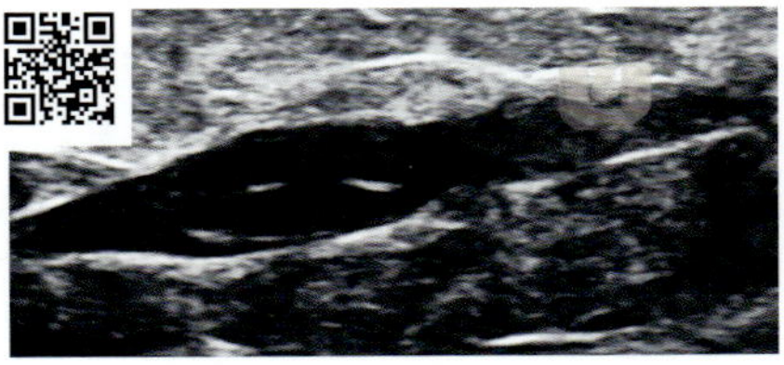

Fig. 11-88. *Treatment failure: Recanalization displayed in grayscale using the longitudinal view.*

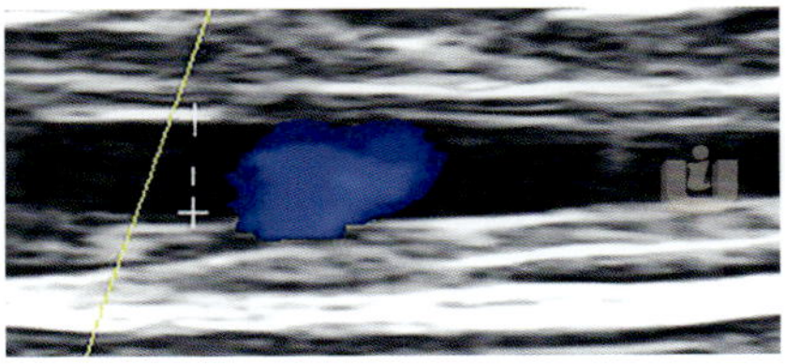

Fig. 11-89. *Treatment failure: Recanalization displayed in color using the longitudinal view.*

Diameter measurements of the incompetent perforating vein should be taken at the location where the vein perforates the deep fascia and at the largest diameter below the fascia. Epifascial diameters are taken as needed.

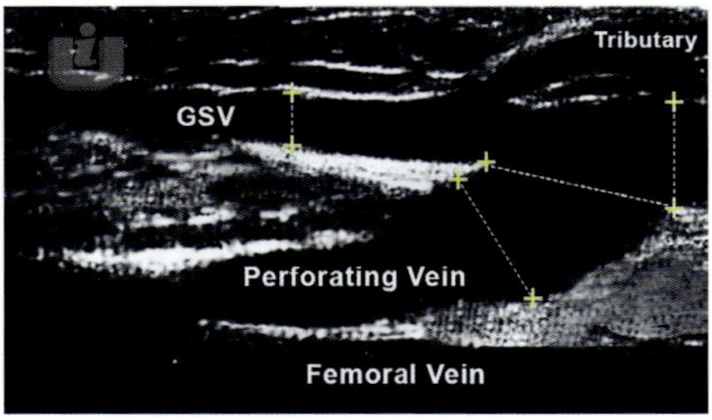

Fig. 11-90. *Mid-thigh perforating vein measuring 26mm at the muscular fascia and 21mm in diameter. The great saphenous vein diameter measures 4.8mm central to the PV and 10.4mm peripherally.*

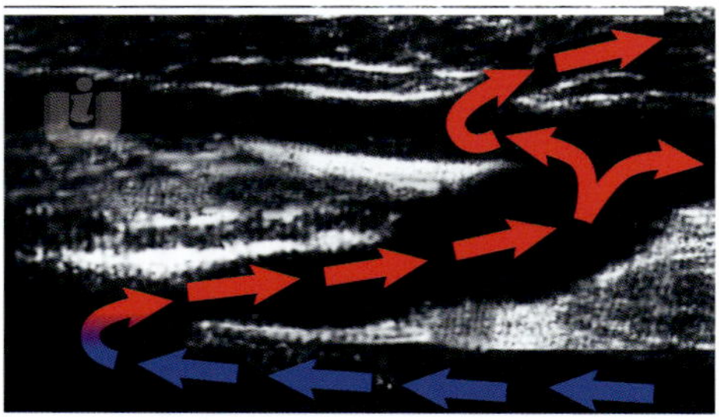

Fig. 11-91. *Incompetent mid-thigh perforating vein resulting in incompetence of the GSV and GSV tributary at the mid-thigh.*

Long-Term Ultrasound Post-Procedure Follow-up

Long term follow-up ultrasound will consist of a complete bilateral lower extremity duplex ultrasound.

Points to Remember

- The patient must be comfortable and appropriately positioned.
- A quick scan should be performed immediately prior to the procedure.
- Ensure all protective barriers are in place.
- Measure saphenous vein diameter and depth at the proposed access site. Veins less than 5mm from the skin surface are at higher risk of skin discoloration and dermal injury. [18]
- Document all areas that may hinder device navigation. [18]
- Marking the course of the vessel will improve accuracy while tracking.
- Adjust the table accordingly during access, tumescent administration and post procedure imaging.
- Keep your eyes on the monitor at all times during access. Turning your head will undoubtedly move your hand, making it more difficult to remain on your target. This may delay access and even worse, dislodge the needle.
- Recheck placement of the device tip prior to activation.

References

1. Gibson, K., Elias. S., Adelman, M., Hager, E.S., Dexter, D.J., Vayuvegula, S., Chopra, P., Kabnick, L.S. (2020). A prospective safety and effectiveness study using endovenous laser ablation with a 400-µm optical fiber for the treatment of pathologic perforator veins in patients with advanced venous disease (SeCure trial). *Journal of Vascular Surgery :Venous Lymphatic Disorders, 8*(5), 805-813. https://doi: 10.1016/j.jvsv.2020.01.014. Epub 2020 Mar 21. PMID: 32205128.
2. Labropoulos, N., Tiongson, J., Pryor, L., Tassiopoulos, A.K., Kang, S.S., Mansour M.A., Baker, W.H. (2003). Definition of venous reflux in lower-extremity veins. *Journal of Vascular Surgery, 38*, 793-798.
3. neuroangio.org. (2022, May 5). Venous sinuses. neuroangio.org/venous-brain-anatomy/venous-sinuses
4. Wittens C., Davies A.H., Bækgaard N., Broholm R., Cavezzi A., Chastanet S. (2015). Management of chronic venous disease: clinical practice guidelines of the European Society for Vascular Surgery (ESVS). *Journal of Vascular and Endovascular Surgery, 49*, 678-737
5. Tzogias, L., Labropoulos, N., Amaral, S.I., Antoniou, G.A., Giannoukas, A.D. (2011). Distribution and clinical impact of phlebosclerosis. *International Angiology,* 3, 212-220. PMID: 21617604
6. DePopas, E., Brown, M. (2018). Varicose Veins and Lower Extremity Venous Insufficiency. *Seminars in Interventional Radiology, 35*(1), 56-61. doi: 10.1055/s-0038-1636522. Epub 2018 Apr 5. PMID: 29628617; PMCID: PMC5886767
7. Gloviczki, P., Comerota, A.J., Dalsing, M.C., Eklof, B.G., Gillespie, D.L., Gloviczki, M.L., Lohr, J.M., McLafferty, R.B., Meissner, M.H., Murad, M.H., Padberg, F.T., Pappas, P.J., Passman, M.A., Raffetto, J.D., Vasquez, M.A., Wakefield, T.W., (2011). Society for Vascular Surgery; American Venous Forum. The care of patients with varicose veins and associated chronic venous diseases: clinical practice guidelines of the Society for Vascular Surgery and the American Venous Forum. *Journal of Vascular Surgery, 53*(5), 2S-48S. doi: 10.1016/j.jvs.2011.01.079. PMID: 21536172
8. Min, R.J,, Khilnani, N., Zimmet, S.E. (2003). Endovenous laser treatment of saphenous vein reflux: long-term results. *Journal of Vascular Interventional Radiology, 14*(8), 991-996.
9. Yao, P., Mukhdomi. T. Varicose Vein Endovenous Laser Therapy. [Updated 2022 Jan 15]. In: StatPearls [Internet]. Treasure Island (FL): StatPearls Publishing; 2022 Jan-. Available from: https://www.ncbi.nlm.nih.gov/books/NBK557719/

10. Coleridge-Smith, P., Labropoulos, N., Partsch, H., Myers, K., Nicolaides, A., Cavezzi, A., (2006). Duplex ultrasound investigation of the veins in chronic venous disease of the lower limbs: UIP consensus document: part I. Basic principles. *European Journal of Vascular and Endovascular Surgery, 31*, 83-92.
11. Labropoulos, N., Leon, L.R. (2005). Evaluation of chronic venous disease. In Mansour, M.A., & Labropoulos, N., (Eds.), *Vascular Diagnosis*. Philadelphia: Elsevier Saunders; (447–461).
12. Cina, A., Pedicelli, A., Di Stasi, C., Porcelli, A., Fiorentino, A., Cina, G., Rulli, F., Bonomo, L. (2005). Color-Doppler sonography in chronic venous insufficiency: what the radiologist should know. *Current Problems in Diagnostic Radiology, 34*(2), 51-62. https://doi: 10.1067/j.cpradiol.2004.12.001. PMID: 15753879.
13. Pascarella, L., Mekenas, L. (2006). Ultrasound examination of the patient with primary venous insufficiency, In J.J. Bergan (Ed.) The Vein Book. 171-181. Elsevier.
14. Nyamekye, I.K. (2019). A practical approach to tumescent local anesthesia in ambulatory endovenous thermal ablation. *Phlebology, 34*(4), 238-245. doi:10.1177/0268355518800191.
15. National Cancer Institute at the National Institutes of Health, Incorporated. (n.d.). Thermal Ablation. https://www.cancer.gov/publications/dictionaries/cancer-terms/def/thermal-ablation.
16. Kuyumcu, G., Salazar, G.M., Prabhakar, A.M., Ganguli, S. (2016). Minimally invasive treatments for perforator vein insufficiency. *Cardiovasc Diagnosis and Therapy, 6*(6), 593-598. https://doi: 10.21037/cdt.2016.11.12. PMID: 28123979; PMCID: PMC5220201.
17. Sharif, M.A., Soong, C.V., Lau, L.L., Corvan, R., Lee, B., Hannon, R.J. (2006). Endovenous laser treatment for long saphenous vein incompetence. *British Journal of Surgery, 93*(7), 831-835. https://doi: 10.1002/bjs.5351. PMID: 16673353
18. American College of Phlebology. (2016. February 3). Treatment of Superficial Venous Disease of the Lower Leg. Practice Guidelines: Superficial Venous Disease. American Vein & Lymphatic Society. https://www.myavls.org/assets/pdf/SuperficialVenousDiseaseGuidelinesPMS313-02.03.16.pdf
19. Kostas, T., Ioannou, C.V., Touloupakis, E., Daskalaki, E., Giannoukas, A.D., Tsetis, D., Katsamouris, A.N. (2004). Recurrent varicose veins after surgery: a new appraisal of a common and complex problem in vascular surgery. *European Journal of Vascular and Endovascular Surgery*, 27(3), 275-282. https://doi: 10.1016/j.ejvs.2003.12.006. PMID: 14760596
20. de Maeseneer, M.G.R, Biemans, A.A.M., & Pichot, O. (2013). New concepts on recurrence of varicose veins according to the different treatment techniques. Phlebologie - Annales Vasculaires, 66(4), 54–60. Retrieved from http://hdl.handle.net/1765/84677
21. Elias, S., & Khilnani, N.M. (2008). Treating the Small Saphenous Vein Anatomical considerations and techniques for treating the SSV and junctional tributaries. Endovascular Today, Aug, 60-64
22. Jones, R.T., Kabnick, L.S. (2014). Perioperative duplex ultrasound following endothermal ablation of the saphenous vein: is it worthless? *The Journal of Invasive Cardiology, 26*(10), 548-550. PMID: 25274866
23. Kabnick, L.S., Sadek, M., Bjarnason, H., Coleman, D. M., Dillavou, E. D., Hingorani, A. P., Lal, B. K., Lawrence, P. F., Malgor, R. D., & Puggioni, A. (2021). Classification and treatment of endothermal heat-induced thrombosis: Recommendations from the American Venous Forum and the Society for Vascular Surgery. *Journal of Vascular Surgery: Venous Lymphatic Disorders, 9*(1), 6-22.
24. Passariello, F. (2014). Post-ablation superficial thrombus extension (PASTE) as a consequence of endovenous ablation. An up to- date review. *Vascular Medicine 2*, 62-66
25. Rabe, E., Breu, F. X., Cavezzi, A., Coleridge Smith, P., Frullini, A., Gillet, J. L., Guex, J. J., Hamel-Desnos, C., Kern, P., Partsch, B., Ramelet, A. A., Tessari, L., Pannier, F., & Guideline Group (2014). European guidelines for sclerotherapy in chronic venous disorders. *Phlebology, 29*(6), 338–354. https://doi.org/10.1177/0268355513483280
26. Woźniak, W., Mlosek, R. K., & Ciostek, P. (2015). Assessment of the efficacy and safety of steam vein sclerosis as compared to classic surgery in lower extremity varicose vein management. Videosurgery and Other Minimally Invasive Techniques, 10(1), 15–24. https://doi.org/10.5114/wiitm.2015.48573
27. van den Bos, R. & Maeseneer, M. (2012). Endovenous thermal ablation for varicose veins: Strengths and weaknesses. *Phlebolymphology, 19*, 163-169
28. Niedzwiecki, G. (2005). Endovenous thermal ablation of the saphenous vein. *Seminars in interventional radiology, 22*(3), 204–208. https://doi.org/10.1055/s-2005-921953
29. Kabnick, L., Ombrellino, M., Agis, H., (2005). Endovenous heat-induced thrombosis (EHIT) following endovenous vein obliteration: to treat or not to treat? A new thrombotic classification. Third International Vein Congress: In-Office Techniques
30. Çalık, E.S., Arslan, Ü., Erkut, B. (2019). Ablation therapy with cyanoacrylate glue and laser for refluxing great saphenous veins - a prospective randomized study. Journal of Vascular Access, 48(5), 405-412. doi: 10.1024/0301-1526/a000792. Epub 2019 Apr 24. PMID: 31014200.
31. Sundaresan, S., Migden, M. R., & Silapunt, S. (2019). Treatment of Leg Veins for Restless Leg Syndrome: A Retrospective Review. *Cureus, 11*(4), e4368. https://doi.org/10.7759/cureus.4368
32. Sadek, M., Kabnick, L.S. (2019). Varicose Veins: Endovenous Ablation and Sclerotherapy. In J.L. Cronenwett & K.W. Johnston (Eds.). *Rutherford's Vascular Surgery and Endovascular Therapy*, (9th ed., 2036-2048)
33. Haruta, N. (2018). Recent Progress of Varicose Vein Treatment Especially About Endovascular Heat Ablation, SEPS and Foam Sclerotherapy. *Annals of Vascular Diseases. 11*(1), 66-71. 10.3400/avd.ra.18-00005
34. Hingorani, A. P., Ascher, E., Markevich, N., Schutzer, R. W., Kallakuri, S., Hou, A., Nahata, S., Yorkovich, W., & Jacob, T. (2004). Deep venous thrombosis after radiofrequency ablation of greater saphenous vein: a word of caution. *Journal of vascular surgery, 40*(3), 500–504.
35. Perrin, M. R., Labropoulos, N., & Leon, L. R., Jr (2006). Presentation of the patient with recurrent varices after surgery (REVAS). *Journal of vascular surgery, 43*(2), 327–334. https://doi.org/10.1016/j.jvs.2005.10.053
36. Kelly, D.M., Sanford, D., Stoughton, J. (2019). Arteriovenous Fistula Is a Rare but Significant Finding After Endovenous Thermal Ablation. *Journal for Vascular Ultrasound, 43*(3), 116-122. doi:10.1177/1544316719848630
37. Khilnani, N.M., Min, R.J. (2005). Imaging of venous insufficiency. *Seminars Interventional Radiology, 22*(3), 178-184. https://doi:10.1055/s-2005-921950
38. Goldman, M.P., Bergan, J.J., Guex, J.J., Partsch, H. & Ramelet, A.A. (Eds.). (2007). Role of Surgery in Treatment of Varicose Veins, Sclerotherapy, (4th ed., 285-306). Mosby.https://doi.org/10.1016/B978-0-323-04258-1.50015-9. (https://www.sciencedirect.com/science/article/pii/B9780323042581500159)
39. Reusz G., Csomos A. (2015). The role of ultrasound guidance for vascular access. *Current Opinion Anaesthesiology*, 28(6):710-6. doi: 10.1097/ACO.0000000000000245. PMID: 26539789.
40. Allegra, Claudio & Antignani, Pier & Bergan, J.J. & Carpentier, P.H. & Coleridge-Smith, Philip & Cornu-Thénard, André. (2002). The "C" of CEAP: Suggested definitions and refinements: an International Union of Phlebology conference of experts. *Journal of Vascular Surgery, 37*, 129-131.
41. Caggiati, Alberto & Ricci, S. (1997). The Long Saphenous Vein Compartment. *Phlebology,12*, 107-111. 10.1177/026835559701200307.

Definition

The combination of real-time B-mode ultrasonography with color and Pulsed Wave (PW) Doppler to evaluate the upper extremity veins for evidence of thrombus.

Indications for Exam

- Edema/swelling (especially when unilateral)
- Limb pain/tenderness
- Limb redness
- Suspected injury after venous puncture/ catheterization, especially of the IJV
- Symptoms of pulmonary embolism (PE) (e.g., shortness of breath, chest pain, hemoptysis)
- Repeat evaluation for DVT to monitor for progression in high-risk individuals (e.g., those unable to be anticoagulated)
- Repeat exam before discontinuation of anticoagulation to establish a baseline.
- Evaluation of veins before access creation
- Assessment of veins in patients with dialysis access devices

Contraindications/Limitations

- Anatomical limitations (clavicle and ribs)
- Open wounds prohibiting access by the ultrasound transducer
- Casts that cannot be removed or bandaging that limits access to the scan areas
- Poor visualization due to vessel depth because of obesity or severe edema
- Patients who cannot be adequately positioned

Mechanism of disease [1,2]

Three factors are responsible for the formation of venous thrombosis, as outlined in Virchow's Triad: vein wall injury, hypercoagulability, and stasis of blood flow. A combination of any of these events may increase the risk of venous thrombosis.

- There is a balance between coagulation (process to prevent excessive bleeding after injury) and anticoagulation (process to prevent spontaneous intravascular clotting) in normal blood flow.
- The venous endothelial layer is normally antithrombotic. In response to endothelial injury, leukocytes (white blood cells) attach to the vessel wall. A plasma protein known as prothrombin is activated. Prothrombin activator catalyzes conversion of prothrombin into thrombin. Thrombin acts as an enzyme to convert fibrinogen into fibrin threads, forming a clot.
- Hypercoagulable states result from genetic mutation or acquired deficiencies that accompany certain diseases (e.g., liver disease). In such cases, naturally occurring anticoagulants (antithrombin, protein C, protein S, etc.) are deficient. For example, genetic mutation, factor V Leiden, causes resistance to the natural anticoagulant protein C.
- Non-movement of blood flow (stasis) permits coagulation. Platelets are thought to become trapped by low shear stress (flow) at valve cusps. Platelets adhere to the subendothelial (collagen) layer of the venous wall and may aggregate depending on the amount of coagulation and thrombolysis occurring in the body at that time.
- Increased coagulation factor activation in cancer patients is thought to lead to venous thrombosis. In addition, the levels of coagulation inhibitors normally found in the blood (e.g., proteins C or S) are considered to be reduced in these patients.
- The use of estrogen (in replacement therapy or birth control) alters coagulation and may predispose individuals to thrombosis.
- Venous aneurysms are a rare condition. Research suggests several possible causes; decreased smooth muscle cells and an increase in fibrous connective tissue or an increase or decrease in the fibrous connective tissue and elastic fibers. [3]

- Once a thrombus is formed, it can:
  - **Stabilize:** Stabilization includes adherence of the thrombus to the vessel wall without changing location or propagating. If a thrombus has formed, the most favorable occurrence would be to stabilize. This reduces the risk to the patient.
  - **Propagate:** Propagation includes "growth of the thrombus" in size or location. Examples of propagation may include a thrombus that extends from the superficial system into the deep system.
  - **Embolize:** During embolization, a portion of a thrombus breaks free and travels downstream in the vascular system. The greatest risk to the patient is that the thrombus travels to the lungs and results in a pulmonary embolus.

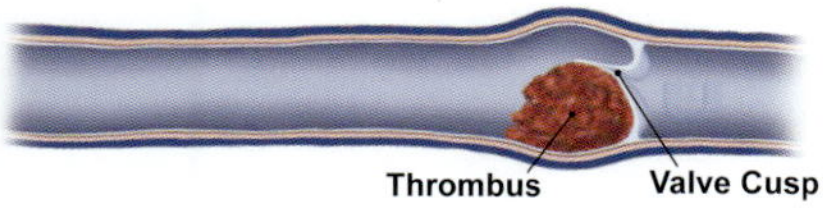

Fig. 12-1. *Thrombosis of vein*

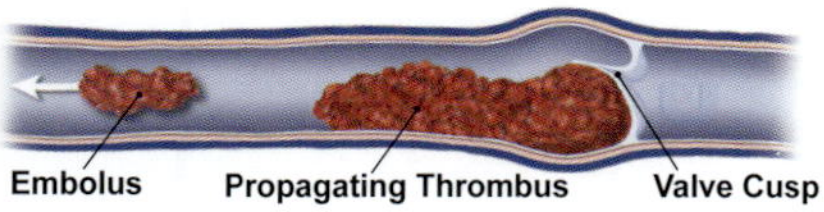

Fig. 12-2. *Venous thrombosis and propagation. In the top vessel, a thrombus has formed behind the valve cusp. This thrombus can stabilize, or as depicted in the bottom vessel, it can propagate. A piece of the thrombus can break off and cause a pulmonary embolism.*

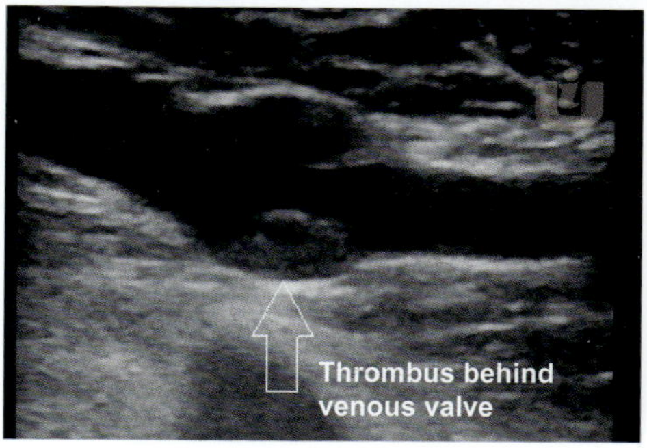

Fig. 12-3. *Longitudinal B-mode image of a thrombus in the brachial vein. Identification of the valve, including the dilation of the vein with echogenic material hanging down from the near wall (valve cusp). A thrombus is located behind the valve cusp.*

Patient History

- Previous DVT
- Recent surgery, postoperative, orthopedic, or neurosurgery (e.g., can occur anytime during surgery or for 6 months thereafter)
- Persistent swelling (usually unilateral, but can be bilateral)
- Clotting issues (including problems regulating anticoagulation therapy, malignant cancer)
- Localized pain, burning, or itching
- Symptoms of pulmonary embolism (PE) (e.g., shortness of breath, chest pain, hemoptysis)
- Difficulties with patient's intravenous catheter

Use venous presets on the duplex scanner; low color and Doppler scales will be needed to detect venous flow.

Physical Examination

- Edema or swelling
- Tenderness
- Limb redness or warmth
- Dark pigmentation, hardened tissue
- Cyanosis (superior vena cava syndrome)
- Excessive collaterals around the area of concern

Location of Disease

Thrombus located within the deep veins is known as deep venous thrombosis (DVT). Thrombus located within the superficial veins is known as superficial thrombosis (SVT).

Any venous site can develop a thrombus. Common origins include:

- Valve sites
- Venous confluences
- Superficial venous system (basilic, cephalic, median cubital)
- Deep venous system:
  - "Central veins" typically refer to the jugular, innominate, subclavian, and sometimes axillary veins
  - Brachial, radial, ulnar veins

Duplex Protocol

- Obtain a patient history to include symptoms and risk factors.
- The patient is examined in the supine position with the head turned slightly to the side and the chin slightly raised.
- Some patients may require the use of a range of transducers, including high-frequency (5 - 7MHz) (8 - 15MHz) transducers and a lower frequency (1 - 4MHz) transducer, which may be useful around the clavicle.

Use the deep transducer to aid visualization around the clavicle.

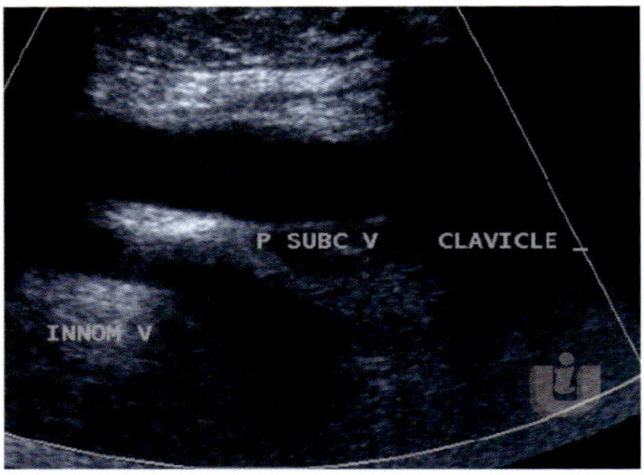

Fig. 12-4. *Longitudinal B-mode image of the subclavian and innominate vein at the clavicle. These veins are 3-6cm below the surface. A low-frequency transducer was used.*

Asking the patient to "sniff" will cause compression of the ScV and sometimes results in flow augmentation.

Transverse Scan and Images

- Perform venous compression in the transverse plane (short axis) every 2 - 4cm along the neck and arm. This is anatomically difficult and may not be possible near the clavicle. Instead of compressions, have the patient inhale *(Fig. 12-7)* or ask the patient to "sniff like you're going to sniff a flower."

Dual Screen Vein Compression

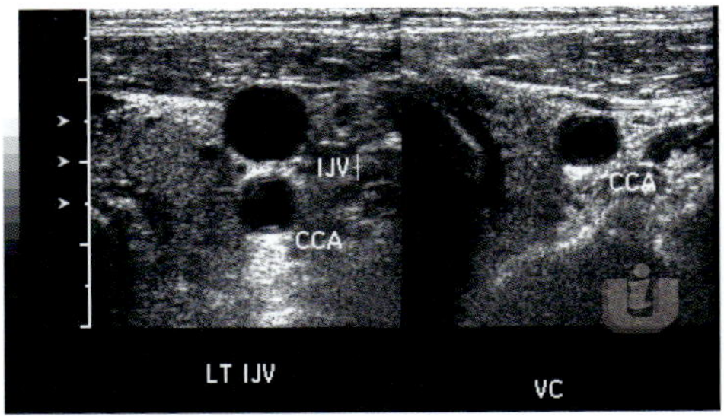

Fig. 12-5. *Internal jugular vein uncompressed (left) and compressed (right).*

Keep the transducer at a 90° angle to the skin for the best grayscale images.

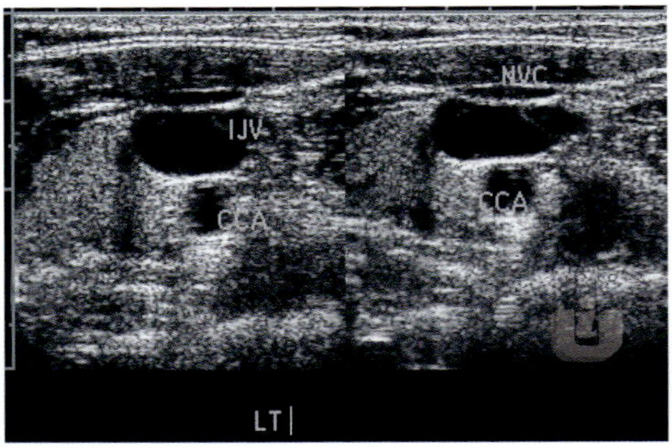

Fig. 12-6. *Compression of a thrombosed internal jugular vein. The internal jugular vein in the right image is completely incompressible.*

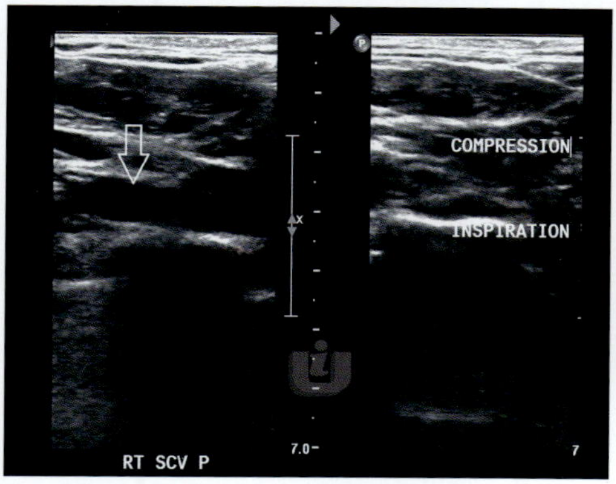

Fig. 12-7. *Collapse of a normal vein by using the "sniff" technique. On the left of the dual-screen image, the non-compressed vein is fully extended. The image on the right was captured immediately after the patient inhaled through their nose ("sniff"). The vein collapsed due to the compressive force that develops with sniffing.*

- Record transverse images using "dual-screen" on the duplex scanner. Obtain and freeze an image without vein compression on the left side of the screen. Capture an image with vein compression on the right side of the screen. Document transverse images of the following veins with and without compressions as described above:
  - Internal jugular vein (IJV)
  - Subclavian vein (ScV) (with compression if possible)
  - Axillary vein(s) (AxV)
  - Brachial veins (BrVs)
  - Basilic vein (BsV)
  - Cephalic vein (CV)
- Additional documentation of compressions can be performed when indicated and anatomically possible to include the subclavian vein junction, brachiocephalic (BcV), also known as the innominate vein (InV), radial, ulnar, or median cubital veins.

The transverse or oblique plane to the body may be better for recording flow in the distal brachiocephalic (innominate) vein.

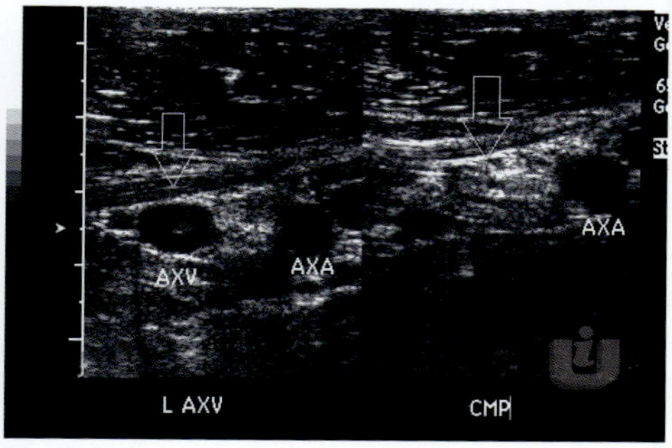

Fig. 12-8. *Compression of the axillary vein. On the left of the dual-screen image is the uncompressed vessel. The axillary vein on the right is compressed.*

Some labs record venous PW Doppler waveforms without setting an angle since actual velocities are usually not important in a venous exam. If your lab chooses to set an angle, use a ≤60° Doppler angle with the cursor placed parallel to the vessel walls in the center of the flow stream.

Longitudinal Scan and Images

- Record pulsed wave venous spectral waveforms with color Doppler in the longitudinal (sagittal axis) view.
- Observe for augmentation of venous flow.
- Documentation should illustrate spontaneity, phasicity, and augmentation. Pulsatility should be noted in the central veins. Record samples of the following veins:
  - IJV
  - ScV
  - AxV
  - BrVs
  - CV
  - BsV
  - Document spectral waveforms of paired veins individually.
  - Additional documentation of patency can be performed when necessary in the distal brachiocephalic, jugular-subclavian junction, radial, ulnar, or median cubital veins.

- Use PW Doppler to analyze the absence of flow by placing the Doppler sample volume in any vein segment suspected to be thrombosed. Doppler flow, or lack of flow, compliments compression, color flow, and B-mode images. Use the adjacent artery to identify an occluded vein when possible.
- Repeat for the contralateral extremity if a bilateral exam is ordered.
- If only a unilateral exam is requested, documentation of the contralateral subclavian venous spectral waveform is performed for comparison.

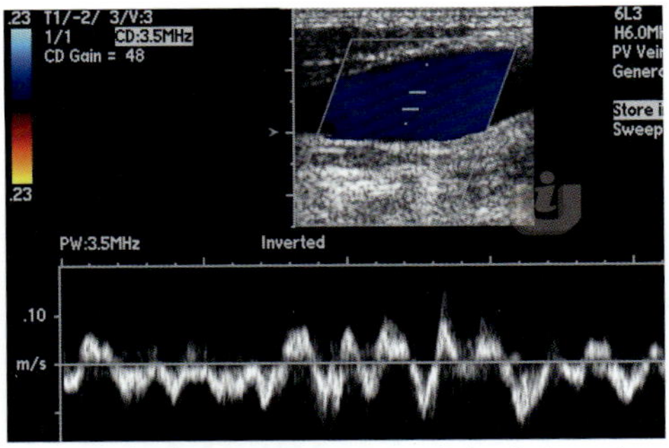

Fig. 12-9. *PW Doppler image of the internal jugular vein. Normal flow is spontaneous and pulsatile in the internal jugular vein.*

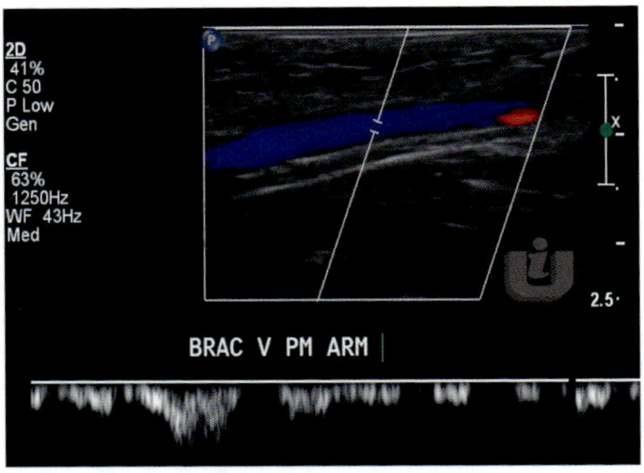

Fig. 12-10. *PW Doppler spectral trace of blood flow in a normal brachial vein.*

Table 12-1. Upper Extremity Venous Protocol Summary

Scan transverse (short axis) with and without color compression

- Internal jugular vein (IJV)
- Subclavian vein (ScV)
- Axillary vein (AxV)
- Brachial vein (BrVs)
- Basilic vein (BsV)
- Cephalic vein (CV)
- Subclavian-jugular confluence (optional)
- Distal brachiocephalic vein (BcV) (optional)
- Radial vein (RadVs) (optional)
- Ulnar vein (UVs) (optional)
- Median cubital vein (MCV) (optional)

Scan longitudinal (sagittal axis) in grayscale and PW Doppler (color Doppler can be used intermediately)

- Internal jugular vein (IJV)
- Subclavian vein (ScV)
- Distal brachiocephalic (BcV)
- Axillary vein (AxV)
- Brachial vein (BrVs)
- Cephalic vein (CV)
- Basilic vein (BsV)
- Subclavian-jugular confluence (optional)
- Radial vein (RadVs) (optional)
- Ulnar vein (UVs) (optional)
- Median cubital vein (MCV) (optional)

Additional documentation

- Compression may be recorded in segments other than those listed during evaluation for thrombus as necessary. (Compressions may be anatomically contraindicated, especially near the clavicle. If so, document patency with color flow and PW spectral waveforms.)
- PW Doppler waveforms in all veins when dual (or more) veins are present.

PRINCIPLES OF INTERPRETATION

Interpretation-Diagnostic Criteria

Collapse of the artery with transducer pressure can be used to confirm the incompressibility of the venous segment.

It is technically difficult to image the neck veins with the patient in a sitting position. The veins sometimes collapse due to compression by atmospheric pressure from the outside.

Normal

B-mode Imaging

Use B-mode imaging to determine if a thrombus is present.

- The vein collapses completely with light transducer pressure.
- No echogenic material is present within the lumen of the vein.
- It is possible for only one vein of a pair to be thrombosed. Make sure all veins are studied carefully. *(Fig. 12-13)*
- The wall-to-wall color flow will fill the vein spontaneously or upon distal limb compression. Confirm there is no filling defect, e.g., turn up color gain.

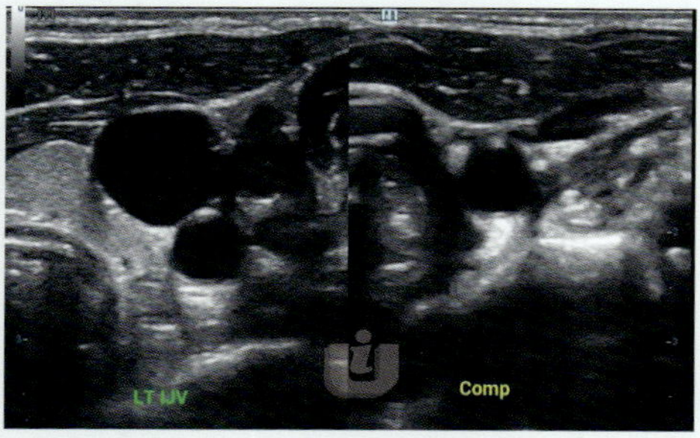

Fig. 12-11. *Normal compression of the internal jugular vein.*

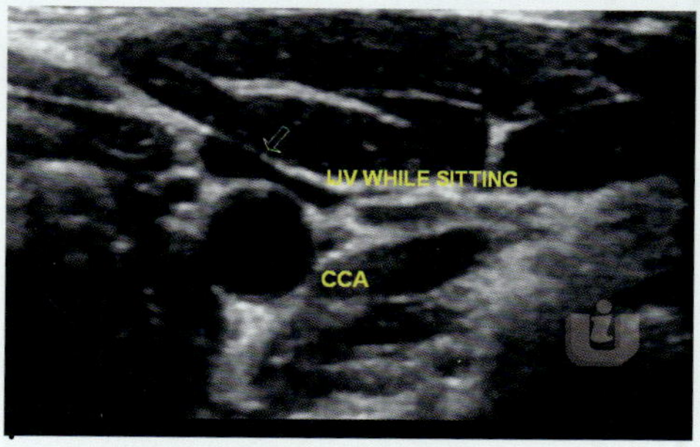

Fig. 12-12. *IJV collapses with the patient sitting up*

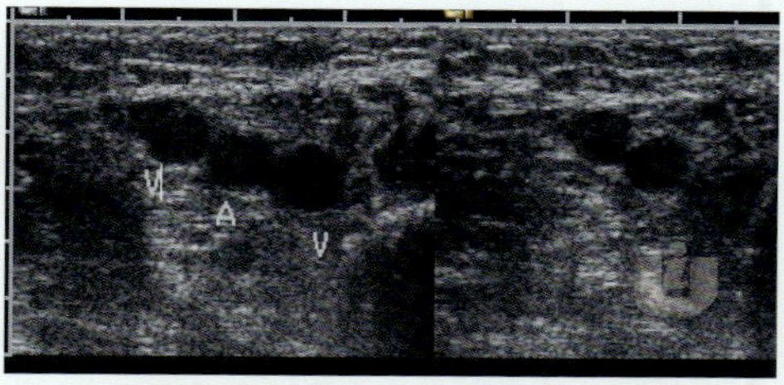

Fig. 12-13. *Dual screen: single brachial vein is non-compressible*

PW Doppler

- **Spontaneity:** The vein demonstrates spontaneous flow, especially in the large veins above the knee. The absence of spontaneous flow can be a normal finding in the forearm veins.
- **Phasicity:** Venous flow is phasic and varies with the respiratory and cardiac cycles. Due to intrathoracic pressure changes during respiration, venous flow increases in the upper extremity during deep inhalation and decreases during exhalation. The absence of phasic flow in the forearm veins is a normal finding..
- **Augmentation:** Compression of the limb distal to the transducer augments (increases) venous flow at the transducer.
- **Pulsatility:** Often present in the upper extremity veins, especially the central veins.

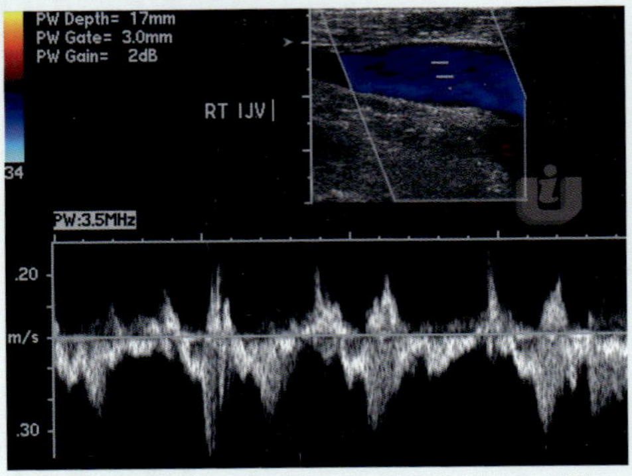

Fig. 12-14. The color Doppler completely fills the internal jugular vein.

> *Normal Doppler signals may be present when the thrombus is partially occlusive.*

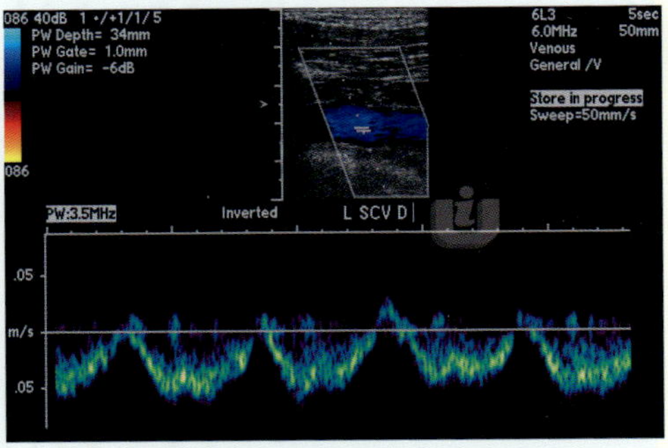

Fig. 12-15. Normal, pulsatile subclavian spectral waveform.

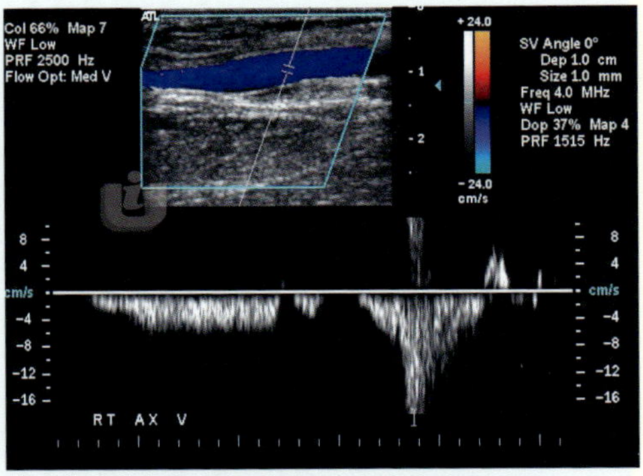

Fig. 12-16. Normal, axillary spectral waveform. Phasic, non-pulsatile flow, which augments upon distal compression.

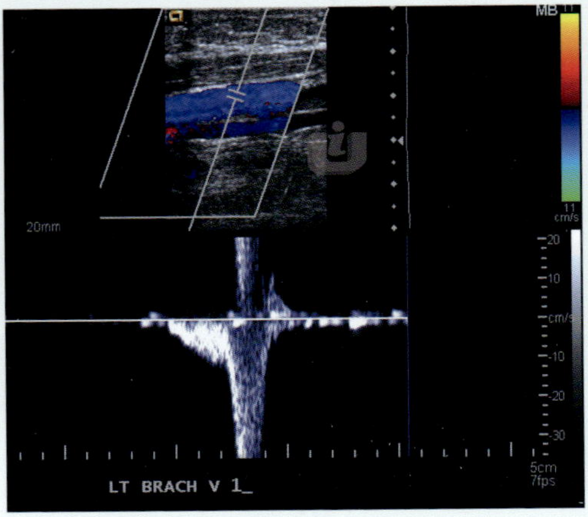

Fig. 12-17. Normal brachial vein spectral waveform. Normal for spontaneity and phasicity to be absent.

Abnormal

B-mode Imaging

- Intraluminal echoes are visualized within the vein, and the vein is not completely compressible
- The vein is partially compressible when the lumen is partially obstructed and incompressible when the lumen is completely obstructed

Thrombus

- If a thrombus is present, determine
  - location (by B-mode)
  - whether the thrombus is partially or completely occlusive
  - extent (by B-mode and color flow)
  - characteristics of the thrombus (echogenicity, acute, chronic, re-canalization; by B-mode)

> *Color flow can obscure a partially occlusive thrombus if the color gain is set too high.*

- Stages of Thrombus
  - **Acute thrombus:** Typical characteristics include medium to lightly echogenic or anechoic; spongy texture appearance and poor attachment of the thrombus to the vein wall or thrombus is noted to be "free-floating" within the lumen *(Fig. 12-19)*. A moving tail may be seen at the end of the thrombus. When a vein is fully thrombosed, the cross-sectional area has usually increased (in an acute event), making the vein larger than the adjacent artery. *(Fig.12-18 and 12-25)*

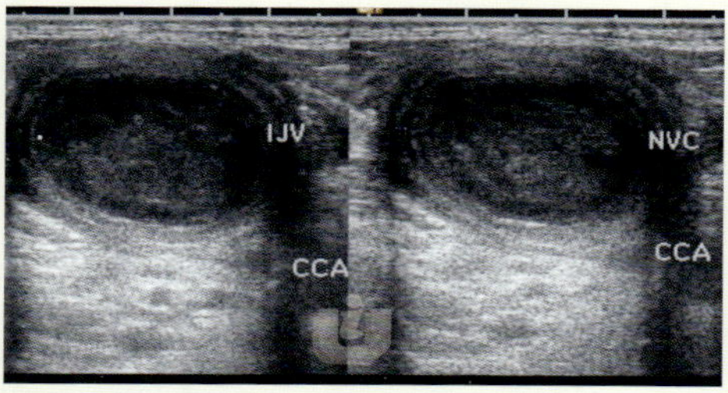

Fig. 12-18. *Acute IJV DVT.*

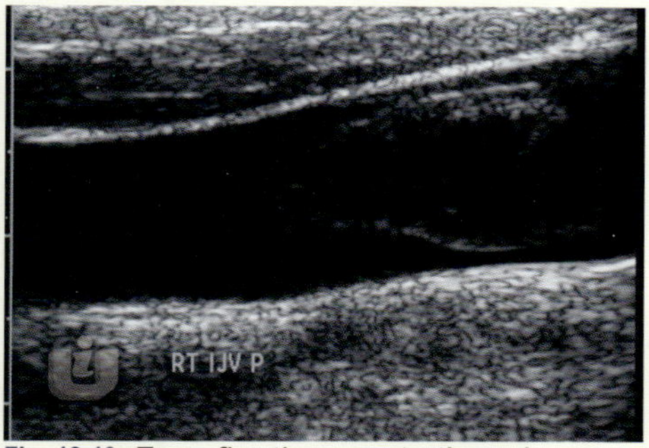

Fig. 12-19. *Free-floating, acute thrombus.*

  - **Chronic thrombus:** Typical characteristics include brightly echogenic or heterogeneous echoes, irregular surface texture, and the thrombus attached to the venous wall with no signs of floating flaps *(Fig. 12-20)*. The vein can stay the same size as the artery but often contracts in diameter over time. Collateral veins may be observed adjacent to the affected vein(s), and small irregular flow channels within the thrombus can sometimes be seen with color flow.

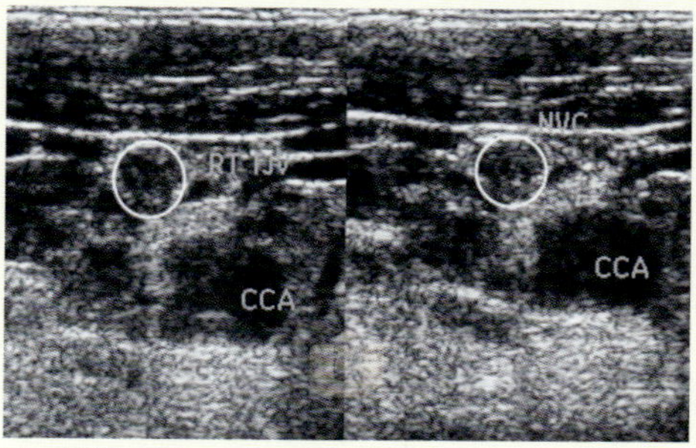

Fig. 12-20. *Chronic IJV DVT.*

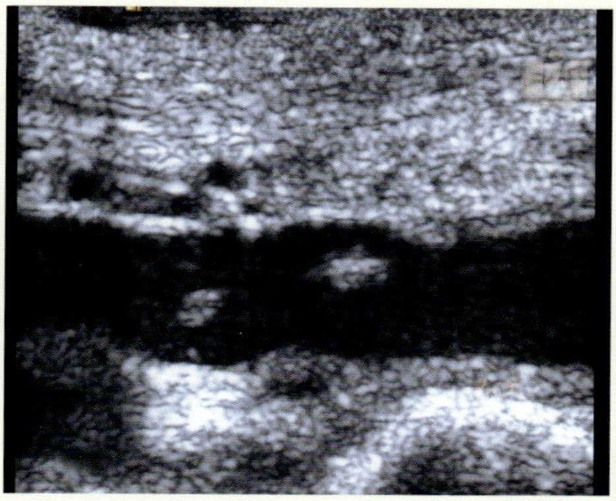

Fig. 12-21. *Chronic thrombus by B-mode.*

  - **Indeterminate age:** Characteristics of both acute and chronic stages may be present, making the age of the thrombus difficult to determine. It is best not to guess. *(Fig. 12-22)*

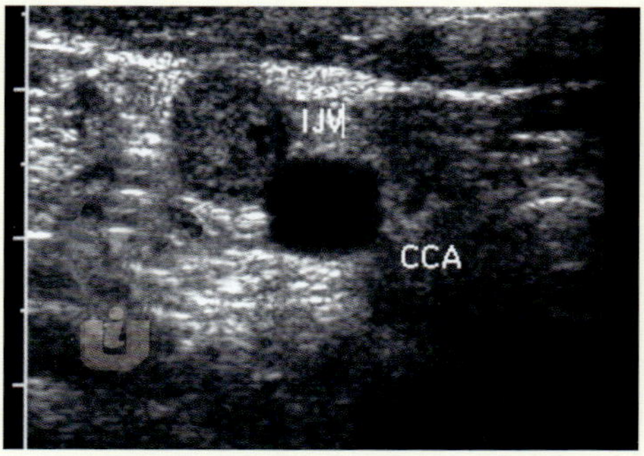

Fig. 12-22. *Indeterminate age: IJV DVT.*

Color Doppler

- If the thrombus does not completely inhibit blood flow, color flow will be seen flowing around echogenic material in the vein, spontaneously or with distal limb compression. *(Fig. 12-23 and 12-26)*

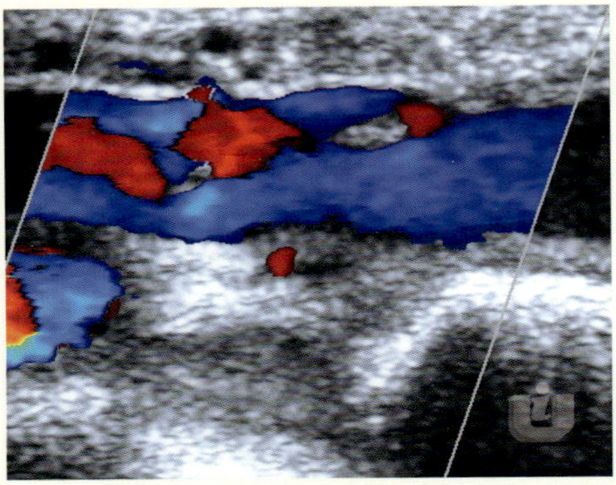

Fig. 12-23. *Longitudinal view-color flows around irregular flow of chronic thrombus.*

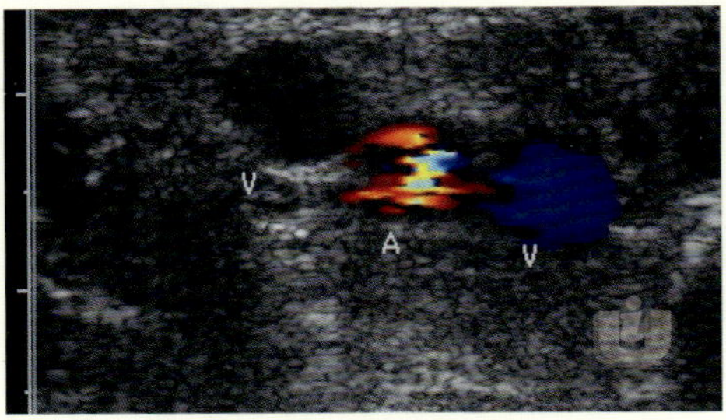

Fig. 12-24. *Single brachial vein without color flow in the transverse plane*

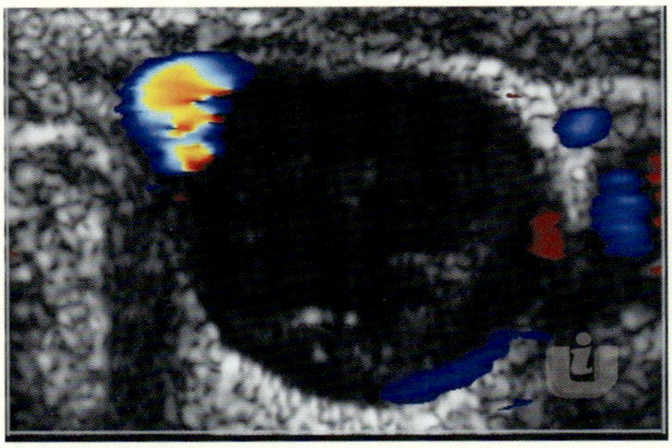

Fig. 12-25. *Transverse view of the occluded brachial vein. The absence of color flow within the vein indicates that the vein has occluded.*

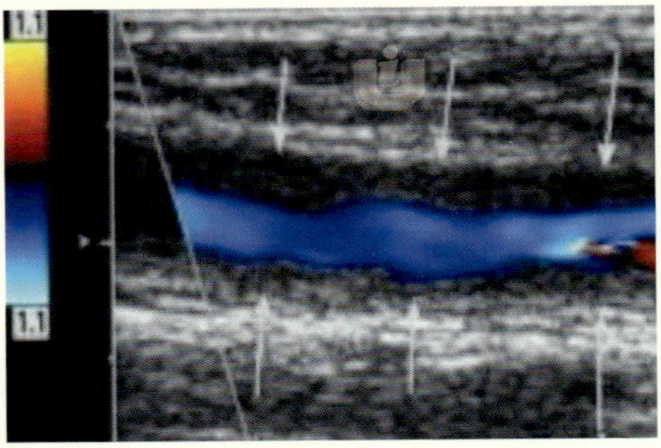

Fig. 12-26. *Longitudinal-partially occlusive thrombus. Partial color flow.*

- If the thrombus completely inhibits blood flow, no color flow will be observed even with distal limb compression using the appropriate low flow machine settings.

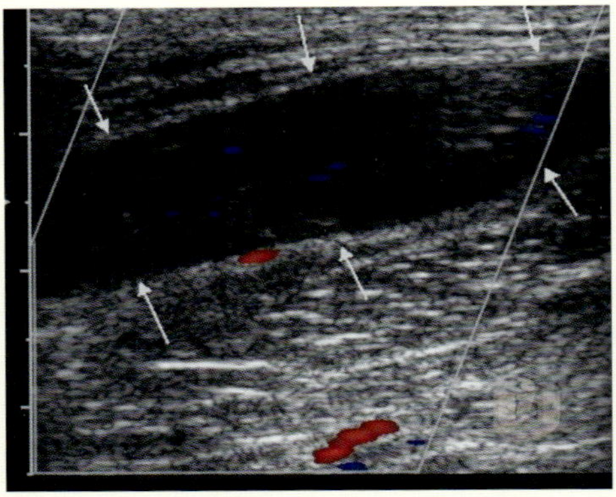

Fig. 12-27. *Longitudinal-totally occlusive thrombus. No color flow, low color scale used.*

PW Doppler

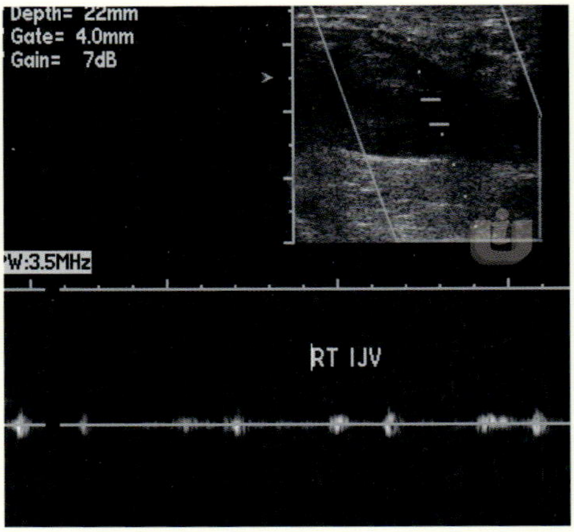

Fig. 12-28. *Absent PW Doppler and color flow.*

- **Spontaneity:** Absence of flow indicates venous obstruction. Use color flow in the adjacent artery as a guide to identifying an occluded vein. But always confirm the absence of flow by placing the sample volume in the vessel while using Doppler. *(Fig. 12-28)*
- **Phasicity:** Continuous venous flow (does not vary with respiratory and cardiac cycles) usually suggests either obstruction from DVT in a proximal venous segment or extrinsic compression of a proximal vein. *(Fig. 12-30)* Partially occlusive thrombus can still produce spontaneous, phasic signals with augmentation.
- **Augmentation:** If distal compression does not produce augmentation of the venous signal, a total obstruction distal to the transducer is suspected. A weak or dampened augmentation also suggests venous obstruction distal to the transducer. It may be helpful to change the patient's position and/or try compressing a more muscular arm area after giving time for a venous refill.
- **Pulsatility:** The absence of pulsatile venous flow suggests obstruction, especially in the central veins.

Table 12-2. **Diagnostic Criteria for Venous Duplex**

Normal	Abnormal
Complete coaptation of vein walls with light transducer pressure	Lack of complete vein compression
Absent intraluminal thrombus	Intraluminal echoes present (acute thrombus can be echolucent)
Color flow fills the lumen completely	Decrease or absence of color flow
Normal venous Doppler spontaneity, phasicity and augmentation	Abnormal venous Doppler spontaneity, phasicity or augmentation
No venous dilatation	Dilated or contracted veins noted

Other Pathology

Extrinsic compression

Continuous venous flow suggests either obstruction in a proximal venous segment or extrinsic compression of a vein. [1]

Venous stenosis

When increased focal venous velocities are noted with or without provocative positional maneuvers (compared to the distal segment of the vein), venous stenosis is suspected. This condition can occur secondary to thoracic outlet syndrome, dialysis access intervention, or extrinsic compression. Some labs use a venous-velocity ratio of ≥2.5 (a velocity increase of at least 2.5 times the immediate distal venous segment) to diagnose hemodynamically significant stenosis. [12]

Effort thrombosis

Effort thrombosis or Paget-Schroetter syndrome usually involves the subclavian venous segment. In this syndrome, the ScV is compressed between the first rib and scalene muscle (the thoracic outlet), which results in formation of venous thrombus and flow obstruction. [11,13]

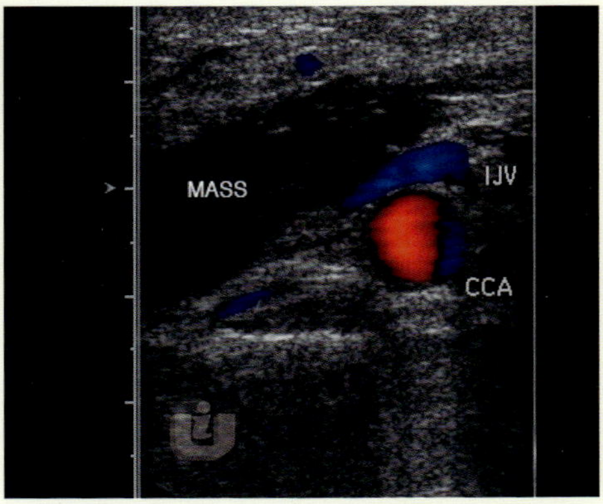

Fig. 12-29. *Extrinsic compression of IJV suspected-transverse view*

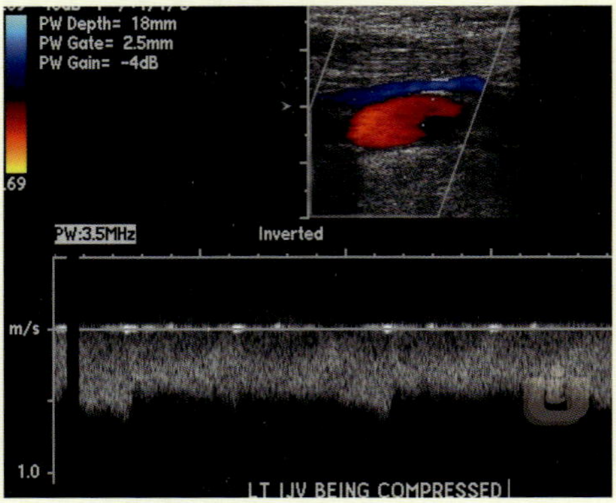

Fig. 12-30. *Venous compression of the jugular vein confirmed by PW Doppler. (continuous flow/lacks pulsatility).*

Superior vena cava syndrome versus BcV obstruction

When comparing the distal BcVs the absence of pulsatile flow on both sides suggests a proximal obstruction in both BcV or in the superior vena cava (SVC syndrome). If the decrease in pulsatility is unilateral, obstruction of that brachiocephalic vein proximally is suspected. [8]

Venous aneurysm

Venous aneurysm is diagnosed when there is an area of significant venous dilatation compared to the adjacent venous segment. Common locations for upper extremity venous aneurysms include the IJV and AxV. Document the presence of any mural thrombus. [14]

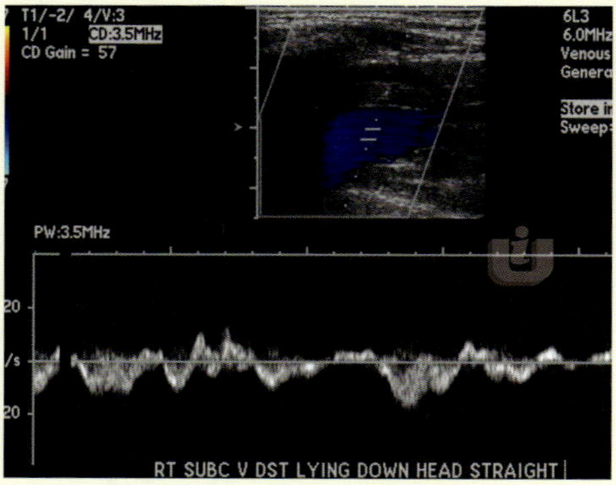

Fig. 12-31. *Normal ScV waveforms at rest.*

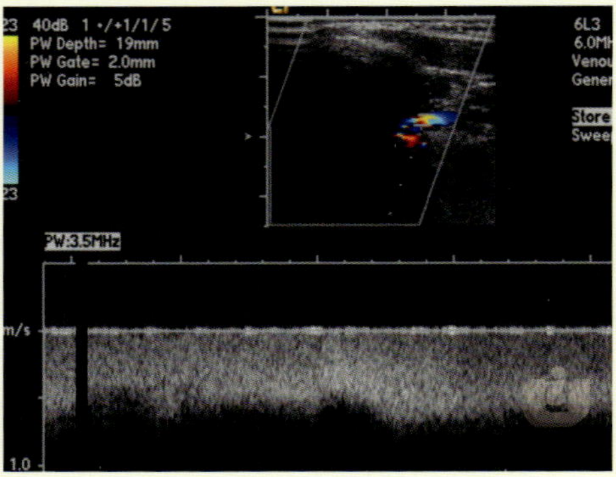

Fig. 12-32. *Abnormal ScV PW Doppler waveforms at rest.*

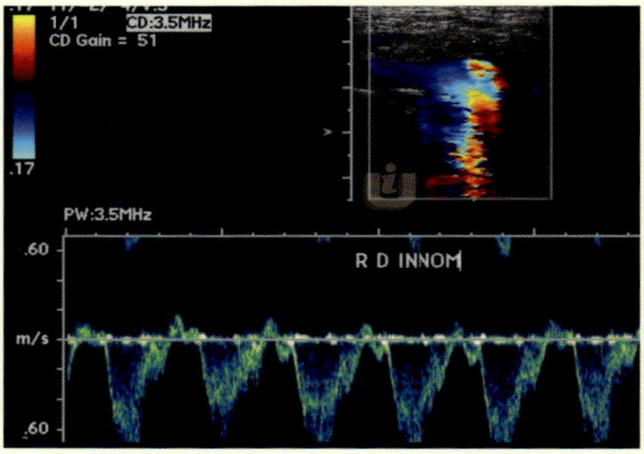

Fig. 12-33. *Normal innominate vein PW Doppler.*

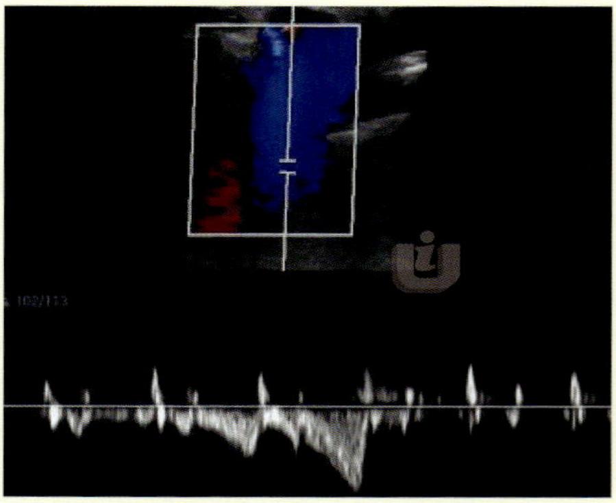

Fig. 12-34. *Abnormal innominate vein: PW Doppler with decreased pulsatility.*

Edema

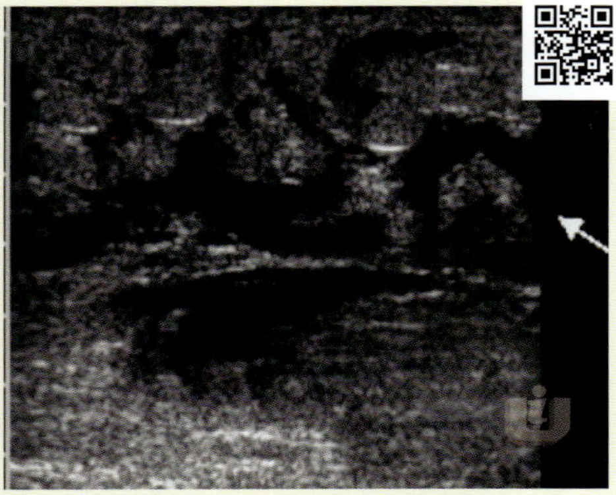

Fig. 12-35. *Upper extremity superficial tissue edema.*

Differential Diagnosis

- Arterial disease
- Lymphedema
- Cellulitis
- Cysts
- Extrinsic compression
- Hematoma
- Muscle tear
- Joint effusion
- Adenopathy
- Arteriovenous fistula
- Heart failure
- Direct injury to an extremity
- Vascularized mass
- Collagen vasculitis
- Abscess

Correlation

- CT scan
- MRI
- Venogram

Medical Treatment and Prevention

- Anticoagulation therapy (e.g., heparin, warfarin)
- Promote venous drainage (e.g., elevate arms, wear elastic/support sleeves)

Surgical Treatment

- IVC filter (acute DVT)
- SVC reconstruction (using PTFE or cryopreserved grafts)

Endovascular Treatment

- Catheter-directed thrombolysis with urokinase (e.g., acute DVT)
- Mechanical thrombectomy such as Angiojet (acute DVT)
- Percutaneous transluminal angioplasty and stenting (SVC syndrome or axilla-subclavian issues).

Central Venous Catheters [8]

- A central venous catheter is placed in one of the central veins and used to administer medication, nutrition, dialysis, or chemotherapy treatments. The use of central venous catheters has greatly increased in recent years. These lines increase the risk for venous thrombosis. [11, 17]
- There are several different types of central venous catheters:
  - **Tunneled catheters:** A catheter that is "tunneled" under the skin makes it more discrete and keeps it in place before the catheter exits through the skin. Common tunneled catheters include *Hickman* and *Groshong* catheters.
  - Implanted ports remain under the skin, and medications are injected through the skin into this type of catheter. Though these ports can be used for hemodialysis patients, they are primarily used for cancer treatment.
  - PICC line (*peripherally inserted central catheter)* is a line inserted in an arm vein with a tip that lies in one of the large veins in the chest. It can remain in position for up to six months.
- Observe the surface of any visualized intravenous catheters for thrombus development. It is possible for the thrombus that forms anywhere along these lines to extend into the more central veins. *(Fig. 12-37)*

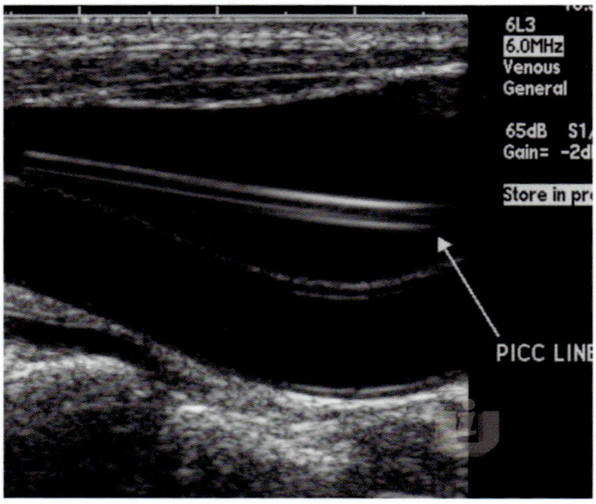

Fig. 12-36. *Upper extremity IJV PICC line without thrombus.*

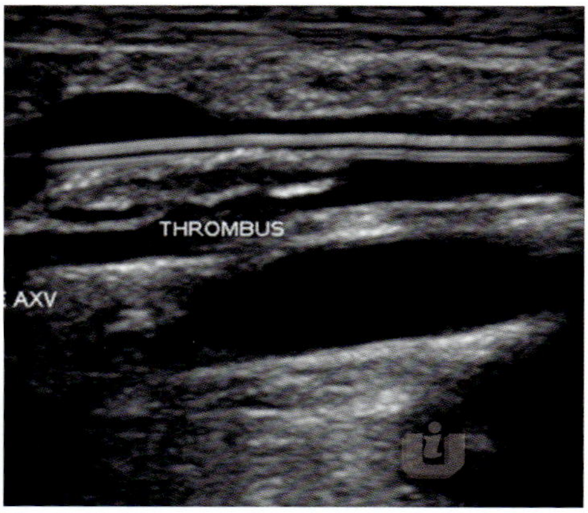

Fig. 12-37. *Upper extremity IJV PICC line with thrombus.*

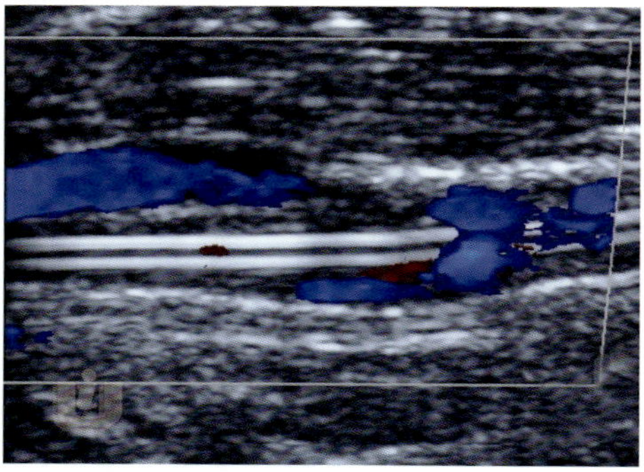

Fig. 12-38. *Color Doppler image of a subclavian vein with thrombus due to a PICC line. The two white stripes within the lumen are the PICC line. The absence of wall-to-wall color flow and the presence of echogenic material along the PICC line indicates that a thrombus has formed around the line.*

Points to Remember

- Venous duplex ultrasound can identify the presence, exact location, extent, and severity of venous thrombosis. The course of the veins, collaterals, and thrombus can be visualized using B-mode and color, while the analysis of Doppler flow patterns can yield further information regarding flow direction of both local and remote obstructions.
- Compressions should always be performed in the transverse plane to ensure full compression, so duplicated veins are not missed.
- The superficial veins of the upper extremity are the primary route of drainage for the arm.
- Upper extremity veins contain far fewer venous valves than lower extremity veins.
- Upper extremity venous thrombosis is less likely to embolize and cause a symptomatic pulmonary embolism than DVT in the lower extremities. [8]
- Upper extremity AxV and ScVthrombosis are divided into two categories:
  - **Primary venous thrombosis:** also known as *Effort thrombosis or Paget-Schroetter syndrome,* results from compression and repetitive trauma to the venous segment in the thoracic outlet.
  - **Secondary venous thrombosis:** occurs due to other causes (e.g., insertion of catheters, hemodialysis ports, pacemakers, immobilization, etc.). Secondary thrombosis is more common (80% of cases). [15]
- Most thrombotic events in the upper extremity veins are due to intravenous catheters. [17]
- Upper extremity venous aneurysms are more common than lower extremity venous aneurysms, although both are rare. [14]
- Incidental findings, such as superficial tissue edema, may be helpful in the report for the clinicians to understand swelling/edema in the absence of a thrombus.

References

1. Wakefield TW. (2005). Bleeding and clotting: fundamental considerations. In Rutherford Vascular Surgery 6th edition. (493 - 511). Philadelphia. Elsevier Saunders.
2. Guyton AC. (1986). Hemostasis and blood coagulation. In Textbook of Medical Physiology 7th edition. (76 - 86). Philadelphia: WB Saunders.
3. Gillespie DL, Villavicencio JL, Gallagher C, Chang A, Hamelink JK, Fiala LA, O'Donnell SD, Jackson MR, Pikoulis E, Rich, NM. (1997). Presentation and management of venous aneurysms. *Journal of Vascular Surg*ery, 26(5):845 - 52.
4. Thrush A, Hartshorne T. (2005). Duplex assessment of deep venous thrombosis and upper limb venous disorders. In Peripheral Vascular Ultrasound, How Why and When, 2nd ed. (189 - 206). Edinburgh: Elsevier Churchill Livingstone.
5. Zwiebel, WJ (2005). Ultrasound Diagnosis of Venous Thrombosis. In Zwiebel WJ, Pellerito JS (Eds.), Introduction to Vascular Ultrasonography 5th ed, (449 - 465). Philadelphia: Elsevier Saunders.
6. Meissner MH. (2005). Venous duplex scanning. In Rutherford Vascular Surgery 6th edition. (254 - 270). Philadelphia. Elsevier Saunders.
7. Myers K, Clough A. (2004). Venous thrombosis in the lower limbs. In Making sense of vascular ultrasound: A hands on guide. (181 - 197). London: Hodder Arnold.
8. Caps MT, Mraz BA. (2010). Upper extremity venous thrombosis. In Zierler RE (Ed.), Strandess's duplex scanning disorders in vascular diagnosis 4th ed. (199 - 221).Philadelphia Wolters Kluwer Lippincott Williams & Wilkins.
9. Sumner DS, Mattos MA. (1993). Diagnosis of deep vein thrombosis with real-time color and duplex scanning. In Vascular Diagnosis 4th edition. (785 - 800). St. Louis. Mosby.
10. Lohr, J (2005). Upper Extremity Venous Duplex Imaging. In Mansour MA, Labropoulos N. (Eds.), *Vascular Diagnosis*, (469 - 477). Philadelphia: Elsevier Saunders.
11. Green RM. (2005). Subclavian-axillary vein thrombosis. In Rutherford Vascular Surgery 6th edition. (1371 - 1392). Philadelphia. Elsevier Saunders.
12. Leon, LR, Labropoulos, N, Mansour MA. (2005). Hemodynamic principles as applied to diagnostic testing. In Mansour MA, Labropoulos N. (Eds.), *Vascular Diagnosis*, (7 - 21). Philadelphia: Elsevier Saunders.
13. Kreienberg PB, Shah, DM, Darling III, RC, Change BB, Paty SK, Roddy SP, Ozsvath KJ, Manish M. (2005) Thoracic outlet syndrome: In Mansour MA, Labropoulos N. (Eds.), *Vascular Diagnosis*, 517 - 522. Philadelphia: Elsevier Saunders.
14. Gillespie DL, Villavicencio JL, Gallagher C, Chang A, Hamelink JK, Fiala LA, O'Donnell SD, Jackson MR, Pikoulis E, Rich, NM. (1997). Presentation and management of venous aneurysms. *Journal of Vascular Surgery, 26*(5), 845 - 52.
15. Spiezia L, Simioni P. (2010). Upper extremity deep vein thrombosis. *Internal and Emergency Medicine, 5*(2):103 - 9. Epub 2009 Sep 26.
16. AIUM Practice Parameter for the Performance of a Peripheral Venous Ultrasound Examination, *Journal of Ultrasound in Medicine* 2020; 9999:1–8
17. Chopra, VC. (2020, May 11). Catheter-related upper extremity venous thrombosis. Up to Date. uptodate.com/contents/catheter-related-upper-extremity-venous-thrombosis

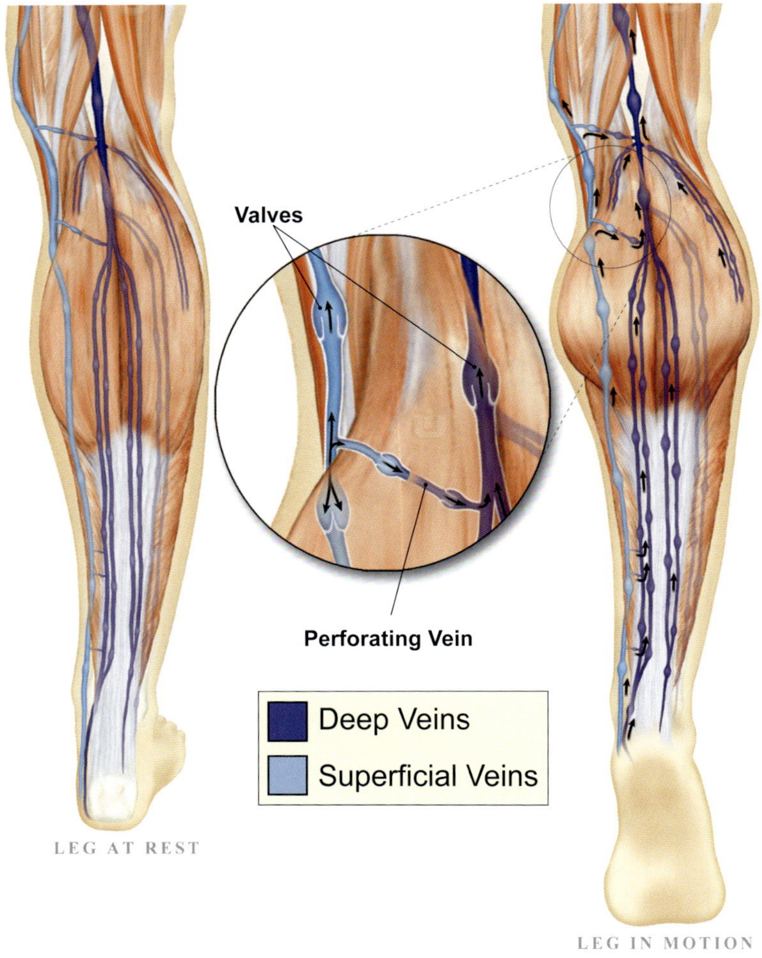

Fig. 13-1. *The calf muscle pump drives venous flow. While walking, muscle contractions squeeze the veins initiating venous blood flow. Venous flow opens the venous valves allowing the blood to flow towards the heart. As the muscle relaxes, valves close to prevent the backwash of blood (reflux).*

Definition

Venous photoplethysmography (PPG) is an indirect method used to evaluate the lower extremity veins for evidence of valvular incompetence. Venous PPG can also help differentiate between primary and secondary venous insufficiency to plan treatment options.

Chronic venous disorders are caused by incompetent valves in the superficial, perforators, and/or deep venous systems, resulting in venous hypertension and stasis.

Venous PPG testing involves exercise or manual calf compressions to cause contraction of the calf muscles. These contractions empty the blood out of the veins in the lower leg.

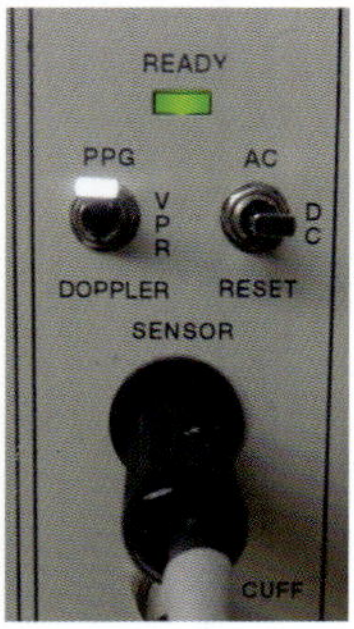

The venous or DC mode on the PPG instrument is used to monitor slow venous changes. The arterial or AC mode is used to monitor the faster volume changes that occur with arterial pulsations.

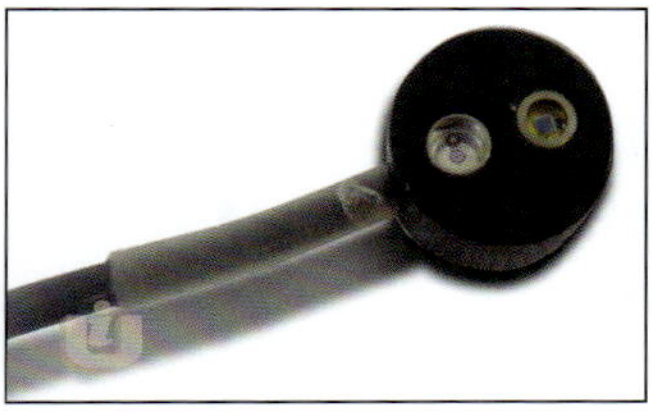

Fig. 13-2. *PPG sensor*

Principle

PPG equipment can monitor and display blood volume changes over time.

A PPG sensor consists of infrared light and a receiver attached to the skin in the gaiter area with double-sided tape or a Velcro strap, approximately 5cm (2in) above the medial malleolus. Infrared light is transmitted into the superficial tissues, and the sensor receives the reflected light. The reflected signal relates to the quantity of red blood cells in the cutaneous circulation.

The calf muscles normally compress the veins during exercise or manual compression. A rapid decrease in venous blood volume is followed by a slow refilling of the veins via the arteries and capillaries.

After obtaining a baseline for the PPG tracing during testing, the calf veins are emptied through exercise or manual compression, and the leg is rested so the veins can refill.

The PPG tracing demonstrates the volume changes during this venous emptying and filling. The venous filling index (a.k.a., Venous Recovery Time or VRT) can be calculated from this tracing.

Valvular incompetence results in a faster VRT than normal since veins refill via immediate backflow of venous blood past the incompetent valves rather than through the normal course; from artery, arteriole, capillary, venule, and then vein.

Indications for Exam

- Varicose veins
- Chronic edema/swelling which worsens at the end of the day (especially when unilateral)
- Pain, which may be localized to a specific varix or described as a "dull ache."
- Discoloration at the gaiter area
- Ulceration (e.g., gaiter area)
- Venous claudication

Contraindications/Limitation

- PPG testing is a subjective test. Although an actual number is calculated (VRT), it is an overall measurement of venous refill and not specific to a particular vein.
- Patient's inability to maximally point/flex their foot (manual compression can be used in such cases).
- Patient's inability to sit and hang their limb over the bedside.
- Ulcerations and lack of intact skin prohibits placement of the PPG sensor.
- Patients with extensive bandages or casts

Mechanism of Disease

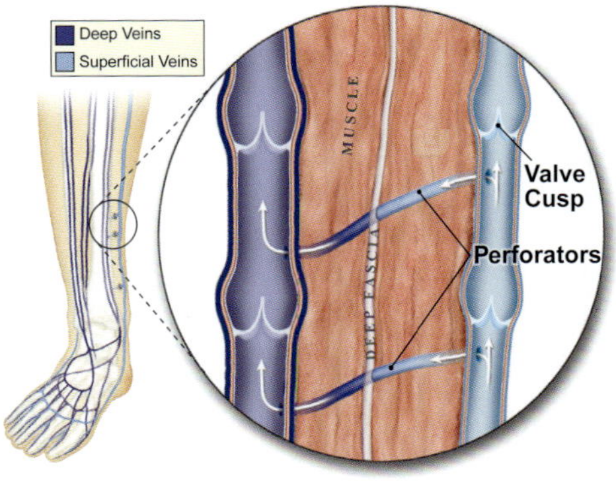

Fig. 13-3. *Blood normally flows from the superficial veins via perforators to the deep veins.*

Venous Flow with Normal Valve Function

- The direction of normal blood flow in the deep and superficial veins is toward the heart. In the perforating (communicating) veins, blood normally flows from the superficial to the deep veins. [1]
- At various times, the blood may encounter pressure to move backward from the heart, e.g., in response to gravity. Normally, flow reversal is prevented by the venous valves, which close in response to pressure from the reversed flow. [1]
- Upon exercise, the action of the calf muscles typically sends blood flow up the leg away from the calf. This action empties the calf veins, reduces blood volume, and reduces venous pressure. [1]

Venous Flow with Abnormal Valve Function

- Valvular damage and dysfunction (valvular incompetence) result in venous reflux, which is venous flow in the wrong (or opposite) direction, away from the heart and back into the leg.
- In the perforating veins, blood flows in the wrong direction from the deep to the superficial system.
- Venous reflux creates a high blood volume in the veins distal to the incompetent valve(s). [1]
- High blood volume in a vein causes ambulatory venous pressure or venous hypertension. [1]
- Hypertension will be greatest upon standing due to the effect of hydrostatic pressure from gravity, adding to the increased pressure from volume. [1]
- Normally venous blood volume and pressure are reduced by activating the calf muscle pump upon walking. When the valves are not working, the venous volume and resulting pressure do not decrease sufficiently, and the patient suffers from ambulatory venous hypertension. [1]
- Venous hypertension also increases pressure within the venules and capillaries. This high-pressure system encourages fluids to escape into the tissues causing edema. [1]
- Local edema results in a decrease in fluid and protein reabsorption. Fibrinogen and red blood cells (RBC) in the capillaries escape back into the tissues. Proteins organize and form tissue fibrosis, causing hardening of the skin. The RBCs break down and cause hyperpigmentation (causing hardening of the skin). Oxygen intake is decreased in the tissues, causing tissue malnutrition/hypoxia. Ulceration may follow. [1,2,3,4]

Varicose Veins

- Histological studies describe an increase in collagen and fibrous tissue within the layers of the venous wall in varicose vein patients. Collagen bundles disrupt the typical, orderly configuration of smooth muscle cells (SMC) in the medial layer. These SMC are thought to contain an excessive amount of granules, which may secrete collagenase and elastase, resulting in weakening of the venous wall and dilatation. Weakened venous walls allow for dilatation and elongation. [5]
- Varicose veins demonstrate decreased ability to contract normally, and the valves of varicose veins become stretched. [1]
- Tributaries of the great saphenous vein (GSV) are thought to varicose before the main trunk of the GSV because they contain less muscle in their vessel walls and lack support in the subcutaneous fat layer under the skin where they are commonly located. [1]

Pregnancy

- Pregnancy increases the amount of blood circulating in the body and causes veins to enlarge. The pressure of the fetus on the veins can decrease the blood flow back through the pelvic venous system. [1,6,7]

Patient History

- Persistent leg/calf swelling (usually unilateral)
- Previous DVT
- Localized pain, burning, or itching
- Tired, heavy legs after prolonged standing
- Varicose veins
- Skin changes and skin ulcers

Physical Examination

- Edema
- Tenderness, warmth, or redness along the course of a superficial vein or varicosity
- Varicose veins
- Hyperpigmentation, hardened tissue around the ankles
- Ulceration (usually the gaiter area)
- Dermatitis in the gaiter area or area along the course of a superficial vein
- Noticeable telangiectasia
- Venous claudication – severe symptoms of CVI (including those listed above) with pain/aching that worsens when walking and is relieved by elevation of the leg.

Location of Disease

Incompetent valves may be located at any segment of the deep, perforating, or superficial veins but are more commonly found in the superficial venous tributaries. [2]

- Most common location for incompetent perforating veins is the gaiter area – just above the medial malleolus.
- Saphenofemoral junction (SFJ)

Venous PPG Protocol

- Obtain a patient history to include symptoms and risk factors.
- Ensure that the patient is not vasoconstricted (cold).
- Explain the procedure to the patient and ensure they understand their role during the examination.
- Position the patient at the edge of the bed/stretcher with their legs dangling over the side in a non-weight bearing position. Be sure the bed is not compressing the back of the calf.
- Set the PPG monitor to the DC (venous) mode.
- Adhere the PPG sensor to the ankle about 5cm (2") above the medial malleolus (gaiter area) with double stick transparent tape or a Velcro strap. Try not to touch the tape surface under the PPG sensor since fingerprints can degrade the skin/PPG sensor coupling and reduce the signal amplitude. Ensure there will be no movement between the PPG sensor and the skin during the exercise.

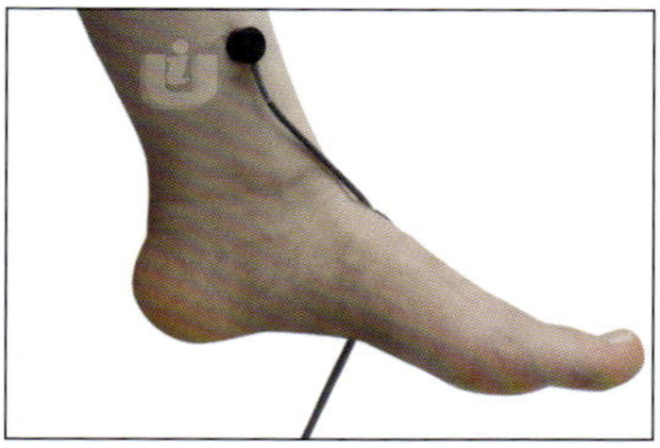

Fig. 13-4. *Resting venous PPG position*

> *Skin integrity must be checked before placing the PPG sensor. Choose a location that is free of ulceration or hardened skin. Do not place sensor directly on a varicose vein.*

- Turn on the PPG strip chart recorder at a speed of 5mm/sec. Adjust the PPG gain to the machine's midpoint. Set the tracing near the top portion of the chart and establish a stable baseline.
- Ask the patient to begin cycles of plantarflexion (pointing their foot downward) and dorsiflexion (pointing their foot upward). This type of exercise causes contraction of the calf muscles and empties the blood out of the veins in the lower leg. *(Fig. 13-5 and 13-6)*

> *Demonstrating the exercise for the patient often helps to obtain maximum flexion and correct timing.*

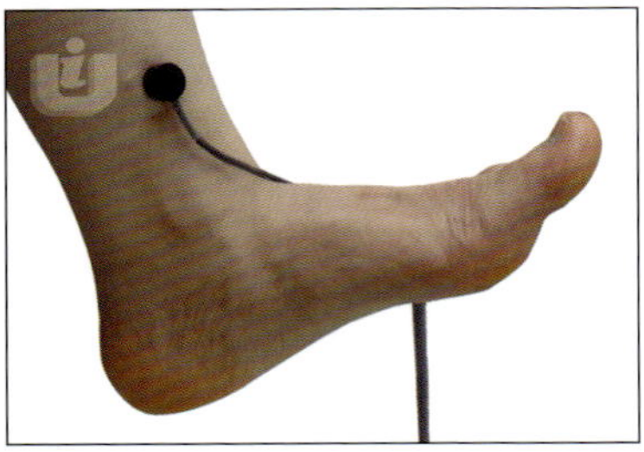

Fig. 13-5. *Dorsiflexion of the foot with a PPG sensor.*

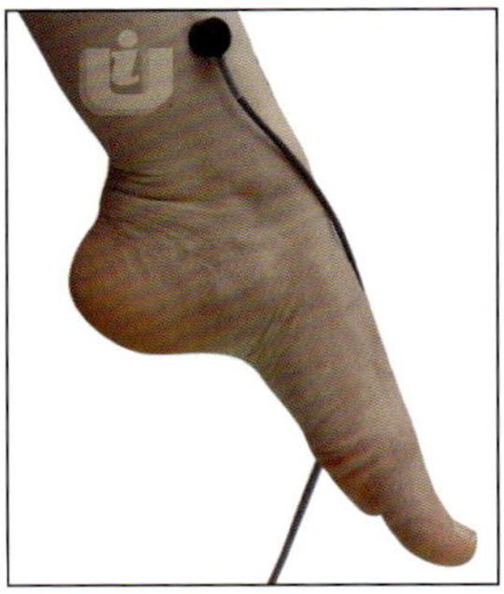

Fig. 13-6. *Plantarflexion of the foot with a PPG sensor.*

- If the tracing starts to drift off the page during exercise, readjust the gain and position of the trace.

> *As an alternative to dorsi- and plantarflexions, manual compressions of the gastrocnemius muscle will empty the blood out of the calf veins. With the patient's legs dangling off the bed, place your thumbs along each side of the tibia and squeeze the back of the patient's calf upward with your remaining fingers. Compress the calf for 1 second, then release the compression for 1 second. Five of these compressions are typically performed.*

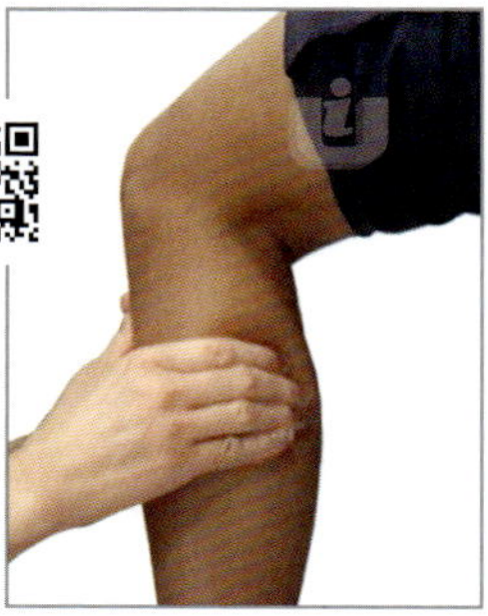

Fig. 13-7. *Manual augmentations*

- The PPG tracing should drop with exercise and then slope slowly upwards once the exercise is completed.
- Let the patient know they can relax while the recording is being taken and analyzed.
- On the tracing, note when the PPG slope either stabilizes by flattening out for at least 5 seconds or peaks and falls slightly. If the tracing is still rising after 20-30 seconds, you can stop the recording since this is past the threshold for reflux.

> *Remember to keep the speed of the PPG strip chart recorder at 5mm/sec.*

- Determine the VRT by calculating the time between the end of the exercise or manual compressions and the peak or beginning of the plateau.

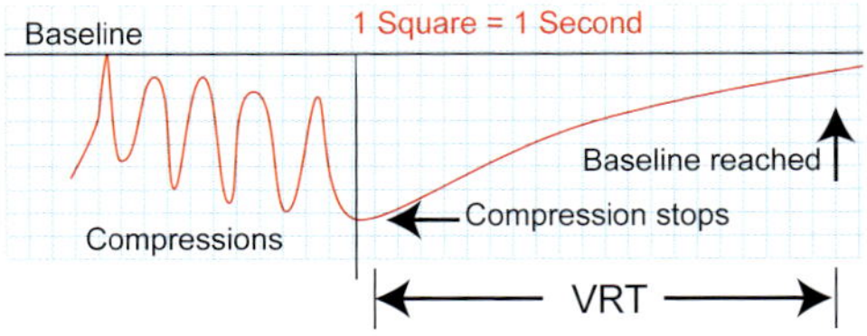

Fig. 13-8. *Calculation of a normal VRT*

- Repeat the exam several times on each leg, with a 1-minute rest period between each attempt. Report the average or mean VRT. The author suggests collecting VRT from three exercises, calculating the sum, dividing this value by 3, and reporting the number as the mean VRT.

The next steps of the exam are based on initial VRT results:

- **If the VRT is ≥20 seconds:** Valvular function is normal, and testing is complete.
- **If the VRT is <20 seconds:** Apply a 10 - 12cm straight pressure cuff (or tourniquet) to the distal thigh to be used to occlude the superficial venous system.
  - Inflate the pressure cuff (or tourniquet) to approximately 50mmHg. This should occlude the GSV in the sitting position while the deep system remains patent.
  - Repeat the exercise and recalculate the VRT.

» **If the VRT is ≥20 seconds:** testing is complete.

» **If the VRT is <20 seconds:** use duplex scanning to further evaluate for reflux or apply a 10 - 12 cm straight pressure cuff (or tourniquet) just below the knee to occlude the small saphenous venous system. Repeat the exercise and recalculate the VRT.

Table 13-1. **Photoplethysmography Protocol Summary**
• Hang the leg over the bedside in a non-weight bearing position. Keep the calf from touching the bed.
• Place the PPG transducer about 5cm (2") above the medial malleolus using double-stick transparent tape or a velcro strap.
• Turn the recorder on DC (venous) mode and run the PPG tracing at a speed of 5mm/sec.
• Ask the patient to perform 5 cycles of the plantarflexion/dorsiflexion exercise. (Or perform manual compressions if the patient is unable to exercise independently.)
• Wait for the tracing to either rise and plateau, or run for 30 seconds, whichever comes first.
• Calculate the VRT on the recorded trace by counting from the end of the exercise/compression cycle until the tracing reaches a stable baseline or runs for 30 seconds.
• Repeat the exam several times on each leg in order to calculate a mean VRT. Resting about 1 minute between cycles.
• The exam is finished if the mean VRT is ≥20 seconds.
• Continue with additional testing or use duplex imaging to further evaluate reflux if the mean VRT is <20 seconds.
• Inflate a pressure cuff (or tourniquet) placed on the distal thigh to 50mmHg.
• Repeat the exercise/compression several times and calculate the mean VRT.
• The exam is completed if the mean VRT is ≥20 seconds. Continue with additional testing or use duplex imaging to further evaluate reflux if the mean VRT is <20 seconds.
• Inflate a pressure cuff (or tourniquet) placed on the proximal calf to 50mmHg.
• Repeat the exercise/compression several times and calculate the mean VRT.

PRINCIPLES OF INTERPRETATION

Some labs may use normal VRT values as low as 17.

Normal

VRT ≥20 seconds is considered normal; the venous refill time via the arterial system is within normal limits.

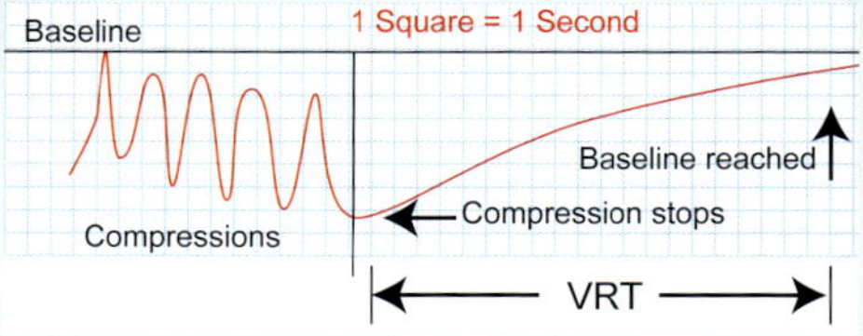

Fig. 13-9. *Calculation of a normal VRT*

Abnormal

VRT <20 seconds is associated with chronic venous insufficiency (CVI). The calf veins do not empty or fill properly due to venous obstruction and/or incompetent venous valves allowing for retrograde flow (backflow).

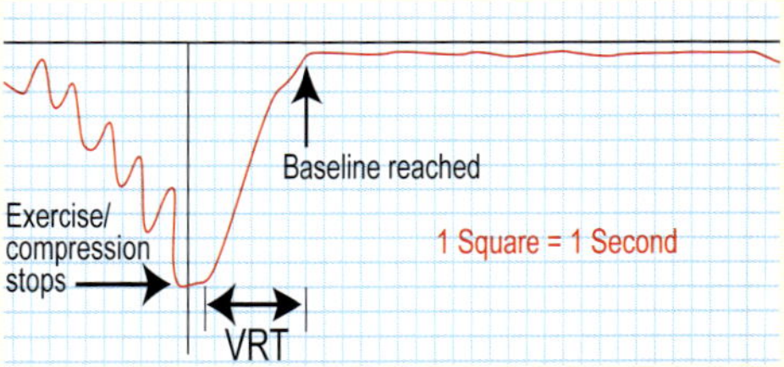

Fig. 13-10. *Calculation of an abnormal VRT (7sec)*

VRT with use of a thigh cuff

- If the mean VRT is <20 seconds without a pressure cuff (or tourniquet) and ≥20 seconds after application of a cuff on the thigh, the diagnosis is primary venous insufficiency or incompetence of the great saphenous system.

Venous Photoplethysmography (PPG)

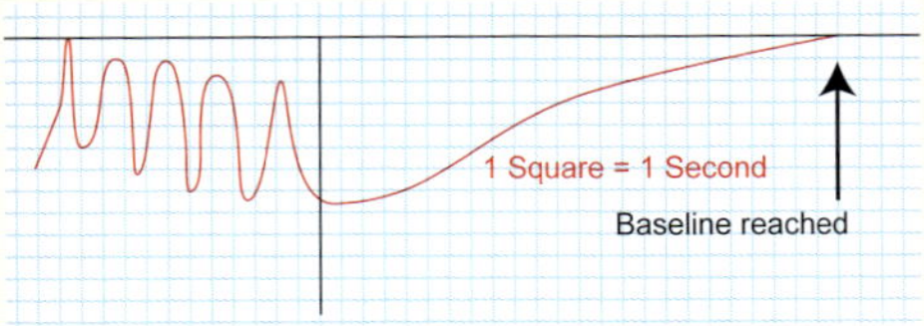

Fig. 13-11. *VRT normalizes with placement of a thigh cuff (20 sec).*

- If the mean VRT remains abnormal <20 seconds with a pressure cuff (or tourniquet) on the thigh, the diagnosis is secondary venous insufficiency or incompetence of the superficial and deep systems.

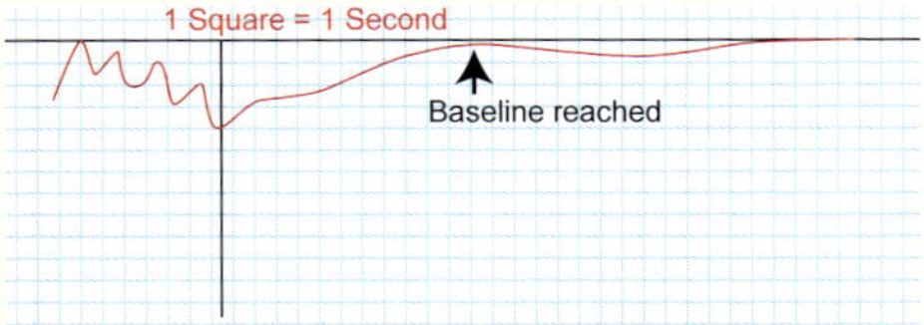

Fig. 13-12. *VRT remains abnormal with placement of a thigh cuff (10 to 11 sec).*

VRT with use of a cuff below the knee

- If the mean VRT <20 seconds with the pressure cuff (or tourniquet) below the knee but ≥20 seconds above the knee, this finding suggests reflux in the small saphenous vein.
- If the mean VRT is <20 seconds with the pressure cuff (or tourniquet) above AND below the knee, venous incompetence is present in the deep venous, great saphenous, and small saphenous.

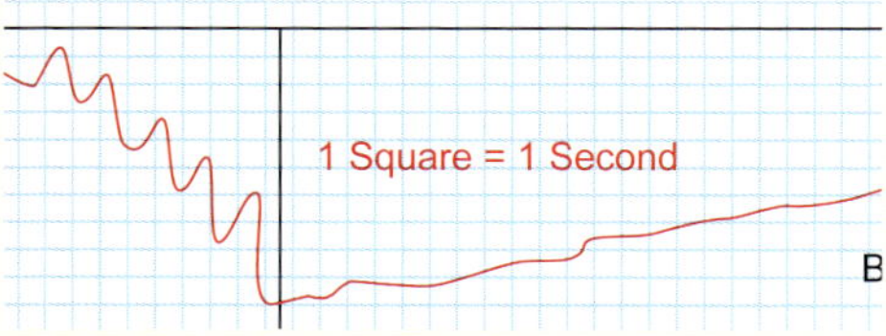

Fig. 13-13. *VRT normalizes after placement of a proximal calf cuff (22 sec)*

Table 13-2.
Diagnostic Criteria for PPG

Position of pressure cuff or tourniquet	Mean VRT	Location of venous incompetence
None	≥20 sec	None
	<20 sec	Incompetence present (*Test further to determine if superficial or deep)
Distal thigh	>20 sec	Great saphenous
	<20 sec	Deep and superficial venous system
Proximal calf	≥20 sec	Small saphenous
	<20 sec	Deep and superficial venous systems

Differential Diagnosis for CVD

- Lymphedema
- Cellulitis
- Deep venous thrombosis
- Adenopathy
- Arteriovenous fistula
- Direct injury to an extremity
- Mass (including vascularized mass)
- Arteriovenous malformation (AVM)
- Collagen vasculitis
- Abscess
- Peripheral neuritis
- Stasis dermatitis
- Klippel-Trenaunay
- Skin cancer
- Arterial disease

Correlation

- Lower extremity duplex scan for venous insufficiency
- PW Doppler reflux testing
- Descending venography

Medical Treatment for CVD

- Promote venous drainage (e.g., elevate legs, wear elastic stockings/support hose)
- Limit long periods of inactivity
- Compression bandaging (for ulceration)
- Proper skin care

Surgical Treatment for CVD

- Ligation (e.g., of saphenofemoral junction)
- Vein stripping
- Subfascial ligation of perforators
- Ambulatory phlebectomy (a.k.a. stab avulsion phlebectomy)

Endovascular Treatment for CVD

- Thermal venous ablation
- Mechanochemical ablation
- Chemical ablation (with visual or ultrasound-guided sclerotherapy)
- Visual or ultrasound-guided sclerotherapy
- Adhesive ablation

Points to Remember

- If the trace does not oscillate during testing, let the patient rest for about 1 minute and try increasing the gain settings while repeating the exercise. Expect the trace to show "pendulum" flow during exercise.
- Primary venous insufficiency is thought to have a congenital etiology and involves the superficial more than the deep venous system.
- Secondary venous insufficiency is typically an acquired condition (e.g., after venous thrombosis) and can involve the superficial, perforating, and deep venous systems.[8]
- Secondary venous insufficiency can result from a congenital condition such as an extrinsic compression of an iliac vein by an overlying iliac artery.

References

1. Sumner DS, Zierler RE. (2005). Vascular physiology: essential hemodynamic principles. In Rutherford *Vascular Surgery 6th edition.* (75-123). Philadelphia. Elsevier Saunders.
2. Labropoulos N, Leon LR. (2005). Evaluation of chronic venous disease. In Mansour MA, Labropoulos N. (Eds.), Vascular Diagnosis, (447-461). Philadelphia: Elsevier Saunders
3. Zwiebel, WJ (2005). Ultrasound diagnosis of venous insufficiency. In Zwiebel WJ, Pellerito JS (Eds.), Introduction to Vascular Ultrasonography 5th ed, (479-499). Philadelphia: Elsevier Saunders.
4. Meissner MH. (2010). Chronic venous disorders. In Zierler RE (Ed.), Strandess's duplex scanning disorders in vascular diagnosis 4th ed. (223-229).Philadelphia Wolters Kluwer Lippincott Williams & Wilkins.
5. Browse NL, Burnand, KG, Thomas, ML (1988). Disease of the Veins; Pathology, Diagnosis and Treatment, Edward Arnold, a division of Hodder & Stoughton.
6. Meissner MH, Strandess DE. (2005). Pathophysiology and natural history of acute deep venous thrombosis. In *Rutherford Vascular Surgery 6th edition.* (2124-2142). Philadelphia. Elsevier Saunders.
7. Min RJ, Rosenblatt M. US Department of Health and Human Services, Office on Women's Health (2010). Varicose Veins and Spider Veins. Retrieved from http://www.womenshealth.gov/faq/varicose-spider-veins.cfm. (7-7-2010).
8. Eberhardt RT, Raffetto JD. (2005). Contemporary Reviews in Cardiovascular Medicine. Circulation. 111: 2398-2409.

Additional References

9. Barnes RW, Garrett WV, Hummel BA, et al: (AAMI 13th Annual Meeting, March 1978) Photoplethysmographic assessment of altered cutaneous circulation in the post-phlebitic syndrome. In Technology in Diagnosis and Therapy. (25). Washington, DC.
10. Abramowitz HB., Queral LA., Flinn WR., et al. (1979). The use of photoplethysmography in the assessment of venous insufficiency: a comparison to venous pressure measurements. *Surgery 86*, 434 – 441.
11. Li JM., Anderson FA., Wheeler HB. (1983). Non-invasive testing for venous reflux using photoplethysmography: Standardization of technique and evaluation of interpretation criteria. *Bruit [J Vasc Technol]* 7, 25 – 29.
12. Needham TN., Jury P., Hoare M. (1983). Photoplethysmographic refilling time: The relationship between the initial rate of refilling and venous incompetence. *Bruit [J Vasc Technol]* 7, 18 – 21.

All images in this chapter are courtesy of ACI Medical

Definition

Air plethysmography (APG)® quantifies the physiological components of chronic venous disease, including; chronic obstruction, valvular reflux, calf muscle pump function, and venous hypertension.

Rationale

APG® uses a calibrated air chamber to measure small volumetric changes of the calf in response to positional changes and exercise by measuring absolute volume changes of blood in milliliters (ml). Lower extremity venous function is measured by quantitating venous valve reflux and the efficiency of the calf muscle pump function by measuring venous filling (measured as the patient stands from a supine position), calf ejection (following one tip-toe exercise), and residual volume (following a series of tip-toe exercises). *(Fig. 14-6)*

Indications for Exam

- Venous insufficiency
- Varicose veins
- Muscle pump evaluation
- Venous ulcerations
- Post-treatment, follow-ups

Contraindication/Limitations

- Patients with acute venous thrombosis
- Excessive bandaging or casts
- Patients must be able to stand
- Patients must be able to follow directions for exercise

Mechanism of Disease

Normal Venous Flow

- Normally, venous blood volume and pressure are reduced by activating the calf muscle pump upon walking. When the valves are not working, the venous volume and resulting pressure do not reduce sufficiently, and the patient suffers from ambulatory venous hypertension.
- Normally, blood is propelled from the superficial veins via perforators to the deep venous system and toward the heart.
- Venous outflow in the lower extremities depends upon:
  - Vein patency
  - Valve competence
  - Adequate calf muscle function

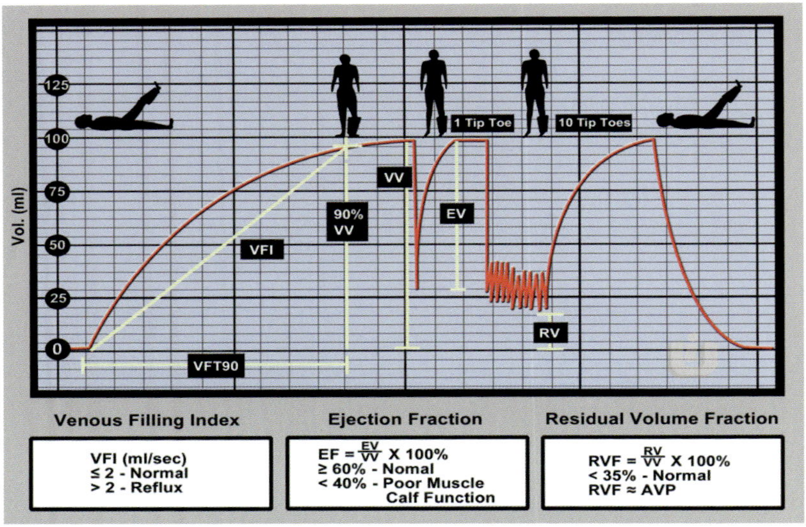

Fig. 14-1. *Graph displays volume changes during the standard testing procedure*

Abnormal Venous Flow, Abnormal Valve Function, and the Calf Muscle Pump

- Severe chronic venous insufficiency is often caused by calf muscle pump failure.
- Calf muscle pump failure is common in patients with venous leg ulcers.
- Valvular damage and dysfunction (valvular incompetence) result in venous reflux, which is venous flow in the wrong direction, away from the heart.
- In the perforating veins, blood flows in the wrong direction from the deep to the superficial system.
- Venous reflux creates a high blood volume in the veins distal to the incompetent valve(s).
- High blood volume in a vein causes increased venous pressure (venous hypertension). [1]
- Hypertension will be greatest upon standing due to the effect of hydrostatic pressure from gravity, adding to the increased pressure from volume. [1]
- Venous hypertension also increases pressure within the venules and capillaries.
- This high-pressure system encourages fluids to escape into the tissues causing edema. [1]

Patient History

- Leg edema or swelling
- Varicose veins
- Pain
- Itching
- Aching
- Throbbing
- Tired, heavy legs
- Fatigue
- Restlessness
- Night cramps

Physical Exam

- Leg edema or swelling
- Tenderness
- Varicose veins
- Venous hyperpigmentation
- Venous ulceration
- Venous claudication

Location of Disease

- Incompetent valves may be located at any segment of the deep, perforating, or superficial veins and their tributaries [2]
- Perforating veins in the gaiter area medial aspect of the leg, just above the medial malleolus (most common location)
- Areas affected by calf muscle pump failure

Calf Muscle Pump

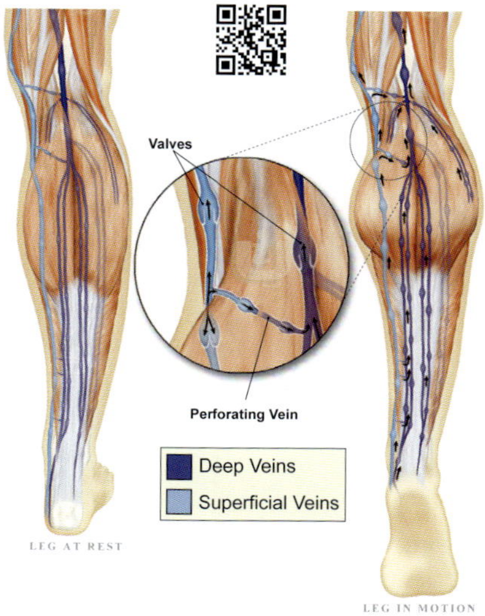

Fig. 14-2. *The calf muscle pump drives venous flow. While walking, muscle contractions squeeze the veins initiating venous blood flow. Venous flow opens the venous valves allowing the blood to flow towards the heart. As the muscle relaxes, valves close to prevent the backwash of blood (reflux).*

Air Plethysmography Protocol

(for reflux, calf muscle pump function, and venous hypertension testing)

- Obtain a patient history to include symptoms and risk factors.
- Patient is placed in the supine position; the leg is externally rotated, resting on a foam foot support.
- The sensing cuff is placed around the calf, ensuring that the cuff only touches the leg.
- The cuff is attached to a pressure transducer, amplifier, and recorder and is calibrated.
- The patient is asked to rest for approximately 3-5 minutes so the cuff can be stabilized and there is equilibration of arterial inflow.

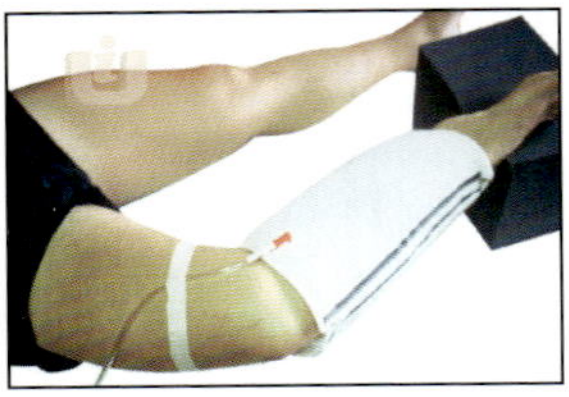

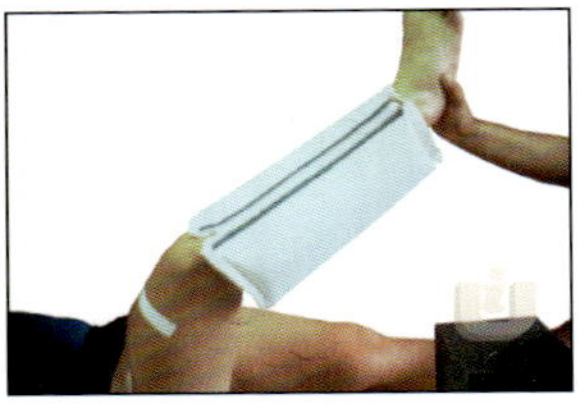

Fig. 14-3. *Patient resting with calibrated cuff and elevation of the leg to empty the venous system*

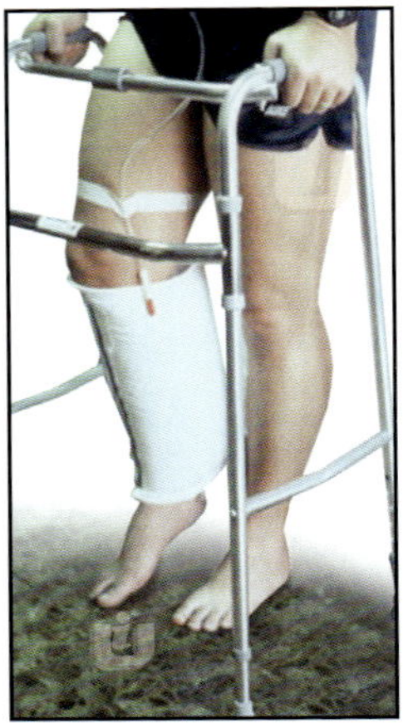

Fig. 14-4. *As the patient stands, the leg fills with resting arterial inflow and venous flow. (if reflux is present)*

Reflux

- Elevate the leg 45° with your hand for approximately 15 seconds, making sure the patient's leg is relaxed while being held. *(Fig. 14-3)*

- After a stable zero baseline is obtained while ensuring no disturbance to the cuff, ask the patient to stand and hold onto a frame for support. The purpose is to examine the limb while it is non-weight bearing.

> *Hint: You must demonstrate the testing sequence a few times to ensure maneuvers are understood.*

- Ask the patient to remain standing with no weight bearing on the leg being examined. *(Fig. 14-4)* Obtain a stable baseline trace while standing. The leg begins filling with resting arterial inflow and venous flow if reflux is present. This volume change is called the Venous Volume (VV). The normal VV is 80 - 150ml.

- The Venous Filling Index (VFI) is calculated using the VV. The VFI is the average filling rate of the veins to 90% of the VV. A normal VFI is < 2ml/sec. with slow filling from the arterial supply.

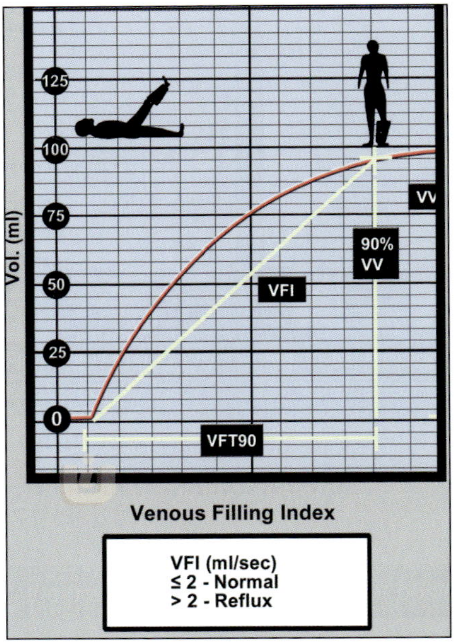

Fig. 14-5. *Graph representing the increase in leg volume upon standing. (venous volume, VV). The VFI is then calculated from this maneuver.*

Calf Muscle Pump Function

- After obtaining a stable plateau, the patient is asked to stand on both feet and perform one tip-toe maneuver. *(Fig. 14-6)* A decrease in volume (ml) is observed during the exercise due to venous emptying from calf muscle contraction. This volume change from one tiptoe is the Ejection Volume (EV).
  - This maneuver can be repeated until two or three consistent calf EV are obtained.

- The Ejection Fracture (EF) is calculated from this EV and the VV.

$$EF = EV/VV \times 100$$

- A normal EF is 60% or greater.

Venous Hypertension

- The patient is asked to stand on both feet once again and perform a series of 10 rapid tip-toe exercises at a rate of one per second. The patient then returns to the original position with no weight bearing on the leg being examined. A diminishing calf volume is recorded with the exercises.
- Once a plateau in the tracing is obtained from the 10 tiptoe maneuvers, the patient is returned to the supine position, ensuring no weight bearing on the leg being examined. The leg is once again elevated. A new zero baseline is obtained, which will be used to measure Residual Volume (RV).
- The value of the Residual Volume Fraction (RVF) has been shown to correlate directly to Ambulatory Venous Pressure (AVP). The RVF is calculated as follows:

$$RVF = RV/VV \times 100$$

- This entire exam can be repeated with a tourniquet, cuff, or stockings.

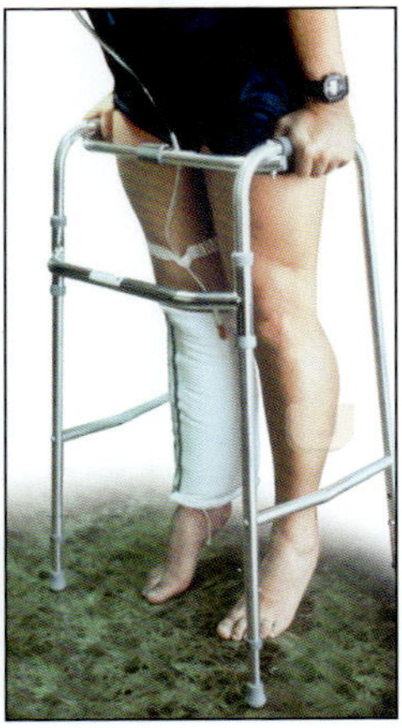

Fig. 14-6. *Patient performs a series of ten tip toe maneuvers. As the patient stands, the leg fills with resting arterial inflow and venous flow (if reflux is present)*

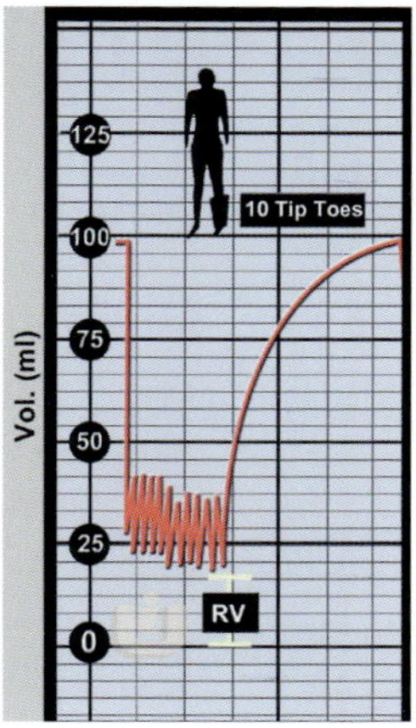

Fig. 14-7. *Graph representing diminished calf volume (RV) from the 10 tip toes*

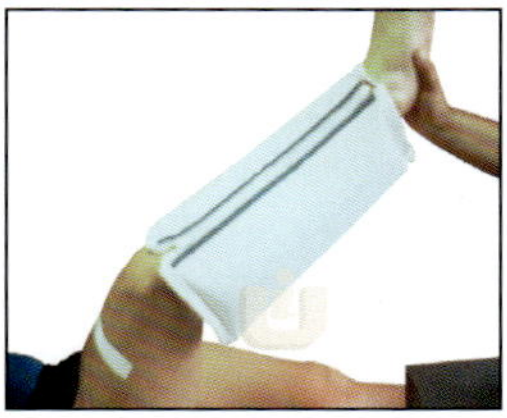

Fig. 14-8. *Elevating the leg to empty the venous system*

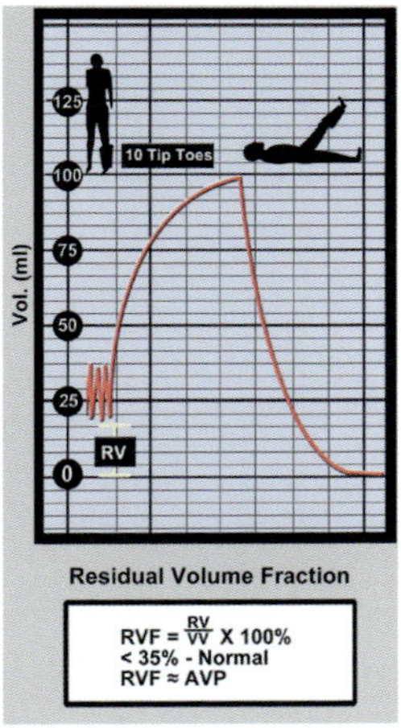

Fig. 14-9. *Graph representing re-establishing the zero functional venous volume*

Table 14-1. **APG Protocol Summary**

Reflux

1. The patient's leg is elevated to empty the veins.
2. The patient stands, and the leg begins to fill to their venous volume (VV) with resting arterial inflow and reflux resent.
   - The Venous Filling Index (VFI) is the average filling rate of the veins to 90% of Venous Volume.
   - Normal legs fill with less than 2ml/sec.
   - This measurement can be repeated with a tourniquet occluding the superficial veins to quantify deep versus superficial reflux or with compression stockings.

Calf Muscle Pump Function

3. The patient performs one tip-toe movement. The Ejected Volume (EV) is the amount of blood in ml expelled by the calf muscle pump. Ejection Fraction is calculated as EF = EV/VV x 100%. A normal leg exhibits 60% or greater ejection fractions.

Venous Hypertension

4. The patient performs 10 tiptoe maneuvers
5. The patient returns to the supine position with the leg elevated to reestablish the zero functional venous volume upon which the residual volume is measured.

Residual Volume Fraction (RVF) is calculated as RVF= RV//VV x 100% and has been shown to correlate directly to Ambulatory Venous Pressure (AVP)

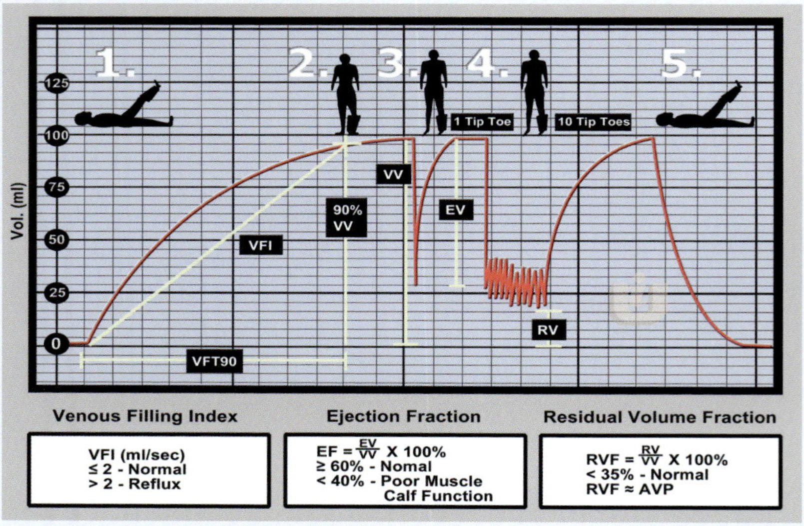

Fig. 14-10. *Reflux, calf muscle pump function and, venous hypertension*

Principles of Interpretation

Changes in calf volume during the examination provide quantitative information regarding the venous system. A series of direct and derived measurements are calculated and recorded. The non-invasive equivalent of venous reflux, calf muscle pump function, and ambulatory venous pressure are determined.

Table 14-2. **Air Plethysmography Normal Values**

Direct Measurements	Normal Values
Functional Venous Volume (VV) *(the increase in leg volume on standing)*	100 - 150ml
Venous Filling Time (VFT90) *(time taken to reach 90% of VV)*	70 - 170sec
Ejected Volume (EV) *(decrease in leg volume from one tiptoe movement)*	60 - 150ml
Residual Volume (RV) *(volume of blood left in the veins after 10 tiptoe movements)*	2 - 45ml
Derived Measurements	**Units**
Venous Filling Index *(VFI) (average filling rate: 90% VV/VFT90)*	ml/sec
Ejection Fraction *(EF=(EV/VV) x 100)*	%
Residual Volume Fraction	%

Table 14-3. **Diagnostic Criteria for Venous Filling Index**

VFI (ml/sec)	Interpretation
≤2	Normal
>2 - 5	Mild reflux
>5 - 10	Moderate reflux
>10	Severe reflux

Venous Filling Index

The Venous Filling Index (VFI) indicates the degree of valvular insufficiency.

- The VFI represents the increased volume changes from the supine position to the standing position.
- The VFI is the average, gravity-induced filling rate defined as the ratio of 90% of the VV divided by the time taken to achieve 90% of venous filling. This measures average filling rate and is expressed in milliliters per second (ml/sec).
- The beginning baseline from the VFI test could be used to get a more accurate RVF measurement when poor outflows exist.
- Not elevating the leg high enough for an adequate ending baseline will cause false results.

Ejection Fraction

The Ejection Fraction (EF) is a measure of calf muscle pump function and is measured as a percentage (%) of functional calf volume.

- EF is calculated by dividing the volume of blood ejected (EV) by the calf during one tip-toe exercise and dividing it by the functional Venous Volume (VV):

$$EF = EV/VV \times 100$$

Residual Volume Fraction

The Residual Volume Fraction (RVF) indicates the overall efficiency of the calf muscle pump.

- The RVF compares the volume changes between the 10 tip-toe exercises and the zero baseline. It is reported as a percentage of the functional calf volume.

- A good linear correlation exists between RVF and AVP.
- RVF is calculated by dividing the Residual Volume (RV) by the functional Venous Volume (VV).

$$RVF = RV/VV \times 100$$

- The ending baseline (after the RVF test) may be higher or lower than the baseline value at the beginning of the VFI test.

Calf Muscle Pump

Possible causes of poor calf muscle pump are:

- Non-venous related problems, including arthritis.
- Proximal obstruction that prevents blood flow from traveling out of the calf.
- Incompetent calf perforator veins
- Calf varicosities retain a large venous volume not expelled with calf .muscle contraction.

Interpretation-Diagnostic Criteria

Normal

Venous Filling Index

- Venous filling should increase the leg venous volume by 100 - 150ml in normal limbs.
- A VFI of 2ml/sec or less indicates absence of significant venous reflux and normal slow filling of the veins from the arterial inflow circulation.

Ejection Fraction

Normal ejection fractions are >60%.

Residual Volume Fraction

Because most of the blood in the calf will be ejected during exercise, normal extremities will have an RVF of 35% or less.

Abnormal

Venous Filling Index

- In limbs with chronic venous insufficiency, venous filling increases the leg venous volume between 100 to 350ml.
- A VFI >7ml/sec is associated with a high incidence of skin changes, chronic swelling, and ulceration.

Ejection Fraction

Table 14-4. **Diagnostic Criteria for Ejection Fraction (EF)**

EF (%)	Interpretation
>60%	Normal
30 - 55%	Primary varicose veins (average 50%)
20 - 55%	Deep venous insufficiency (average 40%)
18 - 50%	Deep venous obstruction (average 35%)

Venous valvular insufficiency results in lower ejection fractions, usually due to reflux in the deep venous system.

Table 14-5. **Diagnostic Criteria for Residual Volume Fraction (RVF)**

RVF (%)	Interpretation
<35	No significant hypertension
>35	Venous hypertension

The greater the RVF%, the greater the incidence of CVI and ulceration

RVF% is equivalent to the ambulatory venous pressure in mmHg

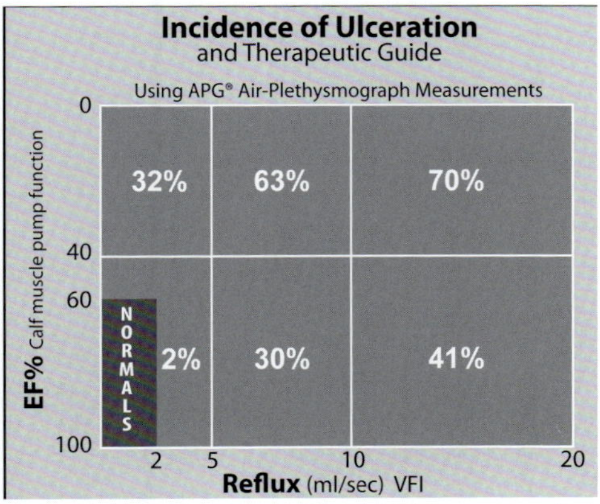

Fig. 14-11. *Plotting the VFI and EF can predict the likelihood of ulceration Source: Christopoulos and Nicolaides, St Mary's Vascular Laboratory, London, England.*

Residual Volume Fraction

An RVF >35mmHg indicates venous hypertension. Extremities with chronic venous insufficiency usually have reflux and have less efficient calf muscle pumps, creating an RVF >35%.

In cases of venous obstruction, arterial inflow may be greater than the obstructed vein's capacity for outflow, and the calf cannot be completely emptied. The RVF is unreliable in these cases since it will be an artificially low "normal" value due to the elevated obstruction baseline.

Differential Diagnosis *(for obstruction, abnormal valve, and calf muscle pump function)*

- Deep venous thrombosis
- Lymphedema
- Cellulitis
- Arteriovenous fistula
- Arteriovenous malformation

Correlation

- Venous photoplethysmography for reflux testing
- Descending venography

Medical Treatment

- Promote venous drainage (e.g., elevate legs, wear elastic stockings/support hose)
- Limit long periods of inactivity
- Compression bandaging (for ulceration)
- Injection sclerotherapy
- Ultrasound-guided sclerotherapy

Surgical Treatment

- Ligation (e.g., of saphenofemoral junction)
- Venous ablation
- Stab avulsion phlebectomy
- Vein stripping
- Subfascial endoscopic perforator vein surgery
- Transverse repair of incompetent valves
- Subfascial ligation of perforators
- Ambulatory phlebectomy

Endovascular Treatment

- Radiofrequency ablation
- Laser thermal ablation

Points to Remember

- APG® provides a global measurement of venous function.
- The more efficient the calf muscle pump, the lower level of pressure in the venous system.
- Failure of the calf muscle pump interferes with healing.
- Failure of the calf muscle pump in some patients is related to decreased ankle joint mobility due to painful venous ulceration in this area.
- The EF can be >100%, suggesting exercise empties more blood than gravity, indicating an excellent calf muscle pump function.
- APG® can be used to monitor pre and post-op venous changes.
- Negative ending baseline values may be due to cuff slippage during the ten toe-up exercises.
- Selecting the zero volume too early in the trace will result in underestimated VFI values.

- The differential diagnosis of peripheral edema discriminates venous insufficiency from cardiac disease, lymphedema, and cellulitis.
- The VFT 90, or the amount of time required to fill 90% of the venous volume, is more accurate to use than the VV.

References

1. 1. Nicolaides, A. et al. Investigation of Patients with Deep Venous Thrombosis and Chronic Venous Insufficiency. (1993). Med-Orion Publishing Co. 39–43.
2. Christopoulous DG., Nicolaides AN., Szendro G. (1987). Air-plethysmography and the effect of elastic compression on venous hemodynamics of the leg. *J Vasc Surg 5*(1),148-159.
3. Christopoulous DG., Nicolaides AN., Galloway JMD. (1988). Objective noninvasive evaluation of venous surgical results. *J Vasc Surg 8*(6), 683-687.
4. Katz M., Comerota A., Kerr R. (1991). Air-plethysmography (APG): A new technique to evaluate patients with chronic venous insufficiency. *J Vasc Technol 15*(2).
5. Nicolaides, A. et al. (1993). *How air plethysmography (APG) influences patient management.* ACI Medical.

Purpose

Ergonomics is the study of factors that affect humans in their workplace with a focus on design and the arrangement of physical spaces so that people and things interact efficiently and safely.

As ultrasound exams become more complex and physically demanding and volumes increase, more sonographers report experiencing workplace injury and chronic pain. As vascular testing becomes more popular and space in offices and hospitals is limited, you may be required to perform exams in tighter spaces. The demand for portable exams in intensive care units for example makes it more difficult for the technologist to use ergonomically friendly exam rooms and maintain proper posture. The percentage of sonographers experiencing musculoskeletal pain at work has increased from 84% in 1997 [1] to 90% in 2009 [2] according to published studies. When rest is not enough, some sonographers undergo surgery to relieve their symptoms while others are forced to leave the field of vascular sonography altogether.

The term "Work Related Musculoskeletal Disorders (WRMSDs)" is used to describe the numerous conditions that are caused by repetitive use and performing difficult activities in the workplace. Back-to-back abdominal exams or venous exams on obese patients are often part of the regular schedule in many vascular labs. WRMSDs occur over time and affect the muscles, nerves, ligaments, and tendons of those in our profession. Often, the pain and discomfort of WRMSDs will linger throughout the day well after you put the transducer down and finish scanning your patients.

Work-related injuries cost up to $20 billion/yr in medical expenses and worker's compensation benefits, with even more money being lost due to absenteeism, lost productivity, and the time needed to hire and train new staff. [3] In contrast, the approximate cost to set up an ergonomically friendly work area for the sonographer is $188,205. [6]

There is substantial physical effort needed for vascular scanning beyond the force required to compress vessels, including pushing, pulling, and gripping the transducer. Vascular exams call for the sonographer to stay in an awkward posture, sometimes for an extended amount of time to obtain the information needed to diagnose the patient's issue/disease. Wrist and shoulder flexion/extension, reaching, bending and twisting are common to vascular testing.

Location of Disease

The most common WRMSDs injuries involve the following areas of the body:

- Shoulder
- Hand/wrist
- Back (upper > middle and lower)
- Neck

Patient History

The physical symptoms of Musculoskeletal Disorders (MSDs) include:

- Pain
- Numbness, tingling
- Loss of control (unable to grip or feeling like you will drop the transducer, for example)
- Blurred vision, headaches
- Inflammation
- Joint stiffness and decreased range of motion

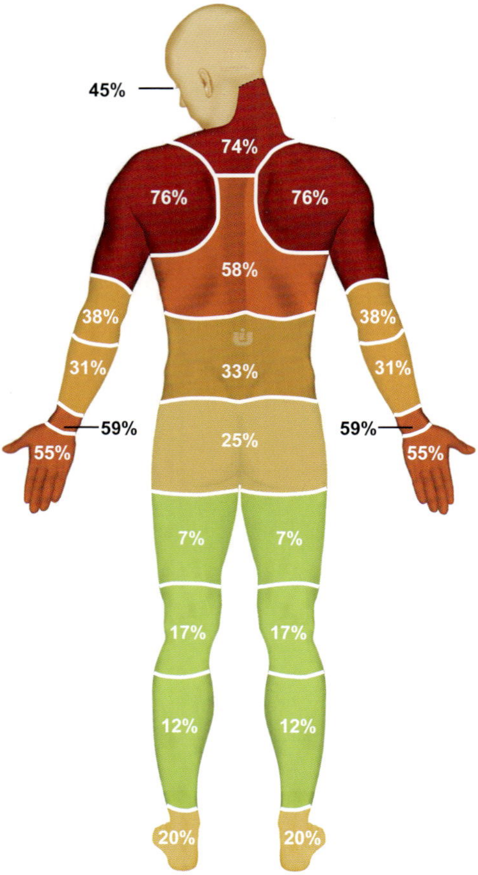

Fig. 15-1. *Percentage of injuries reported by area*

Modified from J. Baker "Musculoskeletal Injury and Sonography: The American Experience Statistical Evidence of Risk Factors" www.sonoworld.com

Common Conditions Diagnosed as a Result of a WRMSD

- Carpal tunnel syndrome
- Tendonitis/Tenosynovitis
- Bursitis (especially of the shoulder)
- Thoracic Outlet Syndrome
- Epicondylitis (tennis elbow)
- Trigger Finger- inability to extend the finger

Optimization Goals for Vascular Labs Pre, During, and Post Scan

Scheduling

- Scheduling templates for vascular lab exams should include time for indirect (exam room set-up, time to allow the patient to change, and patient assessment), as well as direct patient care (actual scan) and the time needed afterward to clean, complete worksheets and bill.
- Some of the recommended exam times for vascular studies are listed below: [9]
  - » 70 minutes for a bilateral CVI exam
  - » 45 minutes for a unilateral CVI exam
  - » 92 minutes for a complete renal exam
  - » 67 minutes for a complete carotid exam
- Scheduling templates should allow for breaks between patients complying with local, state, and federal labor laws and workplace policies for breaks/meal periods.
- Limit the number of portable exams performed to those that are truly necessary (critically ill patients, for example) versus bedside exams just for convenience. Make sure providers know that the patient will probably receive a better-quality scan if they can travel to your department, where you have all your equipment and additional resources.
- Try to rotate tasks between staff sonographers or try to schedule different exam types each hour if you are working alone. It is better to schedule a carotid exam in between two abdominal exams to give your body a break. Varying the type of exam(s), you perform daily allows you to use different muscle groups while you rest others. This variation will reduce the risk of repetitive use injury.

Moving Patients/Equipment

- Do not bend over when moving a patient cart.
- Raise the cart to allow your arms to be at a 90° angle. This will facilitate pushing with the arms instead of the back.

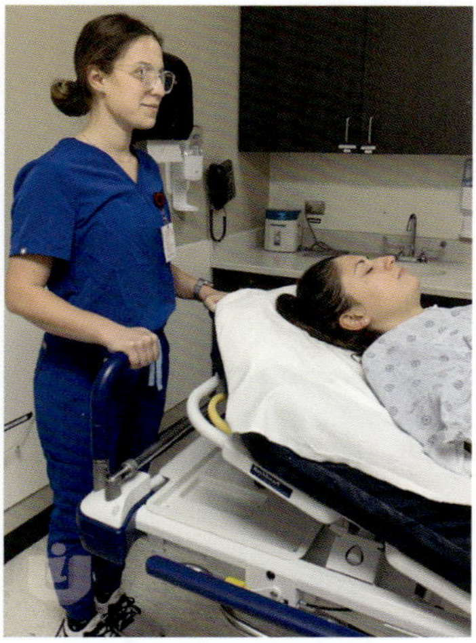

Fig. 15-2. **CORRECT POSTURE**
Raise cart, so arms are at 90°.
Use your arms (not your back) to push.

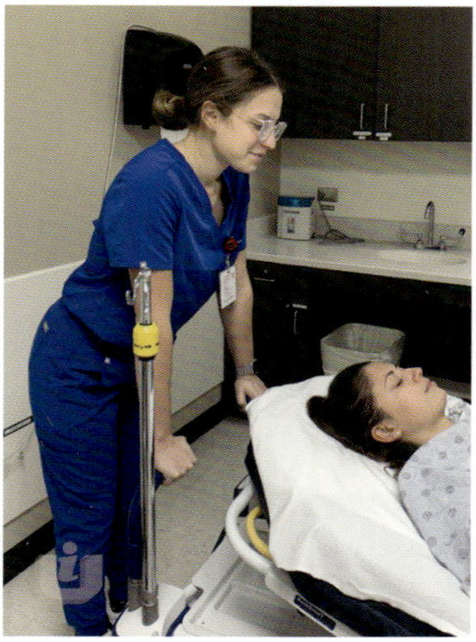

Fig. 15-3. **INCORRECT POSTURE**
Cart is too low and arms straight, which requires the use of your lower back to push.

Moving Ultrasound Machines

- Lower the monitor so you have an unobstructed view as you move through the doorways and halls.
- Do not bend over when moving equipment.
- Raise the equipment to allow your arms to be at a 90° angle. This will facilitate pushing with the arms instead of your back.
- If your machine has a "2-way steer" option, make sure it is engaged, so you will have better control when traveling long distances. If you leave the machine engaged in "all-wheel drive" it will be more difficult to control and stop.

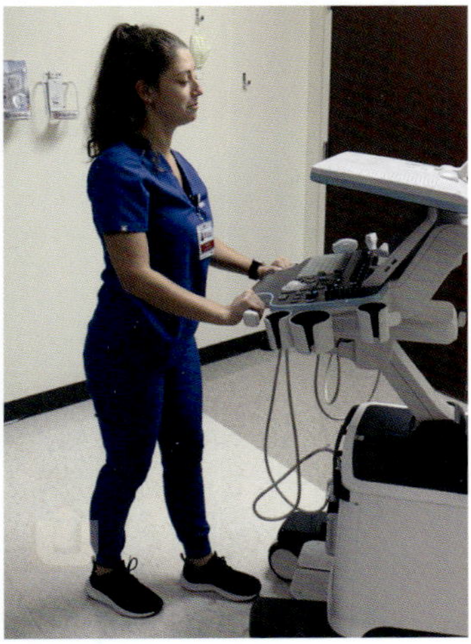

Fig. 15-4. **CORRECT**
The lowered screen allows for better visibility, and the machine height allows for a 90° arm angle to avoid using your back.

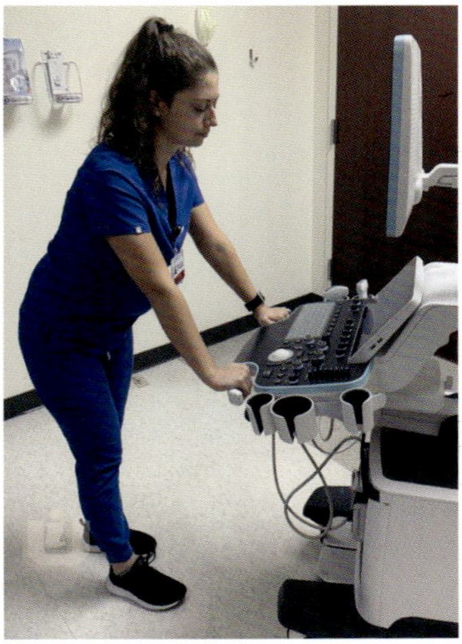

Fig. 15-5. **INCORRECT**
The raised screen may obstruct the view. The low height of the machine does not allow for a 90° angle of the arms, causing the use of your lower back.

Scanning

- Make sure to wear the proper size gloves for your hand to maintain a proper grip on the transducer.
  - A proper transducer grip will be more comfortable for you and should ensure a steady image.
- Once the patient has been safely positioned, the table should be raised to allow for the use of proper ergonomics.
  - Electronically controlled tables are preferred.
  - Stand in front of pedal controls used to raise the bed up/down instead of trying to make adjustments with your body at an angle.
- Take the time to position the patient properly, as close to you as possible, and at an appropriate height. Try to minimize reaching, bending, or twisting during the scan.
- Adjust window coverings and exam room lights so there is no glare on the monitor during the scan.
- Before the start of the scan, adjust your chair, monitor, exam table, and keyboard to the best level for you.
- Your machine's monitor should be 10-15° below your eye level and an arm's length away from your eyes (about 18-30 inches). Make sure to keep the screen of your monitor clean. Refocus your eyes occasionally during the scan to give them a break.
- Keep your arm as close to your side as possible to avoid overreaching.
- Grip the transducer as lightly as possible while remaining steady.
- Hold the transducer as close to the patient's skin as possible.
- Rest the side of your hand, from the tips of your pinky finger to the outside of the wrist on the patient's leg.
- Keep your wrist as straight as possible when scanning, and try not to have too great of an angle between your wrist and forearm.
- Stop and pay attention to your body if you feel pain during the scan. Just as you would try to reposition your patient during the scan if they were uncomfortable, you should do the same for yourself. Try to keep your shoulders, arm, and wrist relaxed. Try to move your chair. Grab a cushion or roll up a blanket to use as a support for your arm if needed.
- Take "micro-breaks" during the scan, where you ease up on your transducer grip for a moment and then return to a tighter grip.
- Make use of equipment available to you to aid in the proper positioning to achieve good ergonomics.
  - Adjustable exam beds
  - Height adjustable stools/chairs
  - Support blocks and cushions
  - Raised platform or steps tool.
  - Automated cuff augmentation device for lower extremity venous insufficiency duplex exams.
- You are ultimately responsible for using proper form while scanning.
- Work as a team on difficult patients. Sometimes this might not seem possible, but when you can, try to ask for help from coworkers. For example, one technologist can stand on the opposite side of the bed to scan the contralateral limb, while the other technologist controls the machine.
- Ask the patient for help when you can. An example of this is asking the patient to lie on their side or in the prone position to avoid reaching and twisting to scan the back of the calf.
- Remember that there are limits to ultrasound exams. Maintain reasonable expectations about the images you can get when there are technical limitations such as body habitus, poor patient positioning, or extreme patient discomfort.

Hand and Wrist Ergonomics

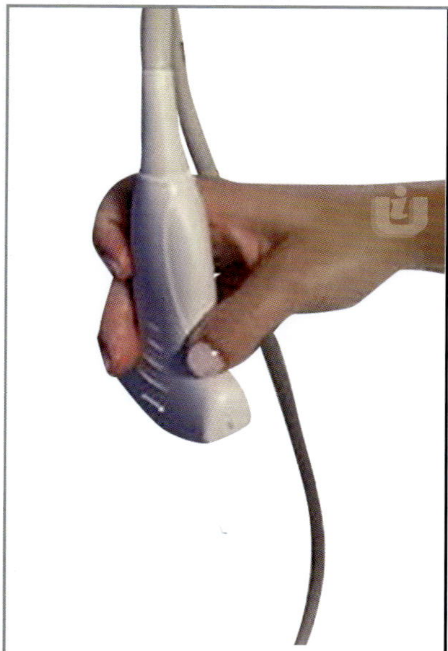

Fig. 15-6. **CORRECT** *The angle between your wrist and forearm should be close to 0°.*

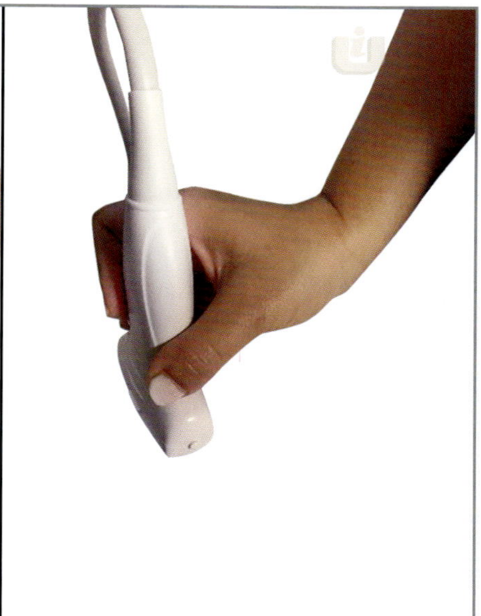

Fig. 15-7. **INCORRECT** *Reduce the angle at your wrist.*

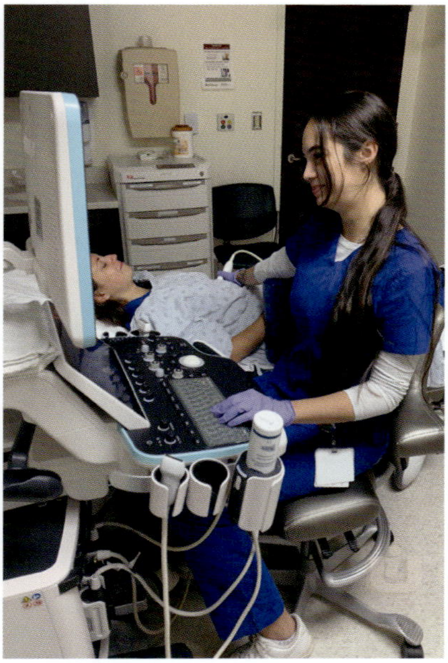

Fig. 15-8. **CORRECT POSTURE** *Adjust the chair for support, adjust the machine height and monitor, support your arm with a cushion/rolled blanket.*

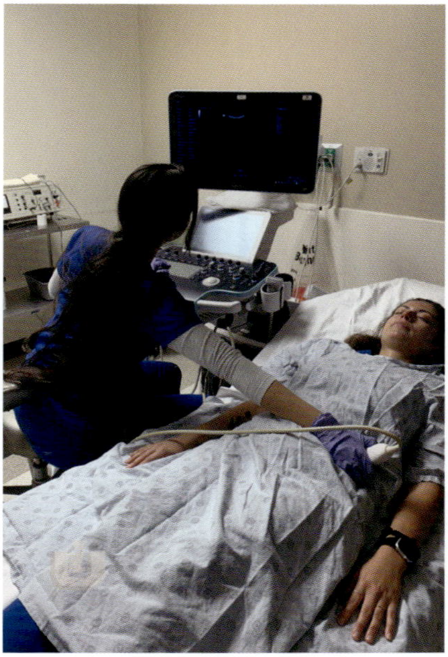

Fig. 15-9. **INCORRECT POSTURE** *Chair, machine and monitor are too high, arm and back are not supported, and not sitting in chair properly.*

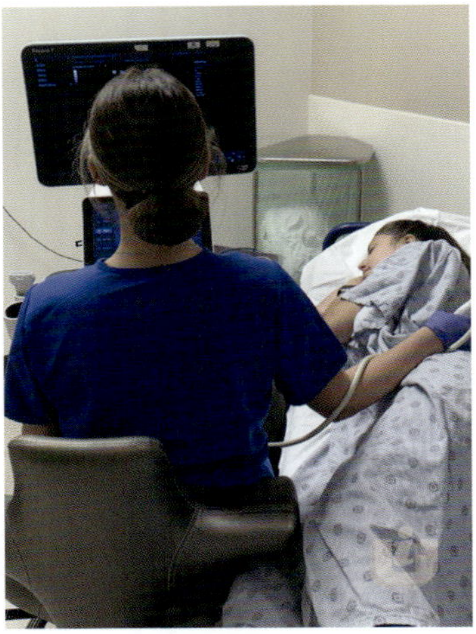

Fig. 15-10. CORRECT POSTURE
Move the patient as close to you as possible, use a chair and adjust its height for support, adjust height of the machine and monitor. Monitor should be at eye level.

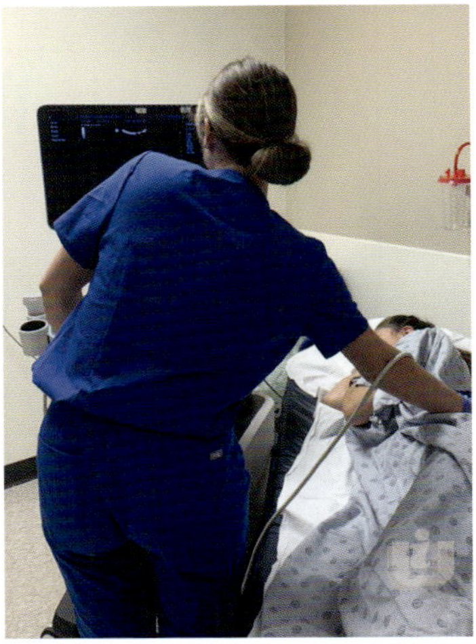

Fig. 15-11. INCORRECT POSTURE
Avoid neck extension/rotation, awkward trunk postures (e.g., leaning sideways) and excessive reach.

Standing Venous Insufficiency

Achieving good ergonomics during a standing venous insufficiency ultrasound requires the use of additional equipment.

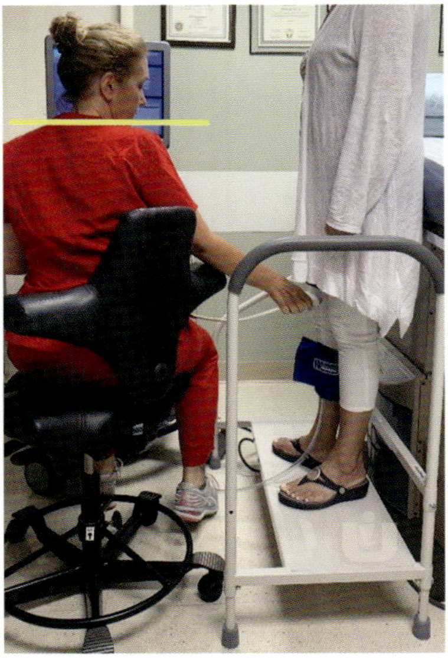

Fig. 15-12. CORRECT
The shoulders should remain parallel when scanning. Use a step or platform to raise the patient to a good height.

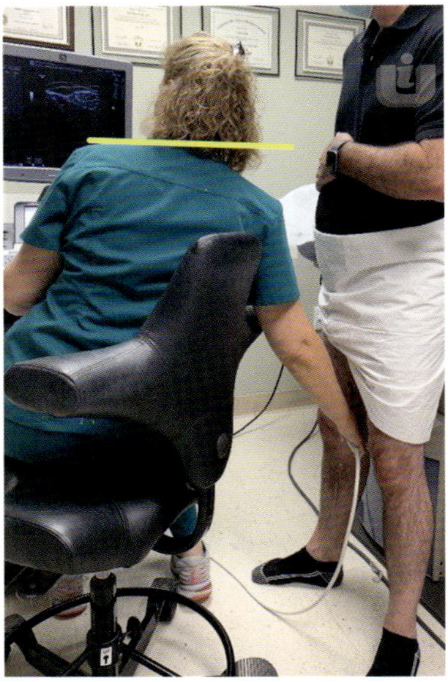

Fig. 15-13. INCORRECT
Right shoulder is much lower than the left shoulder.

Automated Cuff Augmentation Devices

The demonstration of venous reflux or lack of venous reflux most often relies on an augmentation of the calf muscle to propel the blood in the antegrade (normal) direction followed by a rapid release of the muscle to watch for retrograde (abnormal) flow. Automated rapid cuff augmentation devices are available to replace the need for the sonographer to manually augment the calf.

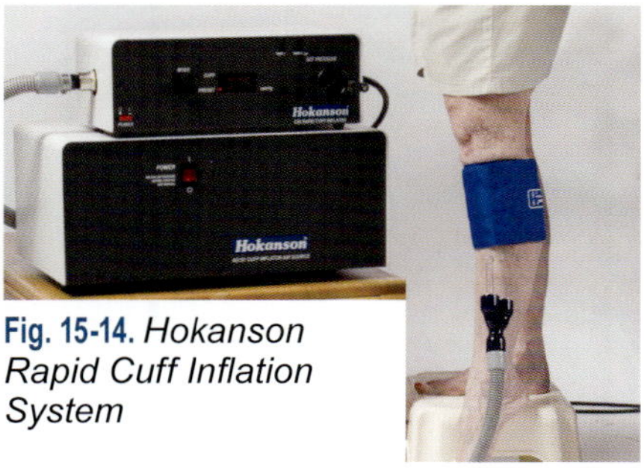

Fig. 15-14. *Hokanson Rapid Cuff Inflation System*

Photo courtesy of Hokanson, Bellevue, WA hokansonvascular.com

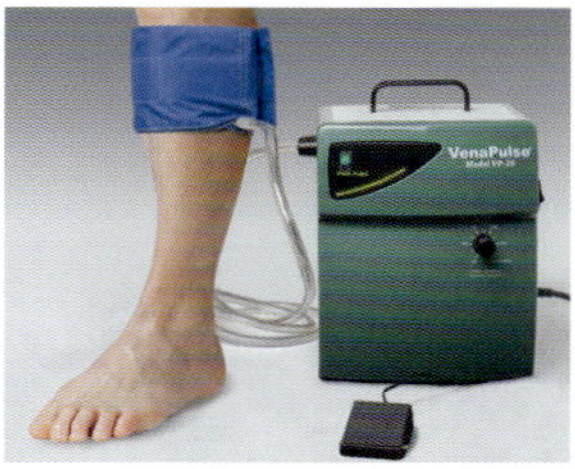

Fig. 15-15. *VenaPulse® Hands-Free Augmentation Device*

Photo courtesy of ACI Medical San Marcos, CA. acimedical.com/products/venapulse

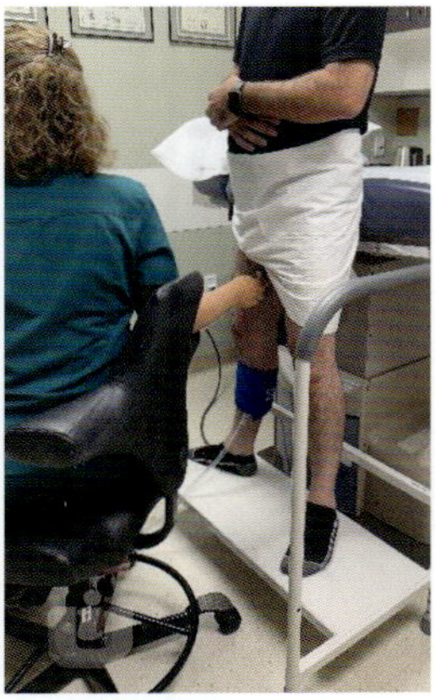

Fig. 15-16. CORRECT *Using an automated cuff augmentation device allows for handsfree augmentation to maintain proper posture.*

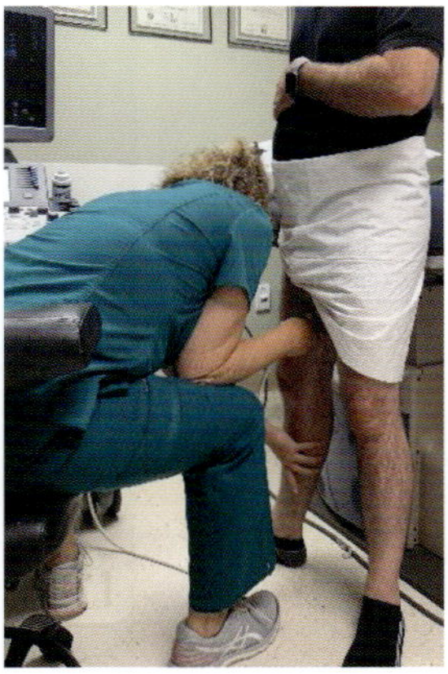

Fig. 15-17. INCORRECT *Hand augmentation of the calf causes strain on multiple parts of the sonographer's body.*

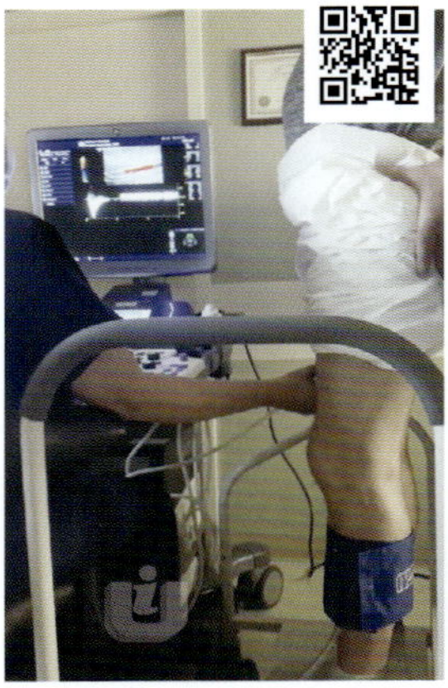

Fig. 15-18. *Cine loop demonstrating the use of an automated cuff augmentation device*

Height Adjustable Table

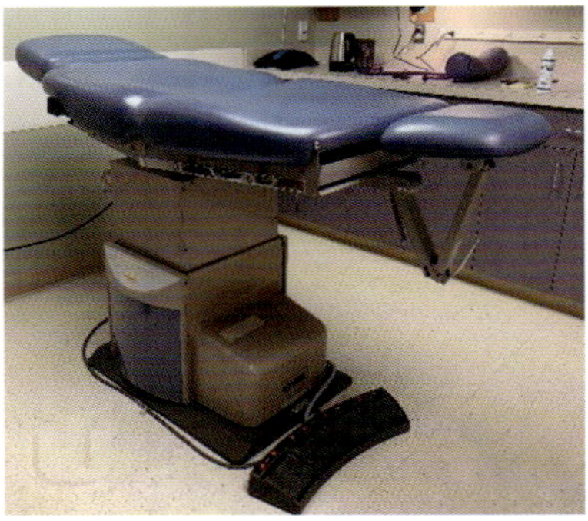

Fig. 15-19. *Motorized height adjustable exam table.*

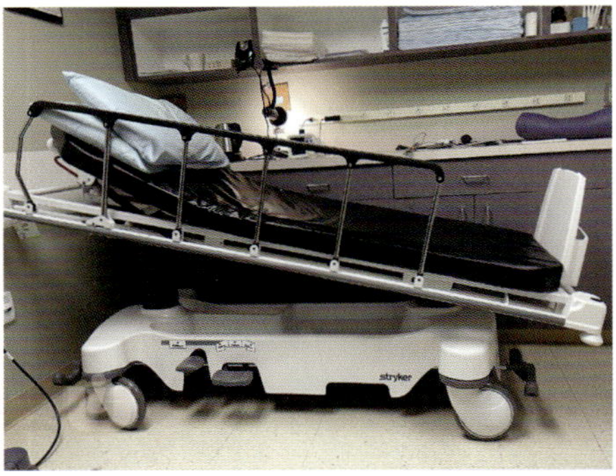

Fig. 15-20. *Manual (foot pump) height adjustable stretcher.*

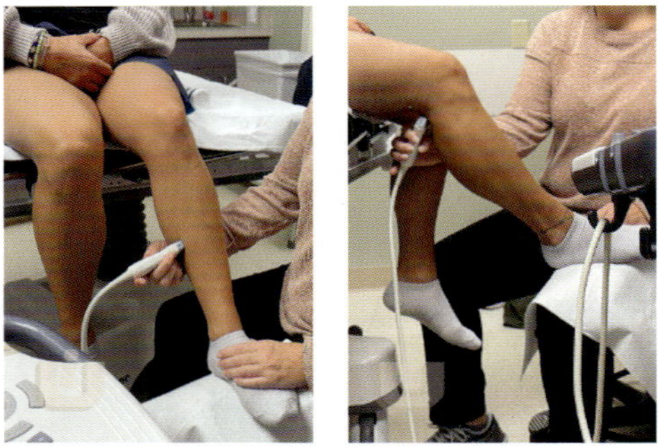

Fig. 15-21. *Alternate positions for evaluation of the calf veins; seated on the side of the bed with leg dependent and foot resting on examiner's lap or stool. When using this position, be sure the back of the leg or knee is not resting against the bed.*

Scanning Chair/Stool

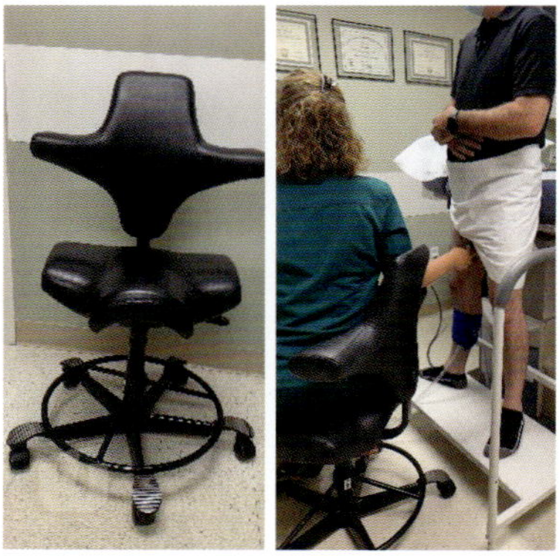

Fig. 15-22. *The ideal stool for this test has a saddle style seat which allows the user to be seated in multiple positions including the position pictured above. Note the seat and the back rest have been turned so the "wing" can support the scanning arm.*

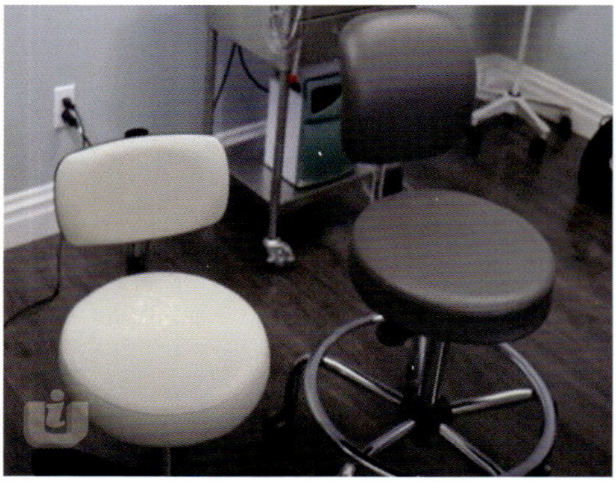

Fig. 15-23. *At a minimum, the sonographer should use a stool/chair that has a pneumatic height adjustment and can easily swivel.*

Sitting at Your Desk

- Use chairs that have wheels, are height adjustable and support the lumbar area (low back) with a tilt feature whenever possible. A footrest is another option. The seat should be deep enough to fit most of the thigh, up to the knee.
- Maintaining a neutral position supports the natural curves of the spine and keeps your body in proper alignment. Sustaining good posture will help you complete tasks essential to job performance. You should concentrate on trying to keep your head, neck, shoulders, elbows and hips aligned when sitting.
- Try to keep your hips higher than your knees to some extent.
- Try not to tense your shoulders, keep them relaxed.
- Keep elbows bent at >100°

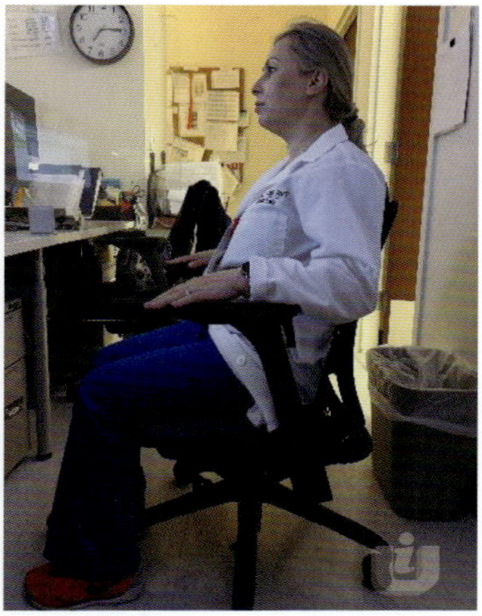

Fig. 15-24. *Neutral position when sitting; head, neck shoulders and hips are aligned, back is supported*

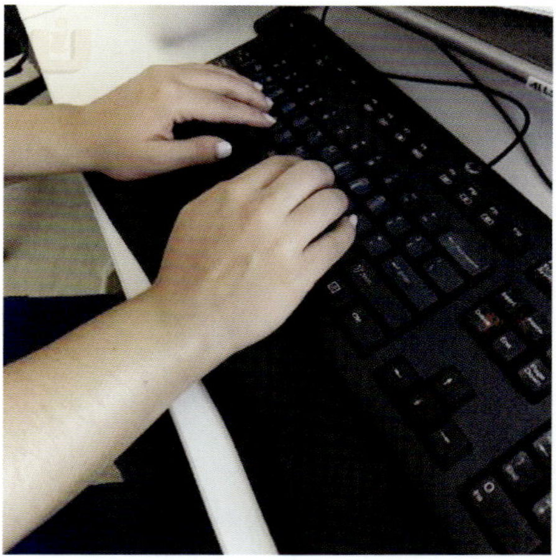

Fig. 15-25. *Keep your wrists straight when typing. Commercially available wrist supports might be helpful.*

After Scanning and Reporting

- Research suggests that there are possible benefits from stretching between patients. Walking or gentle exercise increases blood flow to your joints.[4, 5]
- Rest periods during the workday are seen as essential.[4]
- Work to strengthen all of the muscle groups in the arm, hand and shoulder. Pilates or other exercises that strengthen your core have been suggested as a way to reduce the risk of WRMSDs and promote career longevity.

Important to Note

- Congress passed the Occupational Safety and Health Act of 1970 creating the group known as OSHA (Occupational Safety and Health Administration) to ensure safe and healthy working conditions for employees. OSHA is part of the US Department of Labor and allows employees to file complaints about workplace safety and substandard conditions. If someone believes their employer is not following OSHA standards, they can file a complaint online, via fax, mail/email or in person. Call your local OSHA office for more information at 800-321-6742 (OSHA) [6]
- Sonographers share in the responsibility for complying with OSHA standards. This chapter provides guidance for practicing proper form and scanning techniques.
- Take the time to properly set up the room, position the patient properly and be sure to use any equipment that your employer provides such as support cushions, scanning chairs, etc. Offer input about equipment purchases so that the right equipment is selected.
- Consider regular monitoring between coworkers to support proper body mechanics as a team. Involve sonographers in the writing of safety guidelines and policies for the department.
- Ultrasound manufacturers have made substantial improvements to equipment design over the years including some of the modifications listed here: [5]
  - Central break controls (instead of one brake on every wheel)
  - Height adjustable keyboards and monitors
  - Footrests to encourage neutral positioning, redesigning units so technologists' knees and legs are unobstructed when sitting.
  - Systems designed so transporting takes no more than 50 pounds of force by one technologist to push/pull equipment on bare flooring.
  - Lighter weight transducers that are more slip resistant and encourage better grip
  - Better cable lengths and management systems for transducers
  - Optimization of control layout, options for right- and left-handed users
  - Better font size and type
- Poor staff morale and timely access to patient care are directly related to workforce shortages caused by WRMSDs.
- Encourage students to practice proper body mechanics early in their careers.
- Report symptoms early to your supervisor so you can discuss improvements and get help before it is too late.

References

1. Pike I, Russo A, Berkowitz J, Baker J, Lessoway V. The Prevalence of Musculoskeletal Disorders Among Diagnostic Medical Sonographers. (1997). *Journal of Diagnostic Medical Sonography 13(*5), 219-227.
2. Evans K, Roll S, Baker J. Work-Related Musculoskeletal Disorders (WRMSD) Among Registered Diagnostic Medical Sonographers and Vascular Technologists: A Representative Sample. (2009). *Journal of Diagnostic Medical Sonography, 25*(6), 287-299.
3. Murphey, S. (2017). Work related musculoskeletal disorders in sonography. *Journal of Diagnostic Medical Sonography, 33*(5), 354-369.
4. Harrison G., Harris A. (2015). Work-related musculoskeletal disorders in ultrasound: Can you reduce risk? Ultrasound, 23(4), 224-230.
5. Alaniz J, Veale B. Stretching for Sonographers: A Literature Review of Sonographer-Reported Musculoskeletal Injuries. (2013). *Journal of Diagnostic Medical Sonography, 29(*4), 188-190.
6. *How to File a Safety and Health Complaint. Occupational Safety and Health Administration* (2016). OSHA.gov. Available at: https://www.osha.gov/workers/file_complaint.html. Accessed August 23, 2021.
7. Industry Standards for the Prevention of Work-Related Musculoskeletal Disorders in Sonography. Consensus Conference on Work-Related Musculoskeletal Disorders in Sonography. (2011). *Journal of Diagnostic Medical Sonography, 27*(1), 14–18.
8. *Employer Responsibilities; Work Related Musculoskeletal Disorders in Sonography White Paper.* Society of Diagnostic Sonography. (n.d.). https://www.sdms.org/resources/careers/work-related musculoskeletaldisorders/employer-responsibilities. (Accessed Aug 30, 2021)
9. *Professional Performance Guidelines. Society for Vascular Ultrasound.* (2019.). Society of Vascular Ultrasound. https://www.svu.org/practice-resources/professional-performanceguidelines/. (Accessed Aug 30, 2021)
10. Environment Health and Safety. *Maintain a Neutral Posture.* University of California San Francisco. https://ehs.ucsf.edu/maintainneutral-posture. Accessed 8/23/21.

Definition

Correlative tests are alternative testing modalities used when there is a need to further investigate disease extent and clearly define etiology identified by duplex ultrasound exam. Alternative tests are also useful when clinical correlation is suggested; the vascular exam is limited or non-diagnostic.

Differential Tests

- Computerized Tomography (CT)
- Computerized Tomography Pulmonary Angiogram (CTPA)
- Magnetic Resonance Imaging (MRI)
- Magnetic Resonance Venography (MRV)
- Angiography (Venogram)
- D-dimer blood test
- Ventilation/Perfusion Scan (VQ Lung Scan)

Computed Tomography (CT)

A CT is a widely used diagnostic imaging test for many specialties. Tomography is derived from the Greek word "tomo" for slice. Computed tomography is a computerized x-ray procedure that creates multiple thin cross-sectional images (stacked one on top of the other) through a narrow beam of x-rays and electronic detectors that rotate swiftly around the body in a spiral motion.

The two-dimensional (2D) image provides detailed diagnostic information of the internal organs, bones, blood vessels, other soft tissues, and any abnormalities (e.g., luminal reductions, tumors, foreign bodies, etc.). Multiplanar reconstruction CT and three-dimensional (3-D) rendering techniques use computer software to provide alternative views of the information gathered. During the procedure, the patient will lie supine on a narrow, motorized table that will slide into the donut-shaped device. A special dye called contrast may be used for certain CTs to highlight blood vessels. There are several types of CTs:

Spiral CT/Helical CT: Traditional CT is used for a broad range of diseases, abnormalities, and conditions, with or without contrast.

Computerized Tomography Pulmonary Angiogram (CTPA): Used to obtain images of the pulmonary arteries, mainly to diagnose pulmonary emboli (PE), using contrast.

Computerized Tomography Angiography (CTA): Utilized to obtain images specifically of arteries, veins, associated vascular diseases, and related conditions, using contrast.

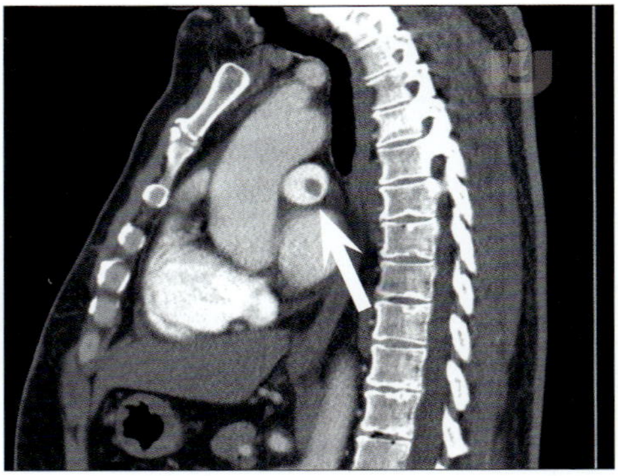

Fig. 16-1. *CTPA image of pulmonary embolus*

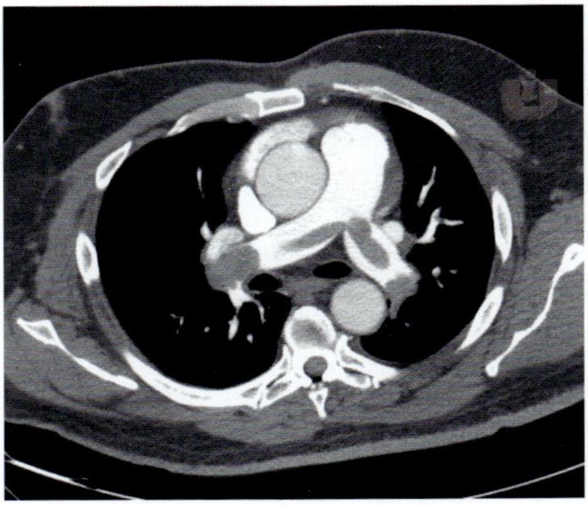

Fig. 16-2. *CPTA image of a saddle embolus. (Scan QR code for pulmonary embolus images in other body parts.)*

Indications

- Cardiovascular-related concerns
  - Initial diagnosis
  - Used to monitor disease progression and effectiveness of treatment
- Musculoskeletal-related concerns
- Neurological-related concerns
- Liver & gastrointestinal related concerns
- Tumors/other diseases of the body
- Procedure guidance
- Internal injuries and bleeding

Contraindications/Limitations

- Allergy to iodinated contrast agent
- Renal impairment
- History of anaphylactic reaction
- Hyperthyroidism
- Pheochromocytoma (benign, adrenal gland tumor)
- Myasthenia gravis (chronic autoimmune disorder)
- Pregnancy and/or breastfeeding
- Arrhythmia
- Body habitus
- Children under two years of age
- Extreme anxiety
- Inability to lie still/flat

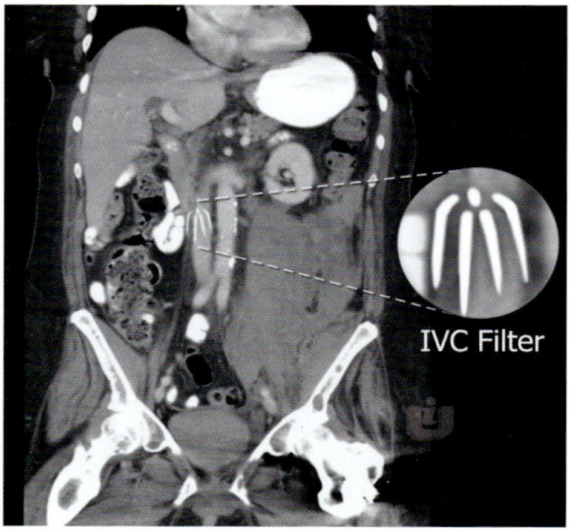

Fig. 16-3. *CT imaging of an IVC filter*

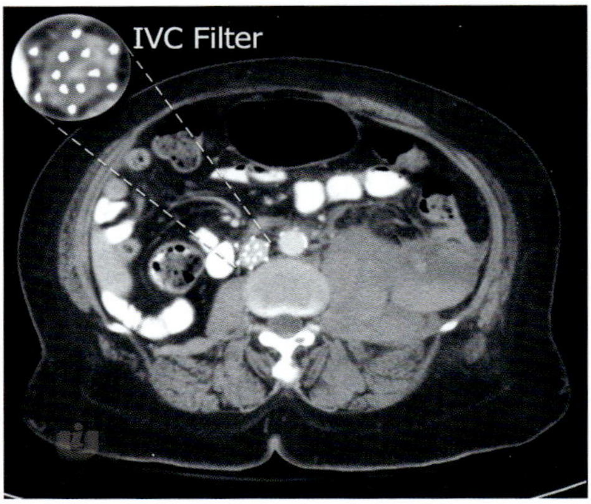

Fig. 16-4. *CT imaging of an IVC filter*

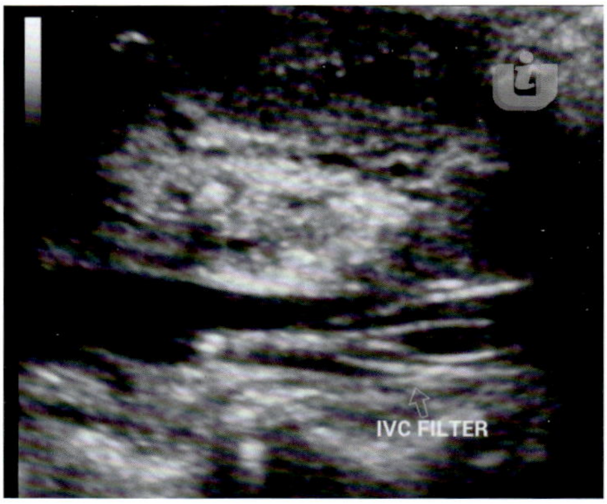

Fig. 16-5. *IVC filter on duplex scan*

Magnetic Resonance Imaging

MRI is a diagnostic imaging test of the body's anatomy and physiological processes using magnetic components of our own natural elements. The MRI scanner is a large tube that uses a strong circular magnet, radio wave frequency, and the hydrogen atoms in the body to create detailed multiple cross-sectional images (2D/3D) of internal organs, bones, blood vessels, other soft tissues, and any abnormalities. When the hydrogen atoms and their protons are exposed to the magnetic field, different tissues will appear darker/lighter depending on the number of protons.

During the exam, the patient is placed on a narrow, motorized table that moves into the scanner. The scanner can be open or closed. The MRI scan itself is non-invasive, but IV or oral contrast may be used, depending on the information needed. Since MRI uses radiation in the "radiofrequency" range, there is little risk of developing cancer, even with repeated exposure.

Magnetic Resonance Venography (MRV): A study of veins in the body, including the organs, neck, chest, abdomen, pelvis, and extremities. Contrast agents can be used for image enhancement.

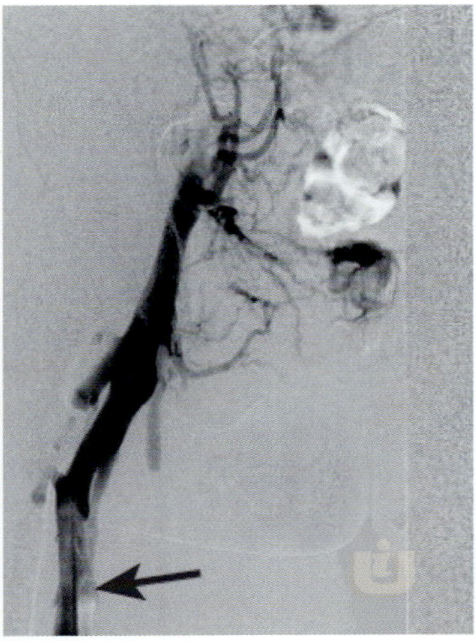

Fig. 16-6. *MRV of an iliac vein thrombosis. Note the filling defect (at arrow) and collateral network toward midline.*

Indications

- Cardiovascular-related concerns
- Neurological-related concerns
- Musculoskeletal-related concerns
- Liver and gastrointestinal related concerns
- Clinical correlation with angiogram
- Tumors/diseases of the body

Contraindications/Limitations

- Metal implants in the body (total replacement joints, clips, stents, pacemakers, defibrillators, cochlear implants)
- Oxygen-dependent breathing
- Pregnancy
- Claustrophobia
- Body habitus
- Renal impairment (non-dialysis patient)
- Extreme anxiety
- Inability to lie still/flat

Angiography (Venogram)

Angiography is derived from the Greek word "angio" for vessel. An angiogram is used to image the two main kinds of blood vessels; arteries (arteriography) and veins (venography or phlebography).

Venogram

There are two types of venograms, ascending and descending. Venograms are no longer used as screening studies and have mostly been replaced by duplex ultrasound imaging. During this invasive angiographic imaging technique, a radio-opaque contrast material is injected into the veins with a needle.

Descending Venography

Descending venography is used to assess for chronic venous insufficiency. The contrast is injected into the common femoral vein (or into a superficial vein in the upper extremity). On the x-ray film, the contrast in the veins either:

- Returns to the heart (indicating that valves are competent).
- Appears to "pool" in the extremity (indicating that valves are incompetent).

Ascending Venography

Ascending venography images the veins of patients with suspected Deep Vein Thormbosis (DVT), venous malformations, venous aneurysms, and incompetent perforators. Contrast material is injected into a vein on the dorsum aspect of the foot or a segment distal to the area of interest.

- If intravenous thrombus is present, there will be partial or complete lack of contrast material that appears as a deficit on the x-ray image.
- Contrast helps highlight the dilated size of the vein in cases of a venous aneurysm.
- Venous malformation will be highlighted on the image as an area with larger diameter veins that often appear "tangled."

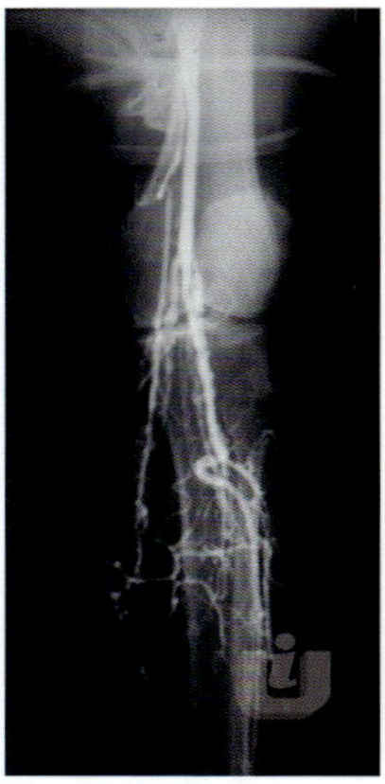

Fig. 16-7. *Popliteal and tibial veins on venogram.*

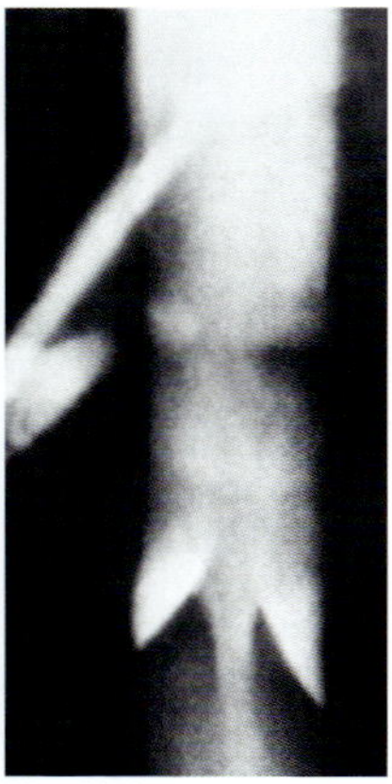

Fig. 16-8. *Venous valve on descending venogram.*

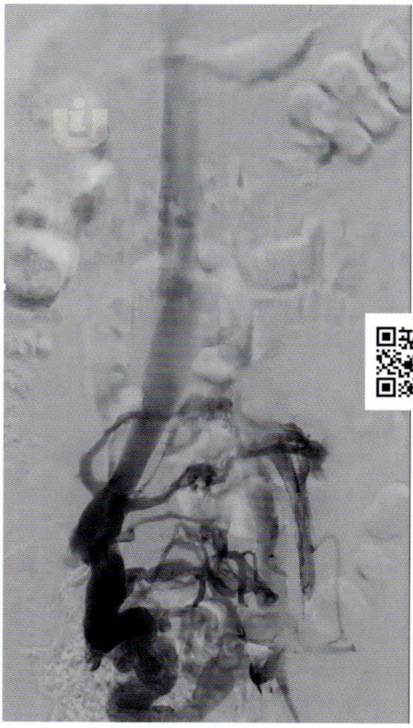

Fig. 16-9. *Cine loop using fluoroscopy with contrast demonstrating the absence of filling of the left CIV. The next cine loop shows post-stenting filling.*

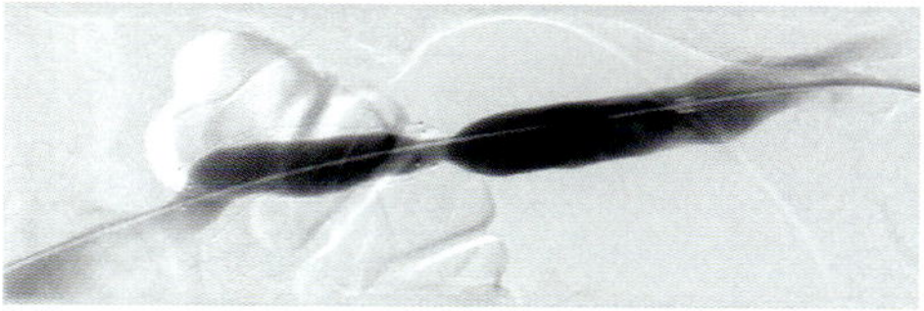

Fig. 16-10. *Venogram of a stented left iliac vein with partial thrombosis.*

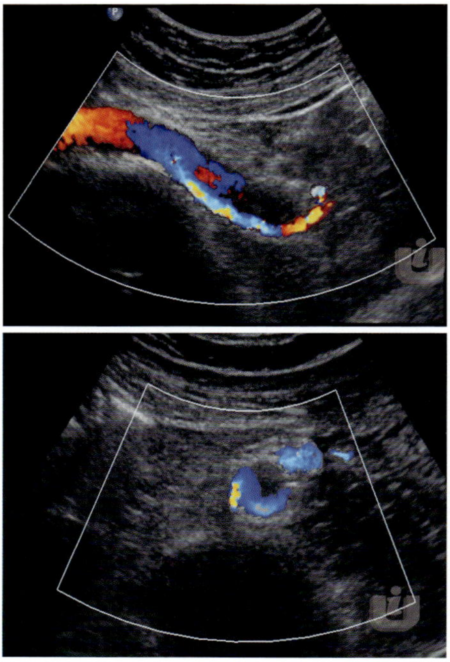

Fig. 16-11. *Longitudinal and transverse views of a partially thrombosed iliac vein stent demonstrating a lack of wall-to-wall color filling with visualization of the thrombus.* *Images courtesy of Aleta Rigsby RVT, RPhS VeinCare Centers of Tennessee*

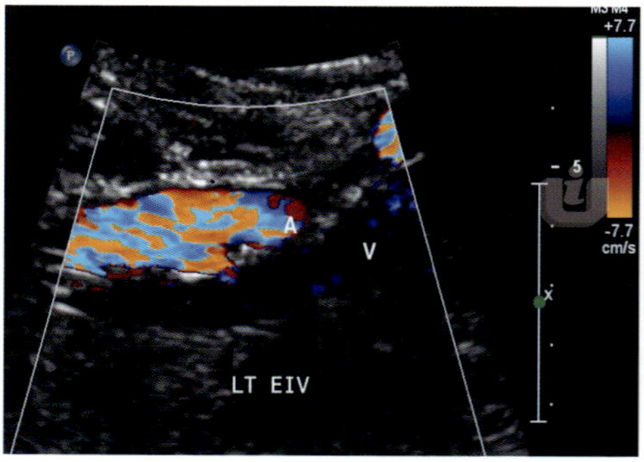

Fig. 16-12. *Occluded left iliac vein stent.*

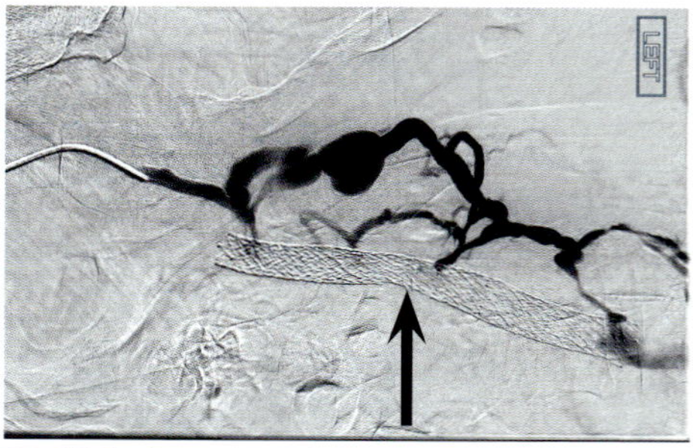

Fig. 16-13. *Imaging of an occluded left iliac vein stent using venography.*

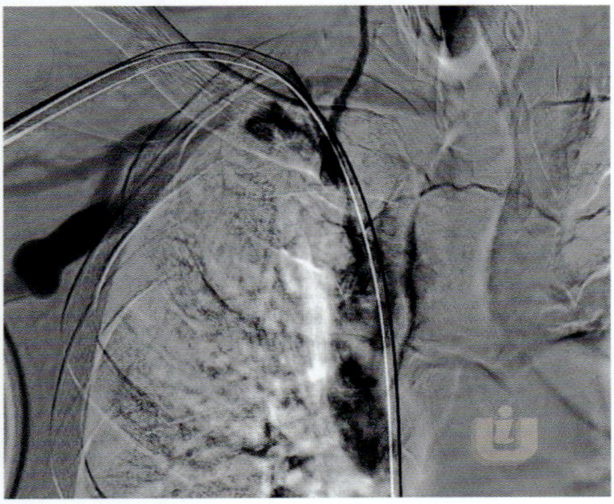

Fig. 16-14. *Innominate vein stenosis on venography*

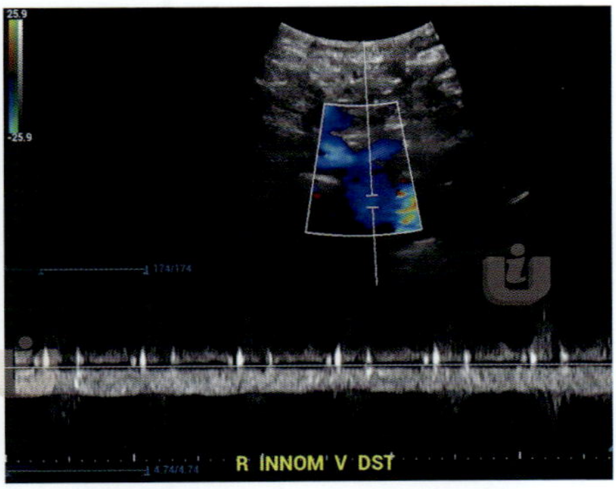

Fig. 16-15. *Continuous venous Doppler waveform pattern in the distal innominate vein from the digital subtraction venogram in Fig. 16-14.*

Digital Subtraction Venography (DSV) may be used to obtain a more intense image of the veins. Bones and tissue are digitally subtracted, allowing the veins to be seen with greater clarity and detail.

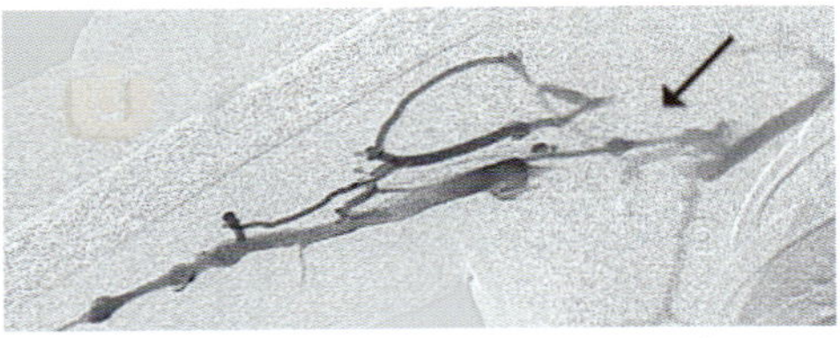

Fig. 16-16. *Digital subtraction venography*

Indications

- Deep vein thrombosis (DVT)
- Venous insufficiency
- Venous stenosis
- Adjunct imaging during venous thrombolysis
- Venous anomalies
- Venous vascular malformation
- Venous hypertension
- Venous aneurysm
- Vein mapping (preoperative planning)

Contraindications/Limitations

- Active cellulitis (involving the extremity to be imaged)
- Allergy to iodinated contrast agent
- Renal impairment
- Antiplatelet/blood thinning medication
- Coagulopathy
- Extreme anxiety
- Inability to lie still/flat

Intravascular Ultrasound

Intravascular Ultrasound (IVUS) is a medical imaging modality using a specially designed catheter with a miniaturized ultrasound transducer attached to the distal end of the catheter. The proximal end of the catheter is attached to computerized ultrasound equipment. It allows for the use of ultrasound technology to see from inside blood vessels through the surrounding blood column, visualizing the endothelium (inner wall) of blood vessels.

IVUS is typically used in conjunction with arteriogram/venogram with the intent to treat significant lesions if they are identified. An example of treatment would be Percutaneous Transluminal Angioplasty (PTA).

Vessel access is obtained using ultrasound guidance. A needle is inserted into the vessel, and a guide wire is introduced. A sheath is inserted into the vessel to allow for the introduction of the IVUS catheter.

IVUS of the vein is useful for the morphologic diagnosis of iliac venous outflow obstruction and is an invaluable tool in the accurate placement of venous stents after venoplasty. IVUS can accurately determine lumen size, including cross-sectional area stenosis. It identifies intraluminal lesions, wall thickness, delineates diseased or compressed vein segments, identifies the confluence of the iliac vein and IVC, identifies normal vein segments for landing sites of stents, and helps estimate the stent diameter needed for a vein.[14] *(Figs. 16-17 through 16-19)*

Indications

- Edema/swelling (especially when unilateral)
- Limb pain/tenderness
- Ulceration (venous or arterial)
- Discoloration in the gaiter area
- Iliac vein compression indicated during noninvasive testing

Contraindications/limitations

- Obesity
- Severe edema
- Inability to lie still
- Inability to be anticoagulated

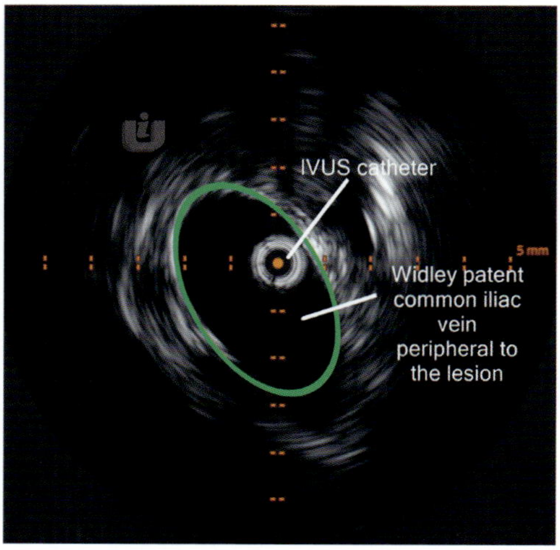

Fig. 16-17. *Visualization of the widely patent lumen of the peripheral left CIV.*

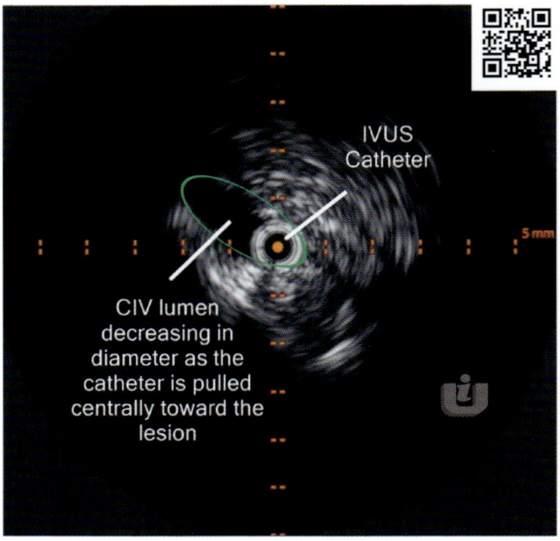

Fig. 16-18. *Visibly narrowed left CIV lumen as the catheter is moved centrally toward the lesion.*

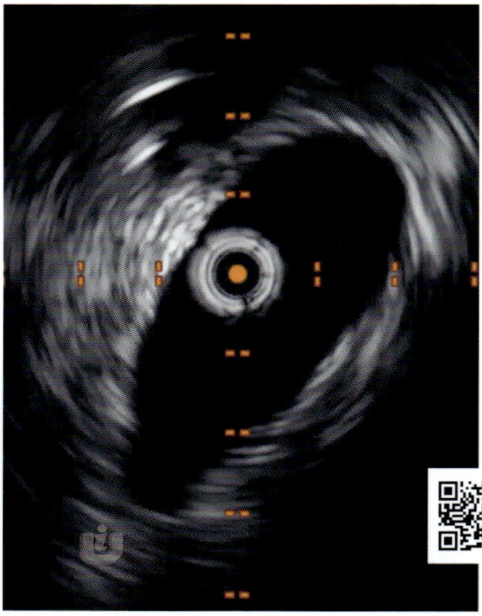

Fig. 16-19. *Cine loop of IVUS visualizing the Lt CIV post stenting.*

VQ scan

A VQ scan is a scintigraphic nuclear diagnostic technique that detects radiation emitted from radioactive tracers that are inhaled and injected intravenously, constructing a physiologic map of the lungs, representing air and blood flow patterns. The primary utilization of the scan is to help diagnose thrombus that has traveled to the lungs, known as a Pulmonary Embolus (PE). The test comprises two nuclear scans that can be performed simultaneously or one after the other. The first part of the exams is known as the ventilation scan, and the second is the perfusion scan.

Ventilation Scan

A radio-isotope labeled aerosol will be inhaled into the lungs for a few minutes through a non-rebreathing mask. The inhaled micro aerosol particles extend to the distal-most aspects of the lungs. A nuclear scan using a gamma camera is then used to identify the areas of the lungs that are not receiving any or adequate air. Scans at different angles are obtained. The scan has three phases: initial breath, equilibrium, and washout.

Perfusion Scan

An intravenously injected radioactive contrast travels throughout the lungs, illuminating areas that do not receive adequate blood flow. Similarly, a nuclear scan is performed where multiple images of the patient's chest are taken at different angles.

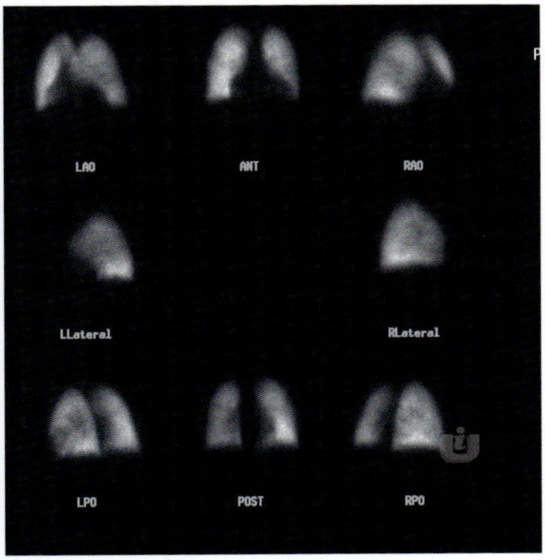

Fig. 16-20. *Normal VQ scan.*

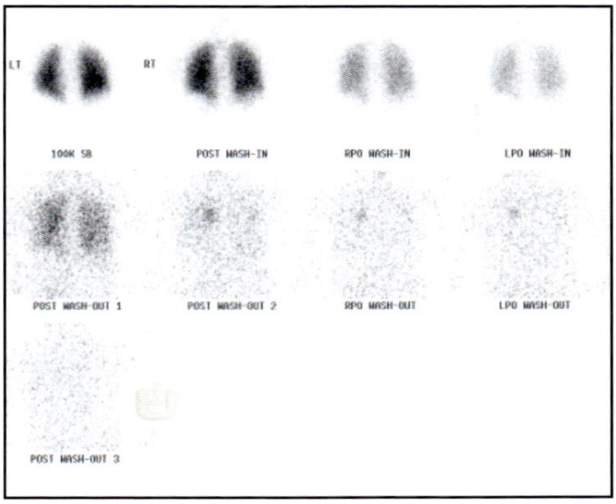

Fig. 16-21. *Abnormal VQ scan*

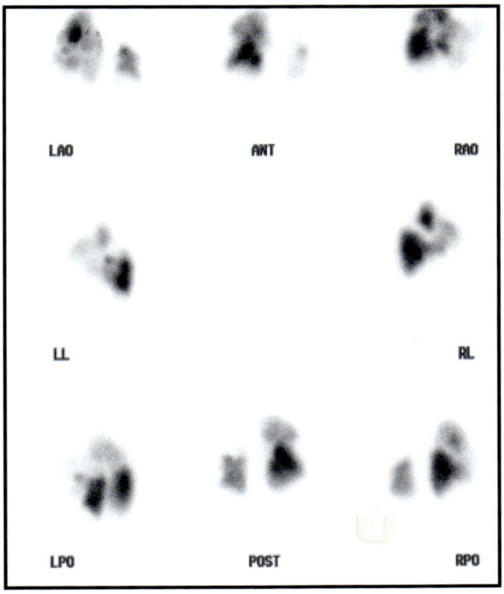

Fig. 16-22. *Abnormal perfusion scan.*

Indications

- CTPA for suspected PE is contraindicated or inconclusive
- Identification of chronic or acute PE
- Determining PE resolution
- Pregnancy with PE suspicion and normal chest radiograph
- Congenital pulmonary diseases
- Congenital cardiac diseases
- To confirm the presence of bronchopleural fistulae
- To evaluate the cause of pulmonary hypertension
- Evaluation of lung transplant
- Measuring lung function (preoperative/ monitoring)

Contraindications/Limitations

- Potential fetal exposure: risk versus benefit should be assessed. Low-dose, perfusion-only imaging technique may be indicated.
- Lactating patients should stop breastfeeding for 24 hours after the scan.

Table 16-1. Pioped Criteria (Prospective Investigation of Pulmonary Embolism Diagnosis)

The **p**rospective **i**nvestigation **o**f **p**ulmonary **e**mbolism **d**iagnosis (PIOPED) criteria states ranges for diagnosing the likelihood of a pulmonary embolism (PE) by VQ scan:

Probability	Likelihood of PE
High	80 - 100%
Intermediate	20 - 80%
Low	0 - 20%

Source: Medoff, B. (9-13-2008). Pulmonary ventilation/perfusion scan-overview. Retrieved from http://www.umm.edu/ency/article/003828.htm

Table 16-2. Clinical Prediction Criteria for Pulmonary Embolism

Condition	# Points Assigned
Clinical DVT symptoms	+ 3
Alternative diagnosis as likely or more than DVT	+ 3
Heart rate >100 beats/min	+ 1.5
Major surgery/trauma within the past four weeks	+ 1.5
History of DVT/PE	+ 1.5
Hemoptysis	+ 1
Malignancy	+ 1
Interpretation of risk according to point total	
High	≥ 6 pts
Moderate	2 - 6 pts
Low	≤ 2 pts

Source: Line JA, Wells PS. (2003). Methodology for a rapid protocol to rule out pulmonary embolism in the emergency department. *Annal Emerg Med; 42*, 266 - 275.

D-dimer

D-dimer is an adjunct intravenous blood test used to help rule out abnormal blood clotting. However, it is not used independently for a diagnosis. The test identifies the presence and the amount of a protein product in the blood called D-dimer. The moment the clotting cascade is activated and thrombus formation occurs, the body begins slowly breaking down the protein releasing the protein fragment into the blood. An enzyme called plasmin dissolves the thrombus into small pieces for removal. The thrombus is partly made up of threads of cross-linked fibrin. As the thrombus lysis, the subsequent fibrin fragments are called Fibrin Degradation Products (FDP), and one of the final products is D-dimer. The level of D-dimer detected is dependent on the amount of cross-linked fibrin that is lysed; as thrombus formation increases, D-dimer production is higher.

The D-dimer blood test is low cost, easy to obtain, and can be an initial screening for deep vein thrombosis and Venous ThromboEmbolism (VTE). When a positive D-dimer test is combined with a high clinical probability for DVT, further imaging tests are obtained (e.g., venous ultrasound exam, CT, direct pulmonary angiography, or ventilation-perfusion scan). Elevated D-dimer levels are also seen in other conditions that cause the production and dismantling of fibrin (not just DVT).

- A D-dimer value is reported in units of parts per million (ng/ml or ug/ml).
- D-dimer is also known as fragment D-dimer and fibrin degradation fragment
- Fibrinolytic activity in the blood reflects the breakdown of fibrin.
- D-dimer test results can be used as a predictive value for active blood clotting. Therefore an elevated level suggests blood clot formation, whereas a low level (within normal range value) indicates there is likely no significant activity of blood clot formation in the body.

- A normal D-dimer result, indicating a lack of fibrinolytic activity, is more valuable than a positive D-dimer value. See the "Contraindications/Limitations" section.
- Following an initial encounter of unprovoked DVT and treatment of at least six months, a D-dimer test can help predict the likelihood of recurrent venous thrombosis.
- D-dimer levels can also be measured while a patient is on anticoagulant therapy. If normal, the anticoagulants can be stopped, and the test may be repeated in 30 days. If the test result remains normal, the risk of recurrent thrombosis is low (about 3% per year). If the test result is positive, the risk of re-occurrence is >10% per year. The test should be repeated in 3 months.

Indications

Suspicion of DVT

- Lower/upper extremity or tenderness
- Lower/upper extremity swelling or edema
- Lower/upper extremity discoloration
- Disseminated Intravascular Coagulation (DIC): a rare but serious condition where blood vessels clot throughout the body

Suspicion of PE

- Acute shortness of breath or labored breathing
- Lung-related chest pain
- Rapid heart rate
- Acute coughing with or without hemoptysis
- Fainting
- Stroke

*See also **TABLE 16-3:** Risk Factors for Acute Deep Venous Thrombosis (Caprini Risk Score) on page 250*

Contraindications/Limitations

Note: Patients may have elevated D-dimer levels due to conditions other than DVT.

- Trauma
- Infection
- Recent surgery
- Heart attack
- Some cancers
- Liver disease (fibrin will not clear)
- High rheumatoid factor, trauma
- Pregnancy
- Advancing age

References

1. Medoff, B. (9-13-2008). Pulmonary ventilation/perfusion scan-overview. Retrieved from http://www.umm.edu/ency/article/003828.htm.
2. Dunn KL, Wolf JP, Dorfman DM, Fitzpatrick P, Baker JL, Goldhaber SZ. (2002). Normal D-dimer levels in emergency department patients suspected of acute pulmonary embolism. *J Am Coll Cardiology, 40,* 1475-1478.
3. American Association for Clinical Chemistry. (June 18, 2010) *D-dimer.* Retrieved from http://www.labtestsonline.org/understanding/analytes/d_dimer/test.html
4. Wells PS, Anderson DR, Rodger M, et al. (2003). Evaluation of D-dimer in the diagnosis of suspected deep-vein thrombosis". *N. Engl. J. Med. 349* (13): 1227–35.
5. Kutinsky H, Blakely S, Roche V. (1999). Normal D-dimer levels in patients with pulmonary embolism. *Arch Intern Med.* 159, 1569-1572.
6. RadiologyInfo.org (March 15, 2010). Retrieved from http://www.radiologyinfo.org
7. Medical Journal of Australia.www.mja.com.au/public/issues/180_11_070604/dic10124_fm.html
8. McKenzie J, Goergen, S. (2017, Sept. 15). Computed Tomography (CT). Inside Radiology. https://www.insideradiology.com.au/
9. computed-tomography-hp/
10. Berger A. (2002). Magnetic resonance imaging. BMJ (Clinical research ed.), 324(7328), 35. https://doi.org/10.1136/bmj.324.7328.35
11. Cronenwett, J.L. (2014). Venography. In Rutherford Vascular Surgery (8th ed., pp. 307-311). Philadelphia. Elsevier Saunders
12. Bradley, A.M., Loscalzo, J. (2007) The Role of Platelets in Fibrinolysis. Science Direct. https://www.sciencedirect.com/topics/medicine-and-dentistry/fibrinolysis#:-:text=Fibrinolysis%20 describes%20the%20process%20of,trauma%20or%20in%20pathological%20thrombosis.
13. Mirza H, Hashmi MF. Lung Ventilation Perfusion Scan (VQ Scan) [Updated 2020 Oct 24]. In: StatPearls [Internet]. Treasure Island (FL): StatPearls Publishing; 2021 Jan-. Available from: https://www.ncbi.nlm.nih.gov/books/NBK564428/
14. Philips Volcano. (2017, June). The Value of Intravascular Ultrasound Use in Hemodialysis Arteriovenous Access. A panel of experts addresses how and why clinicians today are increasingly reaching for IVUS during AV access evaluations. With Bart Dolmatch, MD; Rick de Graaf, MD, PhD; Jeffrey E. Hull, MD; and Edward Pavillard, MD. Endovascular Today. https://evtoday.com/articles/2017-june/the-value-of-intravascular-ultrasound-use-in-hemodialysis-arteriovenous-access
15. Neglén, P., & Raju, S. (2002). Intravascular ultrasound scan evaluation of the obstructed vein. Journal of vascular surgery, 35(4), 694–700. https://doi.org/10.1067/mva.2002.121127.)
16. Romaric, L., Falvo, N., Galland, C., Fréchier, L., Ledan, F., Midulla, M., Chevallier, O. (2020). Intravascular Ultrasound in the Endovascular Treatment of Patients With Peripheral Arterial Disease: Current Role and Future Perspectives. Frontiers in Cardiovascular Medicine, 7, 1-8. https://www.frontiersin.org/article/10.3389/fcvm.2020.551861. DOI=10.3389/fcvm.2020.551861

Table 16-3. **Risk Factors for Acute Deep Venous Thrombosis (Caprini Risk Score)**

Download this form or take the assessment online at capriniriskscore.org

Illinois State Medical Society

Are You at Risk for DVT?

FOR PATIENTS Complete this risk assessment tool to find out.

Be CLOT Aware — Know Your Caprini Score And Save Your Life

❑ Male
❑ Female

Name ______________________ Today's Date ______________

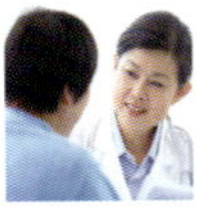

Only your doctor can determine if you are at risk for Deep Vein Thrombosis (DVT), a blood clot that forms in one of the deep veins of your legs. A review of your personal history and current health may determine if you are at risk for developing this condition. Take a moment to complete this form for yourself (or complete it for a loved one). Then be sure to talk with your doctor about your risk for DVT and what you can do to help protect against it. Your doctor may want to keep a copy in your file for future reference.

Directions:

1. Check all statements that apply to you.
2. Enter the number of points for each of your checked statements in the space at right.
3. Add up all points to reach your total DVT Risk Score. Then, share your completed form with your doctor.

Add 1 point for each of the following statements that apply now or within the past month:

- ❑ Age 41– 60 years ____
- ❑ Minor surgery (less than 45 minutes) is planned ____
- ❑ Past major surgery (more than 45 minutes) within the last month ____
- ❑ Visible varicose veins ____
- ❑ A history of Inflammatory Bowel Disease (IBD) (for example, Crohn's disease or ulcerative colitis) ____
- ❑ Swollen legs (current) ____
- ❑ Overweight or obese (Body Mass Index above 25) ____
- ❑ Heart attack ____
- ❑ Congestive heart failure ____
- ❑ Serious infection (for example, pneumonia) ____
- ❑ Lung disease (for example, emphysema or COPD) ____
- ❑ On bed rest or restricted mobility, including a removable leg brace for less than 72 hours ____
- ❑ Other risk factors (1 point each)*** ____

****Additional risk factors not tested in the validation studies but shown in the literature to be associated with thrombosis include BMI above 40, smoking, diabetes requiring insulin, chemotherapy, blood transfusions, and length of surgery over 2 hours.*

For women only: Add 1 point for each of the following statements that apply:

- ❑ Current use of birth control or Hormone Replacement Therapy (HRT) ____
- ❑ Pregnant or had a baby within the last month ____
- ❑ History of unexplained stillborn infant, recurrent spontaneous abortion (more than 3), premature birth with toxemia or growth restricted infant. ____

Add 2 points for each of the following statements that apply:

- ❑ Age 61–74 years ____
- ❑ Current or past malignancies (excluding skin cancer, but not melanoma) ____
- ❑ Planned major surgery lasting longer than 45 minutes (including laparoscopic and arthroscopic) ____
- ❑ Non-removable plaster cast or mold that has kept you from moving your leg within the last month ____
- ❑ Tube in blood vessel in neck or chest that delivers blood or medicine directly to heart within the last month (also called central venous access, PICC line, or port) ____
- ❑ Confined to a bed for 72 hours or more ____

Add 3 points for each of the following statements that apply:

- ❑ Age 75 or over ____
- ❑ History of blood clots, either Deep Vein Thrombosis (DVT) or Pulmonary Embolism (PE) ____
- ❑ Family history of blood clots (thrombosis) ____
- ❑ Personal or family history of positive blood test indicating an increased risk of blood clotting ____

Add 5 points for each of the following statements that apply now or within the past month:

- ❑ Elective hip or knee joint replacement surgery ____
- ❑ Broken hip, pelvis or leg ____
- ❑ Serious trauma (for example, multiple broken bones due to a fall or car accident) ____
- ❑ Spinal cord injury resulting in paralysis ____
- ❑ Experienced a stroke ____

Add up all your points to get your total Caprini DVT Risk Score ☐

What does your Caprini DVT Risk Score mean?

- Risk scores may indicate your odds of developing a DVT during major surgery or while being hospitalized for a serious illness.
- Airplane passengers who fly more than five hours may also be at risk for DVT.
- Studies have shown if you have 0-2 risk factors, your DVT risk is small. This risk increases with the presence of more risk factors.
- Please share this information with your doctor who can determine your DVT risk by evaluating all of these factors.

For more information call ISMS at 1-800-782-4767, ext. 1678

www.isms.org

Adapted with permission. Our thanks to ISMS member, J. A. Caprini, MD, associated with NorthShore University HealthSystem

February 2013

Purpose

Optimizing your image is a way of putting your stamp of approval on a study. Many factors come together in image optimization.

General Optimization

- Ensure the comfort of your patient in terms of environment and positioning. Results of certain vascular studies, such as preoperative vein mapping, can be affected by the environment and patient comfort.
- Choosing the transducer that is most appropriate for the study.
  - Abdominal studies should be performed using one of the low-frequency transducers, such as a curved transducer.
  - Evaluate the patient's body habitus and any edema in the extremities to be examined. Then estimate the depth of the veins before choosing a transducer, as these factors may affect which frequency is optimal; a low-frequency transducer may be required for the exam.

Optimization of Settings

Depth

- The depth is shown by the scale on the side of the screen *(Fig. 17-1)*.
- The vessel or structure of interest should be adjusted, so the vessel or structure of interest is in the center of the screen, eliminating any excess space above or below the image.
- The depth is directly related to the Pulse Repetition Period (PRP).
- The PRP is the time between the start of a set of ultrasound signals (pulse) and the start of the next set of signals. This equals the amount of time needed to send the pulse (pulse length), plus the amount of time the transducer is listening for a return signal. The transducer cannot send and receive at the same time.
- The wavelength cannot be changed in ultrasound. The sonographer cannot change the number of signals in a pulse. Thus, the length of a pulse (= wavelength period X number of pulses) cannot be changed by the sonographer.
- The sonographer can change how long the transducer listens in between pulses. If they increase the listening time, they increase the PRP. If they decrease the listening time, they decrease the PRP.
- When the transducer listening time is increased, echoes from further away have time to reach the transducer. When the transducer listening time is decreased, only echoes reflected off of closer objects have time to reach the transducer before the transducer stops listening.
- The sonographer changes the transducer's listening time, by changing image depth. Increasing depth increases the listening time, increasing the PRP. Decreasing depth decreases listening time, decreases PRP.

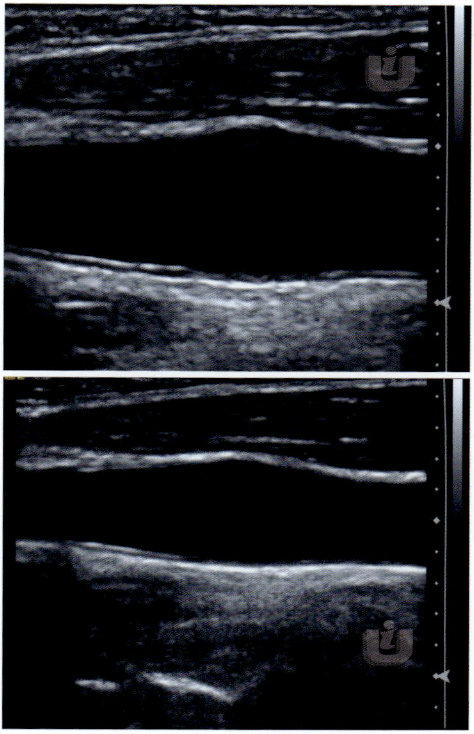

Fig. 17-1. *Increased depth. The effect of depth on resolution. The same vessel was imaged at two different depths.*

Gain

- The overall "brightness" of the image is adjusted by changing the gain.
- An image with the gain set appropriately will depict the area of interest without obscuring it with too many echoes *(Fig. 17-2).*

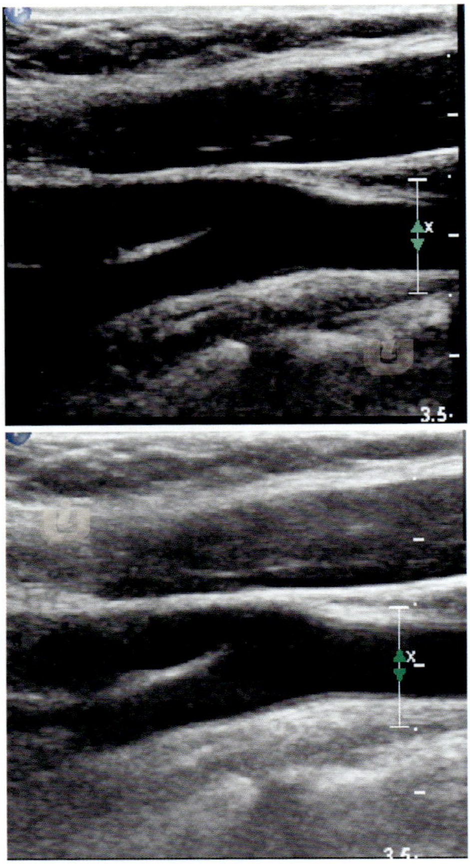

Fig. 17-2. *Effect of gain on image brightness. The same vessel was imaged using two different gains. The appropriate gain was used for the image on the top, whereas the gain for the image on the bottom was too high (sometimes referred to as over gaining). The structure of interest is frequently obscured by over gaining.*

Time Gain Compensation (TGC)

- Time gain compensation increases the signal intensity to adjust for attenuation (loss of signal intensity) with distance traveled.
- The greater the distance to a reflecting object, the more tissue the signal travels through. The more tissue the signal travels through, the greater the attenuation.
- The greater the distance to a reflecting object, the longer it takes for the Doppler signal (soundwave) to reach the reflecting object and for the echoes to reach the transducer.
- The longer it takes for the signal to return, the greater the distance traveled, and the greater the attenuation. Thus, time can be used to determine how much the signal needs to be increased (gain) to compensate for distance traveled.
- Proper adjustment of the TGC controls will result in an image with a homogenous brightness from top (skin) to bottom.

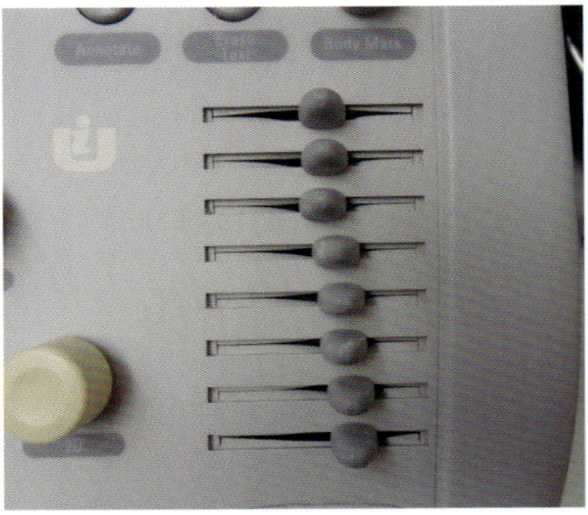

Fig. 17-3. *Typical TGC controls on a duplex machine. The top knob controls the time gain for echoes reflecting off objects near the surface. Going down, each subsequent knob controls the gain for echoes returned from objects a little deeper. The bottom knob controls the time gain for echoes reflected off objects at the maximum depth of the image. Thus, going from top to bottom, each knob sits a little further to the right, increasing time gain as the distance of the signal increases.*

Focus (focal zones)

- The focal zone(s) should be placed beside or just below the vessel or structure of interest. This is the depth at which the ultrasound beam is the narrowest and most intense and, thus, where image resolution will be the best.
- This feature is adjustable, so the beam will be in "focus" at a particular depth within the image and provide the highest quality detail possible at this location *(Fig. 17-4)*.

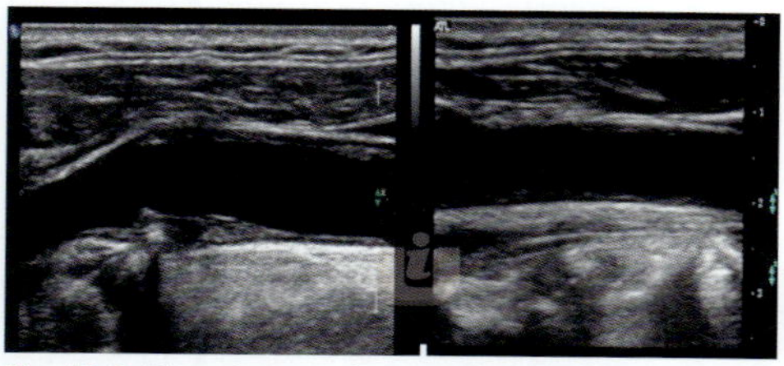

Fig. 17-4. *Focal zone in an ultrasound image. The image on the left has one focal zone. The focal zone marker (double-headed green arrow) is located next to the vessel of interest in the left image. The image on the right has two focal zones (two green arrowheads). The use of two focal zones increases lateral resolution but also decreases temporal resolution.*

Image courtesy of Philips Healthcare

> *Tip: if imaging moving objects, use only one focal zone*

Active Gain PW Doppler

- It is important to demonstrate the silhouette of the PW Doppler waveform. Over-gained waveforms usually overestimate flow velocities, and under-gained waveforms usually underestimate the velocity *(Figs. 17-7 and 17-8)*.

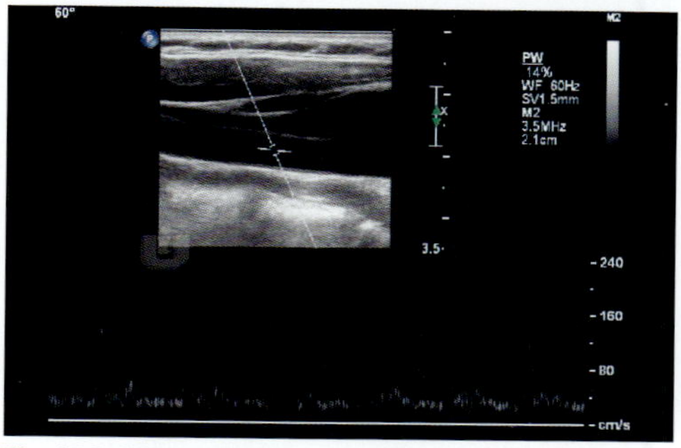

Fig. 17-5. *Under gained PW Doppler spectral waveform. The PW spectral waveform is very light because the gain was set too low. This makes estimating flow velocities from the waveform difficult, and the estimates are usually lower than the actual velocity.*

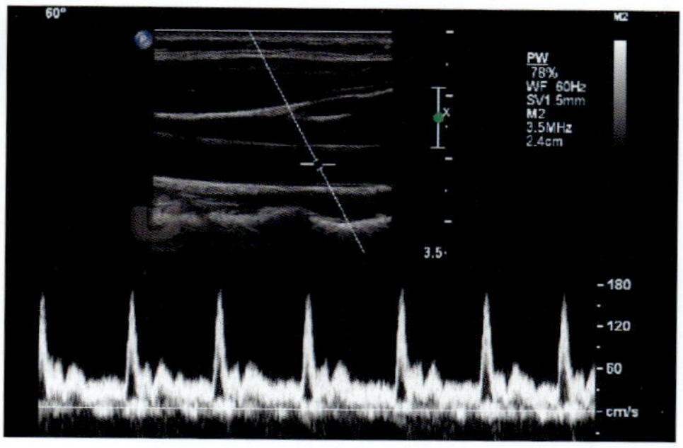

Fig. 17-6. *Over gained PW Doppler spectral waveform. There is spectral broadening of the waveform because the image was over-gained. Flow velocities estimated from over-gained PW Doppler spectral waveforms are usually higher than the actual velocity.*

- Aliasing occurs when the sampled velocity is too high in comparison to the setting of the scale.
- The top of the Doppler waveform appears at the bottom of the Doppler scale, making the measurement inaccurate *(Fig. 17-9)*.
- If aliasing is present, the scale needs to be increased until the top of waveform is no longer present on the bottom of the Doppler scale.
- Lowering the baseline is also another option to fix this issue.

> *In many cases where aliasing occurs, a combination of increasing the scale and adjusting the baseline is necessary to optimize the PW Doppler waveform.*

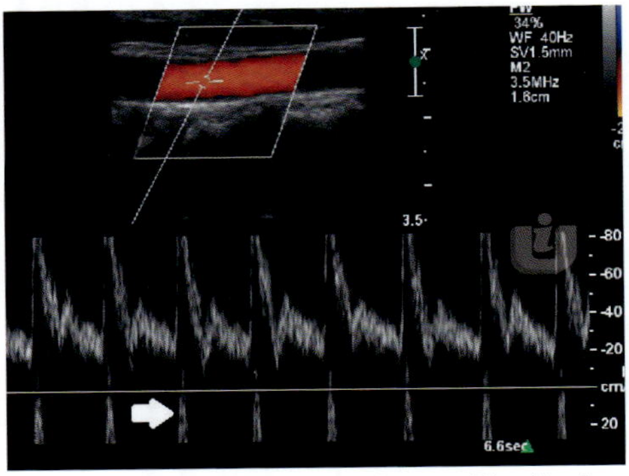

Fig. 17-7. *PW Doppler waveform with aliasing. The arrow points to the top of the waveform that is present below the baseline due to aliasing.*

Active Gain Color Doppler

- Color should fill the lumen of the vessel or structure without "bleeding" outside of the vessel. *(Fig. 17-8)*
- Adjusting the wall filter to decrease the depth can eliminate any low-frequency Doppler shifts due to tissue movement outside the vessel wall. This will allow the vessel wall to be visible and not obscured by color.
- It is important to be able to visualize any irregularities that are present on the luminal surface of the wall.
- While it is important to eliminate excess color outside the vessel wall, it is equally important to ensure the vessel's lumen is filled with color. *(Fig. 17-9)*
- It may be necessary to decrease the scale to fill in low-velocity flow regions or increase the scale to delineate regions with different flow velocities when high velocities are present.
- A lumen that does not fill with color is an obstructed lumen. A lumen that contains no color is probably occluded. However, in these cases, it is important to evaluate the vessel using PW Doppler and look for low flow before concluding the vessel is occluded.

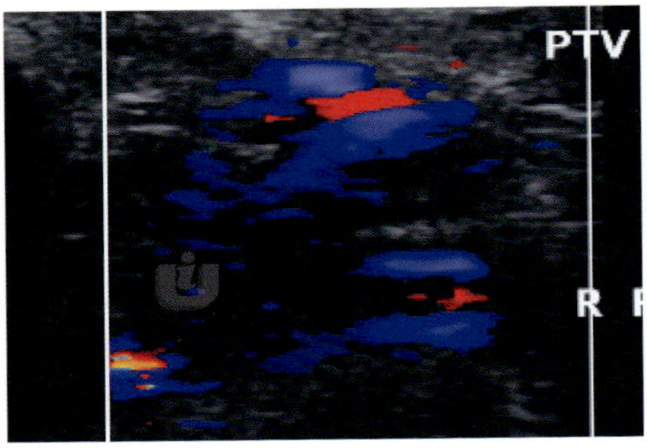

Fig. 17-8. *Color Doppler images showing the effect of over-gaining the vessel with color spilling over the vessel wall*

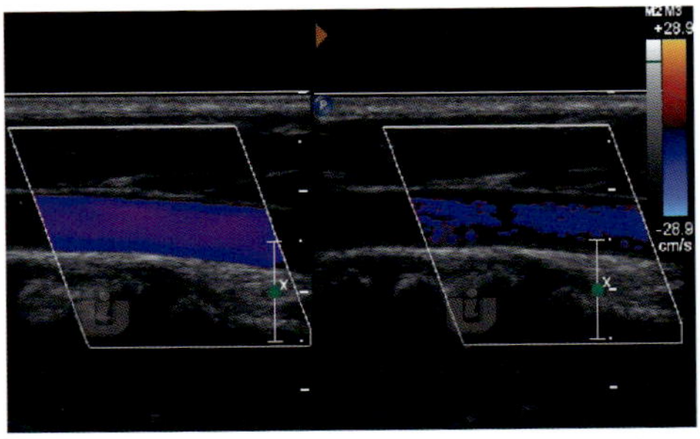

Fig. 17-9. *Color Doppler images showing the effect of under gaining. The vessel in the properly gained image has wall to wall color (left image). The color in the vessel in the under gained does not reach the wall, and there are several small regions within the lumen with no or very light color (right image).*

Frame Rate

This is the rate at which the image is updated. A desirable image has a high frame rate. The higher the frame rate, the better the temporal resolution. Low Doppler frame rates can easily be detected by moving the transducer; this will blur the image when low frame rates are being used. Frame rate is affected by multiple factors: *(Fig. 17-11)*

- Focal zones: increasing the number of focal zones decreases the frame rate.
- Increasing the depth decreases the frame rate.
- Sector width of image: Decreasing the box's width increases the frame rate.
- Color box: decreasing the size of the box increases the frame rate *(Figs. 17-10 and 17-11)*

- The best way to increase frame rate is to decrease sector width, depth, and size of the color box.

Multiple frame rates, larger color boxes, increased depth and width of the image will slow down the frame rate. Try to reduce as many of these as possible.

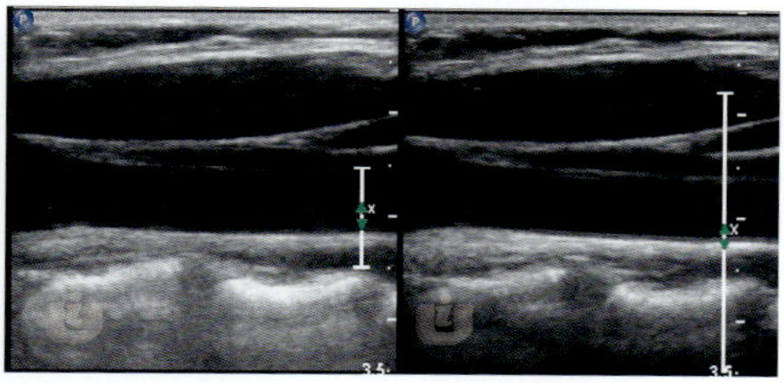

One, smaller focal zone **Multiple, larger focal zones**

Fig. 17-10. *Focal zones. The wider the focal zone or the more focal zones used, the slower the frame rate.*

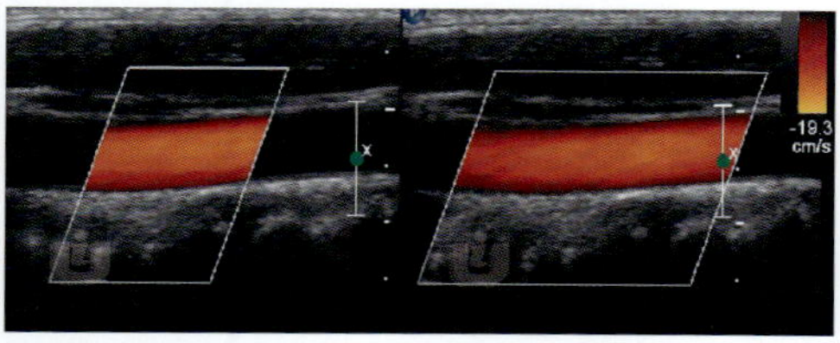

Narrow color box/ sector width *Wider color box/sector width*

Fig. 17-11. *Color Doppler images with different color box sizes. The image on the left has a smaller color box than the one on the right. The sectors are approximately the same size.*

Compression (Dynamic Range)

- Dynamic range is the difference between the highest and lowest signal intensity, expressed in decibels (dB).
- The dynamic range for ultrasound echoes is 60 dB or more. However, the human eye can only differentiate between different shades of grey if they are within a 30 dB dynamic range. Most monitors have a dynamic range between 20 and 30 dB.
- Compression is adjustable by the sonographer. The knob may be labeled "compression," "dynamic range," "contrast," or "curves."
- Usually, the 60 dB dynamic range of the ultrasound signals is compressed into a 20 to 30 dB range for grey scale viewing. Compressions are performed using nonlinear curves.
- Ultrasound machines typically display the dynamic range setting in dB, this will be the dynamic range of the grey levels in the image, but they can display it in curve settings, "C1," "C2," etc.
- High compression produces grayscale images with narrow grayscale ranges.
- An image with a low amount of compression (wide dynamic range, high dB) has a large number of grey shades and high resolution *(more detailed image; Fig. 17-12).*
- A highly compressed image (narrow dynamic range, low dB) has a small number of grey shades and low resolution (less detail) but high contrast *(Fig. 17-12).*

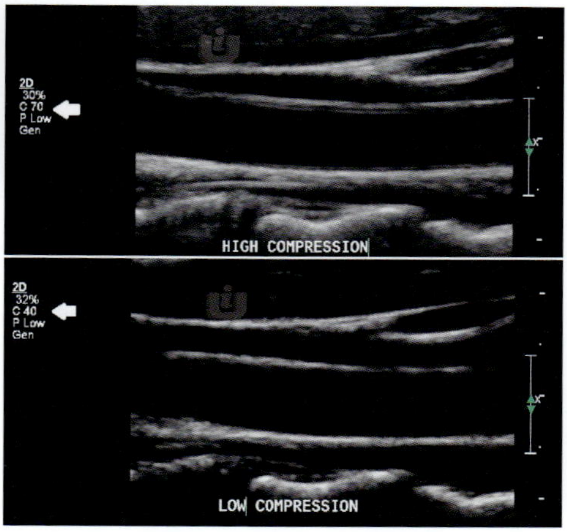

Fig. 17-12. *B-mode images with different levels of compression. The image on top is compressed less than the bottom image. The image on the top is more detailed (notice the intima-media layer), whereas the bottom image has more contrast.*

Doppler Angle

- The Doppler cursor should be placed in the middle of the vessel and be parallel to the flow within the vessel.
- When measuring blood flow velocities, the Doppler (insonation) angle should be 60° by current convention *(Fig. 17-13).*

- A Doppler angle <60°, will result in a lower velocity than when an angle of 60° is used. *(Fig. 17-14)*
- A Doppler angle >60°, will result in a higher velocity than when an angle of 60° is used *(Fig. 17-15)*.
- Angle of the color Doppler box: Due to the cosine of the angle, correct steering of the color box will ensure maximum color fill. *(Fig. 17-16)*
  - The cosine of the angle is in reference to the ultrasound beam and the blood flow.
  - Incorrect steering of the color box prevents complete color fill of the vessel lumen. *(Figs. 17-17 and 17-18)*

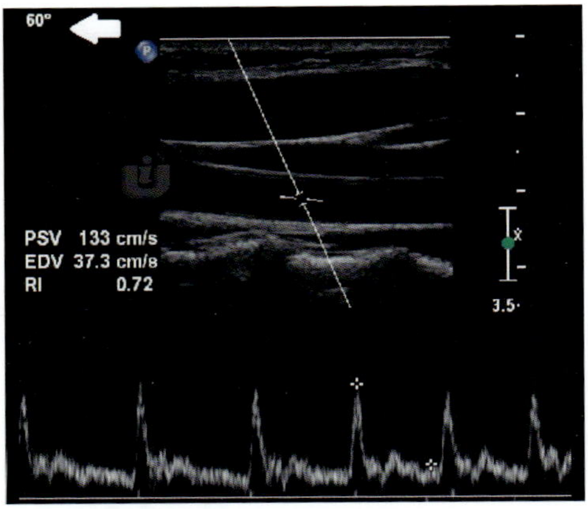

Fig. 17-13. *PW Doppler spectral waveform captured using a Doppler angle of 60°. The peak systolic velocity (PSV) is 133cm/s, and the end-diastolic velocity (EDV) is 37.3cm/s. The arrow points to the value of the Doppler angle.*

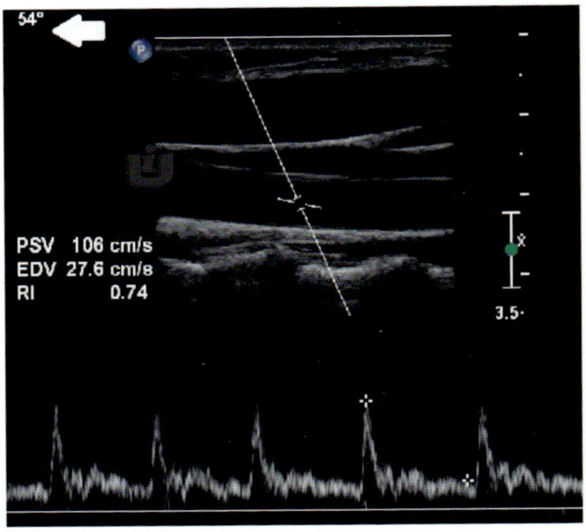

Fig. 17-14. *PW Doppler waveform captured using a Doppler angle of 54°. The measured PSV and EDV are lower than when 60° was used (PSV: 106cm/s verses 133cm/s; EDV: 27.6cm/s verses 37.3). The arrow points to the value of the Doppler angle.*

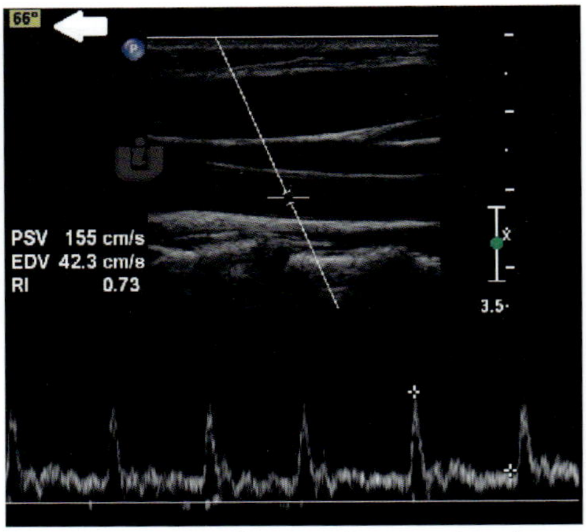

Fig. 17-15. *PW Doppler waveform captured using a Doppler angle of 66°. The measured PSV and EDV are higher than when 60° was used (PSV: 155cm/s verses 133cm/s; EDV: 42.3cm/s verses 37.3). The arrow points to the value of the Doppler angle.*

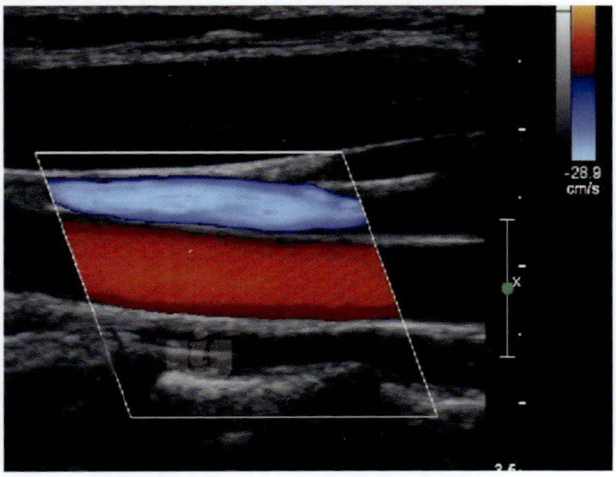

Fig. 17-16. *Color Doppler with optimal color box angle. The angle between the color box and the vessel is the smallest angle that was technically possible. At this angle, the lowest blood velocities are detectable, maximizing the color flow in the vessel.*

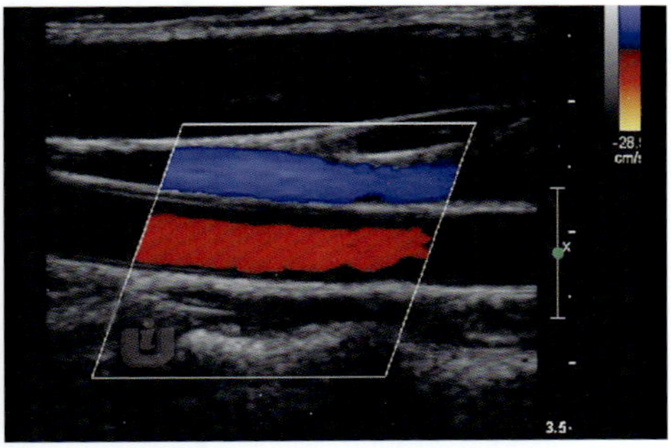

Fig. 17-17. *Color Doppler with suboptimal color box angle. The vessel is not completely filled with color. Blood flowing at low velocities could not be detected. The angle between the color box and the direction of flow needs to be decreased. The regions with no color are low-velocity flow areas.*

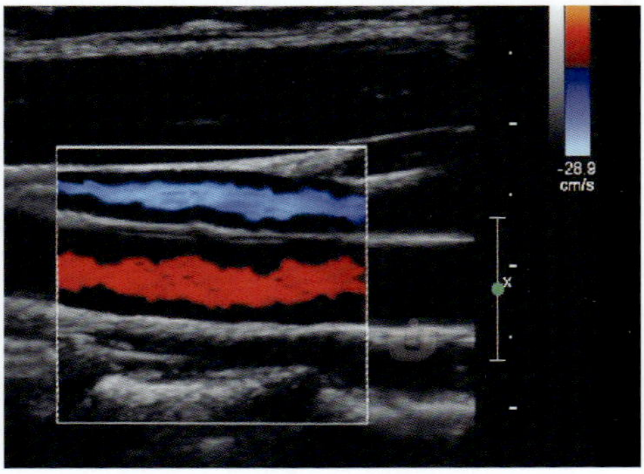

Fig. 17-18. *Color Doppler with color box almost perpendicular to flow. The vessel is not filled wall to wall with color because the color box is almost perpendicular to the direction of flow. Blood flow at any velocity is undetectable when the Doppler angle is 90° (perpendicular) to the direction of flow. Color will be present in regions where blood flow is not perpendicular to the color box, and the velocity is high enough to be detected.*

Points to Remember

- Be familiar with your ultrasound machine and its capabilities, this is essential for image optimization. The ultrasound machine is only as useful as you make it.
- A brief, initial evaluation of your patient and thoughtful deliberations regarding appropriate transducer type and examination presets are the first few steps in ensuring an optimal study.
- Before capturing an image, perform a quick run-through of the ultrasound machine settings, optimizing each one. This will help optimize the images.
- Capturing an accurate velocity is one of the most important tasks in vascular ultrasound.
- Remain perpendicular to your vessel when scanning in B-mode.
- Try to keep the sample volume gate at 1.5-2.0mm and the sample gate centered in the lumen whenever possible.
- If there are reverberations throughout the vessel, decrease the B-mode gain.

- Adequate color flow in the vertebral arteries may be difficult. Try the following adjustments:
  - Increase the color gain
  - Decrease the color scale
  - Increase the color gate
  - Increase the color filter
- A quality image of the distal SFA can be difficult to obtain. Try "harmonics" to make the vessel stand out. Enlarge the image and create a smaller color box. Apply pressure to omit any venous flow interference.
- The subclavian artery and vein can also be difficult to image.
  - Recall your anatomy. The mid-subclavian vessels run underneath the clavicle bone. Start with the transducer in the clavicular area (supraclavicular is suggested).
  - Begin with the transducer in sagittal and with the notch towards the head. The non-notched end of the transducer should touch the clavicle.
  - If an adequate amount of gel is used, a longitudinal view of both the proximal and distal subclavian vessels can often be visualized in a single image.
- If you are not getting adequate color flow through a vessel, try the following adjustments:
  - Turn up the gain. Increase it all the way up till you see color "speckles" and decrease from there.
  - Decrease the scale (especially for calf veins).
  - Decrease the frequency.
  - Increase the color filter.
  - Increase the size of the color gate.
  - Change transducers (use an abdominal transducer for difficult/obese patients or deep vessels).
  - Place the patient in reverse Trendelenburg while imaging lower extremity veins to promote vessel filling.

References

1. AbuRahma AF, Bergan JJ. (2007) *Non-invasive vascular diagnostics, A practical guide to therapy, 2nd edition.* Springer-Verlag London Limited. ISBN-13: 978-1-84628-446-5.
2. Rumwell C, McPharlin M, (2006). *Vascular technology, An illustrated review, 3rd edition*, Davies Publishing, Inc, ISBN-0-941022-69-2
3. Edelman S. (2007). *Understanding ultrasound physics, 3rd edition*, E.S.P. Ultrasound. ISBN 0-9626444-4-7

Richard Palma, BS, ACS, RCCS, RCS, RDCS, FACVP, FSDMS, FASE
Laura J Phillips, BS, RDCS, RVT

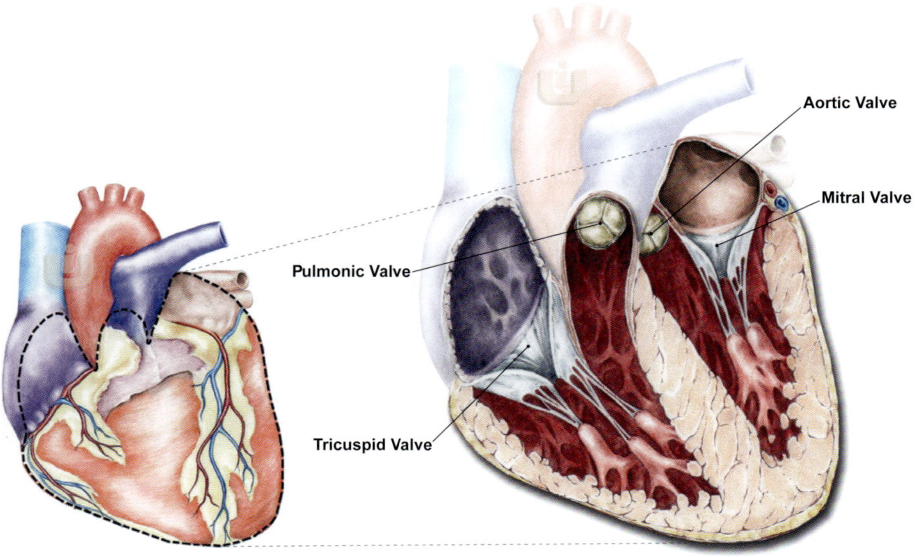

Table 18-1. **Summary of Cardiac Effect on PW Doppler Vascular Waveforms**

Over Estimate Stenosis: High Cardiac Output	Under Estimate Stenosis: Low Cardiac Output
Chronic anemia	Congestive heart failure
Chronic hypercapnia	Cardiac valvular problems
Sepsis	Coronary artery disease
Beriberi heart disease	Cardiac diastolic dysfunction
Sickle cell anemia	Pericarditis
Pregnancy	Congenital heart disease
Obesity	Cardiomyopathy
Hepatic disease	Systemic hypertension
Carcinoid syndrome	Anemia
Paget's disease	Cardiac arrhythmias
Multiple myeloma	Atrial fibrillation
Cardiac arrhythmias	Cardiac tamponade

Introduction

According to the American Heart Association, cardiovascular disease is still the leading cause of death for U.S. men and women and risk factors are on the rise. When performing a vascular exam in the aging population, heart disease must be considered and general knowledge of how heart disease affects the PW Doppler waveform in the vascular examination should be understood. Abnormal Doppler waveforms may not always be associated with vascular disease. Certain conditions can either overestimate or underestimate the stenosis. Use a combination of velocities and velocity ratios, along with an algorithm, weighing the findings for each.

High Cardiac Output

An increase in cardiac output (normal range: 4 to 6 liters per minute (lpm)) may result in an increase in peak systolic velocities. The ICA/CCA ratio may be useful to calculate when the B-mode information does not match the increased systolic velocities. The following disease states are associated with increased cardiac output:

- Chronic anemia
- Chronic hypercapnia
- Sepsis
- Beriberi heart disease
- Pregnancy
- Obesity
- Hepatic disease
- Carcinoid syndrome
- Paget's disease
- Multiple myeloma
- Cardiac volume overload diseases
- Cardiac arrhythmias (compensatory beats)

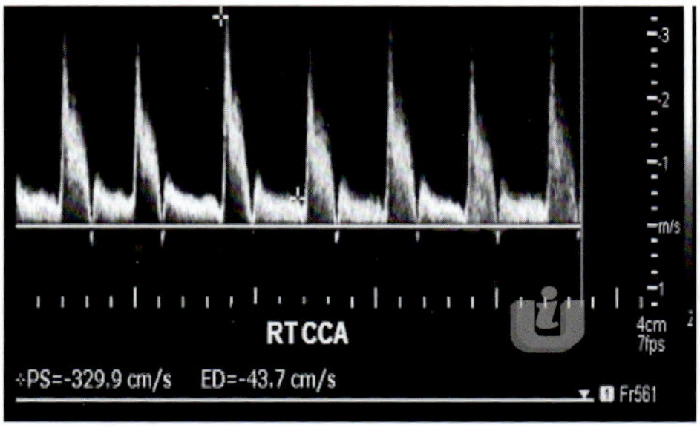

Fig. 18-1. *PW Doppler waveform with elevated velocities of the CCA in a patient with high cardiac output. This waveform will be found bilaterally in the CCA.*

Low Cardiac Output

A reduction in cardiac output may result in a decrease in peak systolic velocities. The ICA/CCA ratio may be useful to calculate when the B-mode information does not match the decreased peak systolic velocity. Low cardiac output is defined as a cardiac output below 4 lpm. The following disease states are associated with low cardiac output:

- Congestive heart failure (CHF)
- Low ejection fraction (EF%)
- Coronary artery disease
- Cardiac diastolic dysfunction
- Pericarditis
- Congenital heart disease
- Cardiomyopathy
- Systemic hypertension
- Anemia

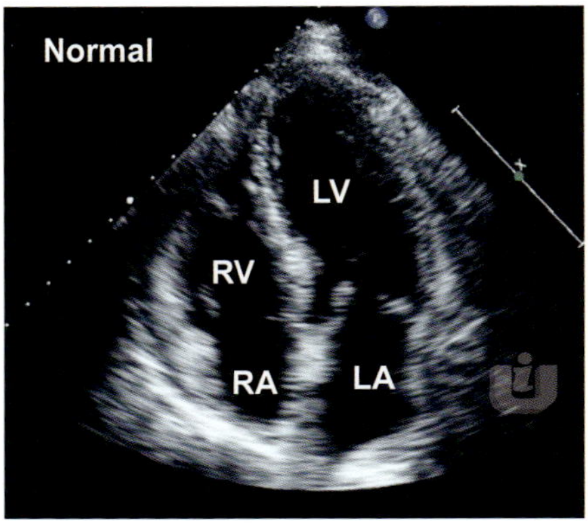

Fig. 18-2. *4-chamber normal ejection fraction*

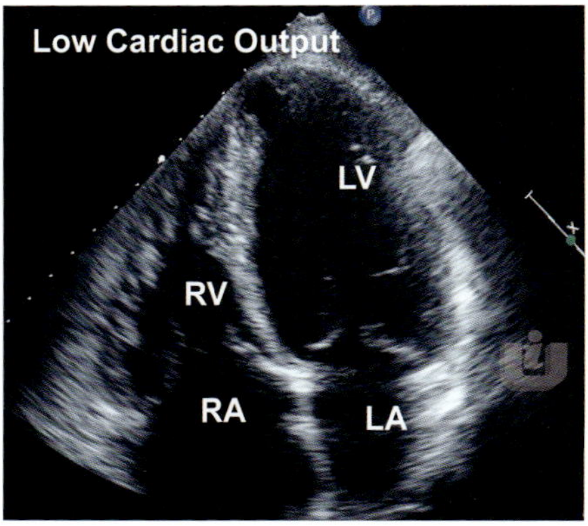

Fig. 18-3. *4-chamber low cardiac output/low ejection fraction*

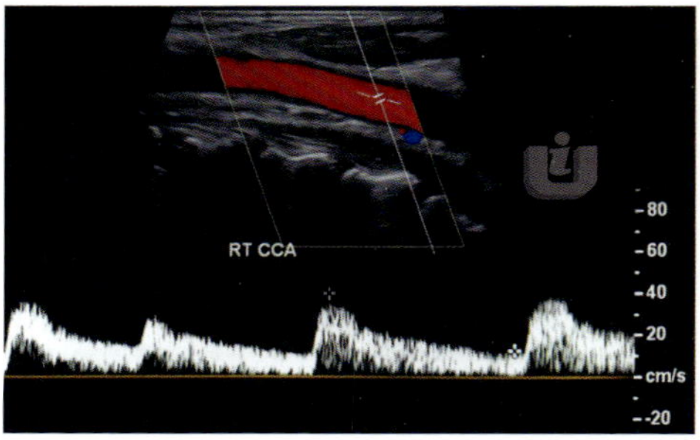

Fig. 18-4. *PW Doppler waveform of low cardiac output with severe congestive heart failure. This waveform will be found bilaterally in the CCA.*

The low cardiac output will be seen in all the vessels examined and should not be confused with proximal high-grade stenosis.

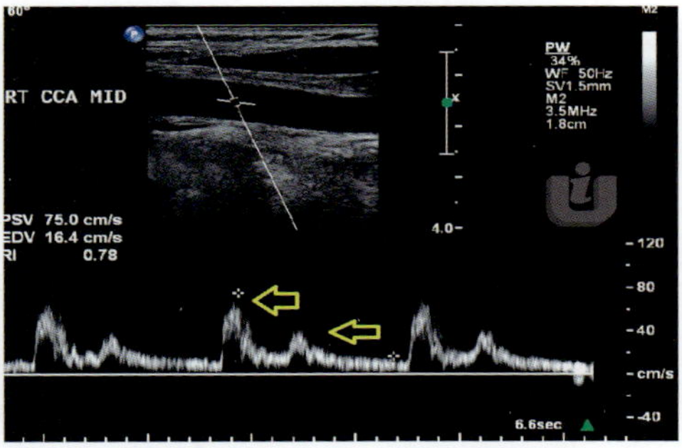

Fig. 18-5. *Pulsus Alternans. The PSV of the vessel alternates between two levels on sequential beats. This rhythm can also be associated with hypocalcemia, or IVC compression.*[1]

When performing vascular exams on patients with significant cardiac disease, the velocity ratio is usually more useful than the peak systolic velocity (PSV) in the exam interpretation when the abnormality is found throughout the cardiac cycle.

Aortic Stenosis (AS)

Aortic stenosis is the narrowing and restriction of antegrade blood flow through the aortic valve.

- The most common etiologies of aortic stenosis are as follows:
  - Congenital (e.g., bicuspid aortic valve)
  - Degenerative and rheumatic. Severe aortic stenosis is defined as the narrowing of the aortic valve area <1.0cm^2.
  - Doppler interrogation of the ascending aorta will usually show increased velocities.
  - In cases of severe aortic stenosis, Doppler interrogation of the common carotid artery may only show a low amplitude, turbulent PW waveform with a prolonged acceleration time. This finding may be most apparent in the proximal common carotid artery PW Doppler tracing.
  - Severe AS is associated with a body surface area (BSA) <0.06cm^2

In a patient with aortic stenosis, the PSV will be underestimated; use the ratio for interpretation of disease.

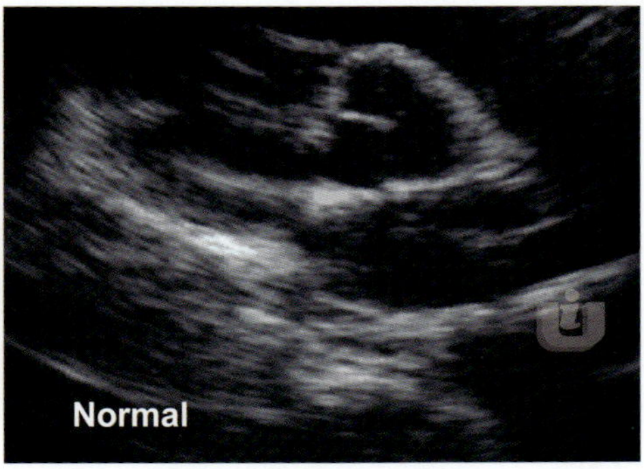

Fig. 18-6. *Normal 2D aortic valve*

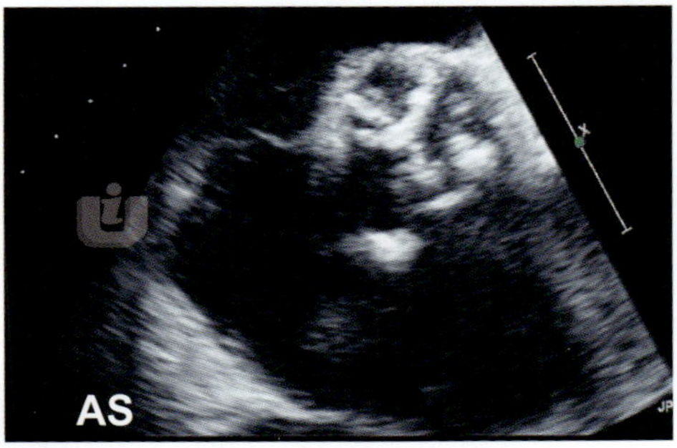

Fig. 18-7. *2D aortic valve stenosis*

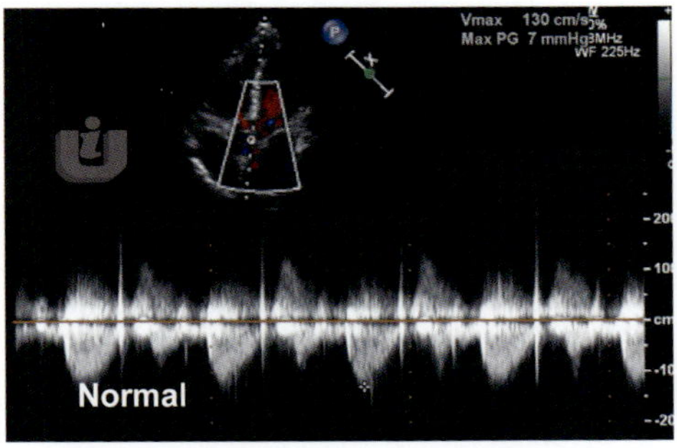

Fig. 18-8. *PW Doppler of a normal aortic valve.*

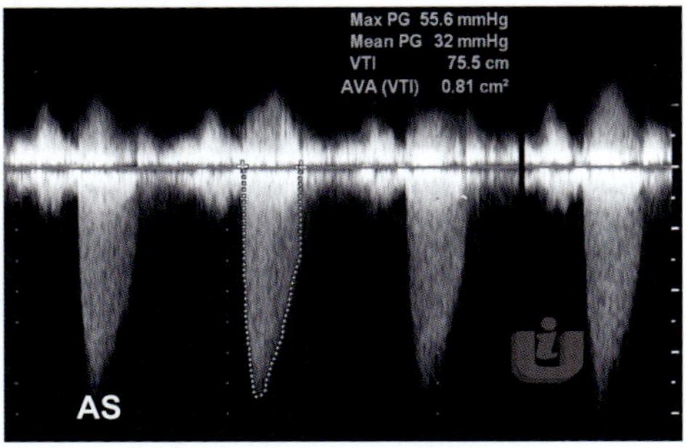

Fig. 18-9. *PW Doppler of aortic stenosis.*

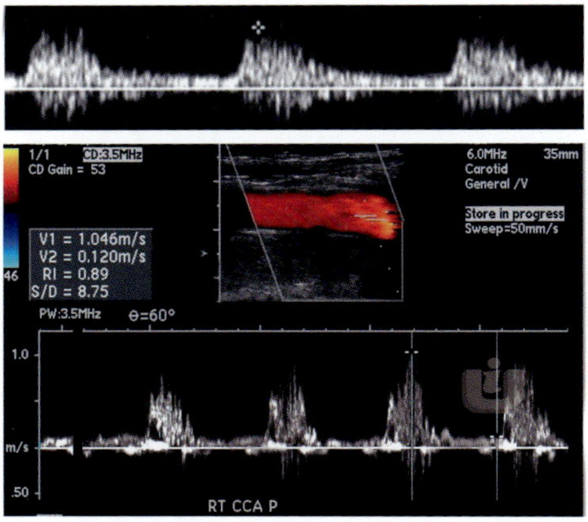

Fig. 18-10. *Low amplitude and turbulent PW Doppler waveforms of the CCA.*

Turbulent waveforms may be found bilaterally in the CCA in cardiac patients and should not be confused with a stenosis.

- The ICA/CCA ratio may be useful to calculate when the B-mode information does not match the decreased PSV.
- Overall systemic circulation will be reduced, and low amplitude signals will be present.
- Low brachial blood pressures may be seen bilaterally.
- If unilateral, you should suspect subclavian stenosis.

Aortic Regurgitation (AR)

Aortic regurgitation is defined as the backflow of blood through the aortic valve during ventricular diastole into the ventricle.

Some labs may refer to aortic regurgitation as aortic insufficiency.

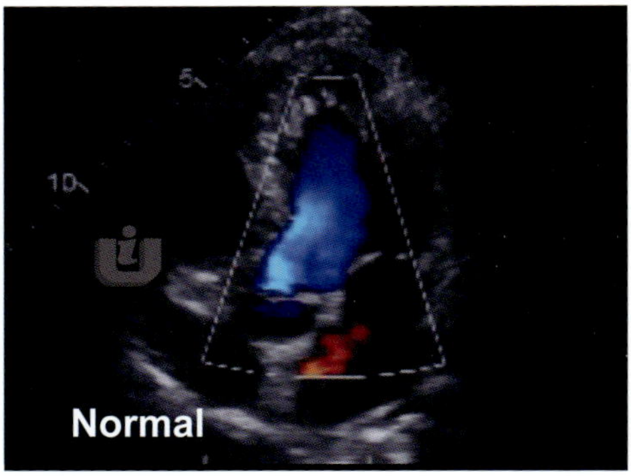

Fig. 18-11. *Color Doppler of a normal aortic valve.*

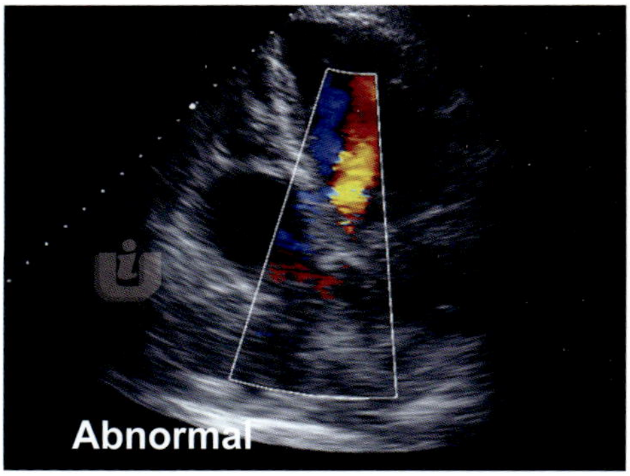

Fig. 18-12. *Color Doppler of aortic regurgitation.*

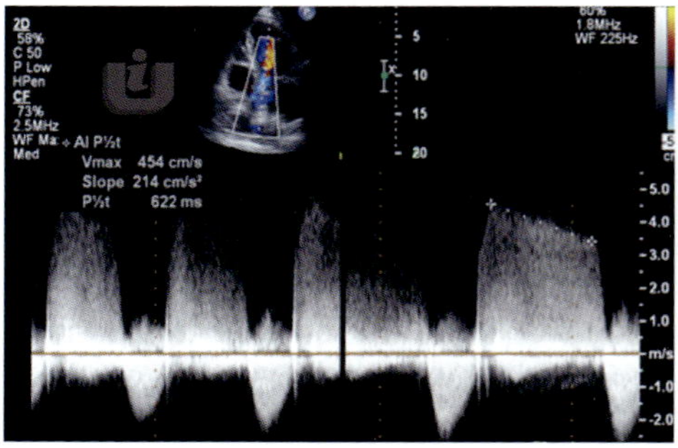

Fig. 18-13. *PW Doppler of aortic regurgitation (Mild is >500).*

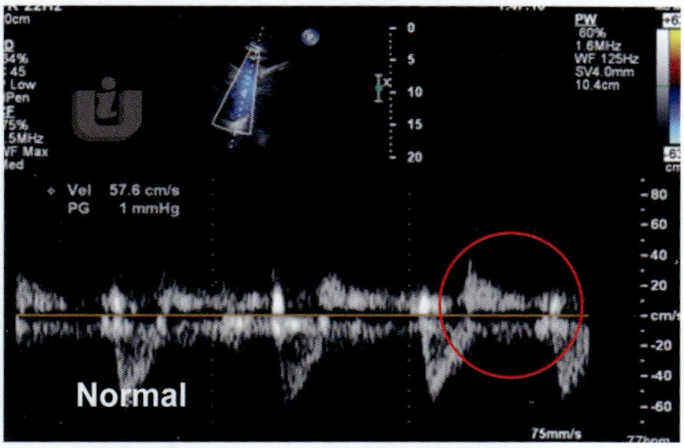

Fig. 18-14. *Normal PW Doppler of early diastolic flow reversal in the arch.*

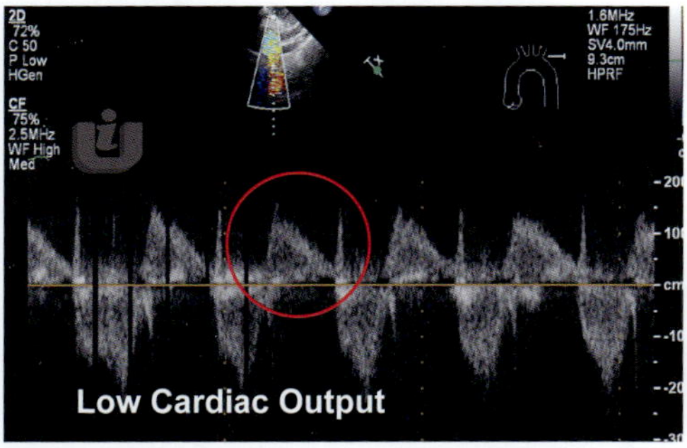

Fig. 18-15. *Holodiastolic flow reversal in the arch.*

Pulsus Bisferiens is seen in approximately 50% of patients with aortic valvular disease and can also be associated with hypertrophic cardiomyopathy.

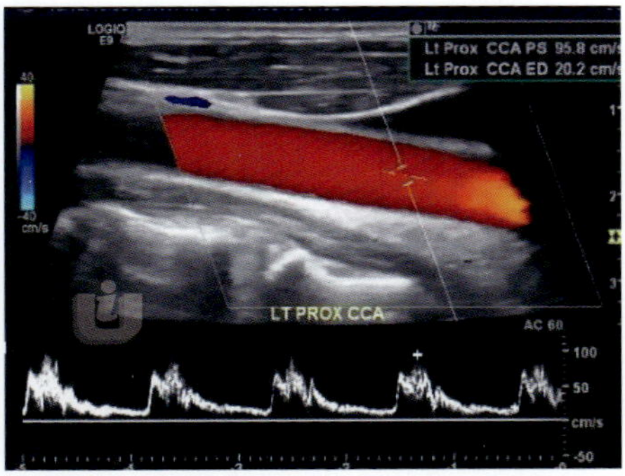

Fig. 18-16. *Color and PW Doppler waveform of pulsus bisferiens.*

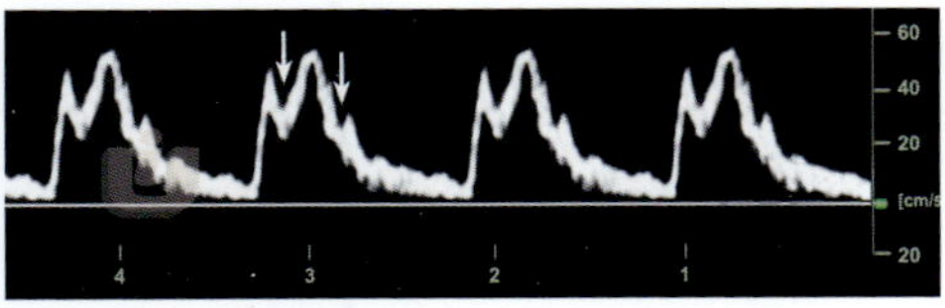

Fig. 18-17. *Note the two peaks per cardiac cycle of pulsus bisferiens.*

- Aortic regurgitation may be acute or chronic.
- An echocardiogram will be required to ascertain the presence, etiology and quantification of aortic regurgitation.
- Severe aortic regurgitation results in a volume overload of the left ventricle.
- Increased pressures may inhibit pulmonary return.
- AR can result in dilation of the left ventricle.
- Doppler waveforms of the aorta and the great vessels may show holo-diastolic flow reversal characteristics.
- A "double peaked" vascular waveform may be seen when aortic regurgitation or stenosis is present.

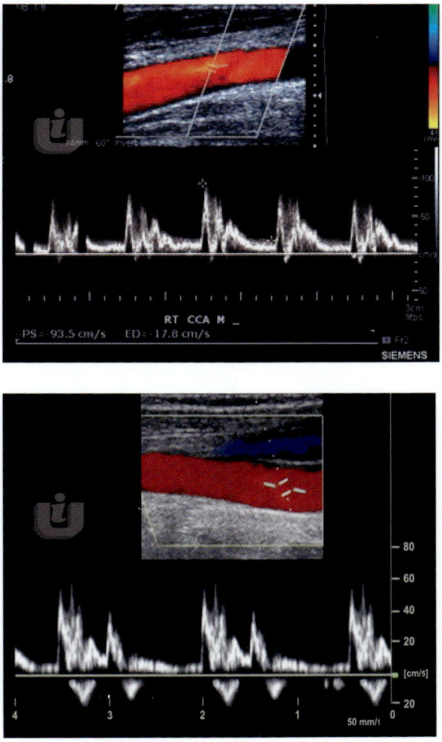

Fig. 18-18. *Bisferiens waveform from two separate patients with aortic valvular disease.*

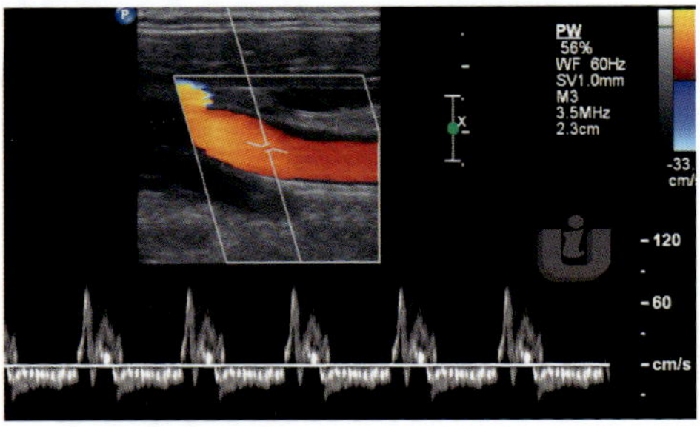

Fig. 18-19. *Water-Hammer Pulse from a patient with severe aortic regurgitation. The end-diastolic flow is reversed due to severe regurgitation.*

Mitral Stenosis (MS)

Mitral stenosis is the narrowing and restriction of antegrade blood flow through the mitral valve.

- Severe MS will cause a pressure overload in the left atrium and reduced filling of the left ventricle.
- Doppler waveforms of the aorta and carotid arteries may show low amplitude signals as a secondary result of MS.

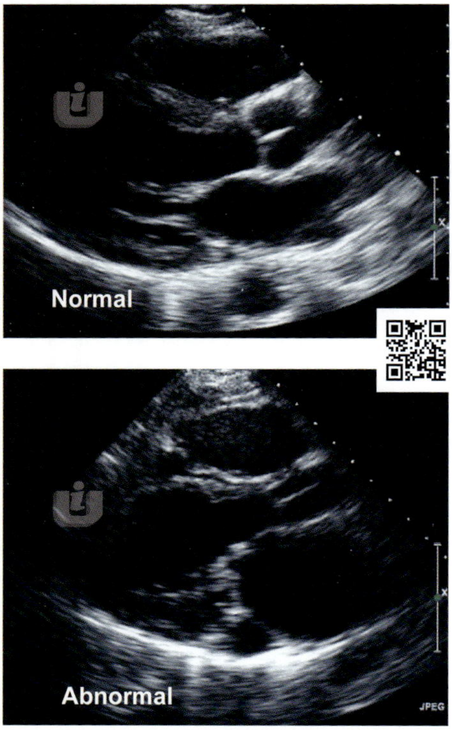

Fig. 18-20. *Normal 2D of the mitral valve vs. mitral stenosis.*

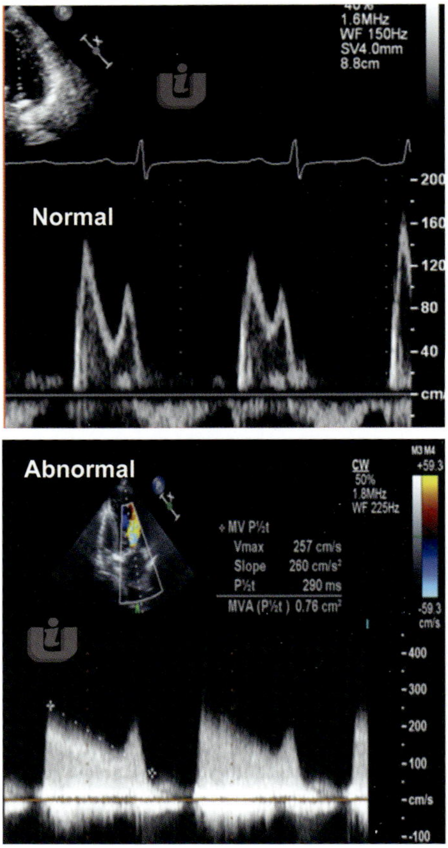

Fig. 18-21. *Normal mitral valve PW Doppler vs. mitral stenosis*

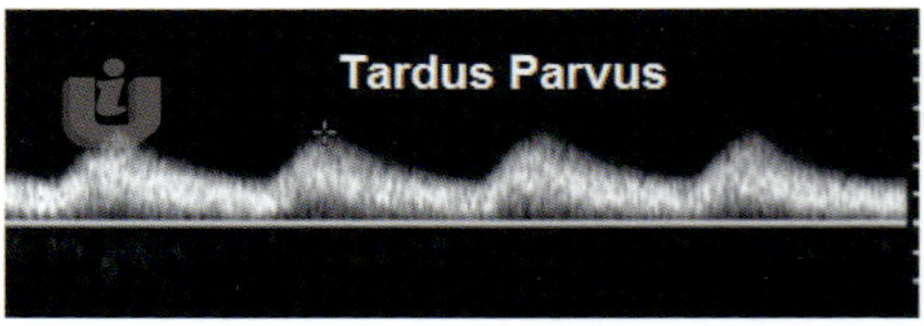

Fig. 18-22. *A low amplitude PW Doppler waveform can result in the CCA secondary to severe mitral stenosis. Note the prolonged peak with diminished amplitude. Parvus tardus waveforms are often identified distal to severe stenosis.*

Mitral Regurgitation (MR)

Mitral regurgitation is the abnormal back flow of blood through the mitral valve.

- Severe mitral regurgitation results in a volume overload of the Left Atrium (LA), resulting in increased pressures in the left atrium and pulmonary capillary wedge.
- Increased pressures will inhibit pulmonary venous return.
- MR can result in dilation of pulmonic veins. (There are 4 pulmonary veins that return blood into the LA.)
- Doppler waveforms of the pulmonary veins show marked reversal characteristics during systole, particularly in the systolic pulmonary vein waveform.
- MR does not usually affect the PW Doppler in vascular exams.

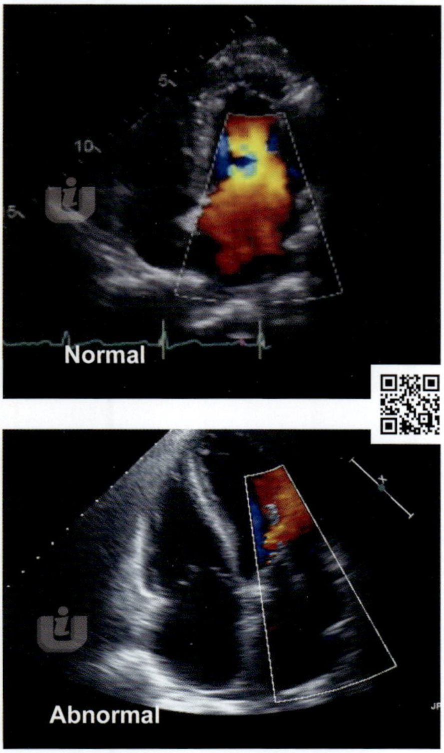

Fig. 18-23. *Normal color Doppler of the mitral valve vs. abnormal mitral regurgitation.*

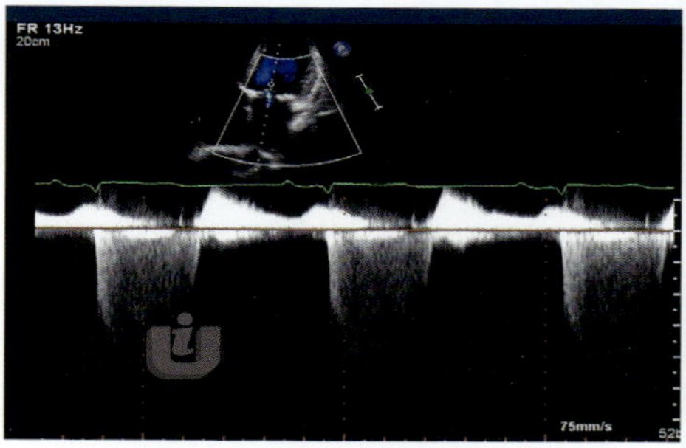

Fig. 18-24. *Mild mitral regurgitation with sparse Doppler profile and parabolic shape.*

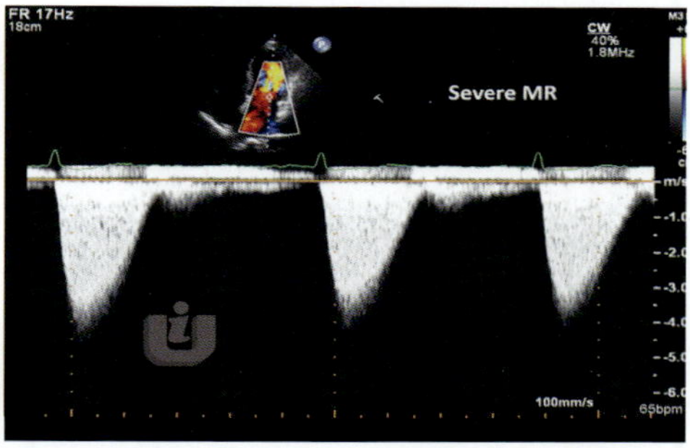

Fig. 18-25. *Severe mitral regurgitation with bright, dense PW Doppler profile and triangular shape.*

Tricuspid Regurgitation (TR)

Tricuspid regurgitation is the abnormal back flow of blood through the tricuspid valve.

- Severe tricuspid regurgitation results in a volume overload of the right atrium.
- Increased pressures in the Right Atrium (RA) will restrict/inhibit venous return.
- TR can result in dilation of the RA, IVC, and hepatic veins.
- PW Doppler waveforms of the hepatic veins and IVC may show marked reversal characteristics during systole.
- Jugular vein distention may also be present.
- Systolic murmur may be present.
- Increased or elevated pressures within the right side of the heart may result in pulsatility of hepatic, portal, internal jugular vein, and peripheral veins.

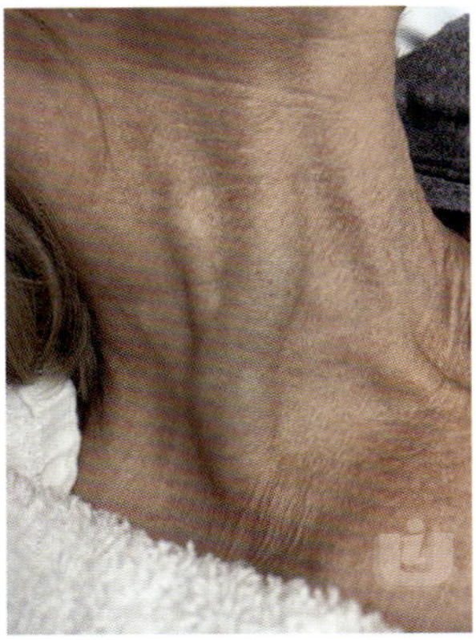

Fig. 18-26. *Jugular vein distention*

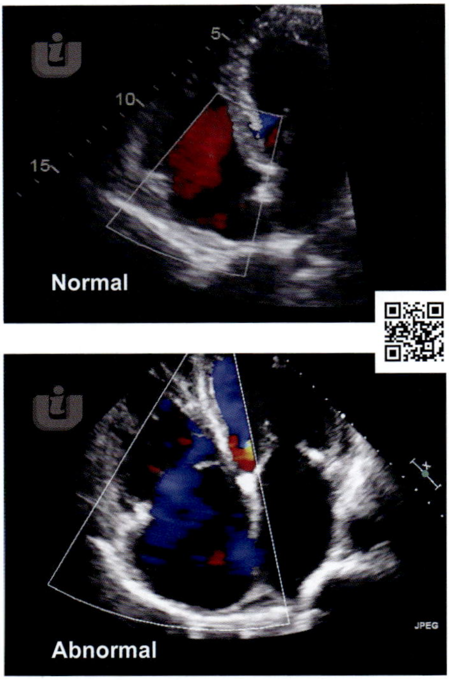

Fig. 18-27. *Normal color Doppler of the tricuspid valve vs. abnormal tricuspid regurgitation.*

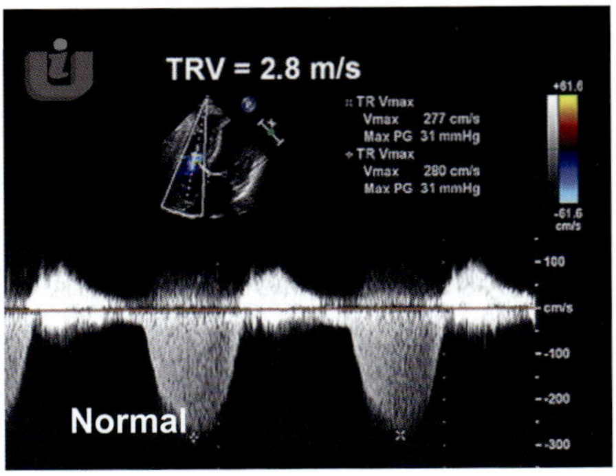

Fig. 18-28. *PW Doppler of tricuspid regurgitation*

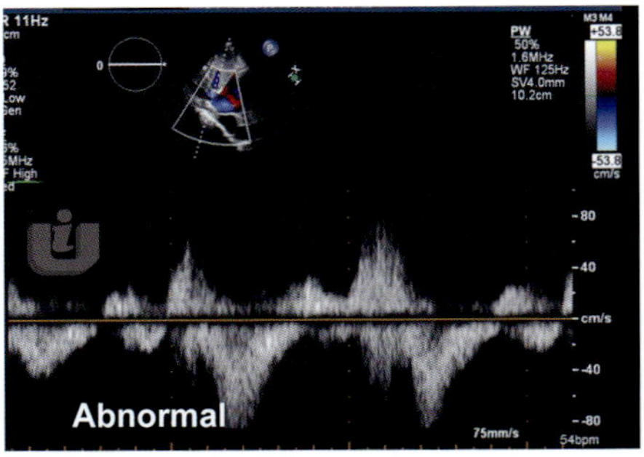

Fig. 18-29. *PW Doppler showing systolic reversal in the hepatic vein from severe tricuspid regurgitation.*

Tricuspid Stenosis (TS)

Tricuspid stenosis is the narrowing and restriction of antegrade blood flow through the tricuspid valve.

- Severe tricuspid stenosis will cause a pressure overload in the right atrium and reduced filling of the right ventricle.
- PW Doppler waveforms of the main pulmonary artery may exhibit a turbulent waveform pattern.
- IVC and hepatic veins may become dilated.

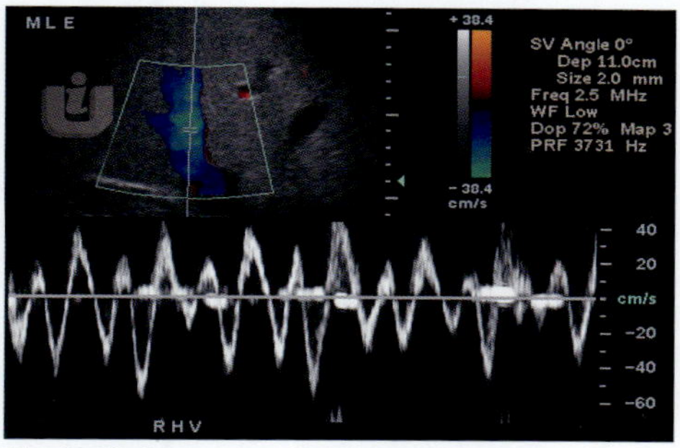

Fig. 18-30. *Increased pulsatility in the hepatic vein.*

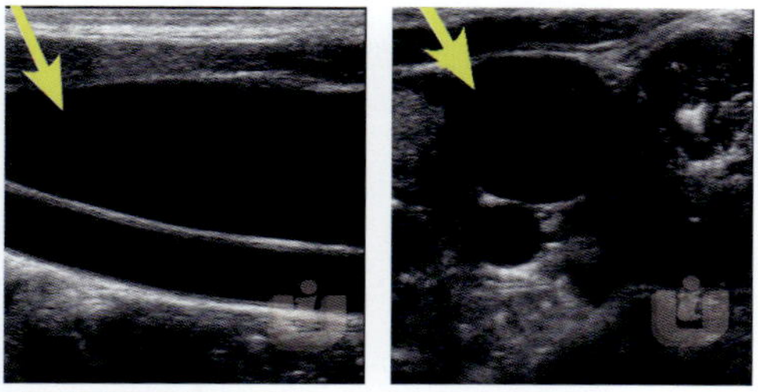

Fig. 18-31. *Dilated internal jugular vein caused from elevated pressure within the right side of the heart*

Pulmonary Regurgitation (PR)

Pulmonary regurgitation is the abnormal back flow of blood through the pulmonic valve.

> *Some labs refer to pulmonary regurgitation as pulmonic insufficiency.*

Severe pulmonary regurgitation results in a volume overload of the right ventricle.

- Increased pressures can inhibit venous return.
- PR can result in dilation of the right ventricle.
- PW Doppler waveforms of the pulmonary arteries may show marked flow reversal components during diastole.
- Increased or elevated pressures within the right side of the heart may result in pulsatility of peripheral veins.

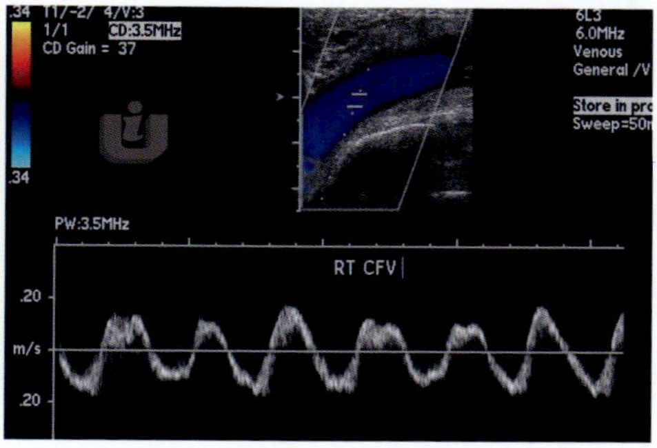

Fig. 18-32. *Increased pulsatility in a common femoral vein caused from elevated pressure within the right side of the heart.*

Pulmonic Stenosis (PS)

Pulmonic stenosis is the narrowing and restriction of antegrade blood flow through the pulmonic valve.

- Severe pulmonic stenosis will cause a pressure overload in the right ventricle and reduced flow to the pulmonary arteries.
- PW Doppler waveforms of the pulmonary arteries may show increased amplitude and turbulent waveform patterns.
- Increased or elevated pressures within the right side of the heart may result in pulsatility of peripheral veins.

Cardiac Tamponade

Cardiac tamponade is an emergent cardiac finding. There is a reduction in diastolic filling of the heart due to increased intrapericardial pressures from the accumulation of fluid or blood around the heart (pericardial effusion).

- Patients with cardiac tamponade are considered to have emergent findings and should be addressed immediately.
- The classic clinical finding for cardiac tamponade is pulsus paradoxus, defined as a drop in systolic blood pressure by greater than 10mmHg upon inspiration. This drop in blood pressure is due to a reduction of left ventricular filling during inspiration.

- Consequently, the carotid PW Doppler tracing will demonstrate a decrease in peak systolic carotid Doppler signal.
- Conversely, an increase in left ventricular filling with expiration results in an augmented peak systolic carotid PW Doppler signal velocity during expiration. This is referred to as respiratory variation.

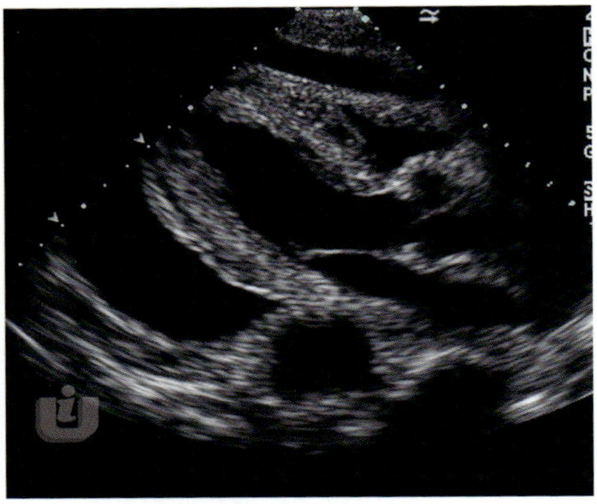

Fig. 18-33. *2D cardiac tamponade right ventricular collapse.*

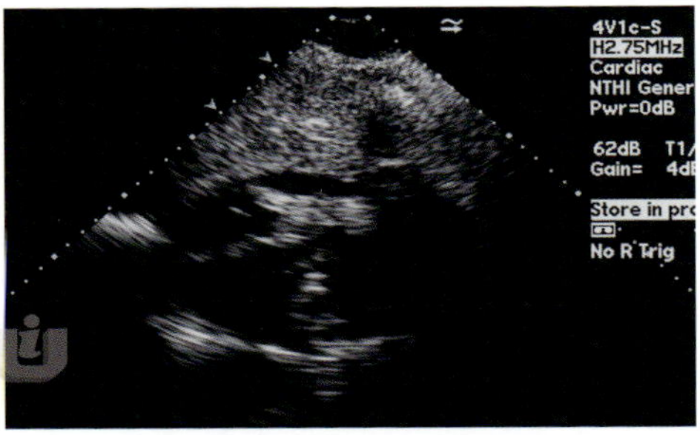

Fig. 18-34. *Right ventricular compression tamponade.*

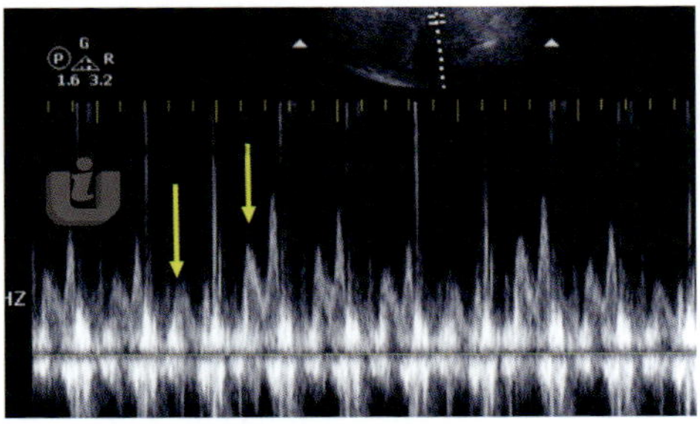

Fig. 18-35. *Respiratory variation of the mitral valve in cardiac tamponade.*

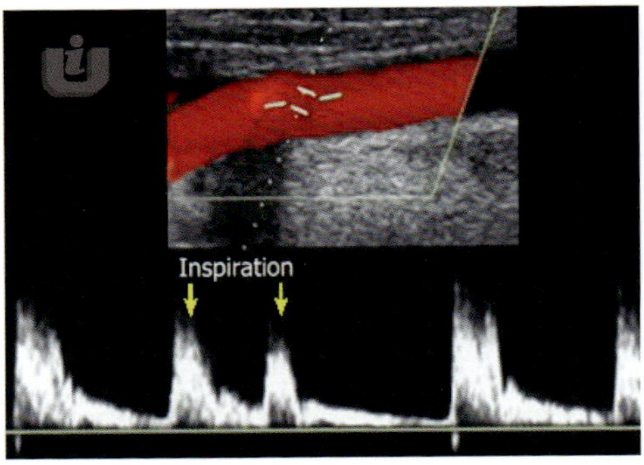

Fig. 18-36. *Decreased PSV during inspiration and increased PSV during expiration.*

Constrictive Pericarditis

Constrictive pericarditis is the thickening of the pericardium due to inflammation which interferes with the diastolic filling of the heart.

IVC dilation without inspiratory collapse is a very helpful sign of constrictive pericarditis.

- Commonly seen in post-cardiac surgery.
- Distension of the internal jugular vein, IVC, and peripheral edema is usually present.
- The resultant carotid PW Doppler tracing will demonstrate a decrease in peak systolic velocity upon inspiration.

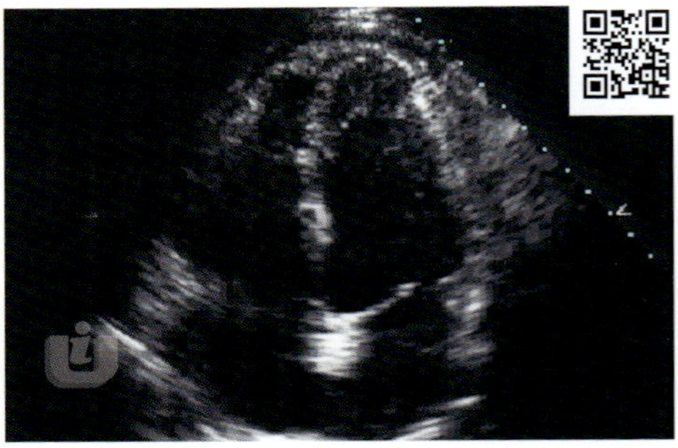

Fig. 18-37. *Constrictive pericarditis respiratory shift.*

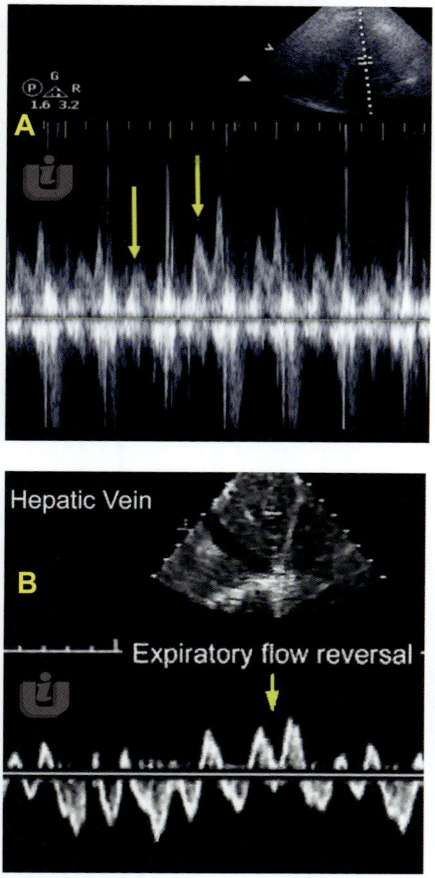

Fig. 18-38. *Constrictive pericarditis: A) PW Doppler of mitral valve inflow demonstrating respiratory variation B) PW Doppler of hepatic vein showing expiratory flow reversal.*

Cardiac Arrhythmias

Cardiac arrhythmias exhibit irregular PW Doppler waveforms that correspond with the heart rhythm and rate.

- Vascular labs have adopted several methods of measuring velocities when arrhythmias are present.
- A common technique used when an irregular rhythm is present is to measure the most consistent beats. This may be a string of three or more.
- In cases where the rhythm present is "irregularly irregular" (no pattern that can be followed), it becomes more difficult. An average of the 3-5 most consistent beats may be taken. This is more subjective, and care should be taken when reporting results using this method. Diameter and area reduction tools may prove extremely useful in cases of irregularly irregular arrhythmias.
- In cases where an intraortic balloon pump is used, it may be difficult to determine the underlying rhythm.

Some physicians will allow the balloon pump to be turned off for brief periods so underlying rhythms can be seen and measurements taken.
This should NOT be done by the sonographer!

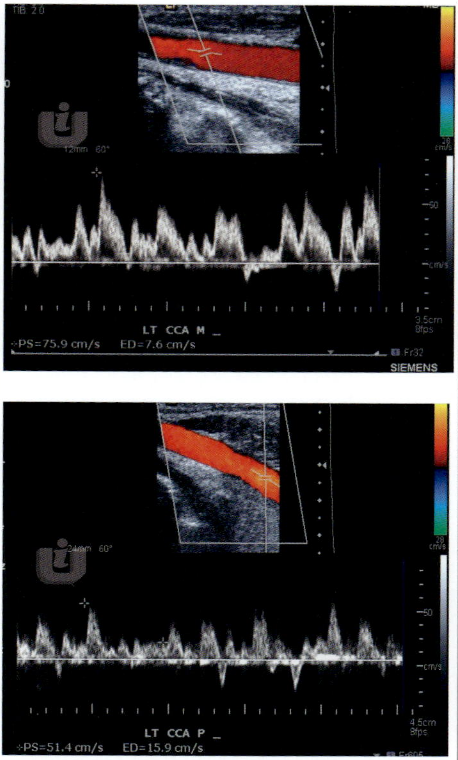

Fig. 18-39. *PW Doppler waveform from a patient on an intra-aortic balloon pump (IABP).*

Sinus Arrhythmia

All waveforms are normal. The heart rate increases and decreases with respiration.

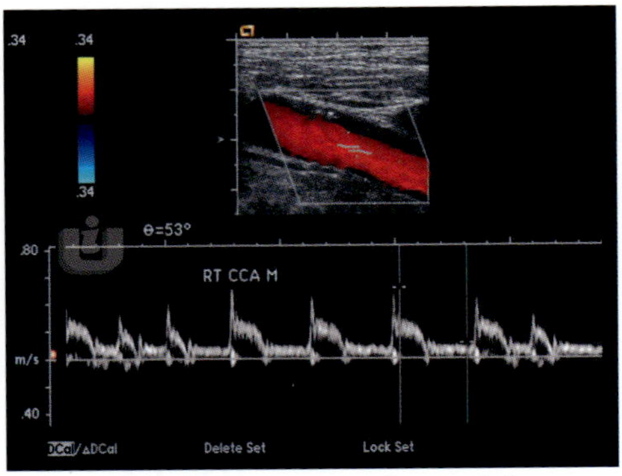

Fig. 18-40. *PW Doppler waveform of sinus arrhythmia*

Sinus Bradycardia

All waveforms are normal, but the heart rate is below 60bpm.

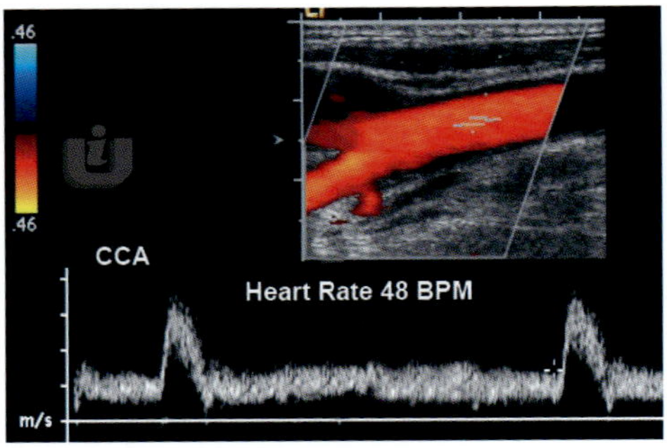

Fig. 18-41. *PW Doppler waveform of Sinus Bradycardia*

Sinus Tachycardia

All waveforms are normal, but the heart rate is above 100bpm.

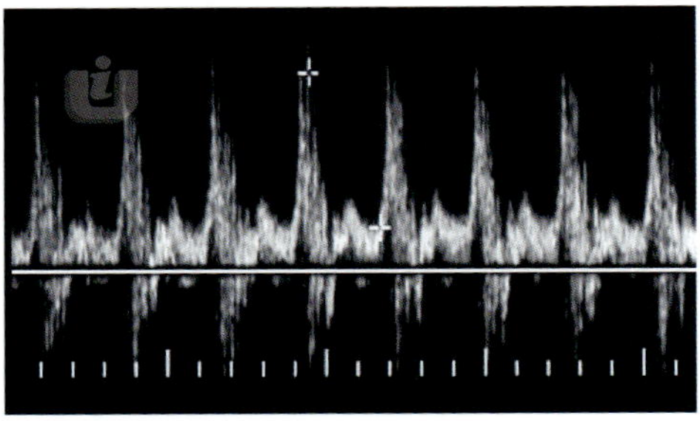

Fig. 18-42. *PW Doppler waveform of sinus tachycardia*

Sinus Pause (Sinus Arrest)

The SA node (natural pacemaker) fails to send out an impulse for a period of time.

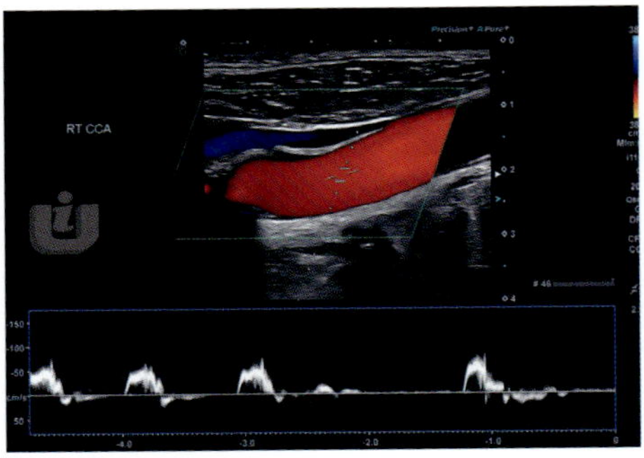

Fig. 18-43. *PW Doppler waveform of sinus pause from a patient with severe congestive heart failure.*

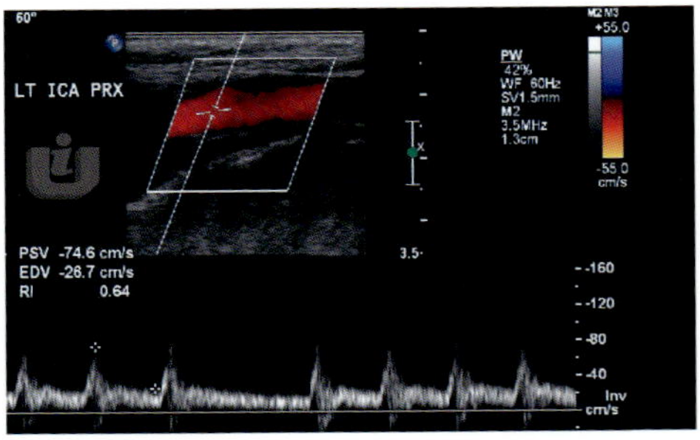

Fig. 18-44. *PW Doppler waveform of sinus pause.*

Atrial Fibrillation/Atrial Flutter

Atrial fibrillation is a common cardiac arrhythmia which may result in a mixture of short and long R-R cardiac cycles. It is the fibrillation of the heart's two upper chambers (atria). The carotid PW Doppler waveform appears to have a variety of peak systolic velocities due to the varying R-R intervals. It is recommended to measure 3 to 5 beats and average.

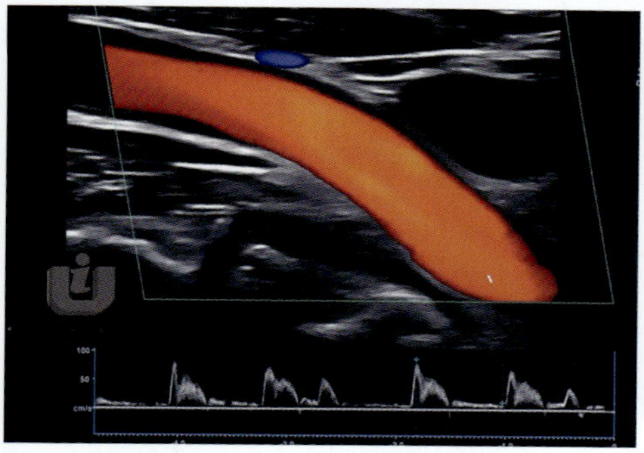

Fig. 18-45. *PW Doppler waveforms and color Doppler depicting atrial fibrillation*

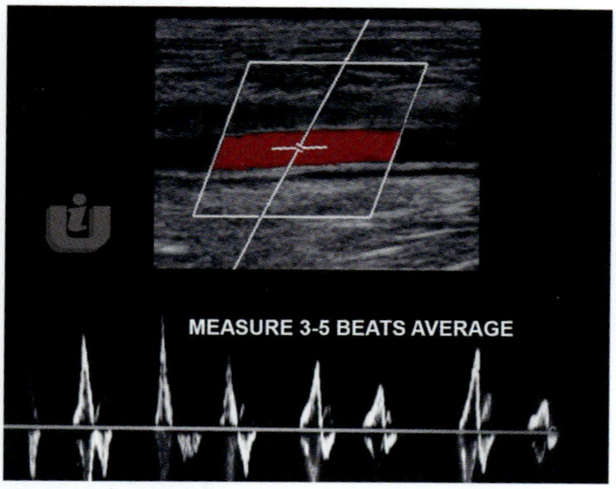

Fig. 18-46. *PW Doppler waveforms of atrial fibrillation*

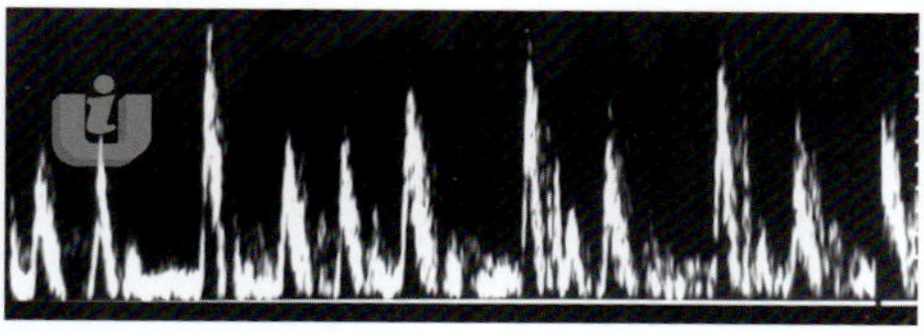

Fig. 18-47. *PW Doppler waveforms of atrial fibrillation*

Premature Ventricular Contraction (PVC)

A PVC originates from an ectopic focus (an abnormal electrical pulse) within the right or left ventricles. PVCs occur earlier than expected and are followed by a delayed beat (compensatory pause). The PW Doppler waveform of a PVC would be lower than normal, and the following delayed beat will be higher than normal. It is recommended not to measure either beat because it doesn't truly represent the velocity when there is a normal sinus rhythm.

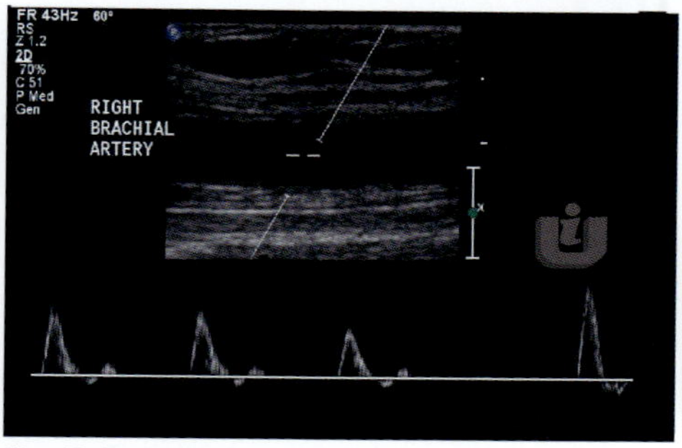

Fig. 18-48. *PVC found in an artery; a repeating pattern of a PVC followed by a normal beat.*

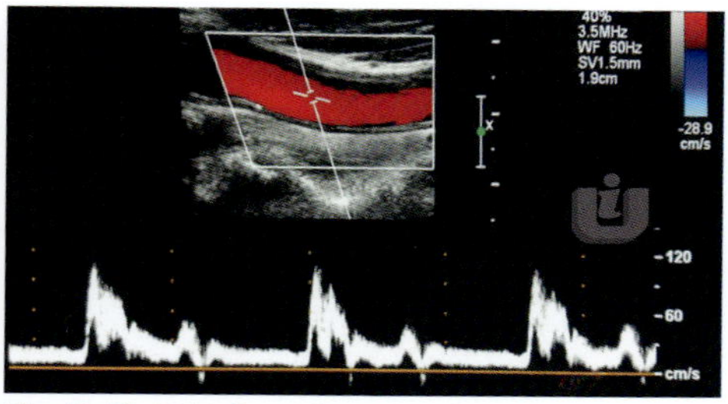

Fig. 18-49. *PW Doppler waveforms demonstrating bigeminy of the common carotid artery*

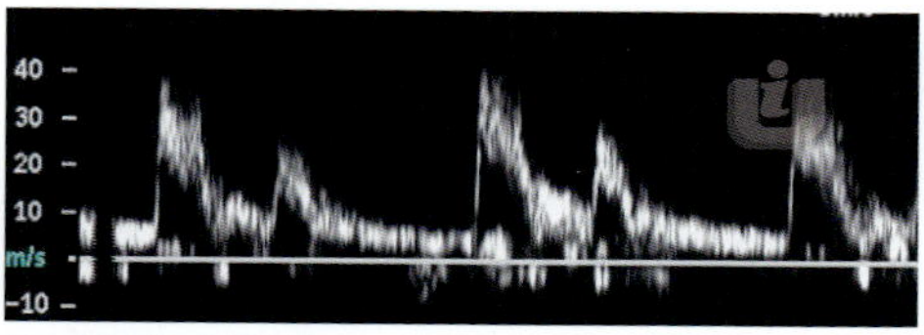

Fig. 18-50. *PW Doppler waveforms demonstrating bigeminy of the common carotid artery*

Trigeminy

A repeating pattern of a PVC following two normal beats.

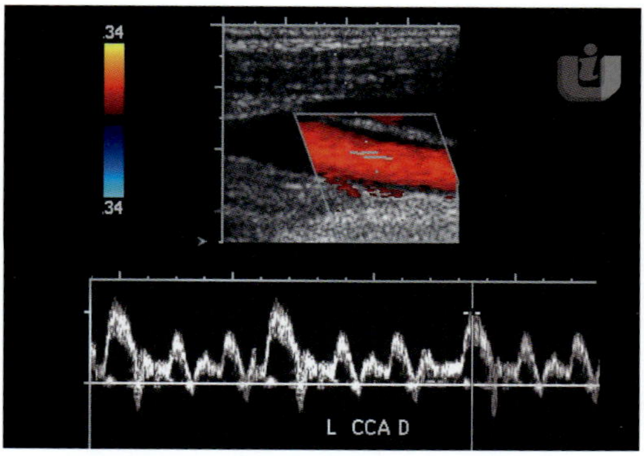

Fig. 18-51. *PW Doppler waveforms of atrial fibrillation of trigeminy of the CCA*

Table 18-2. **Cardiac Diseases and Symptoms**

	Mitral Stenosis	Mitral Regurgitation
General Complaints	Fatigue; DOE; palpations; hemoptysis; hoarseness; orthopnea; PND	Dyspnea; fatigue; exercise intolerance; orthopnea; palpitations
Physical Examination	Resting tachycardia; irregular pulse; jugular venous distention in the presence of RV failure; pulmonary hypertension except in atrial fibrillation	Irregular pulse; sharp upstroke of arterial pulse; jugular venous distention in presence of RV failure; prominent "A" wave in presence of increased RV pressure
Palpation	Diastolic thrill at apex	Apical impulse forceful and downwardly displaced to left
Auscultation	Loud S1; opening snap; low snap; low pitched, rumbling diastolic murmur	Diminished or absent S1; wide splitting of S2; presence of S3; presence of S4 heard in severe regurgitation; holosystolic murmur heard best at apex
EKG	LA enlargement; notched P wave (P Mitral); RV hypertrophy	LA enlargement; LV hypertrophy; atrial fibrillation
Chest X-Ray	LA and RV enlargement; pulmonary venous congestion; pulmonary edema	LA and LV enlargement; pulmonary vascular congestion
Echocardiogram	Decreased excursion of mitral leaflets; diminished E-F slope; enlarged LA	LA enlargement; hyperdynamic LV
Cardiac Cath	Pressure gradient across mitral valve; LA and PAW pressure increased; low cardiac output (fixed)	LVEDP increased; LA pressure increased; angiography with contrast media performed to quantify regurgitation

Table 18-2. **Cardiac Diseases and Symptoms** ***(continued)***

	Aortic Stenosis	Aortic Regurgitation	Mitral Valve Prolapse
General Complaints	Fatigue; dyspnea; orthopnea; angina pectoris; dizziness; syncope	Dyspnea on exertion; palpitation; orthopnea; exertional chest pain	Dyspnea; syncope; palpitations; sharp chest pain unrelated to exercise; fatigue
Physical Examination	Early: normal blood pressure; late-systolic blood pressure decreased; narrow pulse pressure; carotid pulse is slow with small pulse volume	Arterial pulsation; bounding pulse with rapid rise and fall (waterhammer pulse); widened pulse pressure; head bobbing (Musset's sign); skin warm, damp and flushed	May not be any particular signs of cardiac disease unless regurgitation becomes detectable. Most patients are young women.
Palpation	Systolic thrill palpable at base of heart; apical pulse strong and sustained throughout systole	Diastolic thrill along left sternal border; laterally displaced apically; systolic thrill in jugular notch and along carotid arteries	May not be any particular signs of cardiac disease unless regurgitation becomes detectable
Auscultation	Diminished or absent A2; harsh crescendo- decrescendo systolic murmur heart best at base (second intercostal space to right of sternum); aortic ejection sound	Decrescendo diastolic murmur (blowing); high pitched and heard best at base	Systolic click and apical systolic murmur usually high pitched and quite musical
EKG	LV hypertrophy; conduction defects; first degree AV block; LBBB	LV hypertrophy	Normal; may show ST segments and T wave abnormalities, especially in inferior leads or prominent U waves; dysrhythmias; supraventricular tachyarrhymias; premature atrial or ventricular beats
Chest X-Ray	Post-stenotic; dilatation of aorta; aorta valve calcification	Aortic valve calcification; LV enlargement; dilation of ascending aorta	Identifies or confirms presence of skeletal abnormalities
Echocardiogram	Nonrestricted movement of aortic valve; thickening of LV wall	LV dilated; diastolic flutter of anterior leaflet of mitral; vibration of septal wall	Mild to moderate: anterior and/or posterior mitral leaflets separation at the coaptation point of the cusps; enlarged LA size; chordal rupture
Cardiac Cath	LVEDP increased; pressure gradient across the aortic valve	Pulse pressure increased; LVEDP increased; LA pressure increased; angiography with contrast media performed to quantify regurgitation	Normal unless mitral regurgitation present; LV angiogram shows the prolapsed mitral valve

Table 18-3. Effects of Cardiac Diseases on the PW Doppler Waveform

Disease	Effect
High cardiac output	Increased systolic velocity
Low cardiac output	Decreased systolic velocity
Aortic Regurgitation	Double peaked waveform and/or reversal during diastole; diminished or absent dicrotic notch
Aortic Stenosis	Low amplitude and/or turbulent waveform; parvus-tardus
Mitral Stenosis	Low amplitude
Mitral Regurgitation	No effect usually in the vascular exam
Tricuspid Regurgitation	Increased pulsatility in the venous waveform
Pulmonic Regurgitation	Increased pulsatility in the venous waveform
Pulmonary Stenosis	Increased pulsatility in the venous waveform
Tricuspid Stenosis	Increased pulsatility in the venous waveform
Cardiac Tamponade	Decreased peak systolic velocity during inspiration and increased peak systolic velocity during expiration
Constrictive Pericarditis	Decreased peak systolic velocity during inspiration and increased peak systolic during expiration
Cardiac Arrhythmia	Varying peak systolic velocity

Cardiac Rhythm Diagnosis

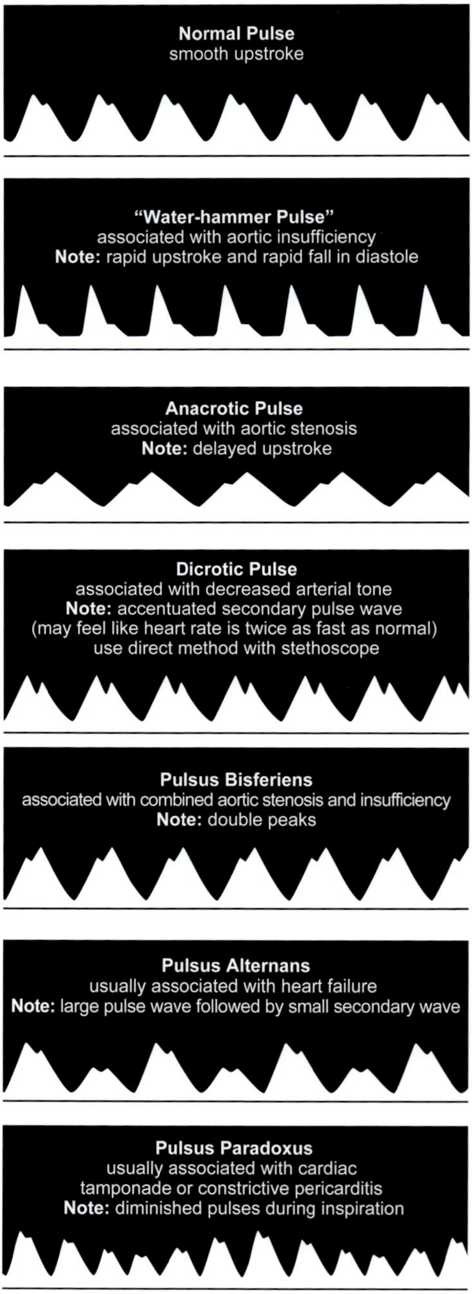

Image courtesy of Rick Duncan

Important to Note

- Left ventricular and aortic valve abnormalities mainly affect arterial hemodynamics (pulse contour and pressure).
- Right ventricular and tricuspid valve abnormalities mainly affect venous hemodynamics.
- If the PW Doppler waveform abnormality stems from cardiac issues, the waveform abnormality is usually seen throughout the vascular exam; it is important to compare waveforms bilaterally.
- Increased cardiac pressures can result in increased recorded velocities (e.g., hyperdynamic left ventricle).
- Decreased cardiac pressures can result in decreased recorded velocities (e.g., low ejection fraction, aortic stenosis).
- Increased or elevated right-sided cardiac pressures may result in pulsatility in peripheral veins (e.g., CHF).
- If pulsatile venous flow is found in the lower extremities, clinical correlation should be considered for pulmonary embolism (PE).
- When a cardiac arrhythmia is encountered, consider waiting for a short time period to begin or continue the exam, as these can be intermittent in some patients.
- Pulsatility of hepatic and subclavian veins is normal due to the proximity to the heart. Peripheral veins will normally exhibit phasic respiratory flow.
- High resistant arterial waveforms with a diminished or absent dicrotic notch indicate aortic valve disease may be present (e.g., AR).
- Paradoxical embolism occurs when an emboli crosses from the right side of the heart to the left through a defect in the septum resulting in a stroke. Septum defects fall into two categories. Atrial septal defect (ASD) is when there is a "hole" in the septum dividing the two atria. Ventricular septal defect (VSD) is when there is a "hole" in the septum dividing the two ventricles. PFO (Patent Foramen Ovale) can also be a source of embolism.
- Cardiomyopathies are diseases that affect the heart's myocardial (muscular) layer. There are several types. This disease can affect the heart globally or segmentally. Cardiomyopathies may affect ejection fraction, cardiac output, and pressures within the heart.
- Any cardiac disease present may affect the vascular system. These effects can be seen in arterial and venous waveforms. Careful examination of patient history will prove useful.
- Cardiac valvular problems can be congenital, genetic, inflammatory, stress, or structural based.

References

1. Rohren E., Kliewer M., et al. (2003). A spectrum of Doppler waveforms in the carotid and vertebral arteries. *AJR, 181*, pages 1695-1704.
2. Bendick P. (2011). Cardiac effects on peripheral vascular Doppler waveforms. *Journal of Vascular Ultrasound, 35*(4), pages 237-243.
3. Palma, R. (2019). *Echocardiographers' Pocket Reference, 5th edition.* Arizona Heart School of Cardiac Ultrasound.
4. Reynolds, T. (1997). *Cardiovascular principles: A registry exam preparation guide.* Arizona Heart School of Cardiac Ultrasound.
5. Kaddoura, S. (2002). *Echo Made Easy*. Elsevier Saunders.
6. Centers for Disease Control and Prevention. (2022, October 14). *Heart Disease Facts.* CDC. gov. http://www.cdc.gov/heartdisease/facts.htm.

Rationale

One of the main objectives for any non-invasive vascular laboratory is to provide accurate test results. Every type of exam performed by the laboratory should have a high degree of reliability and repeatability. Physicians expect that a positive exam truly means that their patient has disease and a negative exam truly means the patient has no significant disease

Gold Standard

The gold standard is the exam (measuring method) that is currently believed to be the most accurate for measuring the variable of interest, e.g. percent stenosis. It is the one to which all other exams are compared. For example, to determine the accuracy of carotid artery stenosis measurements, one would ideally compare results obtained by ultrasound to results obtained by arterial angiograms, the gold standard. However, the current gold standards for many vascular measurements are invasive and rarely performed, e.g. arterial angiograms. So to determine the accuracy of a vascular laboratory's measurements, the results are often compared to those from an exam considered to be either more or as accurate as ultrasound, e.g. CTA. Below are a few ultrasound exams and their "gold standards" for ultrasound comparisons.

- **Abdominal and peripheral arterial:** Angiograms, CT scans, operative findings, MRA and surgical pathology reports
- **Extracranial/intracranial:** CT scans and angiography
- **Peripheral venous:** Venograms, MRV, and repeat venous duplex exams.

Terms used to describe a test result

- **True Positive (TP):** Significant disease is detected and present.
- **True Negative (TN):** Significant disease is not present and is not present.
- **False Positive (FP):** Significant disease is detected but no disease is present.
- **False Negative (FN):** Significant disease is not detected but disease is present.

Terms used to characterize methods of measurement

Compared to the gold standard a measurement method can have a tendency to:

- **Overestimate:** The method over estimates the severity of the exam.
- **Underestimate:** The method underestimates the severity of the disease.

Methods of measuring are evaluated for:

1. **Sensitivity:** The ability of an exam to detect disease among those who have disease.

$$\frac{\text{Have disease \& Test positive}}{\text{All patients with disease}} = \frac{TP}{TP + FN}$$

2. **Specificity:** The ability of an exam to detect the lack of disease in those who do not have the disease.

$$\frac{\text{Without disease \& Test negative}}{\text{All patients without disease}} = \frac{TN}{TN + FP}$$

3. **Positive Predictive Value (PPV):** How often a positive exam is accurate.

$$\frac{\text{With disease \& test positive}}{\text{All patients with positive tests}} = \frac{TP}{TP + FP}$$

4. **Negative Predictive Value (NPV):** How often a negative exam is accurate.

$$\frac{\text{Without disease \& Test negative}}{\text{All Patients with negative tests}} = \frac{TN}{TN + FN}$$

5. **Overall Accuracy (OA):** The percent of exam results that are correct. This number takes into account the sensitivity and specificity and the PPV & NPV

$$\frac{\left[\begin{array}{c}\text{With disease}\\ \text{\& Test positive}\end{array}\right] + \left[\begin{array}{c}\text{Without disease}\\ \text{\& Test negative}\end{array}\right]}{\text{Total number of patients}} = \frac{TP + TN}{TP + TN + FP + FN}$$

Example Calculation

A 2 x 2 table is helpful when organizing data. Typically, the positive and negative results of the gold standard are tabulated by column and the results of the exam being evaluated are organized by row:

		Gold Standard Test Results +	Gold Standard Test Results –
Non-invasive Test Results	+	True Positive (TP)	False Positive (FP)
	–	False Negative (FN)	True Negative (TN)

		Gold Standard Test Results +	Gold Standard Test Results –
Non-invasive Test Results	+	True Positive 11 cases	False Positive 3 cases
	–	False Negative 0 cases	True Negative 136 cases

TN = 136   TP = 11   FP = 3   FN = 0

Count the number of TP, TN, FP and FN.

Then use these numbers to calculate sensitivity, specificity, PPV, NPV and OA.

SENSITIVITY: $$\frac{TP}{TP + FN} = \frac{11}{11 + 0} \times 100 = 100\%$$

SPECIFICITY: $$\frac{TN}{TN + FP} = \frac{136}{136 + 3} \times 100 = 98\%$$

PPV: $$\frac{TP}{TP + FP} = \frac{11}{11 + 3} \times 100 = 79\%$$

NPV: $$\frac{TN}{TN + FN} = \frac{136}{136 + 0} \times 100 = 100\%$$

OA: $$\frac{TP + TN}{TP + TN + FP + FN} = \frac{136 + 11}{136 + 11 + 3 + 0} \times 100 = 98\%$$

References

1. Bower D. (2014) Medical statistics from scratch: An introduction for health professionals, 3rd edition. John Wiley & Son Ltd. West Sussex, UK.
2. Rumwell, C., MCPharlin M. (2015). Test validation, statistics and patient safety. *In vascular technology: An illustrated review, 5th edition.* Davies Publishing, Pasadena, CA.

Arterial (Lower Extremity)

Ankle Brachial Index (ABI)

The ABI is equal to the ratio of the systolic blood pressure at the ankle to the systolic blood pressure of the brachial artery. The TBI is equal to the ratio of the systolic blood pressure at the toe to the systolic blood pressure of the brachial artery. ABIs and TBIs are used to assess arterial blood flow and categorize vascular disease in the lower extremity *(Table 20-1)*. Normally the brachial pressure is approximately equal to the ankle pressure and slightly greater than the toe pressure. When there is a decrease in lower extremity blood flow, both the ankle and toe pressures decrease. When these pressures decrease, the ABI and TBI ratios decrease. Thus, a decrease in the ABI and TBI ratios indicate blood flow in the lower extremity has decreased. The brachial and ankle pressures are measured using CW Doppler and at the toe a digital cuff and photoplethysmography (PPG) is used.

Ankle Brachial Index (ABI)

The ABI is calculated by dividing the higher of the two ankle pressures (posterior tibial artery (PT) or dorsal pedis artery (DP) by the higher of the two brachial pressures (right or left):

Higher Ankle Pressure ÷ Higher Brachial Pressure

Toe Brachial Index (TBI)

The TBI is calculated by dividing the digital pressure by the higher brachial pressure (right or left) to determine the digital brachial index:

Toe Pressure ÷ Higher Brachial Pressure

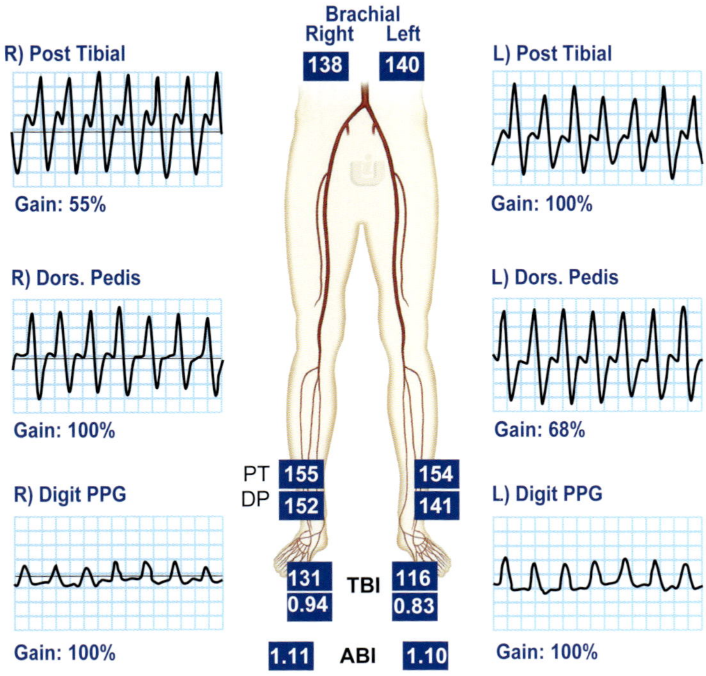

Fig. 20-1. *Pressure measurements of the brachial, posterior tibial, dorsal pedis, and digital arteries in lower extremities with normal blood flow.*

Examples using the data in Fig. 20-1 and 20-2.

A. Normal ABI and TBI (Fig. 20-1)

Right ABI	155 ÷ 140 = 1.11	right extremity is normal
Right TBI	131 ÷ 140 = 0.94	right extremity TBI is normal
Left ABI	154 ÷ 140 = 1.10	left extremity ABI is normal
Left TBI	116 ÷ 140 = 0.83	left extremity TBI is normal

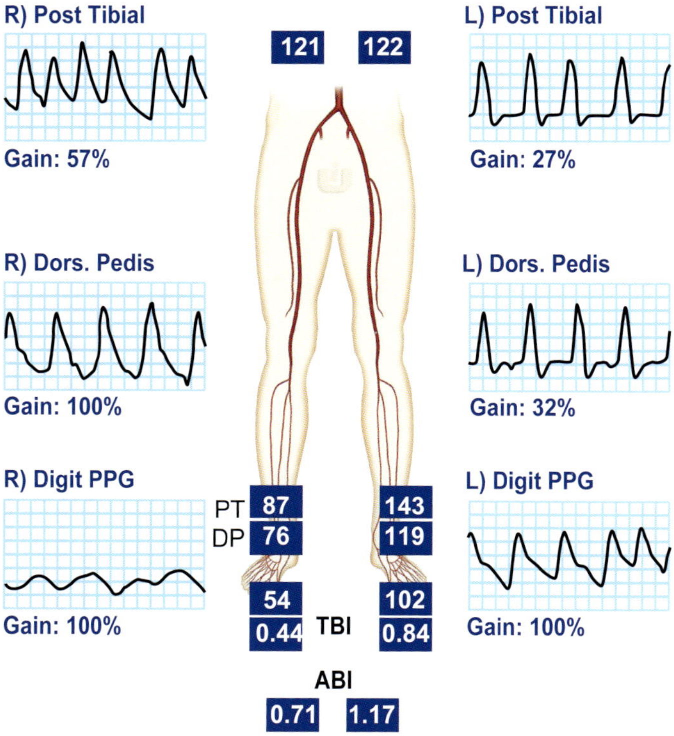

Fig. 20-2. *Pressure measurements of the brachial, posterior tibial, dorsal pedis, and digital arteries in lower extremities with abnormal blood flow.*

B. Abnormal ABI and TBI (Fig. 20-2)

Right ABI	87 ÷ 122 = 0.71	right extremity ABI has moderate disease
Right TBI	54 ÷ 122 = 0.44	right extremity TBI has moderate disease
Left ABI	143 ÷ 122 = 1.17	left extremity ABI is normal
Left TBI	102 ÷ 122 = 0.84	left extremity TBI is normal

Table 20-1. **Disease Categorization for ABI/TBI**	ABI	TBI
Normal	≥ 1.0	> 0.70
Mild	0.90 – 0.99 (right or left)	0.60 – 0.69
Moderate	0.50 – 0.90	0.59 – 0.40
Severe	0.30 – 0.50	< 0.39
Critical	< 0.30	–

BI Data Source: Modified from AbuRahma AF. (2000). Segmental Doppler pressures and Doppler waveform analysis in peripheral vascular disease of the lower extremities. In AbuRahma AF, Bergan JJ (Eds). *Non-invasive Vascular Diagnosis*. (213-229). London: Springer.
TBI Data Source: Internally validated at the University of Chicago Medicine Vascular Laboratory

Table 20-2. **Lower Extremity TBI Symptoms**

TBI Range	Symptoms
0.80-0.90	Normal
0.35 + 15	Claudication
0.11 + 10	Rest pain/ulceration

Source: Zierler, RE, (2005). Nonimaging physiologic tests for assessment of lower extremity arterial occlusive disease. In Zwiebel WJ, Pellerito JS (Eds.), *Introduction to Vascular Ultrasonography 5th ed.*. (275-295). Philadelphia: Elsevier Saunders.

Peripheral Venous

Venous Duplex Evaluation

Venous Insufficiency (diagnosed by measuring reflux): Reflux means to "flow backward." Venous reflux is defined as blood flowing in the wrong direction. Reflux can occur in the deep and superficial venous systems as well as the perforating veins.

- Venous duplex ultrasound can identify the presence, exact location, extent, and severity of venous reflux
- Asses reflux for significance by measuring the duration of backwards blood flow, in seconds, after distal augmentation *(Fig. 20-3)*.

Table 20-3. **Diagnostic Criteria for Venous Reflux**

	Valve Closure Time	
	Normal	Abnormal
Common Femoral Vein (CFV)	<1sec or <1000msec	>1sec or >1000msec
Femoral Vein (FV)	<1sec or <1000msec	>1sec or >1000msec
Popliteal Vein (PopV)	<1sec or <1000msec	>1sec or >1000msec
Calf Veins	<0.5sec or <500msec	>0.5sec or >500msec
Perforating Veins [50]	<0.5sec or <500msec	>0.5sec or >500msec
Superficial Veins	<0.5sec or <500msec	>0.5sec or >500msec

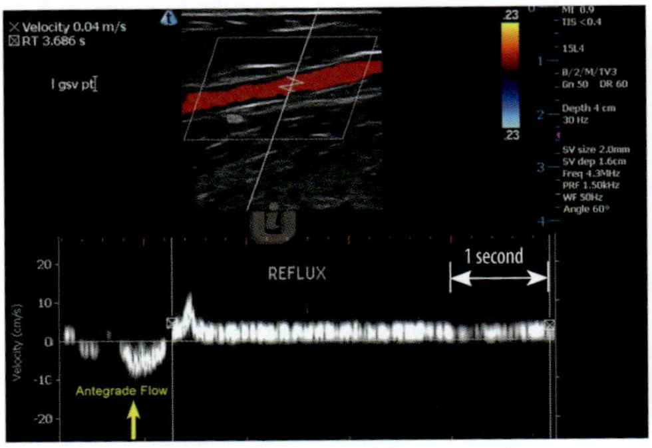

Fig. 20-3. *Duplex ultrasound images for venous reflux. The image reveals venous reflux in the GSV, as venous flow is above the baseline for > 0.5 second.*

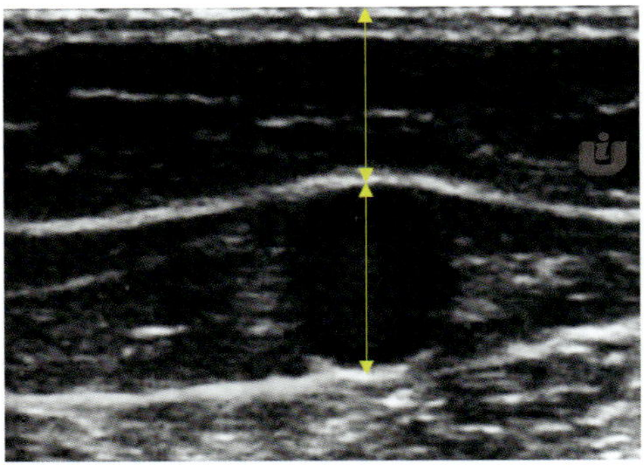

Fig. 20-4. *Diameter and depth measurements of the GSV.*

- Vein diameter should be measured, but not used as a criterion for reflux.
  - Mean diameter GSV: 5.0 ± 2.4
  - Mean diameter SSV: 3.1 ± 1.3
- Perform all measurements in the standing position.
- Using the transverse view, measure the maximum diameter from the anterior outer wall to the posterior outer wall.
- Measure the depth of the vein from the skin surface to help determine treatment options.

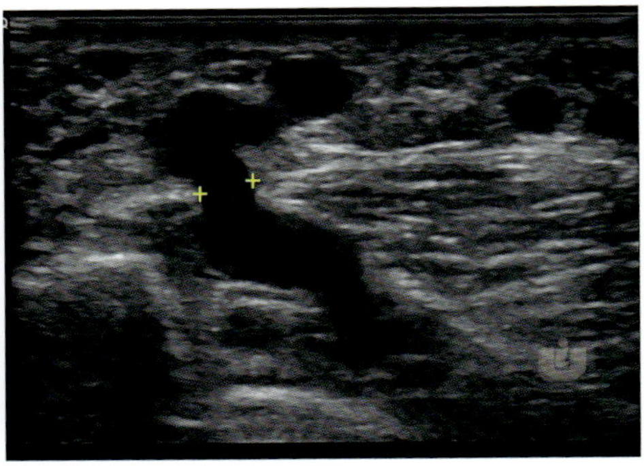

Fig. 20-5. *Perforators are measured at the level that they traverse the fascial plane.*

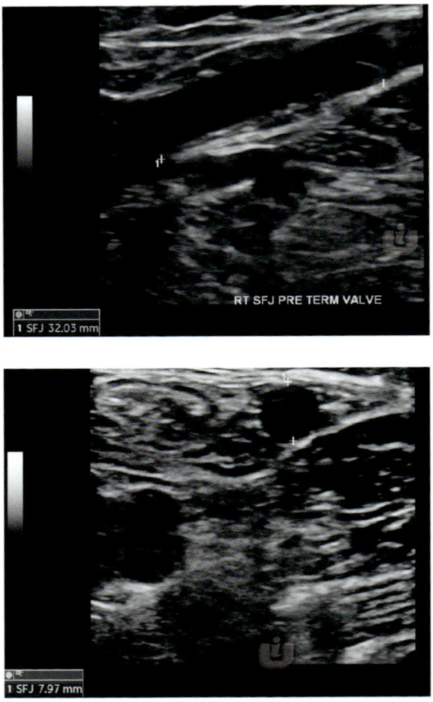

Fig. 20-6. *The SFJ ranges in length from 3-5cm with its most peripheral segment starting at the preterminal valve. The diameter of the SFJ can be obtained at any point between the preterminal valve and the ostial valve. Measure the SFJ diameter in the transverse plane with the calipers placed on the anterior outer wall to the posterior outer wall.*

Pelvic Venous

Table 20-4. Duplex Criteria for Iliac Vein Obstruction

	Doppler Findings	B-mode Findings
Common Iliac and External Iliac Veins	• Velocity Ratio >2.5 (peripheral segment/point of obstruction) • Variability in phasicity from R to L side	• With visible narrowing on B-mode image (intraluminal scarring) • Presence of collaterals
Internal Iliac Veins	• Reflux is noted within the main trunk or its tributaries which can be spontaneous or occur with provocative maneuvers	
Renal Veins	• Peak vein velocity ratio >5	• Diameter ratio >5
Gonadal Veins	• Reflux >1 second in duration; however variable flow patterns have been noted in pathologic gonadal veins.	• Gonadal vein diameter of >6mm (Note: the diameter does not always predict disease; do not base diagnosis on size alone)
Pelvic Varicosities	• Retrograde flow	• Diameter >5mm
Pelvic Escape Points	• At present time, there is no published criteria for diagnosing pelvic escape points. • The presence of varicose veins in the lower extremity that are of non saphenous origin and can be traced toward the pelvis, genitals, perineum and buttocks. More specifically to the defined pelvic escape points.	

Diameter Ratios

Divide the diameter at the level of stenosis by the diameter peripheral to the stenosis *(Example using the CIV diameters in Fig. 20-7)*:

6.9mm ÷ 1.7mm Ratio = 4.1

Diameters of the veins of the pelvic veins are most often taken in a longitudinal view outer anterior wall to outer posterior wall.

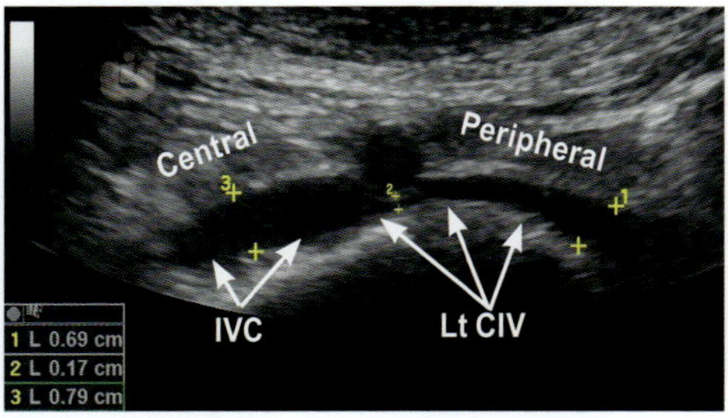

Fig. 20-7. *Diameters are obtained in B-mode to ensure good visualization of the anterior and posterior walls for accurate measurements.*

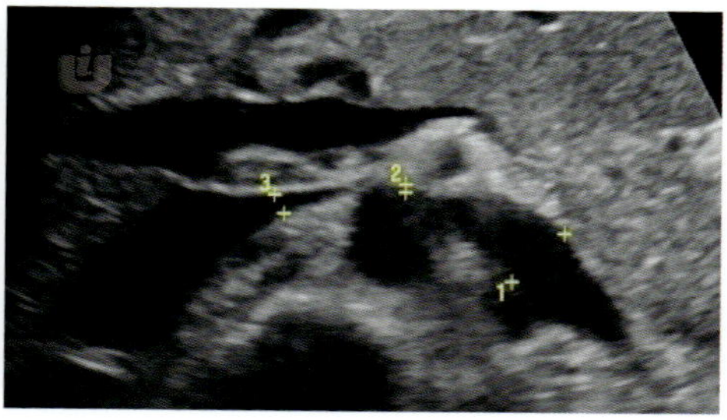

Fig. 20-8. *Compression of the LRV by the overlying SMA in the longitudinal view.*

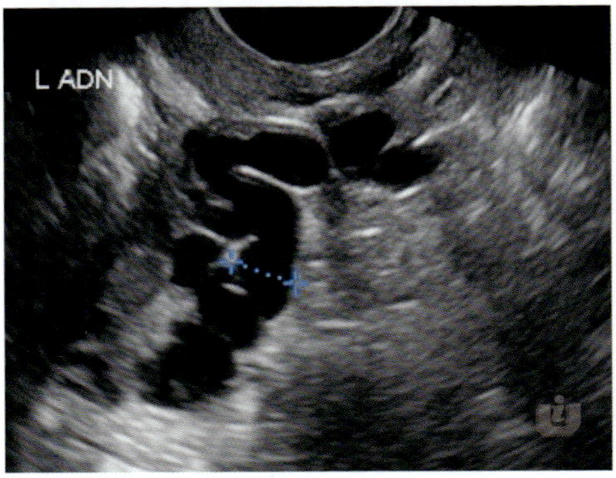

Fig. 20-9. *Endovaginal image of a pelvic adnexa varicose vein.*

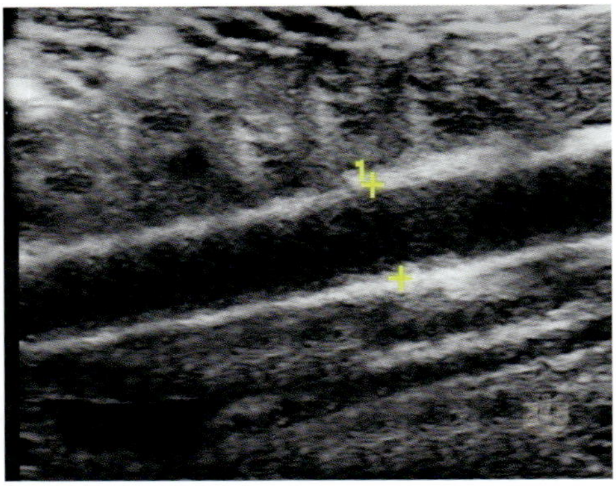

Fig. 20-10. *Longitudinal image of caliper placement for measuring the gonadal vein.*

Velocity Ratios

Divide the peak vein velocity at the site of stenosis by the peak vein velocity within a segment peripheral to the stenosis *(Example using the LRV velocities in Fig. 20-13 and 20-14)*:

121cm/sec ÷ 24cm/sec Ratio = 5.1

Peak vein velocities, when appropriate, are obtained peripheral to the stenosis (inflow), at the level of the stenosis and central to (outflow) the stenosis. The caliper is placed on the highest peak within the PW Doppler waveform.

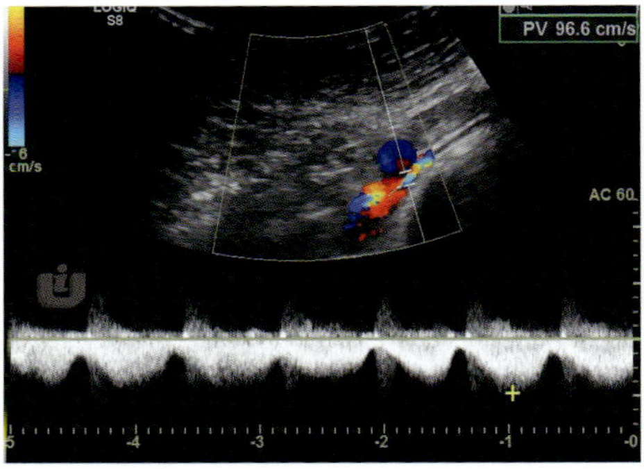

Fig. 20-11. *PW Doppler of the CIV at the level of the compression.*

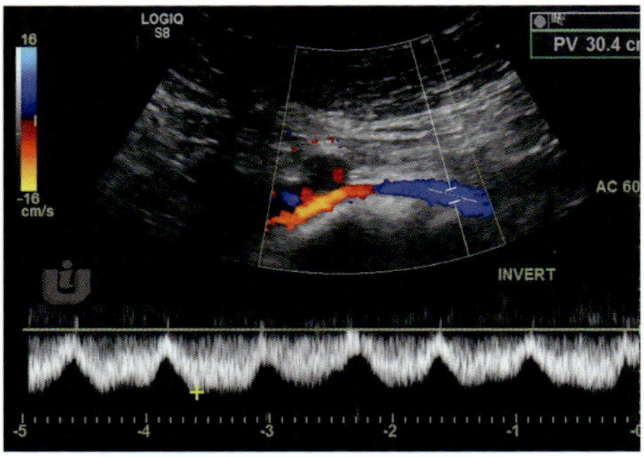

Fig. 20-12. *PW Doppler of the left CIV within the peripheral segment.*

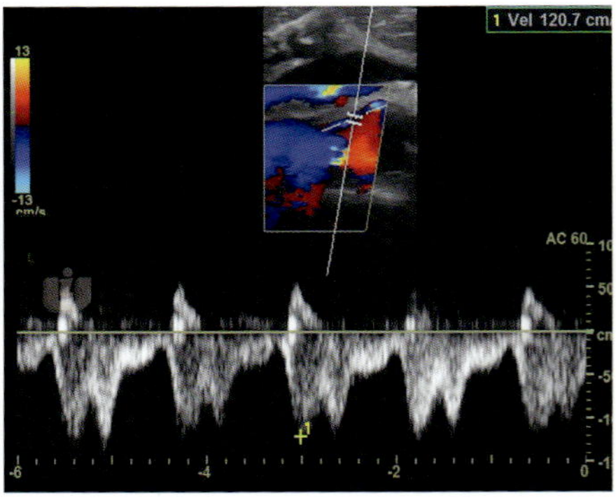

Fig. 20-13. *PW Doppler of the central segment of the LRV with a velocity of 121cm/sec.*

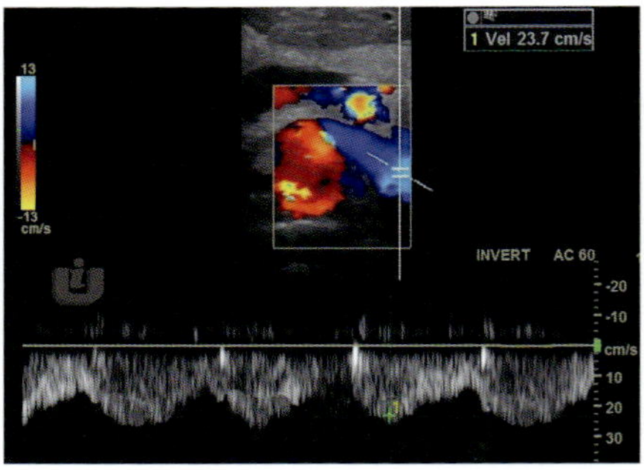

Fig. 20-14. *In the same patient, a peak vein velocity of 24cm/sec is obtained in the peripheral segment of the LRV.*

A

Abduction Drawing away from the midline, opposite of adduction.

Abscess A localized collection of pus surrounded by inflamed tissue.

Acoustic shadow Loss of acoustic properties of targets lying behind an attenuating structure. In the arteries, the most common cause of acoustic shadowing is calcified plaque (see calcification).

Acute Short, severe symptoms of sudden onset or short duration.

Adduction Drawing toward the midline.

Adventitia The outermost layer of a vein or an artery.

Aliasing A phenomenon associated with pulsed Doppler; Doppler shift in a negative direction occurs when the Doppler shift exceeds half the pulse repetition frequency.

Alignment sign Distinguishes the Anterior Accessory Saphenous Vein from the Great Saphenous Vein. The AASV is seated anterior and lateral to the GSV, aligning itself over the deep vessels.

Allen test A test performed to check the continuity of the palmar arch normally supplied by both the radial and ulnar arteries. The test may be performed using a Doppler or PPG.

Ambulatory Phlebectomy (also known as phlebectomy, microphlebectomy, or stab avulsion) A technique to remove varicose veins. In this procedure, several tiny cuts (incisions) are made in the skin through which the varicose vein is removed.

Amplitude The maximum variation in an acoustic variable. It is the difference between the average value and the maximum value of an acoustic variable. Units used with amplitude coincide with the acoustic variable used.

Amputation The cutting off (traumatic or surgical) of all or part of an appendage.

Anastomosis The natural or surgically-created communication between blood vessels or prosthetic graft and blood vessel as in a bypass graft. Anastomosis can then be referred to as proximal or distal.

Anechoic Describes the property of being echo-free or without echoes (i.e., fluid-filled cyst).

Angiogram A series of x-rays taken of a blood vessel following the injection of a radiopaque substance into the vessel (arteriogram).

Angioplasty Dilation of an artery by a balloon tipped catheter. Often referred to as percutaneous transluminal angioplasty (PTA).

Ankle brachial index (ABI) The ratio of ankle systolic pressure to highest arm systolic pressure. The numerical index serves as an indicator of arterial insufficiency. Normal value is 1.0 or greater; the ratio decreases as arterial insufficiency increases. Usually referred to as ABI.

Antecubital fossa A triangular area located at the bend of the elbow that contains the cephalic, median cubital and basilic veins.

Antegrade Proceeding toward.

Antegrade flow Proceeding towards or forward. Opposite of retrograde or reversed.

Anterior Situated in the frontal plane, in the front of.

Anticoagulant Substances which prohibit or delay the normal blood clotting mechanism, e.g., Coumadin and heparin.

Aorta The main trunk of the arterial system with its origin off the surface of the left ventricle. It is usually described in several portions, the ascending

Aplasia Aplasia indicates the lack of development of a vein or of a segment of a vein. The vein is present but diminutive in size. Its structure is similar to the embryo.

Aplastic not exhibiting growth or change in structure

Arrhythmia Abnormal heart rhythm.

Arterial inflow Pertaining to blood flow into the lower extremities proximal to the level of the common femoral arteries.

Arterial insufficiency Reduction in blood flow within the arterial system. Inadequate blood flow results in hypoxia; the symptoms produced by arterial insufficiency vary with the end organ site.

Arterial occlusion Complete blockage of an artery.

Arterial outflow Normally pertaining to the medium size blood vessels, common femoral through the popliteal. Outflow could also pertain to the vessels carrying blood away from a bypass graft.

Arterial runoff The infra-popliteal vessels (tibial and distal vessels).

Arterial ulceration A local defect or excavation which is produced by sloughing of inflammatory necrotic tissue.

Arteriography A radiologic procedure in which an opaque substance is injected into an artery and subsequent x-ray films are taken in order to visualize the arterial system.

Arteriole A minute artery whose distal end leads to a capillary.

Arteriovenous malformation congenital anomalies resulting from faulty development of arterial, capillary, venous or lymphatic structures or any combination thereof. These lesions are thought to be present from birth and do not represent neoplasms.

Artery Any of the blood vessels which carry blood from the heart to the other parts of the body. With the exception of the pulmonary and umbilical arteries, arteries transport oxygenated blood.

Artifact In ultrasound usage, refers to an echo which does not correspond to a real target. In general, refers to any artificial finding which may resemble the expected findings. artifacts may be intrinsic, e.g., reverberation or extrinsic.

Ascites Accumulation of serous fluid in spaces between tissues and organs in the abdominal cavity.

Atherosclerosis Disease of the arterial intima, characterized by intimal proliferation (hyperplasia), deposition of fatty substances and luminal reduction.

Attenuation Reduction in amplitude and intensity as a sound wave passes through a medium. Factors contributing to attenuation include absorption, reflection, refraction, and scattering.

Augmentation To cause to augment or increase. When used in conjunction with Doppler examinations of the venous or cerebral systems, refer to the increased flow velocity which is noted after one or more compression/ release maneuvers.

Avalvulia an absence of valves in the venous trunks of one or more extremities.

B

Basilic vein Large vein on the inner side of the arm (medial), near the brachial veins, a superficial vein.

Bi-directional Doppler A Doppler instrument capable of determining whether the frequency of the Doppler shift is above or below the transmission frequency, permitting determination of blood flow towards or away from the transducer.

Bifurcation That location where an artery branches; a frequent site of atherosclerosis.

Bilateral On both sides.

Biphasic Having two phases or variations having a forward and reverse component.

Blood pressure (BP) Pressure within the arterial system, quantified in millimeters of mercury (mm Hg); includes systolic pressure (during heart contraction), diastolic pressure (during cardiac relaxation) or mean blood pressure. Blood pressure is usually expressed as systolic over diastolic pressure.

Brachial veins A paired set of veins which accompany the brachial artery. They are formed at the elbow by the confluence of the radial and ulnar veins. They drain the same area that the brachial artery supplies.

Brachiocephalic (Innominate) Right artery arising from the arch of the aorta dividing into the right subclavian and right common carotid arteries.

Bradycardia Abnormally low heart rate, generally less than 60 beats per minute.

Budd-Chiari syndrome Venous outflow obstruction or occlusion, located at any level from the hepatic venules to the inferior vena cava (IVC), associated with ascites and liver failure.

C

Calcification Deposition of calcium salts within an organic substance causing hardening. Medial calcification is known as Monckeberg's sclerosis Arterial calcification hampers Doppler ultrasonic evaluation of blood flow because of the high reflectivity of calcium. Calcified structures have a higher acoustic impedance than the surrounding tissues.

Caval Pertaining to the vena cava.

Caudad In a direction toward the feet (or tail), the opposite of cephalad.

CEAP (Clinical-Etiology-Anatomy-Pathophysiology) A classification system for chronic venous disease.

Cellulitis Inflammation of cellular or connective tissue. An infection in or close to the skin is usually localized by the body defense mechanisms.

Central Areas at or near the center of the body.

Cephalad Toward the head.

Cephalic Cranial; superior in position.

Cephalic vein A superficial vein that ascends from the dorsal aspect of the radial border of the forearm, to the anterior surface and subcutaneously up the arm and ends in the axillary vein near the clavicle. Frequently used for arteriovenous fistula formation for dialysis access.

CHIVA The French acronym for "Cure conservatrice et Hemodynamique de l'Insuffisance Veineuse en Ambulatoire" (Conservative and Hemodynamic treatment of Venous Insufficiency in the Office). It is a saphenous-sparing therapeutic approach to lower limb chronic venous disease (CVD) based on hemodynamic concepts proposed by Claude Franceschi in 1988.

Cirrhosis A chronic disease of the liver; dense connective tissue forms, liver cells cease to function.

Claudication Literally, "to limp" symptoms associated with arterial insufficiency of the extremity; intermittent leg pain (ache, cramp, etc.) brought on by exercise and relieved by rest.

Coagulate To become clotted or congealed.

Coagulation To change from a fluid to a semi solid mass.

Coalesce To fuse; to run or grow together.

Coapt To meet or join. When performing a venous duplex exam, with light transducer pressure, the walls of normal veins collapse and come together.

Collateral circulation An alternate, natural circulatory pathway. When there is interference in the arterial supply because of obstruction, communicating channels develop to accommodate blood flow. The peripheral resistance of the collateral vessels is higher because of the smaller diameter of the vessels.

Compartment syndrome This syndrome occurs when increased pressure in the noncompliant fascia compromises circulation and neuromuscular function in that anatomic space.

Competence In the normal vein no retrograde flow is detected, either with Valsalva maneuver, with proximal compression, or with the release of distal compression. Absence of retrograde flow confirms adequate venous valve closure.

Compression The act of pressing or squeezing; the condition of being pressed together.

Confluence A flowing or meeting together; a joining.

Congenital Present at birth.

Congestive heart failure (CHF) A chronic cardiac condition in which the heart is unable to maintain adequate output of blood resulting in congestion of blood in the veins and other organs of the body.

Constriction The narrowing of a vessel opening.

Continuous flow In abnormal veins the respiratory phasicity is lost, resulting in a steady flow signal. When coupled with very low velocity, continuous flow indicates proximal (except in the Portal system) obstruction that is preventing the normal fluctuations in flow that occurs during respiration. It is not always possible to distinguish between extrinsic vein compression and intrinsic obstruction (DVT), most especially in the iliac segments.

Continuous wave Doppler (CW) A Doppler which uses separate transmitting and receiving piezoelectric crystals, each operating without interruption. The reflected sound waves are processed continuously.

Contralateral On the opposite side.

Cord A string like structure. A firm elongated structure consistent with a thrombosed vein.

Coronary artery bypass surgery Surgical establishment of a shunt that permits blood to travel from the aorta to a branch of the coronary artery at a point past an obstruction.

Costoclavicular Pertains to the ribs and the clavicle.

Coumadin anticoagulant One of a group of natural and synthetic compounds that antagonize the biosynthesis of vitamin K dependent on coagulation factors in the liver.

Cramp Spasmodic muscle contraction; term often used by patients to describe claudication pain.

Cuff artifact Refers to abnormally high pressures associated with the use of cuffs which are proportionately too narrow for the limb they are encircling.

Cyanosis A slight bluish, grayish, slate like or dark purple discoloration of the skin caused by reduced amounts of hemoglobin in the blood. Etiology a deficiency of oxygen.

Cyst A closed sac or pouch, with a definite wall, contains fluid, semi fluid, or solid material. A simple cyst is usually spherical, with echo enhancement posterior to cyst. Complex cysts can have internal debris and septations.

D

D-Dimer Formed as fibrin is broken down. Positive levels are suggestive of a thrombotic event such as deep vein thrombosis or pulmonary embolism. Negative levels can virtually rule out the presence of DVT or PE, sparing the patient further expensive, uncomfortable and/or invasive testing

Dead zone The region close to the transducer that cannot be imaged accurately.

Deceleration A decrease in velocity.

Decubitus, lateral Refers to a patient lying on their side.

Deep vein thrombosis (DVT) Obstruction of the deep veins by blood clot. DVT is a non-inflammatory process. The possibility of the loosely attached thrombus dislodging is always present. DVT can lead to valvular destruction, post-phlebitic syndrome, and pulmonary embolism.

Dependent rubor Abnormal redness noted of the toes (filling of the small vessels) and forefoot when the leg is in the dependent position. This is usually noted in patients with severe occlusive disease.

Depth of penetration That depth wherein echoes are no longer detectable; a function of the operating frequency of the transducer.

Dermatitis Inflammation of skin evidenced by itching, redness, and various skin lesions.

Diaphragm A musculomembranous wall separating the abdomen from the thoracic cavity. It contracts and expands with respiration.

Digit A toe or finger.

Dilatation A vessel is stretched beyond normal dimensions.

Dissection Separation of tissues; usually surgically (see aneurysm, dissecting).

Disseminated intravascular coagulation (DIC) A pathological form of coagulation that is diffuse rather than localized. The process damages rather than protects the area involved, and several clotting factors are consumed to such extent that generalized bleeding may occur.

Distal Farthest from the center from medial line, or from the trunk; opposite of proximal.

Doppler A diagnostic instrument which emits an ultrasonic beam into the body. This ultrasound is reflected back from moving structures within the body at a frequency higher or lower than this transmitted frequency (Doppler shift). This shift is amplified and presented as a sound or graphic (chart) display.

Doppler angle The angle between the direction of propagation of the ultrasound and the direction of flow. As an approximation, the angle between the axis of the ultrasound beam and the axis of the vessel lumen is generally used.

Doppler effect Observed frequency change of reflected sound due to reflector movement to the source or the observer.

Doppler shift The frequency shift created between the transmitted frequency and received frequency by an interface moving with velocity at an angle to the sound source.

Dorsal Indicating a position toward the rear part, pertaining to the back opposed to ventral.

E

Ecchymosis A skin discoloration consisting of large irregularity formed hemorrhagic areas.

Echo Reflection of acoustic energy.

Echogenic The acoustic property of a medium which renders it capable of producing echoes.

Ectatic Distended or stretched.

Edema A local or generalized condition in which the body tissues contain an excessive amount of tissue fluid.

EHIT Endothermal Heat-Induced Thrombosis is defined as propagation of a thrombus from a superficial vein into a deeper vein. It is generally considered clinically insignificant if the thrombus does not propagate to the deep venous system.

Elasticity Willingness of a medium to distort from its original size and shape and restore to its original form after the external influence is removed.

Embolectomy Removal of an embolus from a vessel.

Embolism An obstruction in a vessel from a foreign substance or blood clot.

Embolus A mass of undissolved matter present in a blood or lymphatic vessel and carried there by the blood or lymph current.

E Point An ultrasound marker of the Great Saphenous Vein, found 3–5 cm below the saphenofemoral junction where it crosses superficially over the adductor longus muscle. This marker was named "E Point" because it is Easy to identify the Great Saphenous Vein at this point.

Erythema Reddening of the skin.

Erythrocyte A mature red blood cell (RBC) or corpuscle.

Esophageal varices Varicosities of the branches of the azygos vein that anastomose with the tributaries of the portal vein in the lower esophagus; occurs in patients with portal hypertension.

Etiology Study of the causation of disease.

Extravasation Discharge or escape, as of blood or other substance from within a vessel into the tissue.

Extrinsic Originating from without, opposite of intrinsic.

Eye Sign The echographic identification of the Great Saphenous Vein.

F

False aneurysm See aneurysm, pseudo.

False negative rate Rate at which a diagnostic test produces negative results when disease is actually present. False Neg. Rate = FN × 100 = % TP + FN FN = false negative, TP = true positive False positive rate Rate at which a diagnostic test produces positive results when disease is not present.

False Positive Rate The rate at which a diagnostic test produces positive results when disease is actually not present. FP × 100 = % TN + FP TN = true negative, FP = false positive.

Fascia A band or sheet of connective tissue, that surrounds, encloses, and separates muscles, vessels and nerves.

Field of view That plane seen by specific ultrasound transducer.

Fistula, arteriovenous Communication between an artery and a vein. It may be congenital, traumatic, or surgically created for dialysis access.

Frequency Number of cycles per unit of time (usually seconds); expressed in Hertz (Hz) 1 Hz = 1 cycle per second, Kilohertz (KHz) 1 KHz = 1,000 Hz, or Megahertz (MHz) 1 MHz = 1,000,000 Hz or 1,000,000 cycles per second.

G

Gain The ratio of output to input in an amplifying system.

Gaiter area zone The region of the medial lower leg just above the ankle. It is this area where signs of venous stasis are most evident.

Gangrene Tissue death, usually as a result of inadequate blood supply; occasionally due to infection. Lack of blood supply may be due to atherosclerosis, embolism, spasm, frostbite, tourniquets, etc.

Gastrocnemius That large muscle of the posterior portion of the lower leg that propels venous blood up the leg as it contracts. Commonly referred to as the calf muscle pump, this superficial muscle extends the foot and helps to flex the knee.

Gate Electronically controlled device which controls transmission or reception of a signal.

Genicular Venous Plexis The term genicular venous plexus (plexus venosus genicularis) should replace the term genicular veins. At the knee, deep veins do not correspond exactly to the branches of the popliteal artery (articular arteries). They are arranged in a complex plexus of interconnecting veins.

Gray scale A display format in which the intensity information is recorded as changes in brightness. Also known as B-mode.

Great saphenous vein (GSV) One of the two major superficial veins of the lower limb. It originates on the dorsum of the foot, ascends medially along the calf and thigh, and drains into the common femoral vein. It is the longest vein in the body and is the vessel of choice for lower extremity bypass procedures and is also used for coronary artery bypass.

H

Hemangioma A tumor, growth, or abnormal mass composed of blood vessels.

Hematoma A blood-filled swelling.

Hemodynamics Pertaining to the physical principles governing blood flow (i.e., blood pressure, blood flow, vascular volumes, heart rate, ventricular function).

Hemoglobin The iron containing pigment of the red blood cells. Its function is to carry oxygen from the lungs to the tissues. The amount of hemoglobin in the blood averages 14-16 grams per 100ml.

Hemorrhage Escape of blood from a vessel (arterial or venous). Abnormal bleeding.

Heparin Substance used to inhibit coagulation of blood; frequently used in the treatment of deep venous thrombosis.

Hepatic veins Drain blood flow from the liver into the inferior vena cava. There are three main veins, the left, middle and the right.

Hepatofugal flow Directed or flowing away from the liver.

Hepatopetal flow Directed or flowing toward the liver.

Heterogeneous Of different kind or species; used in ultrasound to describe sonographic characteristics of atherosclerotic plaque; opposite of homogeneous.

Homan's sign Pain in the calf muscle resulting from passive dorsiflexion of the foot. Is sometimes indicative of deep venous thrombosis; of limited accuracy.

Homogeneous Uniform in structure, of the same composition.

Hunter's canal A triangular space lying in the distal thigh beneath the sartorius muscle and between the adductor longus and the vastus medialis muscle. It is at this location that the femoral vessels and the saphenous nerve are transmitted.

Hydrostatic pressure A pressure created in a fluid system, such as the circulatory system.

Hyperechoic Producing echoes of higher amplitude than normal for the surrounding medium.

Hyperemia Increased blood in an area. May be active, i.e., caused by increased flow or passive, i.e., increased flow that occurs in response to a previous restriction of flow.

Hypertension Abnormally elevated blood pressure may be essential (etiology unknown) or secondary to another condition (e.g., renal disease, pregnancy). Although there is no universal agreement, 140 systolic and 90 diastolic are considered the upper limits of normal. Control of hypertension is an important consideration; some sequelae of hypertension include stroke, small vessel damage, and congestive heart failure.

Hypoechoic Producing echoes of lower amplitude than normal for the surrounding medium.

Hypoplasia Hypoplasia indicates the incomplete development of a vein or of a segment of a vein. It is less severe in degree than aplasia, and the hypoplastic vein has a reduced caliber with a normal structure.

Hypoplastic Incomplete or underdevelopment of a tissue or organ.

Hypotension Abnormally low blood pressure; may be primary, secondary, or postural.

Hypovolemia Decreased blood volume.

Hypoxia Diminished oxygen content in the tissues.

I

Iliac vein Formed by the confluence of the internal iliac vein which drains the pelvis and the external iliac vein which is a continuation of the common femoral vein. The right and left common iliac veins unite to form the inferior vena cava.

Impedance Electrical resistance; changes in impedance (or resistance) are measured by impedance plethysmography (IPG).

Impedance plethysmography A noninvasive diagnostic technique used in the diagnosis of deep venous thrombosis. Four electrodes are placed around the calf and a small electrical current is sent through the underlying tissues.

Incompetent Unable to perform natural function. Used to refer to venous valves which no longer close completely, permitting blood to flow in a backward direction.

Inflow obstruction Arterial blood flow is severely restricted due to a proximal obstructing lesion.

Inferior Lower than, beneath.

Inferior mesenteric vein (IMV) Is usually small in size and runs to the left of the superior mesenteric vein to join the splenic vein.

Inferior vena cava (IVC) Originates from the confluence of the right and left iliac veins terminating in the right atrium of the heart.

Infrapopliteal Located below the popliteal artery or popliteal space.

Inguinal ligament A fibrous band extending from the anterior superficial iliac spine to the pubis tubercle in the groin.

Innominate vein Formed by the confluence of the internal jugular with the subclavian vein.

Intermittent Occurring at intervals, not constant. Used when describing claudication.

Internal Inside, opposite of external.

Intima Innermost layer of a vein or an artery; comprised of an endothelial lining, a thin layer of connective tissue, and an internal elastic membrane.

Ipsilateral On the same side, opposite of contralateral.

Ischemia Deficient local blood supply to body tissues; due to obstruction of arterial inflow. Symptoms of ischemia include coldness, pallor, pain, impairment of function and ultimately tissue necrosis (gangrene).

J

Joule One joule is defined as the amount of energy exerted when a force of one newton is applied over a displacement of one meter. One joule is the equivalent of one watt of power radiated or dissipated for one second.

Jugular vein Major neck vein subdivided into anterior, external, and internal jugular veins bilaterally.

Jugular vein anterior Originates from the veins draining the lower jaw, descends anteriorly, and terminates in the external jugular vein.

Jugular vein external Drains the exterior of the cranium and deep parts of the face, runs perpendicularly in the neck to empty into the subclavian, internal jugular, or brachiocephalic vein.

Jugular vein internal Continues from the transverse sinus at the base of the skull, runs vertically in the neck to unite with the subclavian vein to form the brachiocephalic vein.

K

Klippel-Trenaunay Syndrome A rare disorder that is present at birth (congenital) and is characterized by a triad of cutaneous capillary malformation ("port-wine stain"), lymphatic anomalies, and abnormal veins in association with variable overgrowth of soft tissue and bone.

L

Lamina A thin layer.

Laminar flow Blood flowing in thin layers in a streamline direction parallel to the vessel wall. The highest velocities are at center stream; slowest along the wall. In laminar flow, red blood cells tend to migrate toward center stream, leaving the less viscous plasma along the wall.

Lateral Away from the mid-line, to the side.

Ligate To tie off, e.g., to tie off a blood vessel at surgery.

Linear Relating to, consisting of, or resembling a line. Linear transducer; multiple elements arranged in a line.

Lipid A broad group of chemicals that include steroids, fats, and waxes characterized by their insolubility in water.

Longitudinal Along the path of a sound beam; or along a lengthwise course, as in a longitudinal scan. (Long axis, LAX)

Lumen The space inside a tube, blood vessel, or duct.

Lymph Transparent fluid, comprised of white blood cells (lymphocytes), conveyed in the lymphatic vessels.

Lymphangitis Inflammation of a lymph vessel.

Lymphedema Fluid retention in the tissues as a result of obstruction in the lymphatic system. Can present symptoms similar to deep venous thrombosis.

Lymphoceles Fluid collections, which result from lymphatic leakage from, disrupted channels along the iliac vessels.

M

Maximum venous outflow Describes the maximum rate of venous emptying which occurs in a limb following rapid cuff deflation post venous occlusion.

Mean Midway between two points or measurements; the arithmetic average.

Media Middle layer of a vein or an artery.

Medial Toward the midline, opposite of lateral.

Median The middle number in a distribution, half of the numbers will be above and half of the numbers will be below it.

Median cubital vein Located in the antecubital fossa and crosses from the medial to the lateral side of the fossa and connects the basilic and cephalic veins.

Membrane A thin lining or covering.

Microphlebectomy (also known as phlebectomy, ambulatory phlebectomy, or stab avulsion) A technique to remove varicose veins. In this procedure, several tiny cuts (incisions) are made in the skin through which the varicosed vein is removed.

Morbidity The ratio of unhealthy individuals to the total population of a given group; a state of being sick/diseased.

Mortality The ratio or total number of deaths to the total number of a given group.

Mottling A condition that is marked by discolored areas.

Mural Refers to the wall of a cavity, organ, or vessel.

Muscle pump A mechanism to direct blood from the lower extremities towards the heart. The contracting muscles of the leg, especially the calf, act as a power source to propel the venous drainage collected in the soleal sinusoids. Competent valves prevent the reflux of blood. When the muscles relax, the space created in the now-emptied deep veins draws blood from the superficial veins into the deep system via the perforators.

N

Necrosis Localized tissue death; when due to arterial insufficiency is called ischemic necrosis; often used interchangeably with the term gangrene.

Negative predictive value The ability of a test to anticipate (predict) normal findings. Neg. Pred. Value = TN × 100 = % TN + FN TN = true negative, FN = false negative

Neointimal hyperplasia The narrowing of an endarterectomized artery by smooth muscle and fibrous overgrowth of the tissue layer that replaces the intima after surgery.

Neovascularization Recurrence through the growth of new vessels.

Neuropathy A functional disturbance or pathological change in the nervous system. Can be related to peripheral vascular disease in the diabetic patient, sensory, motor, autonomic, and mixed varieties.

Nocturnal Occurring during the night. May be used to describe rest pain which causes awakening from sleep.

Nondirectional A Doppler instrument which assesses flow, via frequency shift, without regard for direction of blood flow.

Nonocclusive Not totally obstructed.

O

Obstructive Raynaud's syndrome Episodic attacks of vasospasm resulting in the closure of small arteries and arterioles of the distal extremities in response to cold or stress with obstruction of the palmar and digital arteries.

Occlusion The complete closure of an opening, duct or vessel.

Ohm's law States that voltage equals current multiplied by resistance (impedance). Voltage = Current × Resistance This is the basis for strain gauge and impedance plethysmographic testing. When voltage and current are held constant, the changes in resistance can only be due to changes in limb volume.

Ostial Valve A valve located at the point of entry of a tributary. Ostial valves usually consist of a single cusp.

Overall accuracy Sum of true positive tests and true negative tests divided by the total number of tests performed.

P

Pallor Abnormal paleness or lack of color in the skin.

Pansystolic Extending throughout systole, as in pansystolic bruit. Used interchangeably with holosystolic.

Parasympathetic A division of the autonomic nervous system involved primarily with restorative functions. The parasympathetic nerves are derived from intracranial and sacral nerves and travel via the vagus nerves.

Paraná maneuver A slight push to the waist triggers an isometric contraction of the leg muscle propelling deep venous flow toward the popliteal vein without any ankle movement. Commonly used outside the United States.

Parietal Valve A valve located within the lumen of a vein. Parietal valves are bicuspid, usually consisting of two cusps.

PASTE A Post Ablation Superficial Thrombus Extension into the common femoral vein as a consequence of endovenous treatment of the GSV with laser or radiofrequency.

Patency The state of being open. A venous characteristic assessed in the venous Doppler examination.

Patent Open, not occluded.

Pedal Pertaining to the foot as in pedal pulses, the pulses of the foot.

Perforating veins (communicating veins) Veins that cross the muscular fascia, connecting the superficial and deep venous systems.

Peripheral Areas away from the center of the body.

Peripheral vascular resistance That resistance (or impedance) to blood flow in the systemic arterial system. Resistance to blood flow is determined primarily by the caliber of small arterioles, i.e., the smaller the vessel the greater the resistance. Other factors affecting resistance include the length of the vessel and viscosity. It is vascular resistance which contributes to the brief period of flow reversal in the peripheral vessels.

Perivascular Surrounding a blood vessel.

Phasicity Normal venous flow increases and decreases in response to respiration. In a normal lower extremity, flow will diminish or cease with respiration. Phasicity is reversed in the upper extremity veins.

Phlebectomy (also known as microphlebectomy, ambulatory phlebectomy, or stab avulsion) A technique to remove varicose veins. In this procedure, several tiny cuts (incisions) are made in the skin through which a varicose vein is removed.

Phlebitis Inflammation of a vein.

Phlebography Radiologic procedure in which an opaque substance is injected into a vein; subsequent x-ray pictures are taken in order to visualize the venous system. Synonymous with venography.

Phlebolymphedema is a mixed etiology swelling due to chronic venous insufficiency and lymphatic insufficiency. It is most commonly due to the inability of the lymphatic system to adequately drain the interstitial fluid that accumulates in severe chronic venous hypertension.

Phlebosclerosis refers to the thickening and hardening of the vein walls.

Phlebothrombosis Term used to describe occlusion of vein by clot in the absence of an inflammatory process (see deep venous thrombosis).

Phlegmasia Cerulea Dolens When DVT involves the major veins proximal to the inguinal ligament. Commonly referred to as iliofemoral thrombosis.

Photoplethysmograph (PPG) Infrared light is emitted from a transmitting diode and reflected back to a receiving diode; changes in red blood cell density associated with arterial pulsation are detected by the transducer. PPG detects changes in red blood cell volume; the signal output is in the form of a pulse wave form. PPG is used in a number of noninvasive diagnostic examinations; venous reflux plethysmography, supraorbital plethysmography, digital pressures, Allen's test, and thoracic outlet maneuvers.

Piezoelectric effect Changing of mechanical to electrical energy and vice versa.

Plantar Pertaining to the sole of the foot.

Plaque Generic term used to describe an atherosclerotic lesion. It can consist of platelets, fibrin, lipids, and calcium.

Plasma Fluid portion of the blood.

Platelet A round or oval disk, 1/3 to 1/2 the size of an erythrocyte found in the blood. Platelets number from 150,000 to 450,000 per cc. Platelets play an important role in blood coagulation, hemostasis and blood thrombus formation. When a vessel is injured, platelets adhere to each other and the edges of the injury and form a plug which covers the area. The plug or blood clot formed soon retract and stops the loss of blood.

Plethysmograph Any device, instrument, or transducer which measures volume changes in size or amount. Air plethysmography include volume pulse recordings.

Portal hypertension Increased portal venous pressure, usually due to liver disease. Can cause the dilatation or thrombosis of the portal vein, superior mesenteric vein, splenic vein, and the formation of varices.

Portal system Consists of the portal vein, splenic vein, and inferior and superior mesenteric veins.

Portal vein (PV) Collects blood from the digestive tract and empties into the liver to be detoxified. Formed by the junction of the splenic vein and the superior mesenteric vein.

Positive predictive value The ability of a test to anticipate (predict) abnormal findings. Pos. Pred. Value = P × 100 = % TP + FP TP = true positive, FP = False positive

Posterior Refers to the back; or dorsal side of the body; opposite of anterior.

Postphlebitic syndrome Chronic venous insufficiency secondary to previous deep venous thrombosis. Venous thrombosis damages the valves and renders them incompetent. The physical signs include edema, stasis pigmentation changes, pain, and ulceration.

PREVAIT PREsence of Varices (residual or recurrent) After InTervention

Prone Lying on the abdomen with the face downward, opposite of supine.

Prophylaxis Pertaining to any measures designed to prevent disease development.

Proximal Nearest to a point of reference. Opposite of distal.

Pseudoclaudication Term used to describe a syndrome of symptoms resembling claudication but not of a vascular origin. The most common etiology is neurogenic. Pseudoclaudication can be differentiated from true claudication by the nature of the presenting symptoms. The exercise-pain-rest-relief cycle is not present in pseudoclaudication.

Pulmonary embolus Embolus (blood clot, air, fat) which is carried through the venous system ultimately lodging in the pulmonary vasculature. PE is a serious and occasionally fatal complication of deep venous thrombosis.

Pulse repetition frequency (pulse repetition rate) The rate of repetition of pulses per unit time; in a pulsed system, the number of pulses generated every second. Not to be confused with frequency, PRF is the rate of pulse repetition.

Pulse volume recorder (PVR) Plethysmographic technique in which air-filled cuffs are placed segmentally on an extremity; changes in limb volume associated with arterial pulsation are translated in pulse waveforms. Alterations in the shape of the waveform at each level are associated with obstruction proximal to the cuff.

Pulse wave Doppler (PW) Timed bursts of ultrasound (pulses); a single transducer alternately transmits and receives impulses. Permits more discrete sampling from a select depth and volume. Sample volume is selected through the process of range gating, i.e., receiving reflections after a defined time period has elapsed (see gate, sample volume).

Q

Qualitative A non-objective measurement relating to quality; descriptive assessment of attributes, traits, or characteristics. Measurements in which an exact numerical value cannot be assigned; scales or grades can be used.

Quantitative An observable quantity which can be described in objective, measurable terms, i.e., numbers.

R

Radiography Generic terms referring to any type of x-ray procedure; venography, arteriography are two types of radiographic techniques.

Range The distance between the reflector (target) and the transducer; equal to one half of the total ultrasound path length.

Range ambiguity Occurs when the pulse repetition frequency is too high, causing misrepresentation of echoes ranges.

Recanalization The formation of a new canal or channel of blood flow through an obstruction, such as blood clot or thrombus (deep vein thrombosis).

Reflux Backward flow. A characteristic noted on the venous Doppler examination during peripheral limb compression release maneuver; indicative of valvular dysfunction.

Renal veins Drain the kidney and empty into the inferior vena cava. The left renal vein is longer than the right renal vein.

Renovascular hypertension High blood pressure pertaining to or affecting blood vessels of the kidney, or hypertension produced by renal artery flow reducing stenosis or occlusion.

Rest pain A sign of severe arterial obstruction resulting in pronounced ischemia of an extremity. Arterial compromise is such that pain occurs at rest; often causing night-time wakefulness (due to recumbency and the reduced cardiac output of sleep). The pain is confined to the digit and dorsum of the foot and symptoms are relieved, in part, by dependency of the limb.

Retrograde Proceeding away from or backward; opposite of antegrade or forward.

Retrograde flow Blood flowing moving backwards or against the usual direction of flow.

Revascularization Varicose veins that recur in the saphenous compartment after a saphenous vein procedure.

Rouleaux Flow Stacks or aggregations of red blood cells (RBCs) that form because of the unique discoid shape of the cells.

S

Sagittal In the anterior-posterior plane of the body.

Sample volume With a pulsed Doppler system, describes the site of flow detection; size of the sample volume is determined by beam diameter and length of the ultrasound pulse (see pulsed Doppler, gate).

Saphenous vein There are two veins that serve as the principal superficial venous outflow, the great saphenous and small saphenous. The great saphenous vein runs from the foot to the groin where it joins with the common femoral vein. The small saphenous vein runs from the posterior lateral malleolus (lateral to the Achilles' tendon, near ankle) along the posterior leg and usually joins the popliteal vein in the space behind the knee.

Segmental blood pressures Obtaining blood pressure measurements at different levels of the upper or lower extremities, the comparison of pressure change across each segment of the limb in order to determine the level of occlusive disease.

Sensitivity The ability of a diagnostic technique to identify the presence of disease when disease is actually present. Sens. = TP × 100 = % TP + FN TP = true positive, FN = false negative.

Sequential bypass Arterial bypasses in series; a continuation and/or additional bypass performed to maintain patency of previous surgery.

Shunt Term used to describe a pathway other than the usual to divert blood from one point to another; may be a natural channel, i.e., an arteriovenous fistula or a surgically created channel, i.e., a bypass graft. In carotid endarterectomy a shunt is often used to divert blood from the common carotid artery to the internal system during the procedure. Shunt is synonymous with bypass.

Small saphenous vein (SSV) One of two major superficial veins of the lower limb. Originating on the lateral side of the foot, it extends along the posterior aspect of the calf. The termination of the SSV varies; terminations include the popliteal 2-4 cm/s near knee crease, distal FV, or GSV (either directly or via a perforating vein).

Specificity The ability of a diagnostic technique to identify the absence of disease (normalcy) when no disease is actually present. Spec. = TN × 100 = % TN + FP TN = true negative, FP = false positive

Spectral analysis A method of analyzing and/or displaying the Doppler signal output. Spectral analysis, using a microprocessor, is capable of analyzing and displaying the complete range of frequencies in each waveform. This technique may be used with pulsed or continuous wave Doppler systems. Time is displayed on the horizontal axis, frequency on the vertical axis and amplitude of the signal by the intensity of the gray scale. Spectral analysis provides the most complete assessment of the Doppler waveform and is a useful technique for quantifying degree of arterial stenosis.

Splenic vein Collects blood from the spleen and part of the stomach and joins with the superior mesenteric vein to form the portal vein.

Spontaneity In normal veins flow occurs passively. It should be detectable in all major veins.

Stab Avulsion (also known as phlebectomy, microphlebectomy, or ambulatory phlebectomy) A technique to remove varicose veins. In this procedure, several tiny cuts (incisions) are made in the skin through which the varicosed vein is removed.

Stasis Refers to the stagnation of blood; cessation of normal blood flow. In the venous system of the lower extremity, stagnant blood flow as the result of immobility contributes to venous thrombosis. Stagnation of venous blood in the extremity because of valvular dysfunction (or post-phlebitic syndrome) results in pigmentation changes and ulceration.

Stent A tube made of metal or plastic that is inserted into a vessel or passage to keep it open and prevent closure due to a stricture or external compression.

Streptokinase A protein produced B-hemolytic streptococci. It is used as a thrombolytic agent; used topically on surface lesions or by instillation in closed body cavities to remove clotted blood.

Stricture A narrowing of a tube, usually due to scar tissue formation.

Subclavian vein The direct continuation of the axillary vein at the lateral border of the first rib, it passes medially to join the internal jugular vein and form the brachiocephalic veins bilaterally.

Superior mesenteric vein (SMV) Drains the cecum, transverse and sigmoid colon, and small bowel.

Superior vena cava (SVC) Returns blood from the head and neck, upper limbs and thorax, and is formed by the confluence of the two brachiocephalic veins (innominate veins).

Supine Lying on the back with face upwards, opposite of prone.

Sympathetic A division of the autonomic nervous system involved primarily with emergency responses and muscular activity. It is the sympathetic system which mediates homeostasis and vascular smooth muscle response, i.e., vasodilation and vasoconstriction.

Symptom A subjective manifestation of disease, e.g., pain.

Synechiae (Webbing) Organization and subsequent contraction of a thrombus leading to adherence of thrombus to the vein wall and spontaneous lysis of areas within the thrombus. A fibrous membrane may remain within the lumen of the vein.

Systole The contraction phase of the cardiac cycle.

T

Tachycardia Excessively rapid heart rate, usually over 100 beats per minute.

Thoracic outlet syndrome (TOS) A symptom complex associated with compression of the arteries, veins, or nerves of the upper extremity at the outlet from the thoracic cavity. Symptoms include numbness or pain of the arm associated with activity, elevation, or hyperabduction.

Thrombectomy Surgical removal of a blood clot from a vessel.

Thromboangiitis Clot formation within an inflamed vessel; Buerger's disease was referred to as thromboangiitis obliterans.

Thromboendarterectomy Surgical removal of a blood clot from within an artery.

Thrombogenic Capable of causing blood clotting.

Thrombolysis The breaking up of thrombus.

Thrombolytic Capable of disintegrating a blood clot. TPA, Streptokinase and Urokinase are used to dissolve clots. This agent acts by stimulating the conversion of plasminogen to plasmin (an enzyme which breaks down fibrin). Thrombolytic therapy is used successfully in the treatment of deep venous thrombosis, for acute arterial thrombosis, and graft occlusion.

Thrombophlebitis Inflammation of a vein with secondary thrombosis in the involved segment.

Thrombosis The formation of an intravascular blood clot formation.

Thrombus An intravascular blood clot; plural, thrombi.

Tibio-Gastrocnemious Angle Sign Identifies the Great Saphenous Vein relative to the tibia and medial gastrocnemius muscle below the knee.

Tissue plasminogen activator (TPA) A generic term for a group of substances that have the ability to cleave to plasminogen and convert it to plasmin in its active form; it is used for therapeutic thrombolysis.

Transmetatarsal amputation Toe amputation (across the metatarsals).

Transverse Along the path of a sound beam; or along a cross-sectional course, as in a transverse scan. (Short axis, SAX)

Triphasic Having three phases or variations; forward flow in systole, brief reverse flow, and a third forward flow component (multiphasic).

Trophic Pertaining to nutrition; trophic changes on an extremity (e.g., nail thickening, atrophied skin) are the results of ischemia or lack of nutrition to the skin.

Tunica A coat; lining membrane, as in tunica intima, tunica media, tunica adventitia.

Turbulence The disruption of the normal laminar flow within a tube or vessel; disturbed blood flow in which whirls and eddies occur; usually due to obstruction to blood flow; a source of bruits.

U

Ulcer The most common type of ulcer is a venous ulcer caused by chronic venous disorders. The venous ulcers are typically shallow with granulation tissue and fibrin and are located in the gaiter area over the media malleolus.

Unilateral Pertaining to one side.

V

Valsalva maneuver Forced expiration against the closed glottis impeding blood flow through the pulmonary capillary bed and increasing intrathoracic pressure. This maneuver impedes venous return and is used in the venous Doppler examination to assess venous flow and valvular competency.

Valve A membrane within a tube or vessel allowing flow to move in one direction only. The venous valves are bicuspid and open towards the heart to prevent reflux. Damaged or incompetent valves allow retrograde venous flow.

Varices Enlarged tortuous vessel; the vessels can be veins or lymphatic vessels.

Varicocele Varicosity of the veins of the spermatic cord. A common cause of infertility in the male. Diagnosis can be made by palpation or (in subclinical presentation) by Doppler ultrasound. Venous reflux during Valsalva maneuver is found in the presence of varicocele.

Varicose veins Veins that are distended, lengthened, and tortuous. The superficial veins (saphenous veins) of the legs are most commonly affected. There is an inherited tendency to varicose veins (primary) but obstruction to blood flow or incompetent valves, which permit backflow of venous blood (secondary), also may be responsible.

Vascular Pertaining to the blood vessels.

Vasculogenic Of a vascular origin.

Vasoconstriction Narrowing of the vessel lumen caused by contraction of the muscular vessel wall.

Vasodilation Enlarging of the vessel wall caused by relaxation of the muscular vessel wall.

Vasospasm Spasmodic constricting of a vessel wall.

Vein A blood vessel which conveys blood from the capillaries back to the heart. Veins are composed of three layers, intima, media, and adventitia. The media of the vein is less muscular than an artery. Veins are more compliant than arteries and are equipped with one-way valves to prevent reflux of blood.

Velocity Speed of an acoustic wave per unit time in a specific direction.

Vena cava filter A device placed in the IVC to catch emboli and prevent them from getting to the lungs.

Venography A radiographic procedure in which an opaque substance is injected into the veins. Subsequent x-ray pictures are taken for the purpose of visualizing the venous system (see phlebography).

Venous Pertaining to the veins.

Venous air embolism An air bubble which may enter the venous system during any surgical procedure in which the surgical site is above the level of the right atrium. Doppler ultrasound is the most sensitive method of detection of air emboli in the right atrium.

Venous Aneurysm A localized dilation of a venous segment, with a caliber increase 50% compared with normal.

Venous insufficiency Condition in which faulty or damaged venous valves permit retrograde or backward flow of blood. Stagnant venous blood in the lower extremity may result in pigmentation changes, edema, pain, and ulceration (see post phlebitic syndrome).

Venous outflow Stacks or aggregations of red blood cells (RBCs) that form because of the unique discoid shape of the cells.

Venule A small vein.

Virchow's triad The three mechanisms of thrombosis injury to the vessel wall, decrease in blood flow (stasis), and blood hypercoagulability.

Viscosity Resistance of a fluid to flow when a pressure is applied.

W

Waveform A curve or undulation traced by a recording device and reflecting alterations in electrical activity; the shape of a wave on a graph (see triphasic).

Webbing (Synechiae) Organization and subsequent contraction of a thrombus leading to adherence of thrombus to the vein wall and spontaneous lysis of areas within the thrombus. A fibrous membrane may remain within the lumen of the vein.

X

Xiphoid process The pointed part of cartilage located at the lower end of the sternum.

A

AAA	Abdominal Aortic Aneurysm
AAGSV	Anterior Accessory Great Saphenous Vein
ABI	Ankle-Brachial Index
ACAS	Asymptomatic Carotid Artery Stenosis Study
AFB	Aortobifemoral Bypass
AJV	Anterior Jugular Vein
AK	Above Knee
AKA	Above Knee Amputation
AP	Ambulatory Phlebectomy
AP	Anterior Posterior
APG	Air Plethysmography
ASVAL	Ambulatory Selective Varices Ablation under Local Anesthesia
ATA	Anterior Tibial Artery
ATCV	Anterior Thigh Circumflex Vein
ATVs	Anterior Tibial Veins
AV	Arteriovenous
AVF	Arteriovenous Fistula
AVG	Arteriovenous Graft
AVM	Arteriovenous Malformation
AVP	Ambulatory Venous Pressure
AVVQ	Aberdeen Varicose Vein Questionnaire
AxV	Axillary vein

B

BcV	Brachiocephalic Vein
BKA	Below Knee Amputation
BK	Below Knee
BMI	Body Mass Index
BP	Blood Pressure
BrA	Brachial Artery
BrVs	Brachial Veins
BaV	Basilic Vein

C

CABG	Coronary Artery Bypass Graft
CAD	Coronary Artery Disease
CAS	Carotid Artery Stenting
CCA	Common Carotid Artery
CDI	Color Doppler Imaging
CDT	Complex/Complete Decongestive Therapy
CEAP	Clinical, Etiologic, Anatomic, Pathophysiology
CEA	Carotid Endarterectomy
CFA	Common Femoral Artery
CFV	Common Femoral Vein
CHF	Congestive Heart Failure
CHIVA	Cure conservatrice et Hemodynamique de l'Insuffisance Veineuse en Ambulatoire – Outpatient Hemodynamic Correction of Venous Insufficiency
CIA	Common Iliac Artery
CIV	Common Iliac Vein
CMV	Congenital Venous Malformation
COPD	Chronic Obstructive Pulmonary Disease
CREST	Carotid Revascularization Endarterectomy vs. Stenting Trial
CRP	C-Reactive Protein
CTA	Computed Tomography Angiography
CT	Computed Tomography
CTV	Computed Tomography Venography
CVA	Cerebrovascular Accident
CV	Cephalic Vein
CVD	Chronic Venous Disease/Disorder
CVI	Chronic Venous Insufficiency
CVM	Congenital Venous Malformation
CW	Continuous Wave

D

DBI	Digital Brachial Index
DC	Distal Calf
DES	Drug Eluting Stents
DFV	Deep Femoral Vein
DIC	Disseminated Intravascular Coagulation
DPA	Dorsalis Pedis Artery
DFV	Deep Femoral Vein
DPV	Dorsalis Pedis Vein
DT	Distal Thigh
DUS	Duplex Ultrasound
DVI	Deep Venous Insufficiency
DVS	Deep Venous System
DVT	Deep Vein Thrombosis

E

EAA	Endovenous Adhesive Ablation
EC-IC	Extracranial To Intracranial Bypass
ECA	External Carotid Artery
EDV	End-Diastolic Velocity
EF	Ejection Fraction
EFIT	Endovenous Foam Induced Thrombus
EGIT	Endovenous Glue Induced Thrombus
EHIT	Endothermal Heat Induced Thrombosis
EIA	External Iliac Artery
EIV	External Iliac Vein

EJV	External Jugular Vein
ESRD	End Stage Renal Disease
EVA	Endovenous Ablation
EVAR	Endovascular Aneurysm Repair
EV	Ejection Volume
EVLA	Endovenous Laser Ablation
EVLT	Endovenous Laser Treatment

F

FA	Femoral Artery
Fem-pop	Femoropopliteal
FEVAR	Fenestrated Endovascular Aortic Aneurysm Repair
FMD	Fibromuscular Dysplasia
FP	Femoropopliteal
FV	Femoral Vein

G

GA	Gastric Artery
GCA	Giant Cell Arteritis
GI	Gastrointestinal
GSV	Great Saphenous Vein
GV	Gastric Vein
GVs	Gastrocnemius Veins
GV	Gonadal Vein
GVP	Genicular Venous Plexus

H

HA	Hepatic Artery
HBP	High Blood Pressure
HCT	Hematocrit
HD	Hemodialysis
HDL	High-Density Lipoprotein
HGB	Hemoglobin
HHD	Hand-held Doppler
HHS	Hypothenar Hammer Syndrome
HIT	Heparin-Induced Thrombocytopenia
HITT	Heparin-Induced Thrombocytopenia with Thrombosis
HTN	Hypertension
HV	Hepatic Vein
Hz	Hertz

I

ICA	Internal Carotid Artery
ICS	Iliac Compression Syndrome
IGV	Inferior Gluteal Vein
IIA	Internal Iliac Artery
IIV	Internal Iliac Vein
IJV	Internal Jugular Vein
IMA	Inferior Mesenteric Artery
IMV	Inferior Mesenteric Vein
InV	Innominate Vein
IntSvs	Intersaphenous veins
IPV	Incompetent Perforating Vein
IVC	Inferior Vena Cava
IVUS	Intravascular Ultrasound

J

J	Joule

K

KTS	Klippel-Trenaunay Syndrome

L

LASER	Light Amplification by Stimulated Emission of Radiation
LMV	Lateral Marginal Vein
LDS	Lipodermatosclerosis
LEED	Linear Endovenous Energy Density
LE	Lower Extremity
LGVs	Lateral Gastrocnemius Veins
LLE	Left Lower Extremity
LMWH	Low-Molecular-Weight Heparin
LNVN	Lymph Node Vein Network
LRV	Left Renal Vein
LVS	Lateral Venous System

M

MALS	Median Arcuate Ligament Syndrome
MAV	Median Antebrachial Vein
MC	Mid-Calf
MCV	Median Cubital Vein
MGVs	Medial Gastrocnemius Veins
MHz	Megahertz
MI	Myocardial Infarction
mmHg	Millimeters of Mercury
MMV	Medial Marginal Vein
MRA	Magnetic Resonance Angiography
MRV	Magnetic Resonance Venography
MSD	Musculoskeltal Disorder
MT	Mid-Thigh
MV	Medial Vein of forearm
MVO	Maximum Venous Outflow
MRI	Magnetic Resonance Imaging
MRV	Magnetic Resonance Venography

N

NASCET	North American Symptomatic Carotid Endarterectomy Trial
NIVLs	Nonthrombotic Iliac Vein Lesions

O

OV	Ovarian Vein

P

PAD	Peripheral Arterial Disease
PAGSV	Posterior Accessory Great Saphenous Vein
PASTE	Post Ablation Superficial Thrombus Extension
PC	Proximal Calf
PCRM	Peripheral Compression Release Maneuver
PEP	Pelvic Escape Points
PE	Pulmonary Embolus
PerA	Peroneal Artery
PerVs	Peroneal Veins
PeVD	Pelvic Venous Disorders
PFV	Profunda Femoral Vein
PICC	Peripherally Inserted Central Catheter
PI	Pulsatility Index
PopV	Popliteal Vein
PPG	Photoplethysmography
PPV	Pathologic Perforating Vein
PREVAIT	PREsence of Varices (residual or recurrent) After InTervention
PRF	Pulse Repetition Frequency
PSV	Peak-Systolic Velocity
PT	Proximal Thigh
PTA	Percutaneous Transluminal Angioplasty
PTA	Posterior Tibial Artery
PTCV	Posterior Thigh Circumflex Vein
PTFE	Polytetrafloroethylene
PTS	Post Thrombotic Syndrome
PTVs	Posterior Tibial Veins
PVD	Peripheral Vascular Disease
PV	Portal Vein
PVE	Popliteal Vein Extrinsic Positional Obliteration Syndrome
PVR	Pulse Volume Recording
PVs	Perforating Veins
PW	Pulse Wave

Q

QoL	Quality of Life

R

RadA	Radial Artery
RadVs	Radial Veins
RA	Renal Artery
RAS	Renal Artery Stenosis
REVAS	REcurrent Varices After Surgery
RFA	Radio Frequency Ablation
RLE	Right Lower Extremity
RRV	Right Renal Vein
RVF	Residual Volume Fraction
RV	Renal Vein

S

SA	Splenic Artery
SAV	Superficial Accessory Vein
SCIV	Superficial Circumflex Iliac Vein
SC	Saphenous Compartment
ScP	Sciatic Perforator
ScV	Subclavian Vein
SEPS	Subfascial Endoscopic Perforator Surgery
SEP	Superficial External Pudendal
SEPV	Superficial Epigastric Vein
SFJ	Saphenofemoral Junction
SFJptv	Sapheno-femoral Junction pre-terminal valve
SFJtv	Sapheno-femoral Junction terminal valve
SIEV	Superficial Inferior Epigastric Vein
SMA	Superior Mesenteric Artery
SMV	Superior Mesenteric Vein
SolV	Soleal Vein
SPJ	Saphenopopliteal Junction
SplV	Splenic Vein
SSV	Small Saphenous Vein
SVC	Superior Vena Cava
SVI	Superficial Venous Insufficiency
SV	Soleal Veins
SV	Splenic Vein
SVT	Superficial Vein Thrombosis

T

TAVR	Transcatheter Aortic Valve Replacement
TBI	Toe-Brachial Index
TE	Thigh Extension
TE-SSV	Thigh Extension of the Small Saphenous Vein
TEVAR	Thoracic Endovascular Abdominal Aortic Aneurysm Repair
TGC	Time Gain Compensation
TIA	Transient Ischemic Attack
TMA	Transmetatarsal Amputation
TOS	Thoracic Outlet Syndrome
TPA	Tissue Plasminogen Activator
TV	Terminal Valve

U

UA	Ulnar Artery
UE	Upper Extremity
UGFS	Ultrasound Guided Foam Sclerotherapy
UGS	Ultrasound Guided Sclerotherapy
US	Ultrasound
UVs	Ulnar Veins

V

VA Vertebral artery
VCSS Venous Clinical Severity Score
VCT Valve Closure Time
VertV Vertebral Vein
VFT Venous Filling Time
VM Venous Malformation
VPR Volume Pulse Recording
VTE Venous Thromboembolism
VVs Varicose Veins
VV Varicose Vein
VV Venous Volumev

W

WRMSDs Work Related Musculoskeletal Disorders

Index of all cine clips included in this book

A

B

C

CME Exam Purchase Instructions

Earn up to 15 hours of CME awarded from the Society of Vascular Ultrasound (SVU). This program meets the criteria for SVU-CMEs, which are accepted by the American Registry of Diagnostic Medical Sonographers® (ARDMS®), the American Registry of Radiologic Technologists, Cardiovascular Credentialing International (CCI), the Intersocietal Accreditation Commission (IAC) for laboratory accreditation, and (ARRT) for Category A credit.

To qualify for the purchase of this CME exam, you must be the purchaser of the *Inside Ultrasound Venous Reference Guide*. You are limited to 5 purchases of the online CME Exam per book.

After you purchase the exam, a page will display a download with information about the exam. Within 48 hours of your purchase, you will receive an email with a ULR link for taking the exam with your login and password.

This online exam is based on the information contained in *Inside Ultrasound Venous Reference Guide*. The exam includes 100 multiple-choice questions with a passing grade of 70%. Each candidate will be allowed 3 attempts to complete the exam successfully. The exam does not need to be completed in one session. You may enter and exit the exam as many times as you want. The exam will be available online for 3 months from the registration date.

The CME certificate can be immediately printed from your computer upon passing the exam. The certificate should be uploaded to the appropriate organization CME Bank including the SDMS. Retain the certificate in case of an organization audit. Note: We do NOT forward the CME certificate on your behalf.

To purchase the exam visit this password protected page:

insideultrasound.com/venous_cme

Password: Indications